Anesthesiology

A Comprehensive Study Guide

Anesthesiology
A Comprehensive
Study Guide

Jeffrey Katz, M.D.

Professor and Chairman
Department of Anesthesiology
University of Texas Medical School at Houston

McGRAW-HILL
Health Professions Division

New York   St. Louis   San Francisco   Auckland   Bogotá
Caracas   Lisbon   London   Madrid   Mexico City   Milan   Montreal
New Delhi   San Juan   Singapore   Sydney   Tokyo   Toronto

McGraw·Hill

A Division of The McGraw·Hill Companies

Anesthesiology: A Comprehensive Study Guide

1 2 3 4 5 6 7 8 9 0   MALMAL   9 8 7 6

ISBN 0-07-033986-4

This book was set in Times New Roman by Publication Services.
The editors were M. Wonsiewicz and P. McCurdy;
the production supervisor was Richard C. Ruzycka;
the designer was Greta Sibley; the indexer was Corinne Ferrara.
The project was managed by Hockett Editorial Service.
Malloy Lithographers, Inc. was printer and binder.

This book is printed on acid-free paper.

Library of Congress Cataloging-in-Publication Data

Katz, Jeffrey
    Anesthesiology : a comprehensive study guide / Jeffrey Katz.
       p.   cm.
    Includes bibliographical references and index.
    ISBN 0-07-033986-4
    1. Anesthesiology—Outlines, syllabi, etc.   2. Anesthesiology—
Examinations, questions, etc.   I. Title.
    [DNLM: 1. Anesthesia—adverse effects—outlines.   2. Embolism,
Air—diagnosis—outlines.   3. Embolism, Air—therapy—outlines.
4. Intraoperative Monitoring—outlines.   WO 218.2 K19a 1996]
RD82.4.K38   1996
617.9'6'076—dc20
DNLM/DLC
for Library of Congress   96–15289

Contents

Contributors xiii

Preface xvii

Section I. Review by System 1

A. RESPIRATORY SYSTEM   1

    I. Anatomy 3

    II. Physiology 10

    III. Pharmacology 31

    IV. Physics 35

    V. Disease States 49

B. CARDIOVASCULAR   81

    I. Anatomy 83

    II. Physiology 87

    III. Pharmacology 90

    IV. Physics 100

    V. Clinical Priorities 106

    VI. Aging 140

    VII. Obesity 144

    VIII. Heat Stroke 148

C. CENTRAL NERVOUS SYSTEM   149

    I. Anatomy 151

    II. Physiology 154

    III. Pharmacology 163

    IV. Clinical Entities 166

    V. Pediatrics 185

D. UROLOGIC SYSTEM   192

   I. Anatomy 194

   II. Physiology 196

   III. Diagnostic Evaluation 218

   IV. Pharmacology 224

   V. Clinical Disease States 228

   VI. Perioperative Considerations 237

E. HEPATIC SYSTEM   240

   I. Anatomy 241

   II. Physiology 241

   III. Pharmacology 244

   IV. Clinical Priorities 245

F. ENDOCRINE SYSTEM   251

   I. Anatomy 252

   II. Physiology 254

   III. Pharmacology 274

G. AUTONOMIC SYSTEM   278

   I. Anatomy 279

   II. Sympathetic Nervous System (SNS) 279

   III. Parasympathetic Nervous System (PNS) 281

   IV. Information Transmission in the ANS 282

   V. ANS Pharmacology 284

   VI. Clinical 292

Section II. Pharmacologic Principles 301

A. INTRODUCTION   304

   I. Pharmacokinetics 304

   II. Distribution and Elimination 304

   III. Pharmacodynamics 305

   IV. Characteristics 306

   V. Protein Bindings 306

   VI. Uptake and Distribution 307

B. INHALED ANESTHETICS

309

    I. Halothane 309

   II. Enflurane 311

  III. Isolurane 312

  IV. Desflurane 314

   V. Sevoflurane 315

C. INTRAVENOUS INDUCTION AGENTS

317

     I. Thiopentone 317

    II. Methohexitone 318

   III. Diprivan 319

   IV. Etomidate 321

    V. Ketamine 322

   VI. Diazepam 323

  VII. Midazolam 324

 VIII. Flumazenil 325

   IX. Fentanyl 326

    X. Sufentanil 328

   XI. Naloxone 329

D. INTRAVENOUS ANESTHETICS

331

    I. Opioids 331

   II. Opioid Agonists 333

  III. Opioid Antagonists 336

  IV. Nonsteroidal Anti-inflammatory Drugs 338

   V. Benzodiazepines 339

  VI. Benzodiazepine Antagonists 343

 VII. Antiemetics 343

E. LOCAL ANESTHETICS

346

    I. Structure 346

   II. Mechanism of Action 346

  III. Pharmacokinetics 348

  IV. Side Effects 350

   V. Representative Local Anesthetic Agents 352

F. MUSCLE RELAXANTS   353

   I. Neuromuscular Junction 353

  II. Classification of Neuromuscular Block 354

 III. Nondepolarizing Muscle Relaxants 357

  IV. Depolarizing Muscle Relaxants 373

   V. Reversal of Neuromuscular Blockade 378

  VI. Neuromuscular Blockade Monitoring 381

G. IMMUNOSUPPRESSIVES AND ANTIREJECTION DRUGS   386

   I. Introduction 386

  II. Cyclosporin 386

 III. Steroids 387

  IV. Cytotoxics 387

   V. Doxorubicin (Adriamycin) 388

  VI. Bleomycin 389

H. DRUG REACTIONS: HYPERSENSITIVITY/ALLERGY   390

   I. Drug reactions 390

  II. Anaphylaxis 390

 III. Anaphylactoid Reaction 392

  IV. Clinically Important Reactions 393

Section III. Principles of Technology and Measurement 395

A. DEVICES FOR MEASUREMENT OF FLOW RATES OF FLUID (LIQUID OR GAS)   398

   I. Rotameter 398

  II. Electromagnetic 399

 III. Ultrasonic 399

  IV. Pneumotachometer 400

   V. Spirometer 401

B. BLOOD (DISSOLVED) GASES 402

   I. General 402
   II. Bench-top Analyzer 402
   III. Point-of-care Analyzers 404
   IV. "Ex vivo" Monitors 405
   V. Continuous in vivo Arterial Blood Gas Monitors 405

C. INSPIRED, EXPIRED GASES 406

   I. Mass Spectroscopy 406
   II. Gas Chromatography 407

D. OXYGEN/HYPOXIA MONITORING 409

   I. Pulse Oximetry 409
   II. Transcutaneous P_{O_2} Monitoring 410

E. PRESSURES 412

   I. General 412
   II. Lung 412
   III. Vascular 413
   IV. Intracranial Pressure 417

F. CARDIAC FUNCTION 420

   I. Oscillometry 420
   II. Diagnostic (Echo) Ultrasound 420
   III. Doppler Ultrasound 421

G. PATIENT SAFETY 423

   I. See "Gas Supply" 423
   II. U.S. Food and Drug Administration 423
   III. Patient Electrical Safety 425
   IV. Other Patient Safety Standards and Agencies 428
   V. Explosion and Fire Hazards 428

H. ELECTRICITY, ELECTRONICS, INSTRUMENTATION

I.	Voltage	431
II.	Current	431
III.	Resistance	431
IV.	Capacitance	431
V.	Alternating Current	431
VI.	Basic Concepts	431
VII.	Electronic (Medical) Instruments	434
VIII.	Computer Networks	438
IX.	Wireless Telecommunication	442
X.	Batteries	444
XI.	Medical Imaging Systems	445

I. STATISTICS

I.	Statistical Analysis Programs	448
II.	Descriptive	448
III.	Probability	450
IV.	Inference on Population Means from Quantitative Data	452
V.	Inference on Population Means from Enumeration (or Attribute) Data	457
VI.	Regression and Correlation	459
VII.	Clinical Trials	461

J. OTHER APPLIED MATHEMATICS

I.	Function	463
II.	Asymptote	463
III.	Increment	463
IV.	Derivative of f	464
V.	Definite Integral	465
VI.	Indefinite Integral	466
VII.	Differential Equation	467
VIII.	Transcendental Functions	468
IX.	Infinite Series	469
X.	Complex Variable	470
XI.	Transform Analysis	470
XII.	Biologic Curves	471

Section IV. Special Clinical Situations 475

A. PEDIATRIC ANESTHESIA 479

   I. Introduction 479
   II. Fetal Circulation 479
   III. Neonatal Physiology 481
   IV. Neonatal Emergencies 490
   V. Respiratory Emergencies 496
   VI. Resuscitation of the Newborn 497

B. OBSTETRIC ANESTHESIA 500

   I. Physiology of Pregnancy 500
   II. Maternal–Fetal Physiology 501
   III. Complications of Pregnancy 504
   IV. Assisted Reproductive Technologies 523
   V. Pulmonary Aspiration 525

C. CLINICAL HEMATOLOGY 529

   I. Blood Transfusion 529
   II. Specific Blood Disorders 534
   III. Effects of Anesthetics on Blood System 541

D. PRINCIPLES OF PAIN MANAGEMENT 543

   I. Chronic Pain Theories 543
   II. Chronic Pain Treatment 543
   III. Generalized Pain Disorders 558

E. MISCELLANEOUS CLINICAL ENTITIES 563

   I. Laser Surgery 563
   II. Outside the Operating Room 563
   III. Electroconvulsive Therapy (ECT) 564
   IV. Gamma Knife 567
   V. Burns 568
   VI. Regional Anesthesia for Ophthalmic Surgery 570

F. LEGAL MEDICINE

573

   I. **Legal Liability** 573

  II. **Informed Consent** 573

 III. **Medical Negligence** 574

 IV. **Litigation Issues** 575

  V. **Contracts and Employment** 577

 VI. **Legal Issues Related to HIV** 578

VII. **Ethical Issues at End of Life** 578

Index 581

Contributors

Section Editors

Michelle Bowman-Howard, M.D.
Assistant Professor of Anesthesiology
University of Texas Medical School at Houston
Houston, Texas

Leslie H. Cronau, Jr., M.D., Ph.D.
Professor and Deputy Chairman of Anesthesiology
and Critical Care
University of Texas Medical School at Houston
Houston, Texas

Penelope Duke, M.D.
Assistant Professor and Director
Division of Transplant Anesthesia
University of Texas M.D. Anderson Cancer Center
Houston, Texas

Carin Hagberg, M.D.
Assistant Professor of Anesthesiology
University of Texas Medical School at Houston
Associate Medical Director
Operative Services, Hermann Hospital
Houston, Texas

Jeffrey Katz, M.D.
Professor and Chairman
Department of Anesthesiology
University of Texas Medical School at Houston
Houston, Texas

Stephen M. Koch, M.D.
Assistant Professor of Anesthesiology
University of Texas Medical School at Houston
Houston, Texas

Bruce A. McKinley, Ph.D.
Assistant Professor of Anesthesiology
University of Texas Medical School at Houston
Houston, Texas

Alan S. Tonnesen, M.D.
Professor and Vice Chair
Department of Anesthesiology
University of Texas Medical School at Houston
Houston, Texas

Chapter Contributors

Ezzat I. Abouleish, M.D.
Professor of Anesthesiology
Medical Director of Ob/Anesthesia
University of Texas Medical School at Houston
Houston, Texas

David C. Abramson, M.B., Ch.B., F.F.A.
Assistant Professor of Anesthesiology
University of Texas Medical School at Houston
Houston, Texas

Steven J. Allen, M.D.
Professor of Anesthesiology
University of Texas Medical School at Houston
Associate Hospital Medical Director
Medical Director of Shock Trauma
Intensive Care Unit/Respiratory Care
Hermann Hospital
Houston, Texas

Sheryl Artmann, M.D.
Assistant Professor of Anesthesiology
University of Texas Medical School at Houston
Houston, Texas

Teodulo Aves, M.D.
Assistant Professor of Anesthesiology
University of Texas Medical School at Houston
Houston, Texas

James M. Berry, M.D.
Assistant Professor of Anesthesiology
University of Texas Medical School at Houston
Houston, Texas

Duncan Browne, M.D.
Assistant Professor of Anesthesiology
Medical Director of Day Surgery
Department of Anesthesiology
University of Texas Medical School at Houston
Houston, Texas

Bruce D. Butler, Ph.D.
Professor of Anesthesiology
University of Texas Medical School at Houston
Houston, Texas

Jacques Elie Chelly, M.D., Ph.D.
Professor of Anesthesiology
University of Texas Medical School at Houston
Houston, Texas

Sukhjinder Dhother, M.D.
Assistant Professor of Anesthesiology
University of Texas Medical School at Houston
Houston, Texas

Marie-Francoise Joelle Doursout, Ph.D.
Assistant Professor of Anesthesiology
University of Texas Medical School at Houston
Houston, Texas

Helen Downey, M.D., B.Ch., B.A.O., F.F.A.R.C.S.I.
Assistant Professor of Anesthesiology
University of Texas Medical School at Houston
Houston, Texas

Shannon Hendry Drtil, M.D.
Assistant Clinical Professor of Anesthesiology
    and Program Director of Undergraduate
    Medical Education
University of Texas Medical School at Houston
Houston, Texas

Tiberiu Ezri, M.D.
Visiting Assistant Professor of Anesthesiology
University of Texas Medical School at Houston
Houston, Texas

Hugh Gallagher, M.D.
Assistant Professor of Anesthesiology
University of Texas Medical School at Houston
Houston, Texas

Janet Gilbert, M.D.
Assistant Professor of Anesthesiology
University of Texas Medical School at Houston
Houston, Texas

Mazin Elias, M.B., Ch.B., F.R.C.A.
Assistant Professor of Anesthesiology
University of Texas Medical School at Houston
Houston, Texas

Caroline E. Fife, M.D.
Assistant Professor of Anesthesiology
University of Texas Medical School at Houston
Director
Hermann Center for Hyperbaric Medicine
Houston, Texas

Anita Louise Giezentanner, M.D.
Assistant Professor of Anesthesiology
University of Texas Medical School at Houston
Houston, Texas

Lewis I. Gottschalk, M.D.
Assistant Professor of Anesthesiology
University of Texas Medical School at Houston
Director
Perioperative Anesthetic Care Unit
Hermann Hospital
Houston, Texas

Shareque Haque, M.D.
Private Practice
Houston, Texas

Gordon A. Irving, M.D.
Associate Professor of Anesthesiology
University of Texas Medical School at Houston
Medical Director
University Center for Pain Medicine and
Rehabilitation at Hermann
Houston, Texas

Paul Kenny, M.B., Ch.B.
Assistant Professor of Anesthesiology
University of Texas Medical School at Houston
Houston, Texas

Samia Khalil, M.D.
Associate Professor
Director of Pediatric Anesthesia
University of Texas Medical School at Houston
Houston, Texas

Stephen M. Larson, D.M.D.
Associate Professor of Anesthesiology
University of Texas Medical School at Houston
Medical Director Operative Services
Hermann Hospital
Houston, Texas

Harold S. Minkowitz, M.D.
Assistant Professor of Anesthesiology
University of Texas Medical School at Houston
Houston, Texas

Nha Van Nguyen, M.D.
Assistant Professor of Anesthesiology
University of Texas Medical School at Houston
Houston, Texas

C. Lee Parmley, M.D., J.D.
Assistant Professor and Medical Director Neuro
    ICU
University of Texas Medical School at Houston
Houston, Texas

Evan G. Pivalizza, M.B., Ch.B., F.F.A.
Assistant Professor of Anesthesiology
University of Texas Medical School at Houston
Houston, Texas

Penelope J. Pivalizza, M.B., Ch.B.
Assistant Professor of Anesthesiology
Currently: Resident/Department of Pediatrics
University of Texas Medical School at Houston
Houston, Texas

Veronica Porter, M.D.
Assistant Professor of Anesthesiology
University of Texas Medical School at Houston
Houston, Texas

Mary F. Rabb, M.D.
Assistant Professor of Anesthesiology
University of Texas Medical School at Houston
Houston, Texas

Karel Riha, M.D.
Assistant Professor of Anesthesiology
University of Texas Medical School at Houston
Houston, Texas

Karen S. Thornton Suttle, B.Sc., M.B., Ch.B.
Assistant Professor of Anesthesiology
University of Texas Medical School at Houston
Houston, Texas

Catherine Uzoni-Boecker, M.D.
Associate Professor of Anesthesiology
University of Texas Medical School at Houston
Houston, Texas

R. David Warters, M.D.
Assistant Professor of Anesthesiology
University of Texas Medical School at Houston
Houston, Texas

Lynda T. Wells, M.B.B.S., F.R.C.A.
Assistant Professor of Anesthesiology
University of Texas Medical School at Houston
Houston, Texas

Preface

This book was designed to fill a gap in the current choice of anesthesia texts. It is our firm belief that no soundly researched and referenced comprehensive text in any discipline can be replaced. However, despite the presence of several manuals on anesthesiology subspecialties, there is no comprehensive text that provides short lecture notes for the student of anesthesiology. Indeed, many residents have expressed the need for one volume containing easily available information on the educational continuum in anesthesiology. Our goal was to produce a book that would cover most of the material needed for the written exam of the American Board of Anesthesiology in a readily accessible format.

The book is the work of the faculties of the departments of anesthesiology at the University of Texas Medical School and M.D. Anderson Cancer Center, both in Houston. Its various authors worked independently of each other in the preparation of the material. Thus, during my attempts to edit the full manuscript, it became obvious that, despite careful instructions to each author, some aspects of our knowledge base are appropriately covered in more than one section. The result is some repetition in the book, and in a few cases, the same subject is presented by different authors. It is our belief that in order to facilitate accessibility to a section of material, that material should be retained despite the risk of repetition. Any duplication that does arise can only enhance the reader's ability to access the data he or she is seeking. There also are sections of knowledge that have been omitted because other books are in the planning stage, and there are sections that are relatively brief because of space limitations.

We present this book to all students of anesthesiology as an attempt to provide notes on a broad variety of anesthesiology-related material. We hope that we have accomplished our goal and that medical students, residents, and other students will come to regard it as their first source when quick, but thorough information on the topic is desired.

Acknowledgments

The two essential ingredients of getting this project off the ground were an idea and Michael Houston, and although he did not contribute to the final form of the book, I owe him my gratitude for having had faith in the idea.

Jamie Kircher brought this book to fruition, and I thank her for her wisdom, persistence, and faith.

The body of work for the book was the result of the collective efforts of the faculty members of the departments of anesthesiology at the University of Texas Medical School and the M.D. Anderson Cancer Center, without whose commitment we would still be at the planning stage. My thanks also go to the seven subeditors, who took on a large part of the actual writing and who contributed considerably to the actual organization of this book.

As in all projects, there is one individual who provides the motivation, guidance, and organization that takes an idea through the various stages of production to a mature work. In this case, Kathy Franz was this person, and we all owe her a huge debt of gratitude for her tireless effort. Kathy has been the unsung hero of many projects during her long career in this department, and it is gratifying to be able to acknowledge her in this book.

Jeffrey Katz

Section

I   *Review by System*

A. RESPIRATORY SYSTEM

I. ANATOMY
   a. **Upper airway**
   b. **Lung**
   c. **Pleura**
   d. **Chest x-ray**
   e. **Computed tomography (CT) of chest**

II. PHYSIOLOGY
   a. **Spirometry**
   b. **Mechanics**
   c. **Surface tension**
   d. **Airway resistance**
   e. **Ventilation—perfusion**
   f. **Blood gas; acid base**
   g. **Gas transport**
   h. **Regulation of respiration**
   i. **Nonrespiratory function**

III. PHARMACOLOGY
   a. **Bronchodilators**
   b. **Anti-inflammatory agents**

IV. PHYSICS
   a. **Gas laws**
   b. **Vaporizers**

      1. Background
      2. Copper kettle and derivatives
      3. Temperature-compensated, variable-bypass vaporizers
      4. Pressurized, heated vaporizers

   c. **Oxygen supply**
   d. **Pressures**
   e. **Ensuring proper connections**
   f. **Gas evacuation (scavenging)**
   g. **Solubility and solubility coefficients**

h. **Humidity**

i. **Critical temperature**

j. **Critical pressure**

k. **Breathing systems**

l. **Anesthetic uptake and distribution**

V. DISEASE STATES

a. **Obstructive lung disease**

b. **Restrictive lung disease**

c. **Perioperative management**

d. **Anesthesia ventilators—classification**

e. **Critical care ventilators**

f. **Humidifiers**

g. **Pulmonary edema**

h. **Respiratory disease in pregnancy**

i. **Autoimmune states**

j. **Nervous and muscular diseases**

k. **Altitude physiology**

l. **Obesity**

m. **Hyperbaric and diving medicine**

n. **Near-drowning**

I. ANATOMY

a. Upper airway

1. Nose
   - (a) Turbinates impinge on the nasal cavity
     - (1) May be fractured during passage of tubes
     - (2) Overlying mucosa is often injured, leading to bleeding
     - (3) Increased surface area for humidifying inspired gas
     - (4) Nasolacrimal duct drains under inferior concha

2. Sinuses drain into nasal cavity
   - (a) Sphenoid drains above superior nasal concha
     - (1) Innervated by V, ophthalmic division
   - (b) Ethmoid drains under superior and middle conchae
   - (c) Frontals drain under middle concha
   - (d) Maxillaries drain under middle concha
     - (1) Innervated by V, maxillary division
   - (e) Tubes may impede sinus drainage, leading to secondary infection of stagnant fluid after several days
     - (1) Nasal tubes should be changed to the oral route if more than 2 days of intubation are anticipated

3. Facial fractures
   - (a) LeFort I
     - (1) Horizontal fracture of the maxilla, above the floor of the nose, through lower nasal septum, mobilizing palate
   - (b) LeFort II
     - (1) Pyramidal fracture of midface
   - (c) LeFort III
     - (1) Fracture parallel to skull base, separates midface from skull base, involves ethmoid bone and may involve the cribriform plate, allowing communication from nose to anterior fossa
     - (2) Nasotracheal intubation, nasal airway insertion, bag and mask ventilation are contraindicated in presence of skull base fracture

4. Mouth
   - (a) Innervation
     - (1) V, mandibular division: buccal mucosa, anterior tongue
     - (2) VII: taste of anterior two thirds of tongue
     - (3) IX: tonsils, soft palate, taste, and sensation of posterior one third of tongue, pharynx, eustachian tube
     - (4) X: muscles of soft palate, pharynx
   - (b) Eustachian (pharyngotympanic) tube drains into the superior lateral nasopharynx
     - (1) Tubes may impede drainage, leading to middle ear infection
   - (c) Fractures of zygomatic arch may involve mandibular coronoid process, locking mandible mechanically
   - (d) Mandible
     - (1) Most fractures involve ramus
       - [a] Second most common site is between first and second molar
       - [b] If bilateral fractures occur, the anterior segment may be pulled posteriorly, allowing tongue to occlude pharynx
   - (e) The hard palate is horizontal and forms base of nose
     - (1) The base of the nasal cavity is the widest portion
     - (2) Tubes should be passed parallel to the hard palate

        (3) Innervated by V, maxillary division

    (f) Soft palate is displaced anteriorly to maintain the nasopharyngeal space open in the supine position by active tonic contraction

    (g) Swallowing

        (1) Tensor and levator palati contract, raising the soft palate against the posterior pharynx

        (2) Larynx elevated 2 to 3 cm by infrahyoid muscles, styolphar- yngeus, palatopharyngeus, pushing it against the epiglottis

        (3) Aryepiglottic folds adduct

        (4) Innervation

            [a] Maxillary division of V

  5. Pharynx

    (a) Innervation

    (1) X

---

b. Lung

  1. Epiglottis

    (a) Innervation

        (1) X

  2. Hyoid

  3. Larynx

    (a) Thyroid cartilage

    (b) Cricoid cartilage lies at level of C6 vertebral body

        (1) Complete ring allows application of occlusive pressure to the esophagus to prevent regurgitation

        (2) Marks end of glottis

    (c) Arytenoid cartilages transduce cord movement by laryngeal musculature

        (1) Form synovial joint

        (2) Susceptible to inflammation in rheumatoid arthritis

        (3) Movement may be limited in diabetics

        (4) Can be dislocated during traumatic intubation

    (d) Vocal cords

        (1) Attached to thyroid cartilage anteriorly, arytenoids posteriorly

        (2) Narrowest part of adult airway

        (3) May be damaged by intubation

            [a] Laceration during intubation

            [b] Pressure ulcers with long-term intubation

            [c] Granulomas may form after extubation

            [d] Endotracheal tube lies in posterior half to two thirds

    (e) Innervation of larynx

        (1) Vagus (X) and accessory (XI)

            [a] Recurrent laryngeal nerve

                i) Muscles of phonation

                  a) Thyroarytenoid

                  b) Lateral cricoarytenoid

                  c) Interarytenoid (adductors)

                  d) Posterior cricoarytenoid (abductor)

               ii) Subglottic mucosa sensation

            [b] Superior laryngeal nerve

                i) Internal branch of superior laryngeal nerve

                  a) Sensory of mucosa of larynx from the vocal cords to base of tongue

        ii) External branch
           a) Motor to cricothyroid muscle, which tenses vocal cords

4. Trachea (generation 0)
  (a) Carina represents point of division of right and left main bronchi, at level of fifth thoracic vertebra
  (b) U-, C-, or D-shaped cartilaginous rings lie anteriorly
  (c) Membranous, muscular posterior wall
    (1) Bronchoscopically, longitudinal striations are seen to divide evenly and pass into the right and left main bronchi
  (d) 18 to 20 mm in diameter, 11 cm long in adult male
  (e) Innervation
    (1) Recurrent laryngeal branch of vagus

5. Bronchi (generation 1)
  (a) Right lobar and segmental bronchi (generation 1–4)
    (1) Main stem
      [a] 13 mm in diameter
      [b] Upper lobe takeoff occurs almost immediately below the carina, forming a symmetrical trifurcation
        i) Apical segment
        ii) Posterior segment
      [c] Middle lobe
        i) Lateral
        ii) Medial
      [d] Lower lobe
        i) Apical
        ii) Medial basal
        iii) Anterior basal
        iv) Lateral basal
        v) Posterior basal
  (b) Left lobar and segmental bronchi (generations 1–4)
    (1) Main bronchus bifurcates
      [a] Anterior incomplete cartilaginous rings
      [b] Posteriorly the longitudinal striations of the membranous posterior wall continue into the left lower lobe bronchus, which can help differentiate the left main bifurcation from the tracheal carina
    (2) Upper division subdivides with some variability
      [a] Lingula
        i) Superior
        ii) Inferior
      [b] Upper lobe trifurcates and then subdivides in a variable fashion, as compared with the symmetric trifurcation of the right upper lobe
        i) Apical
        ii) Posterior
        iii) Anterior
    (3) Lower division
      [a] Apical segment arises from the posterior wall at almost the same level as the takeoff of the upper division
      [b] It is directed posteriorly and often becomes occluded with secretions in supine patients
      [c] The remainder of the lower lobe segmental bronchi are somewhat variably arranged and subdivide almost immediately. The following three divisions usually can be identified
        i) Anterior basal arising anteromedially
        ii) Lateral basal arising laterally

         iii) Posterior basal

6. Small bronchi

   (a) Diameter 1–3 mm
   (b) Number 2,000
   (c) Supply secondary lobules
   (d) APUD cells (amine precursor uptake and decarboxylating cells)

7. Bronchioles to terminal bronchioles

   (a) Diameter 0.5–1 mm
   (b) Number 65,000

8. Respiratory bronchioles

   (a) Diameter 0.4 mm
   (b) Number 500,000
   (c) Supply primary lobules
   (d) Nonciliated bronchial epithelial cells (Clara cells)

9. Alveolar ducts

   (a) Diameter 0.3 mm
   (b) Number 4 million
   (c) Supply alveoli

10. Alveolar sacs

   (a) Diameter 0.3 mm
   (b) Number 8 million
   (c) Supply alveoli

11. Alveoli

   (a) Number 200–600 million
   (b) Diameter 0.25 mm
   (c) Varies with position; larger in apical segments
   (d) Septa
       (1) Flat
       (2) Perforated by pores of Kohn
       (3) Occupied mostly by capillaries
          [a] One side extremely thin, 0.3 micrometer (μm)
          [b] Opposite side 1–2 μm thick, containing elastin, collagen, nerves
          [c] Intercapillary space is 0.5 nanometer (nm)
       (4) Site of edema accumulation
       (5) Surface area 126 square meters
       (6) Alveolar epithelial cells, type I
          [a] Line alveoli
          [b] 0.1 μm thick
          [c] Junctions 0.1 nm
       (7) Alveolar epithelial cells, type II
          [a] Precursor to type I cells
          [b] Rounded, found at junctions of septa
          [c] Produce surfactant
       (8) Alveolar brush cells, type III
          [a] Unknown function, rare
       (9) Alveolar macrophages
          [a] Lie on the surface of type I alveolar cells
          [b] Scavenge particles reaching alveoli
       (10) Mast cells
          [a] In alveolar septa

12. Pulmonary vasculature
    (a) Pulmonary artery main branch (~ 5 cm)
        (1) Receives mixed venous blood
        (2) Divides into left and right main branches
    (b) Arteries accompany bronchi to level of terminal bronchioles
    (c) Arterioles
        (1) Initial diameter 100 μm
        (2) Almost no muscle
    (d) Capillaries
        (1) Alveolar inflation decreases diameter and increases resistance
        (2) Passes from one alveolus to another
        (3) Start at about 75 μm, increase to 200 μm
        (4) 300 million
        (5) Short branches
        (6) Diameters larger than in systemic beds
        (7) High flow, low pressure
    (e) Venules
        (1) Minimal to no musculature
    (f) Pulmonary veins
        (1) Small pulmonary veins (between lobules) form into four large veins
        (2) Drain into left atrium
    (g) Lymphatics
        (1) Lymph vessels commence at extra-alveolar level
        (2) Surround air passages of small bronchi back to mediastinum
        (3) Can contain 500 ml
        (4) Responsible for "butterfly" pattern of pulmonary edema
        (5) Left lung enters thoracic duct
    (h) Systemic arterial supply
        (1) Supplies airways down to terminal bronchioles
        (2) Intermingles with pulmonary circulation, causing a left to right shunt

c. Pleura

1. Lined with mesothelium, covered with microvilli
2. Pores communicate with lymphatics
3. Fluid, normally about 10 ml
   (a) Protein = 1.5 g/dl
   (b) 1,500 monocytes/microliter

d. Chest x-ray

1. Anterior–posterior view interpretation
   (a) Evaluate technique
       (1) Chest should be centered on film
       (2) Penetration should allow visualization of the vertebral bodies through the cardiac silhouette
       (3) Position
           [a] Rotation will displace anterior structures in the same direction as the rotation and posterior structures in the opposite direction
           [b] The trachea and the ends of the clavicles should align symmetrically with the vertebral bodies
           [c] Lordotic/kyphotic positioning is recognized by the position of the clavicles in relation to the vertebral bodies. The medial ends of the clavicles should overlie vertebral bodies of T3–4

[d] Kyphotic position will cause the cardiac silhouette to be obscured by the diaphragm and will place the lower anterior lung structures over the diaphragmatic shadow

[e] Lordotic position will place more of the posterior lung bases behind the diaphragmatic shadow, thus hiding pleural effusions and posterior basal pathology, giving the impression of a poor inspiration

  (4) Inspiration is evaluated by noting the levels of the apex of the hemidiaphragm shadows in relation to the vertebral bodies

    [a] The right is normally 1–2 cm higher than the left hemidiaphragm

    [b] A full inspiration should lower the diaphragm to at least T10

(b) Evaluate visible bones for fractures, abnormal lucencies

  (1) Vertebral bodies

  (2) Clavicles

  (3) Scapula

  (4) Proximal humerus

  (5) Ribs

    [a] Standard chest radiograph is not ideal for detecting fractures

  (6) Sternum

    [a] Usually poorly visualized

(c) Position of lines and tubes

  (1) Endotracheal tube

    [a] 3 cm above carina

    [b] Top of cuff 2 cm below cricoid, at top of T1

(d) Identify soft tissues

  (1) Breast and nipple shadows may simulate masses

  (2) Subcutaneous emphysema

  (3) Skin folds may simulate pneumothorax

  (4) Foreign bodies

(e) Identify mediastinal structures

  (1) Heart

    [a] Width

    [b] Right atrium

    [c] Left atrium

    [d] Left ventricle

  (2) Aorta

    [a] Knob should be clearly visible

    [b] Left lateral border can normally be seen as a distinct line from just below the knob almost to the diaphragm

    [c] Arcuate or circular calcium deposits indicate atherosclerosis

  (3) Superior vena cava forms a nearly vertical, slightly curved line concave laterally on the right upper mediastinum

  (4) Azygous vein is an oval density lying on top of the takeoff of the right main bronchus. It is enlarged during vascular overload

  (5) Pulmonary arteries extend horizontally from the mediastinum just below the level of the carina. The right pulmonary artery is often prominent in the right mid to lower lung field

  (6) Pulmonary veins extend horizontally from the mediastinum below the pulmonary arteries

(f) Abnormal densities

  (1) Air

  (2) Tissue

  (3) Calcium

     (g) Trachea

        (1) Width

        (2) Position should be midline

        (3) Subglottic space

           [a] Carina lies at about the fifth thoracic vertebral body

        (4) Angle of right and left main-stem bronchi

     (h) Pleural cavities

        (1) Air

           [a] Characteristics of pneumothorax

              i) Lung markings not visualized in area of pneumothorax

              ii) A thin white line due to visualizing the pleural edge separates lung density from air density

              iii) A skin fold will not show the thin white pleural edge line; the tissue simply seems to disappear

              iv) A skin fold often does not follow the normal contour of collapsing lung and may extend beyond the perimeter of the pleural cavity

              v) Tissue density diminishes as the lung/pneumothorax interface is approached

                  a) Skin folds show increasing tissue density as the interface is approached

              vi) Deep sulcus sign is seen when air separates the lateral border of the diaphragm from the lateral chest wall. This may be seen before other more objective and specific signs of pneumothorax appear

        (2) Fluid density

        (3) Lung parenchyma

           [a] Vasculature

           [b] Opacities

           [c] Lucencies

           [d] Lung lobar anatomy

              i) The lower lobes extend from a few centimeters above the carina to the diaphragmatic shadows

              ii) The upper border of the middle lobe (right) or lingula (left) extends horizontally from just above the carina to the lateral chest wall. The lower border of the middle lobe curves from the lateral chest wall to the heart border, extending inferiorly almost to the diaphragmatic shadow

              iii) The upper lobes extend from the upper border of the middle lobe to the apex of the chest cavity

        (4) Evaluate the upper abdomen for the presence of gastric tubes, air, and abnormal densities

  2. Lateral view

     (a) Evaluate technique

        (1) Evaluate bones

           [a] Vertebral bodies should be visible

           [b] The anterior and posterior borders should form a smooth line

           [c] The heights of the bodies should gradually increase from top to bottom

           [d] The disk spaces should be of uniform height

           [e] Sternum

              i) The cortical borders of the manubrium and body should be intact

           [f] Scapula

     (b) Evaluate mediastinal structures

        (1) Tracheal air column lies about 1 cm anterior to the anterior border of the vertebral bodies

        (2) Pulmonary arteries

        (3) Pulmonary veins

          (4) Aorta
          (5) Evaluate pleural spaces
              [a] Identify two hemidiaphragms
              [b] Fluid meniscus
        (6) Air
        (7) Evaluate lung parenchyma
            [a] Opacities
            [b] Lucencies
            [c] The lower lobes lie inferior and posterior to a diagonal line drawn from the anterior junction of the diaphragm with the chest wall and the upper posterior chest cavity several centimeters above the carina. The middle lobe occupies the area above and anterior to this diagonal line and below a horizontal line roughly at the level of the carina. The upper lobe lies above and anterior to the diagonal line and the horizontal line at the top of the middle lobe

e. Computed tomography (CT) of chest

    1. Good for evaluating
        (a) Mediastinal contents
            (1) Aortic injury with mediastinal hematoma
            (2) Mass lesions, lymph nodes
        (b) Pleural space
            (1) Empyema
               [a] Loculated effusions
            (2) Subtle pneumothorax or loculated pneumothorax
        (c) Lung parenchyma
            (1) Masses
               [a] Abscesses

II. PHYSIOLOGY

a. Spirometry

    1. Measurement of volumes of air moving into and out of lungs
    2. Techniques
        (a) Use of inverted drum with counterbalance in a water bath. Breathing in and out causes drum to rise and fall, precisely recording volume changes
        (b) Pneumotachometer
            (1) Heated element
            (2) Turbine
            (3) Differential pressure
    3. Lung volumes
        (a) Tidal volume (V_T)
            (1) Volume of air inspired or expired breath by breath
            (2) 6–7 ml/kg or 500 ml in 70-kg person
        (b) Inspiratory reserve volume (IRV)
            (1) Volume of air that can be inspired at the end of the inspiratory phase of a normal tidal volume
            (2) ~3,000–3,500 ml
        (c) Expiratory reserve volume (ERV)

        (1) Volume of air that can be expired with extra force after the end of the expiratory phase of a normal tidal volume

        (2) ~1,100 ml

    (d) Residual volume (RV)

        (1) Volume of air remaining in lungs following forceful expiration

        (2) ~1,200 ml

4. Lung capacities

    (a) Functional residual capacity (FRC)

        (1) FRC = ERV + RV = expiratory reserve volume + residual volume

        (2) Volume of air in lungs at the end of normal expiration

        (3) ~2,300 ml

        (4) Determined by passive contraction of lungs due to elastic properties of lungs and tendency of thorax to expand

    (b) Inspiratory capacity (IC)

        (1) V_T + IRV = tidal volume + inspiratory reserve volume

        (2) Begins at normal expiration of tidal volume and entails maximal inspiration

        (3) ~3,500 ml

    (c) Vital capacity (VC)

        (1) VC = IRV + V_T + ERV = VC + ERV = inspiratory reserve volume + tidal volume + expiratory reserve volume

        (2) FVC = forced vital capacity

           [a] Volume of air expelled by a maximal expiratory effort following a maximal inspiration to TLC

           [b] May be smaller than VC in patients with obstructive disease due to airway collapse with forced maneuver prior to complete emptying

        (3) ~4,600 ml

        (4) Maximum volume of air expelled after maximal inspiration

    (d) Total lung capacity (TLC)

        (1) TLC = VC + RV = IC + FRC = vital capacity + residual volume

        (2) ~5,800 ml

        (3) Maximum volume of air within lung after maximal inspiration

    (e) Pulmonary volumes and capacities are 15–30% greater in males than in females and are greater in athletic individuals

    (f) IC, ERC, and VC are reduced with age while RV and FRC increase with age

    (g) Volumes are decreased while supine compared with when standing due to pressure of abdominal contents on diaphragm and increased pulmonary blood volume on recumbency

	Normal value	Obstructive	Restrictive
FRC	50–60 ml/kg	+	–
RV	20–30 ml/kg	+	–
VC	75 ml/kg	0 to –	–
MVV	150–175 L/min	–	–
$FEV_{1.0}$	>70% of FVC	–	0 to –

FRC = functional residual capacity; RV = residual volume;
VC = vital capacity; MVV = maximum voluntary ventilation;
$FEV_{1.0}$ = forced expiratory volume in 1 second; – = decreased; 0 = no change; + = increased.

5. Curves

    (a) Flow/volume: maximal expiratory effort following inspiration to TLC

        (1) Measured with spirometer

        (2) Rapid increase in flow to peak value, decrease over time

        (3) Expiratory flow is limited, i.e., independent of effort

(b) Pressure/volume: airway pressure measured during inspiration or expiration with subject relaxing chest
   (1) At FRC, relaxation pressure of lungs and chest are ambient atmospheric
   (2) Therefore, FRC is volume of equilibrium where lung elastic recoil is balanced by the chest wall's tendency to expand
   (3) At all pressures, the relaxation pressure on the curve for lung and chest wall equals each separate measurement
(c) Volume/time: airway volumes measured with spirometer
   (1) Volume/time curve with chronic obstructive pulmonary disease has decreased rate of expiratory flow and increased RV and TLC, whereas restrictive lung disease has increased rate of expiratory flow and decreased RV and TLC

6. Clinical relevance

(a) Residual volume is air used for oxygenation between breaths, thereby avoiding greater fluctuations in arterial oxygen and carbon dioxide levels
(b) Vital capacity is influenced by body position, respiratory muscle strength, and pulmonary compliance
   (1) Obesity can reduce VC
   (2) Muscular development can increase VC
   (3) Paralysis of respiratory muscles (spinal cord injury, poliomyelitis) can reduce VC
   (4) Decrease in lung compliance (tuberculosis, chronic asthma, lung cancer, chronic bronchitis, fibrotic pleurisy) can reduce VC
   (5) Pulmonary vascular congestion (left heart failure, pulmonary edema) decreases compliance and can decrease VC
(c) Constrictive chest wall lesions (obesity, ankylosing spondylitis, circumferential burns) decrease lung capacities

b. Mechanics

1. Lung expansion and contraction

(a) Diaphragm movement downward lengthens chest cavity or upward shortens chest cavity
   (1) Normal quiet breathing—inhalation primarily involves movement of diaphragm with exhalation determined by elastic recoil of lungs, chest wall, and abdominal structures during passive exhalation
(b) Heavy/exaggerated breathing requires rapid expiration by contraction of abdominal muscles
(c) Rib elevation increases anteroposterior diameter of chest cavity and depression decreases it
   (1) Normal resting position of ribs is slanting downward from posterior to anterior
   (2) When ribs elevate, forward projection increases anteroposterior dimension by about 20%

2. Muscles

(a) Inspiration
   (1) Diaphragm—pulls lower surface of lungs downward, reducing intrapleural pressure
   (2) External intercostals—pull ribs upward and forward
   (3) Accessory muscles
      [a] Scalene muscles—lift first two ribs
      [b] Sternomastoids—lift upward on sternum
      [c] Anterior serrati—lift ribs

   (b) Expiration
     (1) Passive during quiet breathing
     (2) Active expiration requires muscle action
     (3) Abdominal wall muscles
       [a] Rectus abdominous—pulls lower ribs downward and compress abdominal contents upward
       [b] Internal and external oblique
       [c] Transverse abdominous
       [d] Contraction increases intra-abdominal pressure that pushes diaphragm up
       [e] Forceful contraction with coughing, vomiting, and defecation
     (4) Internal intercostal muscles
       [a] Pull ribs downward and inward
       [b] Oppose external intercostal muscles
       [c] Stiffen intercostal space to prevent bulging during straining
     (5) Elastic properties of lungs
       [a] Pressure–volume curve
       [b] Inflation curve different from deflation curve
       [c] Hysteresis
         i) Lung volume at specific pressure on deflation curve is greater than with inflation
     (6) Lung (respiratory system) compliance—expansibility of chest and lungs
       [a] Definition: slope of pressure (*x*-axis)–volume (*y*-axis) curve
       [b] Volume change per unit pressure change
       [c] 150–200 ml/cm water
         i) 1 cm water pressure increase produces 150 to 200 ml lung expansion
       [d] Size dependent
         i) Specific compliance = compliance per unit volume of lung
       [e] Elastic behavior
         i) Pressure around lungs (pleural pressure) is below atmospheric
           a) Due to elastic recoil of lung tending to collapse lung further when chest wall has reached its normal resting position
         ii) Elastic tissue
           a) Elastin
           b) Collagen
           c) In alveolar walls; around vessels and bronchioles
       [f] Surface tension (see below)
 3. Clinical considerations
   (a) Compliance reduced with
     (1) Parenchymal problems
     (2) Pulmonary venous engorgement
     (3) Alveolar edema
     (4) Prolonged nonventilation
     (5) Fibrotic diseases
     (6) Atelectasis
     (7) Pneumonia
     (8) Bronchospasm
     (9) Pulmonary artery obstruction (decreases surfactant)
     (10) Extrapulmonary problems
     (11) General anesthesia
     (12) Ascites
     (13) Pleural effusion
     (14) Pericardial effusion
     (15) Poliomyelitis
     (16) Kyphoscoliosis

I. Physiology (continued)

c. Surface tension

1. Force (dynes) between molecules of liquid acting across imaginary line on surface of liquid
2. Liquid lining of alveoli
3. Molecular forces of liquid exceed those between liquid and gas
    (a) Liquid surface contracts to sphere
        (1) Smallest surface area at given volume
    (b) Laplace's law

$$\text{Pressure} = \frac{(4 * \text{Surface}_{tension})}{\text{Radius}}$$

4. Surface tension contributes to static recoil
    (a) Causes alveoli to collapse
    (b) Accounts for two thirds of lung recoil tendency
    (c) Lung recoil pressure produces negative pleural pressure
5. Surfactant
    (a) Synthesized, secreted by alveolar type II granular pneumocyte
    (b) Lipoprotein molecules
    (c) Synthesized from fatty acids
        (1) Mixture of neutral lipids, protein, carbohydrates, and especially phospholipids
        (2) Lecithins: principally phospholipid
            [a] Dipalmitoyl phosphatidyl choline (DPPC)—principal component of surfactant
        (3) Hydrophobic fatty acid end projects into alveolar air while hydrophilic end projects into water subphase
            [a] DPPC molecule has one hydrophobic end and one hydrophilic end, aligned on alveolar liquid surface
            [b] Opposes normal forces of attraction by intermolecular repulsive forces
    (d) Formed late in fetal development
        (1) Premature babies with inadequate levels can develop hyaline membrane disease
        (2) New treatments involve exogenous surfactant replacement
    (e) Decreased intermolecular force at alveolar liquid and surface tension
        (1) Surface tension is 50 dynes/cm without surfactant
        (2) 75% reduction with surfactant
    (f) Decreased surface tension
        (1) Stabilizes alveoli
        (2) Increases lung compliance
        (3) Decreases work of breathing
        (4) Prevents edema fluid accumulation
        (5) Prevents fluid transudation

d. Airway resistance

1. Air flow types
    (a) Laminar flow
        (1) Occurs at low flow rates
        (2) Airflow streams parallel to sides of tube
    (b) Transitional flow

(1) Occurs at increased flow rate
(2) Separation of flow streams
(3) Development of eddies
(4) Especially at branches
(c) Turbulent flow
    (1) Occurs at high flow rates
    (2) Disorganization of flow stream

2. Pressure/flow relationships
  (a) Flow = $\dot{V}$ = volume/time = velocity × cross-sectional area
  (b) Pressure difference from one end of tube to other is required to produce flow
    (1) Difference depends on rate and type (laminar, transitional, turbulent) of flow
  (c) Described for laminar flow by Poiseuille
    (1) Flow ($\dot{V}$)
      [a] $\dot{V} = \Delta P \, \pi r^4/8nl$
        i) ΔP = pressure gradient or difference
        ii) r = radius
        iii) n = viscosity
        iv) l = length
    (2) Flow resistance: $R = 8nl/\pi r^4$
      [a] $R = P/\dot{V}$
      [b] Velocity profile: flow stream in center two times faster-than-average velocity
      [c] Halving the radius causes 16-fold increase of resistance
      [d] Doubling length doubles resistance
    (3) Laminar flow present in small airways
  (d) Turbulent flow
    (1) Pressure gradient not linearly proportional to flow rate
    (2) Gas density increases pressure drop
    (3) Reynolds number (Re) correlates with onset of turbulent flow in a long straight tube
      [a] Re = $2rvd/n$
        i) Where d = density, v = average velocity, r = radius, n = viscosity
        ii) Turbulent flow occurs when Re > 2,000
        iii) High velocity, large radius, and high density lead to a high Re
        iv) Low-density gas (helium) has less turbulence
    (4) Trachea
      [a] Turbulent flow occurs with exercise

3. Measures of flow
  (a) Peak expiratory flow rate (PEFR)
    (1) Bedside measure of obstruction
    (2) Normal: > 600 L/min
    (3) Severe bronchospasm: < 250 L/min
  (b) Forced expiratory flow rate between 25 and 75% exhaled volume (FEF_{25-75})
    (1) Another measure of obstruction, normal is 4.5–5 L/sec

4. Resistance measurements
  (a) Resistance is pressure difference/flow
    (1) (Alveolar pressure minus mouth pressure)/flow rate
      [a] Inspiration: atmospheric pressure (mouth) − alveolar pressure
      [b] Expiration: alveolar pressure − atmospheric pressure
      [c] Resistance units: cm $H_2O \cdot L^{-1} \cdot sec^{-1}$
  (b) Site of airway resistance
    (1) Principal site: medium-sized bronchi
      [a] Seventh-generation branching

(2) Due to extensive number of and cumulative cross-sectional area of small airways, little contribution to resistance when $r < 1$ mm

(c) Clinical considerations

(1) Resistance increased

[a] Asthma: due to bronchospasm

[b] Emphysema: due to collapse of airways

[c] Airway mucosal buildup

[d] Airway inflammation

    i) Airway edema

[e] Fibrosis

[f] Compression

[g] Intubation

(2) Resistance decreased with increased lung volumes

[a] Increased airway diameter

[b] Tissue resistance

    i) Due to viscous forces within tissues

    ii) ~20% total pulmonary resistance

5. Work of breathing: work $=$ pressure $\times$ volume

(a) Inspiration

(1) Work required to overcome tissue $+$ airway resistance

(2) Overcome elastic forces

(b) Expiration

(1) Stored energy in elastic components

(c) Clinical considerations

(1) Stiff lungs: decreased work with small rapid breaths

(2) Airway obstruction: slow breathing decreases work

---

e. Ventilation—perfusion

1. Pulmonary vascular pressures

(a) Pulmonary artery pressures

(1) Mean $= $ ~15 mm Hg

(2) Systolic $=$ ~25 mm Hg

(3) Diastolic $=$ ~8 mm Hg

(b) Effect of pulmonary tissue pressures

(1) Transmural pressure (TMP) $=$ pressure difference across vessels

[a] TMP $= P_{capillary} - P_{tissue}$

[b] Capillaries surrounded by alveolar pressures: $P_{tissue} = P_{alveolar}$

[c] Extra-alveolar vessels in lung parenchyma

    i) Diameters proportional to lung volume

2. Pulmonary blood flow

(a) Essentially equals cardiac output

(b) Pulmonary vessels usually act as passive tubes

(1) Increased diameter with increased pressure

(c) Inequality of distribution of flow within lung

(1) Regional flow measured with radioactive tracers, angiogram, lung scanning

(2) Influenced by gravity

[a] Flow decreases from bottom to top

    i) Minimal at apex

[b] Influenced by posture and exercise

    i) Supine position equalizes flow from base to apex

[c] Dependent regions receive greater flow

(3) Hydrostatic pressure differences
- [a] Zone 1 (top)
    - i) Alveolar pressure exceeds pulmonary artery and venous pressure
    - ii) No flow
    - iii) Does not occur normally
    - iv) Occurs with hemorrhage or positive pressure ventilation
- [b] Zone 2 (middle)
    - i) Pulmonary artery pressure exceeds alveolar pressure and venous pressure remains lower than alveolar pressure
    - ii) Flow determined by arterial–alveolar pressure difference
        - a) Waterfall effect
        - b) Starling resistor
    - iii) Arterial pressures increased down zone 2, alveolar pressure constant; thus, flow increases from apex to base
    - iv) Venous pressure not transmitted to zone 2
- [c] Zone 3 (bottom)
    - i) Pulmonary artery pressure exceeds venous pressure and venous pressure exceeds alveolar pressure
    - ii) Pressure gradient determined by difference between pulmonary artery and pulmonary venous pressure
    - iii) Capillary distension with increased blood flow
        - a) Capillary recruitment
- [d] Zone 4 (low-flow conditions)
    - i) Narrowing of extra-alveolar vessels
        - a) Low lung volumes
        - b) Increased interstitial pressure

(4) Local hypoxia
- [a] Hypoxic pulmonary vasoconstriction
    - i) Localized smooth-muscle contraction in region of alveolar hypoxia
    - ii) Not dependent upon central nervous system (CNS)
    - iii) Depends on P_{O_2} of alveolar gas, not pulmonary arterial blood
    - iv) Nonlinear stimulus-response curve
    - v) Directs blood flow away from hypoxic region
    - vi) High altitude (global hypoxia)
        - a) Generalized pulmonary vasoconstriction
        - b) Increased pulmonary artery pressure
        - c) Increased work load on right heart

(5) Response at birth
- [a] Fetus has elevated pulmonary vascular resistance due to hypoxic vasoconstriction
- [b] 15% cardiac output flows through lungs
- [c] First breath oxygenates alveoli, decreasing vascular resistance and increasing flow

(6) Clinical considerations: causes of uneven blood flow
- [a] Open hemithorax (surgery)
- [b] Hypotension: vessel resistance increases
- [c] Vessel congestion, heart failure
- [d] Overexpansion of alveoli
- [e] Collapse of alveoli
- [f] Pulmonary edema (alveolar flooding)
- [g] Pulmonary embolism (thrombi, fat, gas)
- [h] Tension cysts
- [i] Atherosclerotic lesions
- [j] Pneumothorax, hydrothorax
- [k] Emphysema, vascular loss, remodeling

[l] Fibrosis
[m] A-V shunts

3. Pulmonary vascular resistance (PVR)
   (a) Resistance = (Pressure [in] − Pressure [out]) / (Blood flow)
   (b) PVR = (MPAP − PAOP)80/CO
        (1) Where MPAP = mean pulmonary artery pressure;
             PAOP = pulmonary artery occlusion pressure;
             CO = cardiac output
        (2) Classical physical terms = $dynes \cdot sec \cdot cm^{-5}$
   (c) Common usage = mm Hg/L/min
   (d) Principal site of resistance to blood flow is in arterioles and capillaries
   (e) Pulmonary vascular resistance ~ one tenth systemic vascular resistance
   (f) Pulmonary vascular resistance will further decrease if pressure rises by
        (1) Recruitment of unperfused vessels
        (2) Distension (↑ radius) of perfused vessels at even higher pressures
   (g) Lung volume influences pulmonary vascular resistance
        (1) Expansion pulls open extra-alveolar vessels, reducing vascular resistance
        (2) Low volumes or collapsed lungs lead to high vascular resistance
   (h) Active influences: (↑ vasomotor tone)
        (1) Chemical
             [a] Alveolar hypoxia
             [b] Alveolar hypercarbia; animals, not humans
             [c] Acidemia
             [d] Hypoxemia
             [e] Left atrial hypertension
             [f] Pulmonary vascular occlusion
             [g] Hypothermia
        (2) Humoral
             [a] Constrictors, ↑ PVR
                  i) Norepinephrine, epinephrine, serotonin, histamine, angiotensin,
                      fibrinopeptides, prostaglandin $F_2\alpha$, leukotrienes
             [b] Dilators, = ↓ PVR
                  i) Acetylcholine, bradykinin, prostaglandin E_1, isoproterenol,
                      prostacyclin
        (3) Neurogenic
             [a] Sympathetic = ↑ PVR animals
             [b] Parasympathetic = ↓ PVR animals
        (4) Other
             [a] *Escherichia coli* endotoxin
             [b] Alloxan
   (i) Passive influences
        (1) Increases in pulmonary artery pressure (decreases PVR)
             [a] Hyperthyroidism
             [b] Fever
             [c] Anemia
             [d] A-V shunts
             [e] Partial pneumonectomy
             [f] Lung volume changes
             [g] Alveolar pressure changes
             [h] Blood viscosity ↑ causes ↑ PVR
             [i] Pulmonary blood volume
             [j] Interstitial pressure ↑ causes ↑ PVR
             [k] Transmural pressure

(j) Clinical pathological conditions
  (1) Embolization
    [a] Thrombi, lipid (fat), air, tumor cells, white blood cells, platelets
  (2) Vascular disease
    [a] Sclerosis
    [b] Endarteritis
    [c] Polyarteritis
    [d] Scleroderma
  (3) Obstructive/obliterative
    [a] Fibrosis
    [b] Emphysema
  (4) Mechanical
    [a] Vessel closure with hypotension
    [b] Compression due to lesion growth
4. Ventilation/perfusion: matching blood flow with alveolar ventilation
  (a) Ventilation/perfusion ratio: ($\dot{V}_A/\dot{Q}$)
    (1) $\dot{V}_A$ = alveolar ventilation
    (2) $\dot{Q}$ = pulmonary blood flow
  (b) Consequences of normal $\dot{V}_A/\dot{Q}$ ratio
    (1) Oxygen absorbed into capillary (venous blood)
    (2) Carbon dioxide diffuses into alveoli for excretion
    (3) Normal
      [a] P_IO_2 = 149 mm Hg, P_ICO_2 = 0 mm Hg
      [b] P_AO_2 = 104 mm Hg, P_ACO_2 = 40 mm Hg
  (c) Consequences of high $\dot{V}_A/\dot{Q}$ ratio
    (1) If $\dot{V}_A$ = > 0 and $\dot{Q}$ = 0, then $\dot{V}_A/\dot{Q}$ = infinity (dead space)
      [a] Ventilation, no blood flow
      [b] No gas exchange
      [c] Physiologic dead space: wasted ventilation to nonperfused areas

$$\frac{Vd}{Vt} = \frac{Paco_2 - P_Eco_2}{Paco_2}$$

      i) Where V_d = physiological dead space; Vt = tidal volume; $Paco_2$ = arterial carbon dioxide; P_Eco_2 = average carbon dioxide in expired air
  (d) Consequences of low $\dot{V}_A/\dot{Q}$
    (1) If $\dot{V}_A/\dot{Q}$ below normal, inadequate blood oxygenation
    (2) Venous admixture includes both shunt and nonzero low $\dot{V}_A/\dot{Q}$ ratios
      [a] Shunt: If $\dot{V}_A$ = 0 and $\dot{Q}$ > 0, then $\dot{V}_A/\dot{Q}$ = 0
        i) No ventilation, blood flow present
        ii) No gas exchange
      [b] Nonoxygenated mixed venous blood "shunted" through unventilated capillaries
      [c] Blood flow through bronchial vessels, nonoxygenated
        i) These are called physiological shunts
      [d] Septal defect in heart = atrial septal defect may cause anatomical shunt
      [e] Shunt effect on Pao_2 is not correctable by increased F_Io_2 or increased ventilation
      [f] Physiologic shunt calculation

$$\frac{\dot{Q}_s}{\dot{Q}_t} = \frac{Cpco_2 - Cao_2}{Cpco_2 - Cmvo_2}$$

      i) Where $\dot{Q}_s$ = shunt, $\dot{Q}_t$ = cardiac output; Cpco = ideal pulmonary arterial oxygen concentration; Cao_2 = measured arterial oxygen concentration; $Cmvo_2$ = measured venous oxygen concentration

        [g] Low V/Q ratio (nonzero, nonshunt)

           i) Uptake of O_2 from alveoli exceeds delivery of O_2 to alveoli

           ii) Low Pa_{O_2} corrected by increasing $F_{I}O_2$. When $F_{I}O_2 = 1.00$, the effect of low, nonshunt V/Q ratio on Pa_{O_2} is eliminated

    (e) Ventilation/perfusion abnormalities are defined as $\dot{V}A/\dot{Q}$ higher or lower than ideal

      (1) Top of lung: high $\dot{V}A/\dot{Q}$ due to decreased $\dot{Q}$

        [a] Dead space in this region

        [b] Blood leaving this region has high P_{O_2} and low P_{CO_2}

      (2) Bottom of lung: too low ventilation to $\dot{Q}$, lower $\dot{V}A/\dot{Q}$

        [a] Physiologic shunt in this region

        [b] Blood leaving this region has low P_{O_2}

f. Blood gas; acid base

    1. Blood gas

      (a) Measurement

        (1) pH: glass electrodes for whole blood

        (2) P_{CO_2} electrode: is a modified pH meter

          [a] Bicarbonate buffer separated from blood by membrane

          [b] Diffusion of CO_2 changes buffer according to Henderson-Hasselbach relation

          [c] P_{CO_2} is calculated from measured pH change

        (3) P_{O_2}: polarographic

          [a] Electrical voltage yields current proportional to dissolved oxygen

      (b) Oxygen (arterial blood tension, Pa_{O_2})

        (1) Dependent on alveolar P_{O_2} ($P_{A}O_2$), which depends on

          [a] $F_{I}O_2$

          [b] Barometric pressure P_B

          [c] Water vapor pressure, which is temperature dependent

          [d] $P_{A}CO_2$ (which is approximately $= Pa_{O_2}$)

          [e] $P_{A}O_2 = F_{I}O_2(P_B - P_{H_2O}) - Pa_{CO_2}/RQ$ (simplified alveolar air equation)

            i) Where RQ = respiratory quotient or respiratory exchange ratio

        (2) Dependent on ventilation–perfusion ratio (see shunt equation)

          [a] Dependent on alveolar ventilation and cardiac output

          [b] Arterial oxygen not necessarily alveolar oxygen due to shape of oxygen dissociation curve

          [c] Reduced with hypoventilation (low V/Q) and vice versa

            i) Low V/Q ratio = ventilation of inadequately perfused alveoli or shunt

            ii) Low Pa_{O_2} not improved with ventilation if $Pa_{CO_2} \leq$ normal

          [d] High V/Q ratio = normal arterial oxygen because dissociation curve flat

    2. Acid base

      (a) Carbon dioxide (CO_2)

        (1) Physiology

          [a] CO_2 formed by metabolic oxidation of carbon

          [b] Diffusion into interstitial fluids and blood

            i) 1.2 millimoles/liter dissolved CO_2 in extracellular fluids

          [c] Carried to lungs in venous blood

          [d] Diffuse into alveoli and excreted via ventilation

            i) Due to steep slope of CO_2 dissociation curve

(2) Pa_{CO_2} (arterial blood CO_2 tension)
    [a] Balance between CO_2 formation (metabolic rate) and pulmonary excretion by alveolar ventilation
    [b] $Pa_{CO_2} \cong P_{A_{CO_2}}$
    [c] $P_{A_{CO_2}}$ proportional to $P_{mv_{CO_2}}$
        i) $P_{mv_{CO_2}}$ proportional to rate of CO_2 production and inversely to cardiac output (CO)
    [d] Pa_{CO_2} inversely proportional to V_A
        i) $V_A = V_t - V_D$
        ii) V_D functionally increased in areas of high V/Q
        iii) Mismatch of regional ventilation

(b) Respiratory alkalosis
  (1) Pa_{CO_2} lower than normal (< 35 mmHg)
    [a] Decrease in CO_2 production or increased ventilation increases pH (alkalosis)
  (2) Doubling V_A
    [a] Decreases Pa_{CO_2} by 50%

(c) Respiratory acidosis
  (1) Elevated Pa_{CO_2} (> 45 mmHg)
  (2) Increase in Pa_{CO_2} (increased production or decreased ventilation) decreases pH (acidosis)
  (3) Reducing ventilation to 25% of normal
    [a] Quadruples Pa_{CO_2}
    [b] Decreases pH by 0.08 unit / 10 mm Hg increase in Pa_{CO_2}
    [c] Acute increase in Pa_{CO_2} increases HCO_3^- concentration by 1 mMol/L/10 mm Hg increase in Pa_{CO_2}
    [d] Chronic increase in Pa_{CO_2} increases HCO_3^- by 2 mMol/L

(d) Hydrogen ion concentration (H^+)
  (1) Acidemia = pH < 7.35
  (2) Alkalemia = pH > 7.45

(e) pH may be normal if there are simultaneous offsetting alkalosis and acidosis
  (1) Can affect rate of ventilation (see "regulation of ventilation")
    [a] 50–75% effective in pH control
    [b] One to two times buffering capacity compared with chemical buffers in the body
  (2) Approximation: [H+] = 80 − last two digits of pH
    [a] e.g., pH = 7.20 is associated with [H+] of 60 nanomoles/L

g. Gas transport

1. Diffusion: occurs from high concentration to low
  (a) Concentration of a gas is proportional to its partial pressure
    (1) Air = 79% N_2 and 21% O_2
    (2) Total pressure = 760 mmHg
    (3) Partial pressures in dry air
      [a] $PN_2 = 600$ mm Hg and $PO_2 = 160$ mm Hg
  (b) Concentration of dissolved gases determined by
    (1) Pressure
    (2) Solubility coefficient
      [a] Henry's law

2. Net diffusion: determined by partial pressure difference
  (a) Net diffusion of gas in a fluid directly proportional to

I. Physiology; g. Gas transport (continued)

        (1) Diffusion gradient = pressure of area of greater concentration minus pressure of area of lesser concentration divided by diffusion distance
        (2) Gas solubility
        (3) Cross-sectional area
        (4) Temperature
        (5) 1/Diffusion distance
        (6) 1/Molecular weight

$$D = \frac{\Delta P * A * S}{d * MW}$$

        [a] Where D = diffusion rate; ΔP = pressure difference; A = cross-sectional area; S = gas solubility; d = diffusion distance; MW = molecular weight
    (b) Diffusion coefficient = S/MW
        (1) At given pressure gradient, temperature, etc., gases diffuse at rates proportional to diffusion coefficient

3. Diffusion from alveolus to capillary
    (a) Barriers
        (1) Fluid surfactant layer on alveolar surface
        (2) Alveolar epithelium
        (3) Epithelial basement membrane
        (4) Interstitium
        (5) Capillary basement membrane
        (6) Capillary endothelial membrane
    (b) Diffusion capacity
        (1) Volume of gas diffusing through membrane each minute at ΔP of 1 mm Hg
        (2) Oxygen = 21 mL/min/mm Hg
            [a] Exercise = 65 mL/min/mm Hg
                i) Capillary recruitment
                ii) Capillary dilation
        (3) Carbon dioxide = ~400–450 mL/min/mm Hg
        (4) Measurement
            [a] Use carbon monoxide technique
            [b] Clinical consideration
                i) O_2 diffusion compromised greater than CO_2
                ii) Pulmonary edema: increases interstitial fluid thickness
                    a) Increases alveolar fluid
                iii) Pulmonary fibrosis increases membrane thickness
                iv) Pneumonectomy: decreases surface area
                v) Emphysema: decreases surface area

4. Transport of oxygen and carbon dioxide
    (a) Oxygen uptake
        (1) Pressure difference: alveolus to capillary (venous blood): 104 − 40 = 64 mm Hg
        (2) → O_2 transport complete by one third distance along capillary
            [a] Safety factor for exercise or gas transport abnormalities
            [b] 98% of blood fully saturated
            [c] 2% of blood passes through bronchial circulation
                i) Shunt
        (3) PO_2 aortic blood = 95 mm Hg
            [a] Oxygenated blood and shunt blood = venous mixture
    (b) Oxygen transport = CO L/min × CaO_2 ml/L

(1) CaO_2
    [a] 3% dissolved in plasma
    [b] 97% in chemical combination with hemoglobin
        i) $O_2 + Hb \rightleftharpoons HbO_2$
        ii) Oxygen–hemoglobin dissociation curve
            a) Increase in O_2 bound to Hb with increased PO_2

PO_2	SO_2
mm Hg	%
27	50
40	75
60	90
80	95
150	100

            b) Shift of oxygen–hemoglobin dissociation curve
              • Shift to right
                —Increased H^+ ($\downarrow$ pH to 7.2)
                —Increased CO_2
                —Increased temperature
                —Increased 2,3-diphosphoglycerate (2,3-DPG)
              • Shift to left
                —Decreased H^+ ($\uparrow$ pH to 7.6)
                —Decreased CO_2
                —Hypothermia
                —Decreased 2,3-DPG
                —Presence of fetal Hb
            c) Bohr effect
              • Increased CO_2, temperature, and H^+ of tissue off load; more O_2 at a given PO_2 in capillary blood
            d) 2,3-DPG: product of red cell metabolism
              • Increased with
                —Chronic hypoxia
                —Chronic lung disease
    [c] Percent saturation
        i) Arterial blood: $\sim$ 97% saturated
        ii) Venous blood: $\sim$ 75% saturated
    [d] 1 gHb binds with 1.34 ml O_2
        i) Therefore, normal arterial blood has 19.4 ml per 100 ml O_2 bound Hb and venous has 14.4 ml
        ii) $19.4 - 14.4$ ml = 5 ml O_2/100 ml blood transported to and used by tissues
(2) Exercise
    [a] Cardiac output increases sixfold
    [b] Increased utilization coefficient
        i) Body consumes 25% of delivered O_2 at rest
        ii) Body can consume 75 to 85% with exercise
        iii) Therefore, $3 \times O_2$ extracted from blood
    [c] Therefore, 18–20$\times$ increase in O_2 use by tissues
(c) Oxygen diffusion into interstitium and cells
  (1) Interstitium
    [a] Normal pressure gradient from arterial blood to interstitial fluid $95 - 40 = 55$ mm Hg
    [b] Decreased Hb concentration same effect as decreased blood flow
        i) $\downarrow$ Hb $\rightarrow$ $\downarrow$ tissue O_2

        (2) Cells

          [a] Intracellular PO_2 ranges from 5 to 40 mm Hg

          [b] 3 mm Hg normally required for cellular metabolism

     (d) Carbon dioxide transport

        (1) CO_2 diffuses from cells into blood primarily in gaseous state

          [a] Cell membrane impermeable to bicarbonate ions

        (2) 4 ml CO_2 dissolved in 100 ml blod

        (3) $Paco_2 \cong 40$ mm Hg, $P_{mv}CO_2 \cong 45$ mm Hg

        (4) 7% total CO_2 in dissolved form

        (5) CO_2 transport as bicarbonate ion

          [a] Dissolved: $CO_2 + H_2O$ forms carbonic acid

          [b] Carbonic anhydrase catalyzes reaction in red cells

            i) Equilibrium within fraction of second

          [c] Accounts for 70% of all CO_2 transported

          [d] Dissociation of carbonic acid to hydrogen and bicarbonate ion

            i) In fraction of second

          [e] H^+ ions combine with Hb in red cells

          [f] Bicarbonate ions diffuse into plasma

          [g] Chloride diffuses into red cell

            i) Via bicarbonate-chloride carrier protein

            ii) Chloride shift: chloride content greater in venous red cells than in arterial

          [h] Acetazolamide (carbonic acid inhibitor) increases tissue Pco_2 to 80 mm Hg

        (6) Carbaminohemoglobin: $CO_2 + Hb \rightarrow Hb \cdot CO_2$

          [a] CO_2 also reacts with Hb

          [b] Reversible loose bond allows CO_2 release into alveoli

          [c] 15–20% of total CO_2 transport

        (7) CO_2 + plasma proteins

          [a] 3.5–5% of total CO_2 transport

        (8) Carbon dioxide dissociation curve

        (9) Normal concentration of CO_2 in blood is 50 volumes percent

          [a] Four volumes percent actually exchanged via blood to alveoli

            i) Haldane effect: binding of O_2 with Hb displaces CO_2

              a) Causes Hb to become stronger acid

              b) CO_2 displacement occurs via

                • More acidic Hb releases more H^+, which binds with bicarbonate ions to form carbonic acid

                • Carbonic acid dissociates into H_2O and CO_2 and CO_2 exhaled

              c) Haldane effect enhances CO_2 uptake in tissues due to O_2 off-loading and release in lungs due to O_2 loading

   5. Respiratory exchange ratio (R)

     (a) Ratio of CO_2 output to O_2 uptake

     (b) Transport of O_2 to tissues is ~ 5 ml/dl and CO_2 to lungs ~ 4 ml/dl

     (c) Therefore, $\sim 80\%$ as much CO_2 exhaled as O_2 taken up

     (d) R varies with metabolic changes

        (1) Carbohydrate energy sources, R = 1.0

        (2) Fat, R = 0.70

        (3) Alcohol, R = 0.6

        (4) Protein, R = 0.8

        (5) Fat production, R = 8.0–9.0

        (6) Normal diet, R = 0.825

h. Regulation of respiration

1. Respiratory center
   (a) Located bilaterally in medulla oblongata and pons
   (b) Consists of dorsal respiratory group, pneumotaxic center, and ventral respiratory group
       (1) Dorsal respiratory group: located in dorsal position of medulla
           [a] Nucleus of tractus solitarius
           [b] Sensory signal transmission into respiratory center from
               i) Peripheral chemoreceptors, baroreceptors
               ii) Nervous signal to inspiratory muscles controls rapidity of lung filling, duration of inspiration
       (2) Pneumotaxic center: located dorsally in nucleus parabrachialis of upper pons
           [a] Controls duration of lung filling
           [b] Limits inspiration
           [c] Increases rate of breathing
       (3) Ventral respiratory group: located in nucleus ambiguus and nucleus retroambiguus
           [a] Remains inactive with normal breathing
           [b] Signals for increased ventilation
           [c] Stimulates both inspiration and expiration
           [d] Provides powerful expiratory force
       (4) Hering-Breuer inflation reflex
           [a] Limits inspiration via bronchi and bronchiolar stretch receptors
           [b] Vagal
           [c] Increases rate of respiration
           [d] Tidal volume greater 1.5 L
       (5) Chemical control of respiration
           [a] Goal of respiration to maintain proper levels of O_2, CO_2, H^+
           [b] Central chemoreceptor—chemosensitive cells on surface of medulla
           [c] Sensitive to H^+ or indirectly to blood CO_2
               i) Direct action of H^+ on respiralveolusatory center in medulla oblongata
               ii) Feedback control: H^+ activates ventilation, reducing CO_2 and H^+
               iii) Vice versa
               iv) CO_2 diffuses through blood–brain barrier (BBB) into cerebrospinal fluid (CSF) and interstitial fluid
               v) Reacts with H_2O to form bicarbonate and H^+
               vi) Increases respiratory rate
           [d] Peripheral chemoreceptor—oxygen's role in control of respiration
               i) Located in carotid and aortic bodies
               ii) Carotid afferent connections to glossopharyngeal nerves and to dorsal respiratory group
               iii) Aortic afferent connections pass through vagus to dorsal respiratory group
               iv) Stimulated by
                   a) Fall in Pa_{O_2} (major effect)
                   b) Rise in Pa_{CO_2}, H^+ (minor effect) serious hypotension
                   c) As P_{O_2} falls and ventilation increases slightly, Pa_{CO_2} and H^+ fall, inhibit excitatory effects of low P_{O_2}
                   d) When Pa_{CO_2} and H^+ are unchanged Pa_{O_2}, ventilation increased
                   e) Gases not exchanged between atmosphere and blood
                   f) Emphysema, pneumonia

(6) Arterial blood
[a] Saturated at normal and hyperventilation
[b] Therefore, blood CO_2 primary influence on respiration
(7) Other factors in control of respiration
[a] Voluntary control
i) From cortex through corticospinal tract to spinal neurons that stimulate respiratory muscles
[b] Vasomotor center
i) Spillover of signals from vasomotor center to respiratory center in medulla
ii) For example, decrease in blood pressure inhibits baroreceptors, increasing vasomotor and ventilatory activity
[c] Temperature
i) Stimulates chemical stimuli indirectly
[d] Irritant receptors (sensory nerves)
i) Epithelium of trachea, bronchi, bronchioles
[e] J receptors
i) In alveolar walls juxtaposed to pulmonary capillaries
ii) Stimuli
a) Irritants in pulmonary blood
b) Engorgement of capillaries
c) Pulmonary edema (congestive heart failure)

2. Clinical implications
(a) High altitude (hypobaric exposure)
(1) Slight increase in respiration, decreases Pa_{CO_2} and H^+
(2) Adaptation to low Pa_{CO_2} causes fivefold ventilation increase
(b) Interaction of P_{CO_2}, pH, and P_{O_2}
(1) As P_{O_2} decreases, blood CO_2 has greater effect on ventilation
(2) As H^+ increases (acidosis), the required P_{CO_2} to stimulate respiratory center decreases
(c) Regulation with exercise
(1) Strenuous exercise increases O_2 utilization and CO_2 production 20-fold
(2) P_{O_2}, P_{CO_2}, and pH remain normal with increased ventilation
(d) Stimuli—neurogenic
(1) Direct
[a] Brain transmits to contracting muscle and likely to respiratory center
(2) Indirect
[a] Body movements stimulate joint proprioceptors that transmit to respiratory center
(e) With anesthesia respiration controlled principally by chemical factors, not neurogenic
(1) Mild depression of respiratory center
[a] Ether, halothane, cyclopropane, ethylene, N_2O
(2) Significant depression
[a] Pentobarbital sodium, morphine
(f) Cerebrovascular disease: respiratory center damage
(1) Hemorrhage, embolic, plaque
(g) Chronic hypercapnia
(h) Cerebral edema
(1) Decreased cerebral blood flow
(2) Cheyne-Stokes breathing: periodic breathing
[a] Waxing and waning respiration
[b] Dampened feedback from chemoreception (Pa_{CO_2})

        i) Cardiac failure: decreased cardiac output
          a) Delay blood flow to brain
          b) Delay CO_2 feedback mechanism
          c) Chronic heart failure patients
    (i) Brain-stem injury
      (1) Increases feedback gain to respiratory center
      (2) Decreases sensitivity of respiratory center
    (j) Hypoxia
      (1) Gain of oxygen control increases
      (2) Gain of CO_2 and pH increases

i. Nonrespiratory function

1. Blood reservoir
   (a) Instantaneous volume depends on balance between blood inflow and outflow ($\sim$600 ml)
      (1) Balance is determined by cardiac output of left and right ventricles and pulmonary vascular distensibility
   (b) Compliance of large vessels in lungs depends on sympathetic activity
      (1) Extra pulmonary receptor
      (2) ↑ Sympathetic activity, ↓ flow efficiency, ↑ reservoir capacity
   (c) Local reactivity (e.g., hypoxia, acidosis) or humoral release can change pulmonary vascular resistance (vasoconstriction) and vascular compliance

2. Intrathoracic reflexes
   (a) Mechanoreceptors
      (1) Reflexes originate in sensory endings in airways
      (2) Usually vagal afferent
      (3) Respond to:
         [a] Stretch (volume)
         [b] Vascular wall tension
         [c] Blood pressure, changes
   (b) Pulmonary artery baroreceptors
      (1) Bainbridge reflex
         [a] Pulmonary artery depressor reflex
         [b] Abrupt ↑ pulmonary artery pressure causes ↓ blood pressure
         [c] Pulmonary venous stretch receptors

3. Water and solute balance
   (a) Conditions inspired air
      (1) Controls heat and water loss
      (2) Humidification aids in ciliary function
   (b) Lungs contain large extracellular fluid volume
      (1) $\sim$60% wet weight
      (2) Interstitial, alveolar, and lymph fluid
   (c) Fluid exchange
      (1) Alveolar water rapidly absorbed due to low capillary pressure
      (2) Low pressure prevents fluid transudation into alveoli from blood
      (3) Aids in aerosol drug delivery
      (4) Alveolar fluid containing protein slowly resorbed
         [a] Pneumonia
   (d) Solute balance, accounted for by
      (1) Hydrostatic forces
      (2) Molecular diffusion
      (3) Excretion of solute by way of CO_2 elimination
      (4) Primarily as bicarbonate in plasma

(5) Excretion of volatile acid (13,000 mEq/day)

4. Defensive mechanism (infection control)

   (a) Air conditioning
      (1) Upper respiratory tract
   (b) Filtration/cleansing
      (1) Gross particulate filter by nasal hairs
      (2) Turbulent flow impinges small particles ($>10\ \mu$m) onto mucosa
      (3) Smaller particles (2–10 μm) settle on walls of nasopharynx, larynx, trachea, bronchi, bronchioles
      (4) Smallest particles ($<0.5\ \mu$m) reach alveoli
      (5) Particulate expulsion via sneezing, coughing, expectoration, cilia migration
   (c) Lower respiratory tract—sterile
      (1) Immunoglobulins (IgA) in bronchial secretions
      (2) Alveolar macrophages are phagocytic and contain bacteriolytic lysozymes
   (d) Defenses adversely affected by
      (1) Hypoxia
      (2) Smoking
      (3) Starvation
      (4) Alcohol
      (5) Cortisone
      (6) Immunodeficiency

5. Blood filter

   (a) Filters venous blood (located between left and right heart)
      (1) Protects against systemic embolism to heart and brain
      (2) Filters blood-borne particles larger than RBCs
      (3) More than 75 μm trapped in small arteries
      (4) Pulmonary arterioles taper in diameter to capillaries (8–15 μm)
      (5) Excess number of capillaries allow filtration (obstruction) and maintenance of gas exchange
      (6) Particulate matter (fibrin, thrombin clots, lipid cells, bone marrow, tumor cells, gas bubbles) are trapped by simple filtration and eliminated by phagocytosis or dissolution
      (7) Transpulmonary passage to left heart via
         [a] A-V shunt
         [b] Atrial septal defect (patent foramen ovale)
         [c] Pulmonary capillaries
   (b) Reflex response to embolic particles
      (1) Vasoconstriction
      (2) Sympathetic
      (3) Histamine, serotonin, bradykinin, prostaglandins, leukotrienes, thromboxanes

6. Oxidative metabolism

   (a) Rate of oxygen consumption increased with infected lungs
      (1) May be increased metabolism or production of oxygen-derived free radicals
   (b) Oxidative phosphorylation
      (1) Major consumption of oxygen is for production of high-energy phosphate compounds
   (c) Cytochrome P-450
      (1) Extrahepatic site for mixed-function oxidation by cytochrome P-450
      (2) Less than liver
      (3) May be involved with biotransformation of drugs
      (4) May be involved in hypoxic pulmonary vasoconstriction

       (5) Detoxification of inhaled substances

    (d) Oxygen-derived free radicals

       (1) Large quantity of oxygen consumed in formation of free radicals and related species derived from molecular oxygen

       (2) Involve marginated neutrophils, macrophages, etc.

7. Protease transport

    (a) Protease released from neutrophils and other phagocytes in lungs

    (b) Elastase

    (c) Trypsin

    (d) Damage potential to alveolar septa

    (e) Injury prevented by

       (1) Mucosal transport of protease toward larynx

       (2) Conjugation by α_1 antitrypsin and removal by circulation and lymph

       (3) Ultimately destroyed by liver after conjugation with α_2-macroglobulin

8. Surfactant synthesis

    (a) Role of surfactant discussed in section on mechanics

9. Processing of hormones and other vasoactive compounds

    (a) Substances largely removed from the circulation

       (1) Noradrenaline

       (2) 5-Hydroxytryptamine

       (3) Bradykinin

       (4) ATP, ADP, AMP

       (5) PGE_2, PGE_1, $PGF_{2\alpha}$

       (6) Leukotrienes

    (b) Substances largely unaffected by passage through the lung

       (1) Adrenaline

       (2) Angiotensin II

       (3) Vasopressin

       (4) Isoprenaline

       (5) Dopamine

       (6) Histamine

       (7) PGI_2, PGA_2

       (8) Oxytocin

    (c) Substances biotransformed by the lung

       (1) Angiotensin I (into angiotensin II)

10. Endogenous vasoactive compounds

    (a) Nitric oxide (NO); endothelium-derived relaxing factor

       (1) Free radical, lipid soluble

       (2) Synthesized in the endothelium from L-arginine in response to several stimuli (histamine, bradykinin, adenosine triphosphate, and acetylcholine)

          [a] Enzyme: nitric oxide synthase (NOS) is activated by calmodulin and the reaction consumes oxygen and NADPH, forming NO and L-citrulline

          [b] Competitive inhibitor: *N*-methyl-L-arginine (NMMA)

       (3) Diffuse rapidly to underlying smooth muscle → relaxation by conversion to GTP to cyclic GMP

       (4) Half-life: few seconds → cannot act as a freely circulating vasoactive hormone

          [a] Inactivated by hemoglobin, myoglobin, and methylene blue

       (5) Potent vasodilator of the pulmonary circulation

          [a] Therapeutic use of inhaled low concentrations of NO for the relief of pulmonary hypertension and as a selective vasodilator of ventilated areas of the lung

       (6) It is also a bronchodilator

I. Physiology; i. Nonrespiratory function (continued)

    (b) Noradrenaline (norepinephrine)
      (1) Half-life: 20 seconds in blood
        [a] About 30% removed in a single pass through the lungs
        [b] Taken up by the endothelium, mainly in the microcirculation, including arterioles and venules
          i) Uptake is not inhibited by monoamine oxidase or catechol-*o*-methyl transferase inhibitors
          ii) Uptake inhibited by inhalation anesthetics
        [c] Rapidly metabolized after uptake
    (c) 5-Hydroxytryptamine (5-HT, serotonin)
      (1) Up to 98% removed in a single pass
        [a] Similar to the processing of noradrenaline; uptake by endothelium, mainly in the capillaries
        [b] Rapidly metabolized by monoamine oxidase
        [c] Half-life in blood: 1–2 minutes and pulmonary clearance plays the major role in the prevention of its recirculation
        [d] Uptake of 5-HT is inhibited (e.g., by cocaine or tricyclic antidepressant drugs)
      (2) Effects
        [a] Bronchoconstriction
        [b] Stimulates respiration
        [c] May be involved in response to pulmonary embolism (as histamine)
    (d) Histamine
      (1) Not removed from the pulmonary circulation because uptake is limited by its transport mechanism across the blood–endothelium barrier
      (2) Enzymatic degradation by oxidative deamination
      (3) Lung is a major site of synthesis of histamine
      (4) Released in response to injury, anaphylactic shock
      (5) May be involved in response to pulmonary embolism
      (6) May participate in local regulation
    (e) Acetylcholine
      (1) Rapidly hydrolyzed in blood
      (2) Half-life of less than 2 seconds
    (f) Angiotensin
      (1) 80% of angiotensin I converted by angiotensin-converting enzyme (ACE) into the vasoactive octapeptide angiotensin II in a single pass through lung
        [a] ACE is free in the plasma and bound to the surface of endothelium in abundance on the vascular surface of pulmonary endothelial cells
        [b] Angiotensin II itself passes through the lung unchanged
    (g) Bradykinin
      (1) A vasoactive nonapeptide
      (2) The half-life in blood is about 17 seconds, less than 4 seconds in various vascular beds
      (3) Very effectively removed during passage through the lung and other vascular beds
        [a] ACE is the enzyme responsible
          i) ACE is inhibited by many substances, some of which (e.g., captopril and enalapril) have a clinical role in the treatment of hypertension; also decreases the degradation of bradykinin by ACE
    (h) Atrial natriuretic peptide (ANP)
      (1) Largely removed by the rabbit lung in a single pass
    (i) Prostaglandins, thromboxanes, and leukotrienes
      (1) The lung is a major site of synthesis, metabolism, uptake, and release of arachidonic acid metabolites

  (2) Eicosanoids are synthesized as required by many cell types in the lung, including
    [a] Endothelium
    [b] Airway smooth muscle
    [c] Mast cells
    [d] Epithelial cells
    [e] Vascular muscle
  (3) Effects
    [a] PGE_1 and PGE_2 are bronchodilators
    [b] $PGF_{2\alpha}$, PGD_2, PGG_2, PGH_2, and thromboxane TXA_2 are bronchial and tracheal constrictors
    [c] PGI_2 and PGE_1 are pulmonary vasodilators
    [d] PGH_2 and $PGF_{2\alpha}$ are pulmonary vasoconstrictors
    [e] Leukotrienes LTC_4 and LTD_4 are mainly responsible for the bronchoconstrictor effects
  (4) Release of eicosanoids, particularly TXA_2, occurs in anaphylactic reactions in response to complement activation
    [a] PGI_2 appears to be continuously released from the lungs of certain anesthetized laboratory animals. In anesthetized humans, blood levels of PGI_2 are subthreshold, but artificial ventilation or extracorporeal circulation causes a 10-fold increase
  (5) Leukotrienes are also eicosanoids derived from arachidonic acid (by the lipoxygenase pathway)

11. Handling of foreign substances by the lungs

 (a) The lungs take up, store, or detoxify foreign substances
 (b) Drugs taken up in the pulmonary circulation include propranolol, lignocaine, chlorpromazine, imipramine, and nortriptyline
 (c) Accumulation of toxic substances in the lung may cause dangerous local toxicity; paraquat is an outstanding example
 (d) The cytochrome P-450 system is active in the lung; certain anesthetics undergo biotransformation

III. PHARMACOLOGY

a. Bronchodilators

1. Agents

 (a) Beta-adrenergic agonists
 (b) Anticholinergics
 (c) Methylxanthine
 (d) Anti-inflammatory drugs
  (1) Corticosteroids
  (2) Cromolyn sodium

2. Beta-adrenergic agonists

 (a) Mode of action
  (1) Bronchodilation by direct stimulation of beta-2-adrenergic receptors in the airway smooth muscle
  (2) Activate adenylate cyclase $\rightarrow$ increases CAMP
  (3) May lower the cytoplasmic concentration of Ca^{++}
  (4) Suppress release of leukotrienes and histamine from mast cells in lung tissue
  (5) Enhance mucociliary function
  (6) Decrease microvascular permeability and possibly inhibit phospholipase A2
  (7) Beta-2-receptors inhibit release of acetylcholine (ACH)

III. Pharmacology; a. Bronchodilators (continued)

                (8) Rank of potency: isoproterenol > epinephrine > norepinephrine (for beta receptors)

       (b) More potent when inhaled versus taken orally

       (c) Adverse effects

                (1) Tachycardia and palpitations

                     [a] Reflex cardiac stimulation secondary to peripheral vasodilation by direct stimulation of the vascular beta receptors

                     [b] Direct stimulation of cardiac beta-adrenergic receptors

                (2) Large doses may cause myocardial necrosis

       (d) Nonselective beta-adrenergic agonists

                (1) Isoproterenol (Isuprel)

                     [a] Route of administration: 0.25% aerosol, intravenous (IV) available, sublingual

                     [b] Mechanism of action

                           i) Stimulates both beta-1 and beta-2 receptors

                         ii) Adverse effects of beta-adrenergic agonists in the treatment of asthma are caused by stimulation of beta-1-adrenergic receptors in the heart

       (e) Selective beta-2-adrenergic agonists

                (1) Albuterol (Proventil)

                     [a] Route of administration: oral, aerosol 0.5% solution

                     [b] Mechanism of action: beta 2 >> beta 1

                     [c] Duration: 4 to 6 hours

                     [d] Therapeutic doses

                           i) Oral (0.10–0.15 mg/kg three to four times daily)

                         ii) Aerosol (0.01 ml/kg three to four times daily)

                (2) Salbutamol (Ventolin)

                     [a] Route of administration: oral, inhalation

                     [b] Mechanism of action: beta 2 >> beta 1

                     [c] Duration: 4 to 6 hours

                     [d] Therapeutic doses

                         i) Oral (2- and 4-mg tablets three to four times daily, total daily dose = 32 mg; syrup [2 mg/5 ml])

                       ii) Inhalation: 90 μg, no more than two inhalations every 4 to 6 hours

                (3) Terbutaline (Brethaire)

                     [a] Route of administration: oral, parenteral, 0.1% solution (subcutaneous [SC]), inhalation

                     [b] Mechanism of action: beta 2 >> beta 1

                     [c] Duration: 4 to 6 hours

                     [d] Therapeutic doses

                         i) Oral: 5 mg, three times a day; 2.5 or 5 mg

                            a) Use in children under age 12 is not recommended

                       ii) SC: 0.25 mg (1 mg/ml), total dose = 0.5 mg in a 4-hour period

                       iii) Inhalation: two sprays every 4 to 6 hours (0.2 mg per spray)

                (4) Metaproterenol (Alupent)

                     [a] Route of administration: oral, aerosol, 5% solution

                     [b] Mechanism of action: beta 2 > beta 1

                     [c] Duration: 3 to 5 hours

                     [d] Therapeutic doses

                         i) Oral: 0.3–0.5 mg/kg three to four times daily

                       ii) Aerosol: 0.01–0.3 ml/kg four times a day

                (5) Isoetharine (Bronkosol)

                     [a] Route of administration: aerosol, 1% solution

        [b] Mechanism of action: beta 2 > beta 1
        [c] Duration: 3 to 5 hours
        [d] Therapeutic doses
            i) 0.02 ml/kg, up to 0.5 ml four times a day
   (6) Formoterenol and Salmetererol (in clinical trials)
        [a] Duration: bronchodilator effects last more than 12 hours
        [b] Alpha and beta receptors
   (7) Epinephrine
        [a] Route of administration: SC, inhaled (aerosol), locally applied
        [b] Mechanism of action
            i) Prominent alpha-adrenergic receptor
            ii) Lack of beta-2 receptors resulting in beta 1
            iii) Cardiac stimulation
        [c] Short duration of action
        [d] Indications
            i) Asthma
            ii) Acute anaphylaxis
        [e] Therapeutic doses
            i) Epinephrine for oral inhalation: 1% aqueous solution of epinephrine hydrochloride
        [f] Metabolic effects
            i) Hypokalemia
            ii) Hypoxemia

3. Anticholinergic agents
  (a) Mechanism of action
    (1) Antagonize muscarinic receptors
        [a] Less effective against antigen challenge, exercise
        [b] Only inhibit reflex cholinergic bronchoconstriction
        [c] Do not significantly block the direct effects of inflammatory mediators (histamine, leukotrienes, on bronchial smooth muscle and vessels)
        [d] No effect on mast cells
    (2) Adverse effects
        [a] Little or no change in heart rate, blood pressure, intraocular pressure, or pupillary diameter
            i) Due to inefficient absorption of the drug from the lungs or the gastrointestinal tract
  (b) Ipratropium bromide (Atrovent)
    (1) Inhaler onset of bronchodilation: slow (30 to 60 minutes)
    (2) Duration: may persist for 8 hours
    (3) Therapeutic doses
        [a] 18 µg per spray, 2 inhalations four times daily, up to 12 inhalations per 24 hours
    (4) Indications
        [a] Less effective than beta-adrenergic agonists in asthmatic subjects, although duration of action is longer
        [b] Chronic obstructive pulmonary disease (COPD)
        [c] More effective in older than in younger patients with asthma
    (5) Adverse effects
        [a] Unpleasant, bitter taste
        [b] No adverse effects on mucociliary clearance
        [c] Less than 1% of an inhaled dose of ipratropium bromide is absorbed systemically, in contrast to atropine and other carminic antagonists; lacks tachycardia, inhibition of salivary secretion, appreciable effect on the CNS
        [d] Greater inhibitory effects on ganglionic transmission

(c) Oxitropium bromide (quaternary anticholinergic)
  (1) Duration: more prolonged effects
  (2) Indications: useful in patients with nocturnal asthma
4. Methylxanthine agents
  (a) Adverse effects
    (1) Modest decrease in peripheral vascular resistance
    (2) Powerful cardiac stimulation
    (3) Increased perfusion of most organs
    (4) Diuresis
    (5) At high concentrations, tachycardia and arrhythmias
    (6) Marked increase in cerebrovascular resistance with a decrease in cerebral blood flow and oxygen tension
  (b) Theophylline
    (1) Mode of action
      [a] Phosphodiesterase inhibition
      [b] Adenosine-receptor antagonism
      [c] Release of endogenous catecholamines
      [d] Prostaglandin inhibition
      [e] Calcium influx
    (2) Metabolized in the liver by the cytochrome P-450 system and the enzyme xanthine oxidase
    (3) Indications
      [a] Asthma, nocturnal asthma, COPD
      [b] Less effective than inhaled beta-adrenergic agonists
    (4) Therapeutic doses
      [a] At therapeutic concentrations weak bronchodilator
      [b] Loading dose is 6 mg/kg over 20 to 30 minutes followed by a maintenance dose of 0.5 mg/kg per hour
    (5) Adverse effects
      [a] Stimulation of CNS
        i) Lethal convulsions
        ii) Headache
        iii) Restlessness
      [b] Cardiovascular
        i) Cardiac arrhythmias
        ii) Modest increases in heart rate
        iii) Increased contractile force
        iv) Decreased preload
      [c] Diuretic
      [d] Nausea, vomiting, abdominal discomfort

b. Anti-inflammatory agents

1. Cromolyn sodium
  (a) Indication: prevents bronchoconstriction
    (1) Ineffective once bronchoconstriction has occurred
    (2) No bronchodilator action
2. Corticosteroid
  (a) Effects
    (1) No direct effect on airway smooth muscle; not bronchodilators

IV. PHYSICS

a. Gas laws

1. Boyle's law

    (a) $P_1V_1 = P_2V_2$

    (b) The volume of a gas is inversely proportional to the ambient pressure, assuming constant temperature. As pressure decreases, volume increases (gas expands)

2. Henry's law

    (a) The volume of gas dissolved in a liquid is directly proportional to the partial pressure of the gas in contact with the liquid

3. Dalton's law

    (a) $P_T = P_1 + P_2 + P_3 \cdots + P_n$

    (b) The total pressure exerted by a mixture of gases is equal to the sum of the pressure of each gas

    (c) Ambient barometric pressure (P_B) is the result of O_2, N_2, CO_2, H_2O, argon, and other trace gases

    (d) $P_B = P_{O_2} + P_{N_2} + P_{CO_2} + P_{H_2O} + P_{argon} \cdots + P_{other}$

4. Pascal's law

    (a) The pressure exerted on a confined liquid at any point is transmitted equally throughout

b. Vaporizers

1. Background

    (a) Vaporizers are used to deliver potent, volatile anesthetic agents in a controlled fashion

    (b) This is done with knowlege of, or control over, the two variables influencing evaporation

        (1) Temperature

        (2) Vapor pressure

    (c) The three types in past or present use illustrate the different approaches to this problem

        (1) Copper kettle and its derivatives (Vernitrol types)

        (2) Temperature-compensated, variable-bypass vaporizers (Tec and others)

        (3) Heated, pressurized vaporizers (Desflurane)

2. Copper kettle and derivatives

    (a) Principles

        (1) Based on bubble-through of variable flow of carrier gas

        (2) This results in saturated carrier gas containing anesthetic proportional to saturated vapor pressure (SVP) of the anesthetic, e.g., halothane in oxygen at 240 mm Hg vapor pressure at 1 atmosphere (760 mm Hg) has a concentration of 240/(760–240) or approximately 50% by volume

        (3) Thus, a flowmeter bubbling 100 ml/min oxygen through halothane would produce 50 ml/min of halothane vapor; this, when mixed into a 5-L/min fresh gas flow, produces a final halothane concentration of 1% by volume

        (4) Temperature compensation is accomplished by calculating the change in SVP for the temperature measured in the vaporizer; circular slide rule–type wheels made calculation of necessary carrier gas flows for a needed agent concentration convenient and simple

    (b) These vaporizers were simple and sturdy; however, they could easily produce toxic concentrations of agent if set improperly

(c) Their use is not currently permitted in the United States under federal regulations

3. Temperature-compensated, variable-bypass vaporizers address the issues of calculation of necessary carrier gas flows by automatically providing a set concentration despite changes in temperature or fresh gas flow

   (a) Principles

   (1) "Variable bypass" means that a constant fraction of the fresh gas flow delivered through the vaporizer is diverted to the vaporizer compartment to be saturated with vapor

   (2) This means that the vaporizer delivers a constant concentration of agent despite changes in fresh gas flow

   (3) Temperature-compensating elements (usually bimetallic strips) change the fraction of the gas flow diverted through the vaporizing chamber to compensate for changes in SVP of the agent with temperature

   (4) Vaporizers are usually quite massive and constructed of material of high heat capacity to minimize cooling as the agent evaporates

   (b) Practice

   (1) These vaporizers are the most common in use today; they allow a concentration to be set directly and provide a predictable dosage over a wide range of temperatures and gas flows

   (2) There is some change in delivered concentration at extremely low fresh gas flows (< 500 ml/min); calibration curves are provided with each vaporizer

4. Pressurized, heated vaporizers

   (a) The only example currently in use is the vaporizer developed for use with desflurane

   (1) This was an innovative solution to the problem of an agent with a very high SVP (near 760 mm Hg at room temperature) and high variability of SVP with temperature

   (2) The vaporizer is heated electrically to a constant 43°C, raising the vapor pressure of desflurane to near 1,500 mm Hg (2 atmospheres)

   (3) At this pressure, liquid and vapor coexist in the vaporizer, much as in a tank of nitrous oxide; the vapor is drawn off through a variable orifice and mixed with the fresh gas flow

   (4) Because the vaporizer is pressurized, a sight glass cannot be used to determine the amount of agent in the vaporizer; an electronic gauge must be used

c. Oxygen supply

1. Liquefied O_2

   (a) Economical only in large institutions and when in constant use

   (b) One cubic foot (0.028 cubic meter) of liquid oxygen at a temperature of $-300°F$ ($-184°C$) will yield 860 cubic feet (24.4 cubic meters) of gas at 70°F (21°C)

   (c) Liquid oxygen cylinder usually stored outside for easy filling by supply trucks

   (1) Should be located where exposure to potential ignition sources is minimal

   (d) To keep it liquefied, oxygen needs to be kept below its boiling point ($-297°F/-183°C$). This is achieved by storing it in a large thermos flasklike container. It may, however, be stored in a liquefied form under pressure at a higher temperature (see "**critical temperature**," below)

   (1) The oxygen is kept cold by the latent heat of vaporization as gaseous oxygen is removed and the temperature of the fluid tends to fall

   [a] If not enough oxygen is drawn off and the fluid rises in temperature, a

pressure-relief valve in the cylinder allows for pressure to be released, with a subsequent drop in temperature

2. Gaseous oxygen is warmed before arriving in the operating room
    (a) Oxygen is usually piped in copper or brass pipes
        (1) Labeled at least every 20 feet
        (2) Labeled at least once in each room so that the identity of the pipes may be known
        (3) Oxygen piping is usually of a different diameter than other gas supply piping to avoid cross-connections
    (b) Appropriately placed shutoff valves should allow the supply to each room to be isolated as required
        (1) This valve must be located outside the anesthetizing location, so that, in an emergency, people may leave the room and cut the supply of oxygen as they leave
    (c) When the central oxygen supply is located outside the building served, an emergency oxygen supply for connection to an auxiliary temporary supply is required
    (d) Oxygen is usually supplied to the operating room at 4 atmospheres pressure
        (1) Other piped gases are usually supplied at slightly different pressures so that cross-connections can be detected

3. O_2 cylinder
    (a) Usually in E cylinders
        (1) 4¼ inches outer diameter by 26 inches in length
        (2) Weigh 14 pounds empty
        (3) 660 liters at a pressure of 1,900 pounds per square inch gauge (psig) (13,100 kPa)
        (4) Oxygen cylinders and oxygen pipelines are always green in the United States
            [a] They are white in Canada and the rest of the world
    (b) Filling of cylinders is controlled by Department of Transportation (DOT) regulations, where the pressure in a filled cylinder at 70°F may not exceed service pressure
        (1) Cylinders are tested to function at 1.66 times service pressure
        (2) The service pressure is stamped on the shoulder of the cylinder in pounds per square inch after the DOT specification number
        (3) The DOT specification number specifies the material used to produce the cylinder

d. Pressures

1. Psi = pounds per square inch
2. Psig = pounds per square inch gauge
    (a) The difference between the measured pressure and the surrounding atmospheric pressure
    (b) Most gauges are set to measure 0 at local atmospheric pressure
3. Psia = pounds per square inch absolute
    (a) Based on a 0 reference point, the perfect vacuum
    (b) Psia = psig plus the local atmospheric pressure
4. Pressure gauges
    (a) Standardized by the American Society for Testing and Materials (ASTM)
    (b) Each yoke on an anesthesia machine must be provided with a gauge
        (1) At least 38 mm in diameter (1.5 inches)
        (2) With the lowest pressure indication between 6 and 9 o'clock
        (3) Clearly and permanently marked with the name of the gas it monitors

IV. Physics; d. Pressures (continued)

    (c) The gauge should be identified by the color assigned to that gas
        (1) The indicator end must contrast with the background
        (2) The tail end should be shorter than the indicator end and blend into the background
    (d) Bourdon tube type

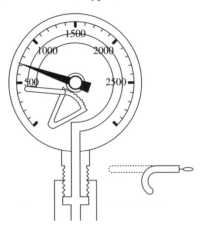

Figure 1. Bourdon pressure gauge. As gas pressure within the flexible tube increases, the tube tends to straighten. The motion is translated through the gearing mechanism so that the indicator shows a higher pressure. The tail end of the pointer is shorter than the indicating end and blends into the background. The lowest pressure indication is between the 6 o'clock and 9 o'clock positions on a clock face.

        (1) A hollow metal tube is bent into a curve, sealed, and linked to a clocklike mechanism
        (2) The other end is connected to the gas source and soldered into a socket
        (3) As the gas increases in pressure, the tube will tend to straighten out, while a pressure drop will allow the tube to resume its curved shape
        (4) Since the open end is fixed, the closed end moves; this motion is translated via the clocklike mechanism into an indicator of the pressures in the gas supply line

e. Ensuring proper connections

    1. On size E and smaller cylinders, a Pin Index Safety System ensures that only the correct cylinder is connected to the appropriate yoke on the anesthesia machine
    2. Unless the pins on the yoke on the anesthesia machine and the holes on the cylinder are aligned, it is impossible to deliver that gas. The pin arrangement on the cylinders follows an internationally agreed upon formula

f. Gas evacuation (scavenging)

    1. Scavenging removes expired anesthetic gases and vapors from the room
    2. Active scavenging systems
        (a) An external source of power draws away the gases
        (b) The simplest active scavenging system is the so-called open system
            (1) The point at which suction is applied to waste gases is also open to the atmosphere without any intervening reservoir bag or valves
            (2) Not very efficient
            (3) Requires high scavenging flow
        (c) Semiclosed system consists of several parts
            (1) An exhaust port from the expiratory port or ventilator
            (2) A transfer system of wide-bore tubing (typically 30 mm in diameter)
            (3) A receiving system consisting of a reservoir and a flow indicator

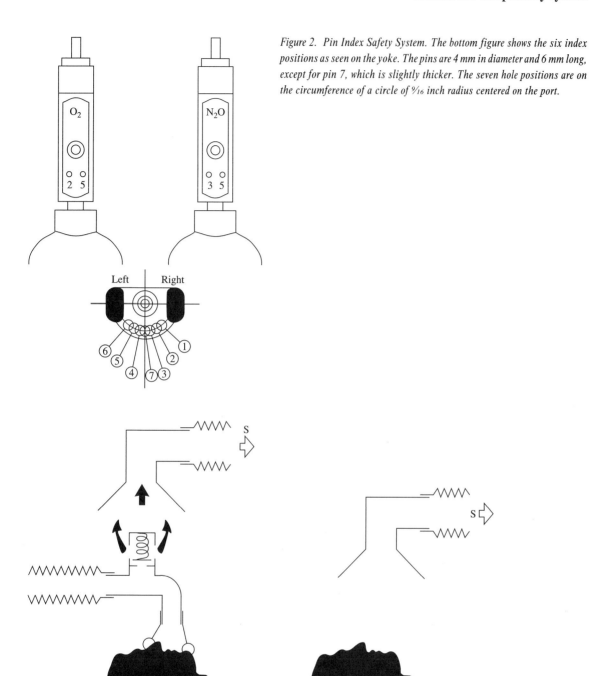

Figure 2. Pin Index Safety System. The bottom figure shows the six index positions as seen on the yoke. The pins are 4 mm in diameter and 6 mm long, except for pin 7, which is slightly thicker. The seven hole positions are on the circumference of a circle of ⁹⁄₁₆ inch radius centered on the port.

Figure 3. Open scavenging systems. Scavenging flow is indicated at S.

    [a] In a simple system, the receiving system is an open-ended reservoir and a flow of about 80 L/min is required for efficient scavenging

    [b] More efficient receiving systems have closed reservoirs, lower scavenging flows, and valves that prevent excesses of positive or negative pressure

    [c] These valves should not exceed a negative pressure of 0.5 cm water and a positive pressure of 10 cm water at 30 L/min flow

    [d] The reservoir may be solid or in the form of a bag, where scavenging may be more accurately visualized

  (d) A disposal system

    (1) May simply be the hospital vacuum system (most common system)

IV. Physics; f. Gas evacuation (scavenging) (continued)

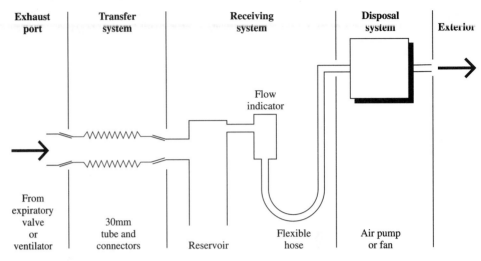

Figure 4. Component systems of the anesthetic gas scavenging technique.

     (2) It has independent fan
     (3) It has passive scavenging
     (4) Gases are driven outside the building by the pressure generated by the patient during expiration
     (5) It is seldom used today
     (6) Wide-bore tubing leading outside the building is involved
  (e) Outlet needs to be at the same level as the anesthetic machine to prevent the dense gases and vapors from applying back pressure on the exhaust system
     (1) Needs to empty into a wind-free area for the same reason

---

g. Solubility and solubility coefficients

  1. When a liquid is placed in a closed container, eventually an equilibrium is established between the vapor and the liquid itself where the number of molecules leaving the liquid into the vapor phase equals that of molecules leaving the vapor phase back into the liquid

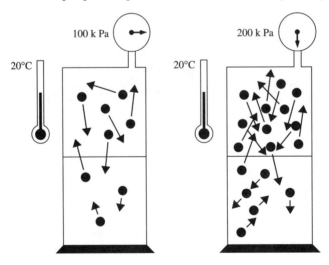

Figure 5. Effect of pressure on the amount of gas dissolved in a liquid.

  (a) At equilibrium, the partial pressure exerted by the vapor is known as the saturated vapor pressure

2. According to Henry's law:

	Solubilities, ml gas/ml H_2O at 37°C, 1 ATA	Relative Solubility
Oxygen	0.024	X
Carbon dioxide	0.57	20X
Carbon monoxide	0.018	
Nitrogen	0.012	
Helium	0.008	

3. At a given temperature, the amount of a gas dissolved in a liquid is directly proportional to the partial pressure of the gas in equilibrium with the liquid
   (a) Concentration dissolved gas = pressure × solubility coefficient
   (b) Thus, as one increases the pressure of a gas above that of a liquid, gas will be more dissolved in the liquid, and vice versa
      (1) Divers, rising too quickly, will allow bubbles to come out of solution, forming bubbles of gas that give them the "bends"
   (c) As a liquid is warmed, less gas dissolves in it
      (1) For example, bubbles form in a solution passing through a blood warmer
   (d) Solubility of solids is described as a given number of moles of solute dissolved in 1 liter of solvent
   (e) Solubility of gases is expressed as volume of gas dissolved in a specific volume of solvent

4. Bunsen solubility coefficient
   (a) Volume of gas, corrected to stp (standard temperature and pressure), which dissolves in 1 unit volume of the liquid at the temperature stated
      (1) Where the partial pressure of the gas above the liquid is 1 standard atmosphere pressure

5. Ostwald solubility coefficient
   (a) The volume of gas that dissolves 1 unit volume of the liquid at the temperature stated
      (1) It is independent of pressure

6. Partition coefficient
   (a) The ratio of the amount of substance present in one phase compared with another, the two phases being of equal volume and in equilibrium
   (b) Temperature must be stated
      (1) For example, at 37°C with the phases of blood and gas, the N_2O partition coefficient is 0.47
      (2) Note that the relative order of the phases must be specified
      (3) Blood-gas coefficient for halothane at 37°C is 2.3
         [a] Halothane is much more soluble in blood than N_2O

h. Humidity

1. Absolute humidity
   (a) The mass of water vapor present in a given volume of air
   (b) Expressed as grams per liter
   (c) As temperature rises, the amount of water that can be present as vapor rises; thus
      (1) At 20°C (room temperature), fully saturated air contains about 17 g/L
      (2) At 37°C (body temperature), fully saturated air contains about 44 g/L

IV. Physics; h. Humidity (continued)

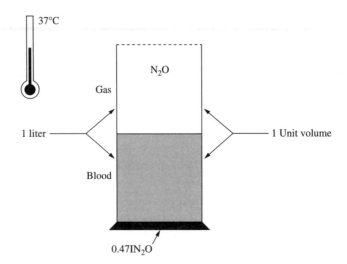

Figure 6. Partition coefficient.

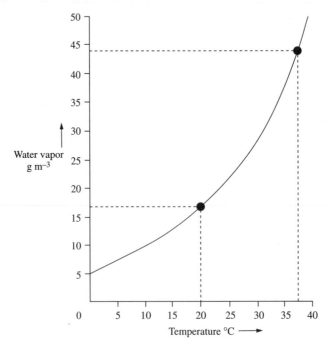

Figure 7. Graph of the humidity of air, saturated at various temperatures.

2. Relative humidity

    (a) Actual vapor pressure ÷ saturated vapor pressure at that temperature

---

i. Critical temperature

1. The temperature above which a substance cannot be liquefied no matter how much pressure is applied

2. Nitrous oxide has a critical temperature of 36.5°C

    (a) Therefore, at room temperature, it can be liquefied

    (b) Nitrous oxide is a vapor at room temperature because its boiling point is lower than room temperature

(c) The pressure gauge on the nitrous oxide cylinder is thus not very helpful since the liquid will constantly vaporize to maintain the saturated vapor pressure in the cylinder, displayed as a constant pressure on the pressure gauge. Only when the liquid in the cylinder is exhausted will the pressure begin to drop. Thus, the only way to tell whether a nitrous oxide cylinder is full is to weigh it

3. Oxygen has a critical temperature of $-119°C$

   (a) At room temperature, therefore, it cannot be compressed into a liquid and so is a gas

j. Critical pressure

1. The vapor pressure at the critical temperature

   (a) For nitrous oxide, for example, it is 73 bar/atmospheres

k. Breathing systems

1. Confusing

   (a) No universally accepted nomenclature
   (b) Complicated by the concept of the degree of rebreathing
   (c) Unless each breath contains only fresh gas (dictated by the fresh gas flow), some degree of rebreathing exists; this implies that some of the exhaled carbon dioxide is inspired in the following breath

2. The degree of "openness" is also confused. The simplest classification is

   (a) **Open:** infinite boundaries, with no restriction to fresh gas flow
   (b) **Semiopen:** the patient's airway is open to atmosphere during both inspiration and expiration
   (c) **Semiclosed:** the patient's airway is closed to atmosphere on inspiration, but open on expiration
   (d) **Closed:** there is no access to atmosphere during either inspiration or expiration
   (e) **Mapleson** breathing systems (probably the most widely used model)
      (1) No valves to direct gas to and from the patient
      (2) No device for absorption of carbon dioxide
      (3) The degree of fresh gas flow dictates the amount of rebreathing
      (4) The Mapleson systems present a confusing set of flow rate choices and most are wasteful of anesthetic gases and increasingly expensive vapors

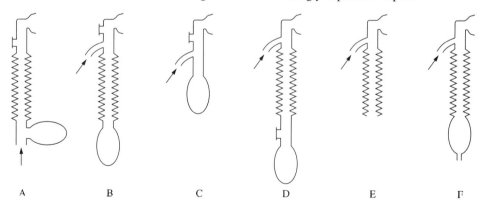

A   B   C   D   E   F

Figure 8. The Mapleson classification. Components include a reservoir bag, corrugated tubing, APL valve, fresh gas inlet, and patient connection. Redrawn from Mapleson WW. The elimination of rebreathing in various semiclosed anesthetic systems. Br J Anaesth *1954; 26:323–332.*

   (5) **Mapleson A, B,** and **C** systems
      [a] An expiratory valve proximally (patient end)

IV. Physics; k. Breathing systems (continued)

[b] Distal reservoir bag (machine end)

[c] **Mapleson A** or **Magill** circuit is the prototype for spontaneous breathing

   i) The flow rate for spontaneous breathing without significant rebreathing may be set at or slightly less than (75%) the patient's minute volume (respiratory rate × tidal volume)

   ii) Not recommended for controlled ventilation

   iii) If used, should be used with much higher flow rates—up to three times the minute volume to prevent rebreathing

   iv) The use of a capnograph will help determine the necessary fresh gas flows

[d] **Lack system** is a modified Mapleson A

   i) The expiratory valve is placed distally (machine end)

   ii) It is connected to the patient by a coaxial tube in the fresh gas supply tube

   iii) It was developed to aid the scavenging of expired gases; it needs to be differentiated from the other common coaxial system, the Bain circuit (see below)

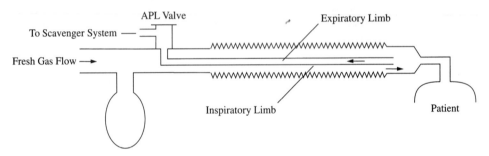

Figure 9. Lack modification of the Mapleson A system. The coaxial version is shown.

(6) **Mapleson B and C** systems are not used much today, but are mentioned as they may be the form of resuscitation bag (e.g., Ambu resuscitator). For the sake of completeness, the suggested gas flows are as follows

[a] **Mapleson B**

   i) Spontaneous: 1.5–2 × minute volume (MV)

   ii) Ventilated: 2–2.5 × MV

[b] **Mapleson C**

   i) Spontaneous: 2 × MV

   ii) Ventilated: 2–2.5 × MV

(7) **Mapleson D, E,** and **F** systems

[a] Fresh gas flow proximal

[b] Exhaust or expiratory valve (if present) distally

[c] All incorporate a T-piece connection proximally (the patient end)

[d] The volume of the expiratory limb and reservoir bag (if present) should exceed the patient's tidal volume

[e] Ideal for anesthetizing the spontaneously breathing infant

   i) Lightweight circuits

   ii) Do not necessitate very high absolute flow rates

   iii) Modifications make scavenging easy

[f] **Bain system** is a modified Mapleson D

   i) Fresh gas supply is provided by a coaxial tube down the center of the expiratory limb

[g] **Mapleson E** is not popular because of concerns about scavenging waste gases

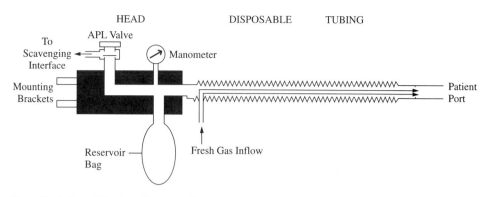

Figure 10. Bain modification of Mapleson D system.

[h] **Mapleson F** system is also called the Jackson-Rees system or the Jackson-Rees modification of the Ayre's T-piece
  i) Flow rates required to prevent rebreathing
    a) There are many opinions about this and formulas written using MV, body weight, and body surface areas as guides
  ii) In terms of safety, the recommendation would be at least 2.5 × minute volume with spontaneous breathing, and slightly less with controlled ventilation
  iii) End tidal CO_2 monitoring should be the guide
3. Circle system with carbon dioxide absorber

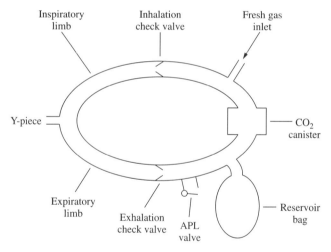

Figure 11. Components of the circle system.

(a) Eliminates any need to set flow rates
(b) Ideal for use as a completely closed breathing system, where flows as low as 250–300 ml oxygen and anesthetic vapor may be safely administered
(c) For ventilated patients, one may use it on the smallest neonate up to the largest adult
(d) For spontaneous respiration, it may present increased resistance to airflow in a small child if used with smaller absorption canisters; it may, however, be safely used in a spontaneously breathing child with a modern adult absorption circuit
(e) Components
    (1) Flow is directed via two one-way valves to and from the patient
    (2) A carbon dioxide absorber is part of the circuit
    (3) An adjustable pressure-limiting valve (APL) is found in the circuit
    (4) A reservoir bag is present (usually 3–5 liters for an adult)

(5) An oxygen sensor is usually located on the inspiratory limb of the circuit
(6) A spirometer should always be located on the expiratory limb
(7) Usually, the circuit has a switching device between the reservoir bag and a ventilator

(f) Carbon dioxide absorber

(1) Most modern absorbers consist of two canisters of absorbent joined in series
   [a] The canisters usually have transparent walls in order to observe whether the absorbent is exhausted (indicated by a color change)
   [b] Carbon dioxide is absorbed mostly in the upper canister; when this is exhausted, the lower canister will be utilized

(2) The most common absorbent is soda lime; barium hydroxide ("baralyme") is also used
   [a] 4% sodium hydroxide
   [b] 1% potassium hydroxide
   [c] 14–19% water
   [d] 76–81% calcium hydroxide
   [e] Small amounts of silica and kieselguhr are added for hardness
   [f] Some form of indicator is included to allow assessment of absorption capacity
      i) Indicator changes its color depending on the pH of the granule

(3) Moisture is essential for the chemical reactions to take place
   [a] $CO_2 + H_2O \leftrightarrow H_2CO_3$
   [b] $H_2CO_3 \leftrightarrow H^+ + HCO_3^-$
   [c] $NaOH \leftrightarrow OH^- + Na^+$
   [d] $Ca(OH)_2 \leftrightarrow 2OH^- + Ca_2^+$
   [e] (f) $2NaOH + 2H_2CO_3 + Ca(OH)_2 \leftrightarrow CaCO_3 + Na_2CO_3 + 4H_2O$
   [f] Heat is generated by this reaction and the temperature of the canisters can help to determine the remaining absorptive capacity of the soda lime (the lower the heat, the less absorptive capacity is left)

(4) The size of the granules of the soda lime determines how easily gases will pass through and around them
   [a] The bigger the granule, the easier it will be for gas to flow around it, but the smaller the overall absorptive area
   [b] Granules are 4 to 8 mesh in size (a 4-mesh strainer has four openings per square inch, and an 8-mesh strainer would have eight), that is, 8-mesh granules are smaller than 4-mesh granules

(5) The only way to reliably detect absorbent exhaustion is by measuring carbon dioxide concentration in the inspired gas

l. Anesthetic uptake and distribution

1. Introduction

   (a) In the progression of anesthetic gases from machine to neural tissue, the most important step to understand is the relationship between inspired and alveolar concentrations
   (b) Alveolar concentration determines (as the limiting factor) the concentrations achievable in the tissues

2. Anesthetic gas concentrations at the alveolar level during gas uptake will always be less than delivered (inspired) concentrations

   (a) The ratio of alveolar to inspired concentration (F_a/F_i) provides a valuable way to compare the behavior of various gases
   (b) Inspired concentration

        (1) Higher concentrations minimize the time needed to reach the desired alveolar concentration

        (2) The concept of overpressure deliberately uses very high concentrations of anesthetic for a brief time during induction to hasten uptake

3. Gas transfer to lung (ventilation)

   (a) The rate of delivery of gas to alveoli is directly proportional to alveolar ventilation V_A

   (b) The anesthetic will be diluted in the FRC

   (c) The ratio of minute ventilation to FRC (time constant) determines the rate of uptake of gas into the FRC

        (1) In one time constant, the concentration of a gas has reached 63% of its new, intended level

        (2) The time constant of a lung can be defined, then, as the ratio of FRC/V_A

   (d) Increased FRC or decreased V_A will slow uptake

        (1) Example: FRC = 2.5 liters, V_A = 5.0 L/min

        (2) Time constant = 2.5 L/(5.0 L/min) = 0.5 min = 30 sec

        (3) 30 seconds after abruptly changing the $F_I N_2 O$ to 0.70, the $N_2 O$ concentration in the FRC will be 0.63 × 0.70 or 0.441

4. Gas transfer to blood

   (a) Uptake V, ventilation

        (1) F_A/F_I is directly proportional to alveolar ventilation V_A

        (2) F_A/F_I is inversely proportional to uptake into the pulmonary arterial blood

        (3) Rapid uptake into blood lowers alveolar concentrations (and thus lowers attainable tissue levels for a given inspired concentration)

   (b) Factors affecting uptake by blood

        (1) Blood uptake is directly proportional to solubility, or blood–gas partition coefficient

           [a] Halothane is moderately soluble

           [b] Nitrous oxide is relatively insoluble

        (2) Blood uptake is directly proportional to cardiac output

        (3) Blood uptake is directly proportional to the alveolar to venous concentration difference

           [a] Venous blood anesthetic is anesthetic that has not been taken up by the tissues

   (c) Uptake from lung to blood (U_L) can be expressed as

$$U_L = \text{solubility} \times \text{cardiac output} \times (C_A - C_v)$$

        (1) Where C_A and C_v are the concentrations of anesthetic in the alveoli and the incoming venous blood, respectively

   (d) Tissue uptake (U_t) is modeled in a way similar to blood uptake

$$U_t = \text{solubility} \times \text{cardiac output} \times (C_a - C_t)$$

        (1) Where C_a and C_t are arterial and tissue concentrations

   (e) The final equation

        (1) This relates alveolar concentration to uptake and ventilation

$$F_A/F_I = 1 - U_L / F_I V_A$$

5. Effects of shunt

   (a) Alveolar ventilation increases alveolar concentration (F_A/F_I), while uptake into the pulmonary arterial blood tends to remove gas from the alveoli (thus decreasing F_A/F_I). Remember that uptake and F_A/F_I are inversely related—high uptake means lower alveolar concentrations (and lower attainable tissue levels for a given inspired concentration)

   (b) Right to left intracardiac or intrapulmonary shunt

        (1) Remaining perfused alveoli are hyperventilated to maintain $P_a CO_2$

           [a] This increases alveolar concentration (F_A) of anesthetic

IV. Physics; l. Anesthetic uptake and distribution (continued)

    (2) Blood bypassing the lung has two implications

        [a] Decreased effective pulmonary blood flow (less uptake, higher F_A/F_I)

        [b] Admixture of venous blood (low in anesthetic concentration) with blood from the lung (high anesthetic concentration)

        [c] Thus, there is a larger difference between alveolar and arterial anesthetic concentrations

        [d] The final effect on induction depends on solubility

    (3) Brain levels depend on arterial levels, thus

        [a] Soluble anesthetics (methoxyflurane)

            i) Hyperventilation increases F_A

            ii) Increased F_A increases delivery to the blood

            iii) High arterial concentrations from normal lung regions are diluted back to near normal by shunted blood

            iv) Thus, soluble anesthetics have normal arterial partial pressures and normal rate of induction

        [b] Insoluble anesthetics (i.e., N_2O)

            i) Low uptake into blood perfusing well-ventilated alveoli

            ii) Hyperventilation only increases F_A slightly

            iii) Thus, hyperventilation increases uptake slightly

            iv) Normal arterial concentrations are diluted to low levels by shunted blood

            v) Thus, shunt lowers arterial partial pressure of insoluble anesthetics and delays induction

6. Systemic shunt (A-V graft or left to right intracardiac shunt)

  (a) Systemic shunt also produces two effects

    (1) A decrease in tissue perfusion

      [a] Reduced peripheral extraction from blood if cardiac output is not increased to compensate for shunt

    (2) Shunted blood does not donate agent to tissues, so venous = arterial concentration

      [a] This effectively lowers the alveolar to venous blood gradient

      [b] This reduces uptake of agent from alveoli

  (b) So, systemic shunt usually has no effect on induction, but can slow induction if brain tissue perfusion is compromised by the shunt

7. Combined pulmonary and systemic shunt (complex congenital defects or septic shock)

  (a) The effects of systemic shunt can partially reverse the slow induction produced by pulmonary shunt

  (b) The recirculation of saturated blood through the lung by the systemic shunt reduces the apparent shunt seen by the lung

8. Summary

  (a) Perfusion of unventilated alveoli may slow the arterial rise in anesthetic concentration, especially with less soluble agents

  (b) Shunts in the body have little effect on induction, except in the presence of a lung shunt (where it lessens the impact of a lung shunt)

9. Concentration and second gas effects

  (a) Concentration effects

    (1) The higher the F_I, the more rapidly F_A/F_I will rise

    (2) No difference in uptake should appear in comparing different anesthetics with similar solubilities; however, for example, in the case of nitrous versus cyclopropane, the nitrous F_A/F_I rises faster

(b) Concentrating effect
  (1) If half of the inspired fraction of a gas is taken up, then the remaining volume of gas is "concentrated" as a fraction of the (now lower) lung volume. The ultimate effect of high inspired concentrations on alveolar concentration is breathing 100% N_2O! The alveolar concentration *cannot* drop below 100% and F_A/F_I is always 1.0
  (2) Augmented ventilation (or gas inflow)
    [a] If a significant volume of gas is taken up during a breath, the lungs do not collapse, but additional gas is drawn in to replace the volume deficit. This effectively increases V_A. This additional anesthetic increases the alveolar concentration faster
  (3) The net combined effect is that if half of the inspired gas (in this example, 80% nitrous) is taken up, the alveolar concentration falls to only 72%. At 100% concentration, the F_A/F_I curves of all anesthetics are the same. At lower concentrations, solubility begins to enter the equation
  (4) The concentration effect is only really significant for nitrous (among the modern agents); others cannot be given in high concentrations because they are too potent
(c) Second gas effect
  (1) Uptake of large volumes of a primary gas (usually nitrous) accelerates the rise of F_A of a second gas
  (2) The uptake of a primary gas decreases the volume in the lung and effectively increases the concentration of all other gases. Since the alveolar concentration of the second gas is now higher, induction is hastened

V. DISEASE STATES

a. Obstructive lung disease

1. Increased resistance to airflow can be caused by pathology in the lumen, in the bronchial wall, or outside the airways
   (a) Chronic obstructive lung (pulmonary) disease (COPD or COLD) is used to describe patients who have either chronic bronchitis, emphysema, or elements of both
   (b) Chronic bronchitis
     (1) "Excessive" sputum production for at least 3 months a year for at least 2 years
     (2) Tend to have increased venous admixture with hypoxia and cor pulmonale
     (3) "Blue bloater"
   (c) Emphysema
     (1) Destruction of lung parenchyma with loss of alveolar walls
     (2) Pathology
       [a] Centrilobular—central part of the lobule
       [b] Panlobular—whole lobule
       [c] α_1-antitrypsin deficiency is a congenital cause
       [d] Bullous
         i) Clinical manifestation
           a) Dyspnea occurs as the patient attempts to correct blood gas abnormalities
           b) "Pink puffer"
2. Reactive airway disease (asthma)
   (a) Definition
     (1) Increased reactivity of the tracheobronchial tree
   (b) Pathology

        (1) Inflammatory reaction characterized by bronchial smooth muscle constriction, mucus production, mucosal edema, leukocyte infiltration, inflammatory mediator release

    (c) Clinical manifestation

        (1) Airflow obstruction, wheezing, sometimes only cough

    (d) Preoperative preparation

        (1) Optimize bronchodilation, consider perioperative course of corticosteroid, severity not always a predictor of intraoperative problems

b. Restrictive lung disease

1. Pulmonary fibrosis

    (a) Pathology

        (1) Alveolar interstitial thickening due to unknown etiology

    (b) Clinical manifestation

        (1) Late-middle-age onset of dyspnea and cyanosis, ground glass appearance on chest x-ray

2. Sarcoidosis

3. Hypersensitivity pneumonitis

4. Systemic sclerosis

c. Perioperative management

1. Preoperative evaluation

    (a) Pulmonary function tests

        (1) On whom?

            [a] Will the answer change anesthetic management?

            [b] Most valuable in patients undergoing lung resection

        (2) Peak expiratory flow rate (PEFR)

    (b) ABGs

        (1) Of use only in patients with significant pulmonary disease, provides insight into patient's baseline status to guide postoperative goals

    (c) Chest x-ray

        (1) Utility of routine preoperative chest x-ray questionable; should only obtain in patients with either pulmonary or cardiac disease or smoking history of more than 20 pack-years

2. Preoperative preparation

    (a) Minimizing bronchospasm is clearly beneficial; other preoperative interventions are of less certain utility

    (b) Smoking cessation

        (1) Needs to have quit smoking at least 2 weeks prior to surgery as more recent cessation leads to increased secretions

        (2) Six to eight weeks required to achieve new baseline function

3. Anesthetic management

    (a) Intubation

        (1) Direct oral—appropriate if intubation difficulty not suspected

            [a] Head (and shoulders in obese patients) elevation

            [b] $F_IO_2 = 1.0$ during induction

            [c] Visualization of glottis and intubation

        (2) Fiberoptic

            [a] Indication: appropriate for difficult airway

　　　　[b] Contraindication: oropharyngeal bleeding generally precludes this approach

　　　　[c] Nasal—topical anesthesia and vasoconstriction, endotracheal tube passed into oropharynx, scope lubricated and passed through the endotracheal tube, cords visualized and may be topically anesthetized, scope passed into trachea, and endotracheal tube passed over scope. Position of endotracheal tube tip with relation to carina confirmed

　　　　[d] Oral—use of an oral airway guide is helpful to direct scope; endotracheal tube placed on scope first, glottis visualized and cords may be topically anesthetized, scope passed into trachea, and endotracheal tube advanced and position confirmed

　　　　[e] Awake

　　　　　　i) Indication: appropriate if difficult airway suspected

　　　　　　ii) High risk for gastric aspiration

　　　　　　iii) Anatomic risk for inadequate cord visualization or mask ventilation after induction

　　　　　　iv) Jaw malformation

　　　　　　v) Head and neck scar tissue

　　　　　　vi) Congenital anomalies of upper airway

　　　　　　vii) Morbid obesity

　　　　[f] Endobronchial

　　　　　　i) Indications

　　　　　　　　a) Appropriate when one lung ventilation desired

　　　　　　ii) Double lumen tube—most widely used, allows independent ventilation of both lungs if desired, passed into trachea in standard fashion and final position confirmed with bronchoscopy. Left-sided tubes are preferred to prevent occlusion of right upper lobe bronchus

　　　　　　iii) Bronchial blocker

　　　　　　　　a) Balloon-tipped catheter advanced into the unventilated lung with the aid of bronchoscopy and then the patient is intubated in the standard fashion. Easy to dislodge balloon and completely obstruct trachea

　　　　　　iv) Univent—retractable bronchial blocker incorporated in an endotracheal tube; positioning can be a problem

(b) Hypercarbia

　　(1) May result in sympathetic stimulation (tachycardia, sweating, hypertension, arrhythmias)

　　(2) Increased cerebral blood flow

　　(3) Usually due to alveolar hypoventilation but could be a sign of increased dead space, such as in pulmonary or air embolism

(c) Hypocarbia

　　(1) May prolong time for resumption of spontaneous ventilation at end of case

　　(2) Decreases cerebral blood flow

(d) Hypoxemia—greatest risk

　　(1) Low F_IO_2

　　　　[a] Anesthesia circuit leak or disconnect

　　(2) Endobronchial intubation

　　(3) Bronchospasm

　　(4) Pulmonary edema

　　(5) Pneumothorax

　　(6) Unplanned extubation

　　(7) Endotracheal tube obstruction

　　(8) Airway obstruction in nonintubated patient

　　(9) Alveolar hypoventilation

V. Disease States; c. Perioperative management (continued)

             (10) Atelectasis

             (11) Worsening of underlying pulmonary disease

             (12) Low cardiac output in patient with underlying pulmonary disease

             (13) Aspiration pneumonitis

          (e) Perioperative changes in gas exchange

             (1) General anesthesia

                 [a] Induction of anesthesia is associated with a 25–30% decrease in functional residual capacity and a concomitant decrease in Pa_{O_2}

                 [b] The decrease occurs immediately, does not change regardless of the depth or duration of the anesthetic, and resolves within 2 hours after the conclusion of anesthesia. Etiology is unclear

             (2) Surgery site

                 [a] On the trunk produces a restrictive type of defect that is not evident until several (more than 8) hours postoperatively, peaks at 72 hours, and is resolved within 2 weeks

                 [b] Site of surgery in increasing order of severity

                    i) Lower abdomen, thoracotomy, subcostal upper abdomen, midline upper abdomen

             (3) Etiology is unclear; neither analgesia nor intraoperative respiratory maneuvers prevent the postoperative changes

     4. Postoperative complications

         (a) Atelectasis—common after some operations (90% following CABG) but only occasionally of clinical importance

         (b) Pneumonia—incidence increased by site of operation and preoperative status. Upper abdominal surgery is associated with the highest incidence of postoperative pneumonia. Postoperative intubation may increase incidence

d. Anesthesia ventilators—classification

     1. Power source

         (a) Compressed gas alone

             (1) Ohio V5 and V5A

         (b) Electricity and compressed gas

             (1) NA Dräger AV-E

             (2) Ohmeda 7000 and 7810

     2. Drive mechanism

         (a) Double-circuit system with compressed gas squeezing the bellows

         (b) Cycling mechanism

         (c) Most are electronically controlled and time cycled

     3. Bellows classification

         (a) Direction of movement during *expiratory* phase determines type. Ascending bellows will not fill if a circuit disconnect occurs whereas a hanging bellows will

e. Critical care ventilators

     1. Sole function is to move gas in and out of lungs

     2. Important concepts

         (a) Tidal volume—set to 8–10 ml/kg

         (b) Positive end expiratory pressure: recruit collapsed alveoli; if effective, should decrease shunt and improve pulmonary compliance

(c) Peak inspiratory pressure: increase related to decreased lung compliance, believed to be critical factor in exacerbating lung injury, avoid over 35 cm H_2O

(d) Mechanical rate: adjusted to maintain Pa_{CO_2} in normal range. However, hypercapnia is acceptable in critically ill patients if it allows lower ventilatory pressures to be used

(e) I:E ratio: normally 1:2–3 but may be altered in pressure control mode to 1:1, 2:1, or even 4:1

(f) Inspiratory flow rate: adjusted to meet patient's demand

(g) Sensitivity: patient has to decrease airway pressure to get gas flow if spontaneous breaths are allowed; sensitivity has be set to minimize the work required to trigger demand valve

(h) Intrinsic PEEP: results from failure to reach 0 expiratory flow rate before next breath is given. Can occur with bronchospasm, mechanical obstruction of endotracheal tube, tachypnea, and emphysema

(i) Modes

(1) Control: patient receives a selected number of breaths of a preset tidal volume (volume limited); no spontaneous breaths allowed

(2) Assist-control: similar to control, but when patient attempts to inspire, ventilator delivers the same preset tidal volume

(3) Intermittent mandatory ventilation (IMV)—patient receives a selected number of mechanical breaths and the tidal volume of the spontaneous breaths is determined by the patient

(4) Pressure support: mode used to decrease the ventilator-imposed work of breathing. When patient takes a spontaneous breath, ventilator injects gas into the circuit at a flow rate sufficient to achieve a preset inspiratory airway pressure (i.e., 5–20 cm H_2O). The ventilator monitors the airway pressure and accordingly adjusts the flow rate every few milliseconds. When the patient approaches end inspiration, the pressure support ceases and the patient is allowed to exhale (pressure limited)

(5) Pressure control: instead of using a preset tidal volume, this mode uses a preset end inspiratory pressure. This mode requires attention to I:E ratio, ventilator rate, and inspiratory flow rate as these parameters determine the tidal volume and minute ventilation. It does not allow spontaneous breaths

(6) Airway pressure release ventilation: the patient is maintained at the positive airway pressure that permits the use of nontoxic F_IO_2. To achieve CO_2 removal, the airway pressure is "released" for less than 2 seconds at a preset rate. Spontaneous breathing is allowed during the "inspiratory" and "expiratory" phases

(7) High-frequency ventilation

(8) High-frequency oscillation: rates over 250 breaths a minute, used in infant respiratory distress syndrome

[a] High-frequency positive pressure ventilation: tidal volumes 1.5–5 ml/kg at rates up to 60–100 breaths per minute

[b] High-frequency jet ventilation: utilizes compressed gas applied to a needle injector to entrain gas into the lungs, tidal volumes 2–3 ml/kg at rates up to 400 breaths per minute. Warming and humidification of gas are a significant consideration

f. Humidifiers

1. Anesthetic gases are anhydrous; water and heat loss not a clinically significant problem; main reason for use is to maintain integrity of mucous blanket

2. Water vaporizers

(a) Passover: gas is passed over heated water reservoir; heated wick types (i.e.,

        Concha) produce 100% humidity even with high flow rates and little additional work of breathing

(b) Bubbler: gas is bubbled through water; not efficient and cools gas

(c) Cascade: generates fine bubbles that are passed through heated water; can provide 100% humidity but imposes substantial work of breathing

(d) Nebulizers deliver particulate water and any contaminants into the inspired air. Thus, infection is a greater risk with nebulizers than with humidifiers operating according to other principles

    (1) Jet: high-velocity gas is passed near the tip of a tube immersed in a liquid to be nebulized. The liquid moves from the tube into the low pressure of the jet stream and is broken into small particles by baffles placed downstream. Larger particles are deposited, leaving 0.5–30 μm particles in suspension. Can suspend up to 50 mg/L

    (2) Ultrasonic: high-frequency vibrations produce particles greater than 5 μm in diameter; water content may exceed 100 mg/L of air

g. Pulmonary edema

1. Cardiac/hydrostatic

    (a) Definition: excess interstitial fluid

    (b) Pathophysiology: edema occurs when the rate at which fluid leaves the capillary exceeds the rate at which the lymphatic can remove it

    (c) Pulmonary capillary hydrostatic pressure (P_c) is the most important factor in edema formation. It may be increased by left heart failure or fluid overload. If permeability is increased, then even small increases in P_c can worsen edema. There is no reliable method to determine P_c as pulmonary capillary wedge pressure is the estimate of the left atrial pressure, not capillary pressure

    (d) Clinical manifestations: fluid in the interstitium decreases lung compliance (becomes stiffer) so patients become tachypneic. When fluid leaks into the alveoli, venous admixture increases so PaO_2 decreases. Fluid leaking into the airways and mucosal edema and vascular engorgement may produce wheezing

    (e) Treatment: decrease pulmonary vascular pressures with diuretics, either with or without venodilators, so that the fluid leaves the capillaries less quickly

2. Neurogenic

    (a) Unusual cause of clinically significant pulmonary edema. Historically, frequently diagnosed before magnitude of aspiration appreciated

    (b) Thought to be due to transient but massive release of catecholamines that raises pulmonary vascular pressures so high that edema occurs; pulmonary vascular pressures have often returned to normal by the time invasive monitoring is placed

    (c) Treatment is supportive

h. Respiratory disease in pregnancy

1. Asthma—definition

    (a) Reversible airway obstruction

    (b) Airway inflammation

    (c) Hyperactive airways

    (d) Large variety of stimulating factors

2. Incidence and progression in pregnancy

    (a) Affects 1% of all pregnancies

  (b) 25% will improve from baseline during pregnancy
  (c) 50% will have no change
  (d) 25% will worsen
  (e) 10–15% will require hospitalization
  (f) Exacerbations are associated with
    (1) Low birth weight
    (2) Preterm birth
    (3) Increased perinatal mortality
  (g) Management in pregnancy similar to standard asthmatic care but exacerbations are more difficult to tolerate owing to the already stressed respiratory system. See Section for physiologic changes of pregnancy

3. Drugs used for asthma in pregnancy
  (a) Prevention of bronchospasm and hypoxia are primary concern
  (b) Sympathomimetic agents
    (1) Unknown teratogenicity potential
    (2) High dose
      [a] Increases heart rate
      [b] Lowers blood pressure
      [c] Acute pulmonary edema
      [d] Uterine relaxation
    (3) Albuterol associated with uterine hemorrhage during spontaneous abortion
    (4) Useful for bronchodilation in pregnant patient
  (c) Corticosteroids
    (1) Direct dilation of large and small bronchi
    (2) Interference with synthesis and action of biochemical mediators of asthma
      [a] Take time to work—should be administered early in course
      [b] Questions of teratogenic potential and possible association with stillbirth, cleft palate, and intrauterine growth retardation
      [c] Efficacy in preventing fetal hypoxia outweighs theoretical concerns
      [d] Beclomethasone inhaler—decreased systemic absorption; if systemic steroids required, use lowest effective dose
  (d) Theophylline
    (1) Falling into disfavor because of side effects
    (2) Need to monitor drug levels to maintain in therapeutic range, especially during pregnancy as clearance may be altered
    (3) Apparently free of teratogenic effects
    (4) Potent relaxant of uterine muscle
    (5) May prolong labor
      [a] Easily crosses placenta
      [b] Fetal heart tracings may have decreased variability
      [c] 10% will have transient tachycardia and jitteriness
      [d] Neonates will have prolonged half-life
  (e) Anticholinergics
    (1) Enhance bronchodilation initiated with beta-adrenergic agonists
    (2) Ipratroprium bromide—aerosol
    (3) No apparent teratogenicity
  (f) Cromolyn
    (1) Mechanism: protects against indirect bronchoconstrictor stimuli
    (2) Does not help all patients
    (3) No significant problems with pregnancy
      [a] If effective, should be continued
  (g) Antihistamines
    (1) Apparently safe in pregnancy; should not be used in last 2 weeks
    (2) May be an association between premature infants with retrolental fibroplasia and antihistamine use in last 2 weeks of pregnancy

4. Acute asthmatic management
   (a) Due to already stressed respiratory system, even slight exacerbations may lead to hypoxemia
   (b) Symptoms
       (1) Chest tightness
       (2) Dyspnea
       (3) Cough
       (4) Wheezing if air movement possible; may be so little ventilation that wheezing is absent
       (5) CO_2 greater than 35 (normal pregnancy 30–35) in pregnant patient may herald a tiring, seriously ill patient
   (c) Treatment
       (1) O_2
       (2) Beta-sympathomimetics
           [a] Metered dose inhaler or nebulizer
           [b] SC epinephrine, 0.3 ml, 1:1,000 solution
           [c] SC terbutaline, 0.25 mg
       (3) Steroids
           [a] Hydrocortisone, 100–200 mg, IV every 4–6 hours
       (4) Aminophylline if unresponsive to above treatment
           [a] Load 5–6 mg/kg over 20 minutes (maximum 400 mg) or bolus; if nontherapeutic, 2.5 mg/kg
           [b] Infusion
               i) 5 mg/kg/hour for a normal patient
               ii) 7 mg/kg/hour for a smoker
               iii) 3 mg/kg/hour for a cardiac patient

5. Obstetric management
   (a) May coincide with induction of labor
       (1) Increased sensitivity to prostaglandin-F_2-alpha's bronchoconstrictor properties
       (2) Prostaglandin E_2—aerosol can provoke bronchoconstriction
   (b) Postpartum hemorrhage
       (1) Drugs used for treatment of hemorrhage, 15-methyl prostaglandin, F_2-alpha, and ergot alkaloids, have been associated with acute bronchospasm
       (2) Oxytocin safe in asthmatic
   (c) Hypertension
       (1) Avoid beta-blockers

6. Anesthetic management
   (a) Opioids
       (1) May inhibit bronchoconstriction
   (b) Epidurals preferred
       (1) Lower stress
       (2) Lower anxiety
       (3) Decreased hyperventilation; in asthmatic patient, may cause bronchoconstriction
       (4) Minimize sedation
       (5) Minimize muscle weakness of respiratory musculature
       (6) May extend coverage to allow for cesarean section
   (c) Labor and vaginal delivery
       (1) Continuous infusion will maintain sensory anesthesia

      (2) Hourly monitoring and low-dose local anesthetic with narcotic (e.g., bupivacaine, 0.125%, with fentanyl, 1–2 μg/cc) will aid in avoiding motor blockade

      (3) Antiasthmatic medications should be continued even though they may decrease uterine contractility and thus prolong labor

   (d) Cesarean section

      (1) Acute exacerbations are more likely to occur following cesarean section than vaginal delivery, especially if endotracheal intubation is required

      (2) Regional anesthesia is preferred

      (3) For general anesthesia

        [a] Preoperative bronchodilation

        [b] Rapid-sequence induction

          i) *Caution*: most bronchodilators also relax uterine muscle and may contribute to hemorrhage; aerosolizing the medications minimizes systemic effects

        [c] Maintenance: routine inhalational agent with nitrous oxide and opioids; inhalational agents are bronchodilators and may relax uterine smooth muscle, and must be used in moderation

        [d] Emergence—awake due to aspiration considerations

          i) Refractory bronchospasm may require prolonged intubation

  7. Respiratory failure

   (a) Incidence and mortality

      (1) Adult respiratory distress syndrome (ARDS), 1 in 3,000 deliveries

        [a] Maternal mortality 50%

   (b) Pathophysiology

      (1) Increased pulmonary capillary permeability

      (2) Loss of lung volume

      (3) Shunting → hypoxemia

   (c) Etiology

      (1) Frequently multiple

      (2) Sepsis

      (3) Hemorrhage

      (4) Preeclampsia

      (5) Aspiration

      (6) Pulmonary embolism

      (7) Shock

      (8) Fluid overload

   (d) Management

      (1) Treatment aimed at maximizing maternal oxygenation

      (2) Cesarean section usually required if mechanical ventilation employed

      (3) General anesthesia with standard monitoring for pulmonary compromised patient

i. Autoimmune states

  1. Systemic lupus erythematosus

   (a) Characterized by antinuclear antibody production

   (b) Affects almost every organ system, including the pulmonary system

      (1) Lungs and pleura are involved in up to 70% of cases

        [a] Most common pathologic findings are pleuritis and pleural fibrosis and interstitial pneumonitis and fibrosis

        [b] Acute lupus pneumonitis is characterized by diffuse pulmonary infiltrates, pleural effusion, dry cough, dyspnea, and arterial hypoxemia

        [c] Radiologic findings

          i) Most common is a pleural effusion, which is frequently bilateral and small

          ii) Nonspecific, poorly defined patchy opacities in the lung bases and situated peripherally

      [d] Pulmonary function tests

          i) Usually show a restrictive pattern with reductions in diffusing capacity and arterial saturation

2. Rheumatoid disease

   (a) Clinical presentation

   (b) Symmetric polyarthropathy

   (c) Frequent systemic involvement

   (d) Most have high titers of antiglobulin antibody (rheumatoid factor)

   (e) Some 5 to 54% of these patients have demonstrable pulmonary disease

      (1) Pleural effusions are the most common manifestation

         [a] Typical features of an exudate

         [b] In half of the cases, it is unilateral and in the other half, it is bilateral

         [c] It usually remains stable for many months or years

      (2) Rheumatoid nodules are rare but do occur in the pulmonary parenchyma and on pleural surfaces. Histologically, the central portion is composed of necrotic material and is surrounded by a layer of palisaded epithelioid histiocytes. Rheumatoid nodules do not usually correlate with symptoms

      (3) Clinical manifestations: dyspnea is the most common presenting symptom. This may also be associated with cough and chest pain

      (4) Pulmonary function tests: restrictive pattern

3. Sarcoidosis

   (a) Systemic granulomatous disease that may involve almost any body organ, including the lymph nodes, lungs, liver, spleen, skin, and eyes

   (b) Etiology unknown, however, both genetic makeup and environmental factors seem to be involved

   (c) Pulmonary involvement is probably the most important manifestation

   (d) Much more common among blacks than among whites in the United States

   (e) The most common age range at the time of diagnosis is from 20 to 30

   (f) Pathology

      (1) The lungs and the intrathoracic lymph nodes are the most common sites of sarcoid reaction. These consist of disseminated nodules and variable fibrosis. Marked scarring with fibrosis and hyalinization, cystic formation, honeycombing, and emphysematous changes are markers of advanced disease. The pathologic hallmark of sarcoidosis is the granuloma, a well-defined collection of epithelioid histiocytes, often containing multinucleated giant cells

   (g) Radiographic findings

      (1) Lymph node enlargement

         [a] Lymph node enlargement is characteristically localized in the hilar regions bilaterally in a fairly symmetrical fashion. Enlargement of the right peritracheal nodes at the angle of the trachea and right main stem bronchus is also characteristic

      (2) Parenchymal lesions

      (3) Both

      (4) The radiographic changes in thoracic sarcoidosis can be classified in five stages

         [a] Stage 0: no demonstrable abnormality

         [b] Stage 1: hilar and mediastinal lymph node enlargement not associated with pulmonary abnormality

[c] Stage 2: hilar and mediastinal lymph node enlargement associated with pulmonary abnormality

[d] Stage 3: diffuse pulmonary disease not associated with node enlargement

[e] Stage 4: pulmonary fibrosis

(h) Clinical manifestations: symptoms develop in about 50% of patients, the remainder being identified in asymptomatic individuals on screening chest roentgenograms. The asymptomatic patients usually have evidence of bilateral hilar lymphadenopathy (BHL). Constitutional symptoms, such as weight loss, fatigue, weakness, and malaise, are often associated with multisystem disease and usually develop insidiously. In a subset of patients with a more acute form, BHL is sometimes accompanied by fever, joint pains, and erythema nodosum (purplish-red indurated rash on the extensor surface of legs and forearms). This type of acute onset occurs most often in young females. Significant pulmonary symptoms develop in only about one fourth of patients, although histologic involvement of the lungs can be demonstrated in the majority. The predictable symptoms include cough and dyspnea. Chest pain is not common and hemoptysis is rare. This finding is important to remember because, in one series, all the asymptomatic patients with BHL had sarcoidosis and all the patients with BHL and symptoms had neoplasms

(i) Pulmonary function tests

(1) Usually show a restrictive pattern with a low diffusing capacity

(j) Variable degrees of hypoxemia

(k) Management

(1) Most require no treatment

(2) Corticosteroids and other immunosuppressive drugs are the only agents known to suppress the active disease

(3) Patients with progressive respiratory involvement, involvement of the eyes, cardiac sarcoidosis, CNS involvement, disfiguring skin lesions, and persistent elevation of serum calcium usually require treatment

j. Nervous and muscular diseases

1. Tetanus

(a) Tetanus is a neurologic disorder caused by the infection of penetrating wounds with *Clostridium tetani*. These bacteria are an anaerobic gram-positive rod that secretes an endotoxin, tetanospasmin, which is taken up by nerve endings and transmitted to the CNS

(b) Pathogenesis: tetanospasmin interferes with the release of acetylcholine at motor end plates, and in the spinal cord, it interferes with the release of inhibitory neurotransmitters

(c) Clinical manifestations

(1) Median time of onset after injury is 7 days and ranges from 3 to 10 days

(2) Muscle tone is markedly increased and the muscle is hyperexcitable, with resulting trismus and severe spasms in response to slight stimuli. Some patients develop paroxysmal, violent, generalized muscle spasms that may cause cyanosis and threaten ventilation. They occur repetitively and may be spontaneous or provoked by the smallest stimulation. Reduced ventilation of laryngospasm is a constant threat during generalized spasm

(3) Disinhibition of the autonomic nervous system leads to labile hypertension, tachycardia, pyrexia, and profuse sweating

(d) Management

(1) Wound debridement, penicillin (questionable benefit), passive immunization with immune globin, and active immunization

(2) Spasms may be treated with high doses of benzodiazepines, such as

diazepam or lorazepam. Neuromuscular blockade and mechanical ventilation are highly effective for treating severe spasms that threaten ventilation

(3) The autonomic cardiovascular changes can usually be controlled by beta-blockade

2. Guillain-Barré (acute idiopathic polyneuropathy)

   (a) Characterized by the sudden onset of proximal lower extremity weakness, which spreads cephalad over a short period to the skeletal muscles of the arms, trunk, and head. It has become the most common cause of acute generalized paralysis, with an annual incidence of 0.75 to two cases per 100,000 population

   (b) Pathogenesis: probably an immunologic basis, but the mechanism is unclear. It sometimes follows infective illness, inoculation, or surgical procedure. There is also an association with preceding *Campylobacter jejuni* enteritis

   (c) Pulmonary manifestations: problems are secondary to intercostal muscle paralysis and pharyngeal muscle weakness, which can lead to difficulty in swallowing and aspiration. Patients should be intubated if their vital capacity falls below 15 ml/kg or if they are unable to handle their secretions. Finally, adult respiratory distress syndrome and pulmonary emboli are common

3. Dystrophies—hereditary diseases characterized by painless degeneration and atrophy of skeletal muscle; there are progressive and symmetric skeletal muscle weakness and wasting, but no evidence of muscle denervation

   (a) Duchenne type muscular dystrophy
       (1) An X-linked recessive disorder sometimes also called pseudohypertrophic muscular dystrophy, it occurs with an incidence of about 30 per 100,000. It usually becomes apparent between the ages of 3 and 5
       (2) Pulmonary manifestations: progressive weakness and contractures, which result in kyphoscoliosis by the age of 12. The chest deformity associated with scoliosis impairs the pulmonary function already demised by muscle weakness. This produces a restrictive pattern on pulmonary function tests. By ages 16 to 18, patients have repeated pulmonary infections and are predisposed to pulmonary aspiration. Death is usually due to recurrent pulmonary infections, respiratory failure, or aspiration pneumonitis

   (b) Becker's muscular dystrophy
       (1) This less severe form of X-linked recessive muscular dystrophy was described in 1955. It is approximately 10 times less frequent than Duchenne, with an incidence of about three per 100,000. The pattern of muscle wasting in Becker's muscular dystrophy closely resembles that seen in Duchenne, except that it presents in adolescence and progresses more slowly. Patients often live into the fourth and fifth decades
       (2) Pulmonary manifestations are very similar to those of Duchenne, except that they present in adolescence

   (c) Myotonic dystrophy
       (1) Myotonic disorders are characterized by sustained contractions of muscles after voluntary or mechanical stimulation. Myotonic contractures often fail to relax, even after neural blockade and administration of nondepolarizing muscle relaxants. Myotonic dystrophy represents the most common adult muscular dystrophy and has an incidence of 13.5 per 100,000 live births. It is an autosomal dominant disorder and involves an equal proportion of males and females
       (2) The disease presents in the second or third decade of life and involves skeletal, cardiac, and smooth muscle. Myotonia is the principal manifestation early in the disease, but as it slowly progresses, muscle weakness and

atrophy become more prominent. Multiorgan dysfunction in some patients is evidenced by presenile cataracts, facial weakness (expressionless face), wasting and weakness of sternocleidomastoids, ptosis, and dysarthria

    (3) Pulmonary manifestations: involvement of respiratory muscles can cause a decrease in vital capacity and a restrictive pattern on pulmonary function tests. Palatal, pharyngeal, and tongue involvement may cause chronic aspiration

k. Altitude physiology

1. Physical principles of environmental changes
   - (a) Gas laws
     - (1) According to Boyle's law, as pressure decreases during ascent, volume increases (gas expands)
       - [a] Physiologic illustrations
         - i) Gas in body cavities expands
           - a) Sinuses
           - b) Middle ear
           - c) Teeth (areas of decay)
           - d) Lungs
           - e) Intestine
         - ii) All gas-filled spaces may cause pain during ascent (gas expansion) or descent (gas volume decreases)
       - [b] Medical considerations
         - i) Equipment
           - a) Endotracheal or tracheostomy tube cuffs
           - b) Foley balloons
           - c) IV bags/bottles
           - d) IV drip chambers
           - e) Pressure bags
           - f) Any air/gas-filled object
         - ii) Implications
           - a) All cuffs, balloons should be filled with saline to prevent volume changes
           - b) IV drip rates and pressure bags must be adjusted if atmospheric pressure increases or decreases
     - (2) Dalton's law
       - [a] Total atmospheric pressure at sea level is 760 mm Hg (P_B = 760 mm Hg)
       - [b] Normal arterial P_{O_2} is 21% of P_B

Composition of Respired Air at Sea Level—Gas Partial Pressure (mm Hg)				
Respired Gas	Tracheal Air	Alveolar Air	Arterial Blood	Venous Blood
O_2	149	100	95	40
CO_2	0.3	40	40	46
N_2	563.7	573	573	573
H_2O	47	47	47	47
Total	760	760	755	706

      (3) According to Pascal's law (see "gas laws")
- [a] Deep tissue compartments experience the pressure changes that occur outside the body
- [b] A bubble deep within the body tissues experiences the pressure applied to the external body

V. Disease States; k. Altitude physiology (continued)

  (4) According to Henry's law (see "gas laws"), more gas will be dissolved in all body fluids when the ambient pressure increases and less when it decreases

2. Physiology of altitude
   (a) Total atmospheric pressure decreases in a nonlinear fashion with increasing altitude (see table, "Respiratory Gas Pressures at Increasing Altitude")
   (b) Normal inspired O_2 tension (P_IO_2) ("normoxia") is 160 mm Hg at sea level
   (c) Normal arterial O_2 tension (PaO_2) is 90–100 mm Hg
   (d) PaO_2 over 60 mm Hg is hypoxemia
   (e) P_IO_2 less than 110 mm Hg will result in hypoxemia, that is, at altitudes of 10,000 feet (equivalent to 10.1 psi or 523 mm Hg; see table, "Respiratory Gas Pressures at Increasing Altitude")

3. Definitions of hypoxia
   (a) Hypoxic hypoxia (low PaO_2)
      (1) A deficiency in alveolar O_2 exchange
      (2) Decrease in partial pressure of inspired O_2
   (b) Hyperemic hypoxia
      (1) Rate of delivery of O_2 to tissue does not meet metabolic demands
      (2) Anemia
      (3) CO poisoning
   (c) Histotoxic hypoxia
      (1) Inability of cell to use O_2
      (2) Metabolic disorders
      (3) Poisoning of cytochrome oxidase system
         [a] CO poisoning
         [b] Cyanide poisoning
   (d) Stagnant hypoxia
      (1) Reduction of cardiac output, pooling of blood, or restriction of blood flow
         [a] *G* forces
         [b] Clot or gas (bubble) embolus
   (e) Subcritical hypoxia: physiologic effects are present but do not affect ability to perform critical tasks
      (1) Beginning of subcritical hypoxia
         [a] 13,000 feet (465 mm Hg)
             i) Atmospheric PO_2 = 97.4 mm Hg
             ii) Alveolar PO_2 = 51.0 mm Hg
   (f) Critical hypoxia: physiologic effects are immediate and affect ability to perform critical tasks
      (1) Beginning of critical hypoxia
         [a] 23,000 feet (P_B = 308 mm Hg)
         [b] Atmospheric PO_2 = 65 mm Hg
         [c] Alveolar PO_2 = 55 mm Hg
   (g) Beginning of need for breathing 100% O_2 with pressure
      (1) 33,000 feet (P_B = 197 mm Hg)
         [a] Atmospheric PO_2 = 41 mm Hg
         [b] Alveolar PO_2 = 32 mm Hg
   (h) Boiling point of bodily fluids (ebullism)
      (1) (Ambient pressure = vapor pressure plasma)
      (2) Armstrong line
         [a] 65,000 feet (P_B = 43 mm Hg)
         [b] Atmospheric PO_2 = 9.0 mm Hg
   (i) Limit of aerodynamic navigation
      (1) 37–49 mm Hg

      (j) Line between atmosphere and space
         (1) 62 miles
      (k) Conversions
         (1) 1 mm Hg = 0.019 psi
         (2) 1 psi = 52 mm Hg

4. Altitude sickness

    (a) Acute mountain sickness
        (1) 15% of resort skiers
        (2) Related to rate of ascent to altitude (fitness not a factor)
        (3) Individual susceptibility varies greatly
    (b) Symptoms
        (1) Headache
        (2) Anorexia
        (3) Nausea
        (4) Dyspnea
        (5) Insomnia
    (c) Signs
        (1) Tachypnea
        (2) Vomiting
        (3) Pulmonary edema
        (4) Cerebral edema
    (d) Etiology
        (1) Hypoxia due to low inspired P_{O_2}
        (2) Impaired gas exchange due to pulmonary edema
        (3) Fluid redistribution and retention
        (4) Increased intracranial pressure (capillary leak syndrome)
    (e) Treatment
        (1) Descend at least 1,000 feet
        (2) Acclimatization
        (3) O_2 (100% if possible)
        (4) Acetazolamide, 125–250 mg, orally every 8 to 12 hours
    (f) Prevention
        (1) Slow ascent
        (2) Avoid respiratory depressants
        (3) Start acetazolamide 1 day before

5. High-altitude pulmonary edema

    (a) 1–2% above 12,000 feet
    (b) Cough, dyspnea, cyanosis, sudden death
    (c) Treatment
        (1) Descend
        (2) Rest
        (3) O_2
        (4) Continuous positive airway pressure (CPAP)

6. High-altitude cerebral edema

    (a) Symptoms
        (1) Ataxia
        (2) Changes in consciousness
    (b) Treatment
        (1) Descend
        (2) O_2
        (3) Other known therapy for cerebral edema

7. Retinal hemorrhages

    (a) Affect vision only if macula involved (rare)

        (b) Hypoxic mechanism
           (1) Bleed in capillary bed
        (c) No treatment known, no prevention known
        (d) Will clear in 7 to 14 days

8. Special considerations during air evacuation
        (a) Environmental factors
           (1) Temperature
           (2) Cold
               [a] Ambient temperature decreases 2°F for each 1,000 feet of altitude
           (3) Noise
               [a] Aircraft are noisy, some more than others. Helicopters are especially noisy. Noise makes taking vital signs and communication very difficult. Noise is also very fatiguing to air crew, caregivers, and patients
           (4) Vibration
               [a] Vibration is especially a problem with helicopters. All of the comments about noise also apply
           (5) Humidity
               [a] As altitude increases, the ambient air is more and more dryIncreased loss of H_2O through lungs
               [b] Need to increase fluid intake (IV or oral), monitor intake and output
           (6) Hypoxia due to low P_IO_2
        (b) Medical considerations
           (1) Give supplemental O_2 for
               [a] Anemia
               [b] Cardiac status
               [c] Pulmonary status
               [d] Pregnancy

9. Physical factors
        (a) Trapped gas (Boyle's law)
           (1) Vent IV chambers and bottles
           (2) Normal saline in all air-containing cuffs/balloons
        (b) Dissolved gas
           (1) If patient has been diving, must allow time for N_2 to come out of solution through pulmonary function (Henry's law)
           (2) Ambient PN_2 is much less than PN_2 in blood (of diver) and N_2 will come out of solution (Henry's law) during ascent
           (3) Recommend no flying 24 hours after last dive
           (4) In some people, the reduction of ambient pressure of flight cabin can produce the "bends" or decompression sickness (DCS), especially with rapid ascent

l. Obesity

1. Introduction
        (a) Affects 25–45% of adult Americans
        (b) Some 5–7% of the obese population falls into the morbidly obese category
        (c) Increases risk of anesthesia + surgery
        (d) Increases risk of body systems impairment
        (e) Cardiovascular
        (f) Pulmonary
        (g) Gastrointestinal (GI) + metabolic

Respiratory Gas Pressures at Increasing Altitude

Breathing Air

| Altitude | | Ambient Pressure | | | | |
Meters	Feet	PSIA	mm Hg	P_AO_2, mm Hg	Pao_2, mm Hg	$Paco_2$, mm Hg
0	0	14.69	759.97	159.21	103.0	40.0
305	1,000	14.17	733.04	153.57	98.2	39.4
610	2,000	13.66	706.63	148.04	93.8	39.0
914	3,000	13.17	681.23	142.72	89.5	38.4
1,219	4,000	12.69	656.34	137.50	85.1	38.0
1,524	5,000	12.23	632.46	132.50	81.0	37.4
1,829	6,000	11.77	609.09	127.60	76.8	37.0
2,134	7,000	11.34	586.49	122.87	72.8	36.4
2,438	8,000	10.91	564.64	118.29	68.9	36.0
2,743	9,000	10.50	543.31	113.82	65.0	35.4
3,048	10,000	10.10	522.73	109.51	61.2	35.0
3,353	11,000	9.72	502.92	105.36	57.8	34.4
3,658	12,000	9.34	483.36	101.26	54.3	33.8
3,962	13,000	8.99	464.82	97.38	51.0	33.2
4,267	14,000	8.63	446.53	93.55	47.9	32.6
4,572	15,000	8.29	429.01	89.88	45.0	32.0
4,877	16,000	7.96	411.99	86.31	42.0	31.4
5,182	17,000	7.65	395.73	84.50	40.0	31.0
5,486	18,000	7.34	379.73	79.55	37.8	30.4
5,791	19,000	7.05	364.49	76.36	35.9	30.0
6,096	20,000	6.76	349.50	73.22	34.3	29.4
6,401	21,000	6.48	335.28	70.24	33.5	29.0
6,706	22,000	6.21	321.31	67.31	32.8	28.4
7,010	23,000	5.95	307.85	64.49	32.0	28.0
7,315	24,000	5.70	294.89	61.78	31.2	27.4
7,620	25,000	5.46	282.45	59.17	30.4	27.0

Breathing 100% Oxygen

10,058	33,000	3.81	197.10	197.10	109	40
10,973	36,000	3.30	170.94	170.94	85	38
11,887	39,000	2.86	148.08	148.08	64	36
12,192	40,000	2.73	141.22	141.22	—	—
12,802	42,000	2.48	128.27	128.27	48	33
13,716	45,000	2.15	111.25	111.25	34	30
14,021	46,000	2.05	105.92	105.92	30	29

Modified from Sheffield PJ, Heimbach RD. In *Fundamentals of Aerospace Medicine.* Edited by RL DeHart. Philadelphia: Lea & Febiger, 1985.

2. Increases incidence of certain medical conditions

    (a) Hypertension
    (b) Diabetes
    (c) Coronary artery disease (CAD), myocardial infarction (MI), sudden death
    (d) Cancer
    (e) Cholelithiasis
    (f) All of the above may be compounded by psychosocial problems

3. Numbers

    (a) There are approximately 30,000 operative procedures done each year just to treat morbid obesity

4. Definition
    (a) Body mass index (BMI)

$$BMI = \frac{Wt_{kg}}{Ht^2_m}$$

    (1) Normal = 22–28
    (2) Overweight = 25–30
    (3) Obese = >30
    (4) Morbidly obese = >40
    (b) Alternative definitions
    (1) Normal = ideal body weight (IBW) for a given age, height, and gender
    (2) Overweight = ≤20% above IBW
    (3) Obese = >20% above IBW
    (4) Morbidly obese = IBW × 2, or 100 pounds above IBW

5. Pathophysiologic changes
    (a) Pulmonary
    (b) Cardiovascular
    (c) Gastrointestinal
    (d) Endocrine
    (e) Airway
    (f) Psychologic
    (g) Pharmacokinetics/dynamic
    (h) Obesity hypoventilation syndrome

6. Pulmonary
    (a) Increase resting metabolic demands (2°) secondary to increase tissue mass
    (1) Increased O_2 consumption
    (2) Increased CO_2 production
    (3) Increased minute ventilation
    (b) Increased work and energy cost of breathing (i.e., decreased efficiency)
    (1) Decreased chest wall compliance
    (2) Decreased FRC and decreased ERV and TLC 2° to decrease compliance
    (c) Closure of basal small airways
    (1) V/Q mismatch during normal resting ventilation
    (2) Increased shunting
    (3) Closing capacity unchanged
    (d) Supine position: these effects are exaggerated
    (1) Further decrease in functional residual capacity (FRC), cephalad shift of diaphragm, and increase in intra-abdominal pressure
    (2) Closure of more basal alveoli
    (3) Further decrease in compliance
    (4) Clinically significant increases in shunting and O_2 consumption
    (e) End result
    (1) Chronic hypoxemia
    (2) With or without hypercapnia

7. Cardiovascular
    (a) Arterial hypertension
    (b) Increased circulating blood volume leads to increased preload
    (1) Increased plasma volume + increased red blood cell (RBC) mass
    (c) Increased resting cardiac output (CO), secondary to increased stroke volume (SV)
    (d) Chronic preload increase leads to left ventricular hypertrophy (LVH) + dilation

(e) Decreased left ventricular compliance

(f) Increased left ventricular end diastolic pressure (LVEDP)

    (1) Increased pulmonary arterial occlusion pressure (PAOP)

(g) High incidence of pulmonary hypertension

(h) Increased incidence of sudden death

(i) Tenfold increase in incidence of PVCs

(j) Supine position

    (1) Significant increase in PAOP and CO

    (2) Increased O_2 consumption (because of increased work of breathing)

8. Gastrointestinal

  (a) Increased gastric volume in fasting state (volume greater than 25 ml)

  (b) Decreased gastric pH (below pH 2.5)

  (c) Increased risk for pulmonary aspiration

  (d) Increased incidence of hiatal hernia

  (e) Increased intra-abdominal pressure

  (f) Increased incidence of hepatic fatty infiltration

9. Endocrine

  (a) Glucose intolerance

  (b) Diabetes mellitus

  (c) Abnormal serum lipid profiles

10. Airway

  (a) Decreased flexion cervical spine

  (b) Decreased mouth opening

  (c) Narrowed airway

  (d) High, anterior larynx

  (e) Breasts or anterior chest wall may interfere with laryngoscopy

11. Psychologic

  (a) Increased incidence of psychopathology in morbidly obese

  (b) Inherent or response to abuse

  (c) Patients can be very demanding emotionally, as well as physically

12. Pharmacokinetics/dynamics

  (a) Obese patients have larger fat compartment

  (b) Biotransformation of drugs may be altered 2° to hepatic disease, or changes in hepatic blood flow

  (c) Renal drug elimination may be affected by changes in glomerular filtration

  (d) Biliary excretion may be altered by presence of cholelithiasis

  (e) High incidence of lipoproteinemia may affect drug binding

  (f) Lipophilic drugs will have increased V_D and increased $T_{1/2}\beta$ (elimination half-life)

    (1) Fentanyl pharmacokinetics unchanged; drug should be given on basis of lean body weight

    (2) Alfentanyl: decreased $T_{1/2}\beta$ due to decreased clearance

    (3) Thiopental: repeat doses lead to accumulation + prolonged clearance

    (4) Hydrophilic drugs (pancuronium have similar V_D, $T_{1/2}$ if dose is adjusted for body surface area (BSA)

    (5) Increased doses of succinylcholine needed because of increased plasma pseudocholinesterase levels

  (g) Increased metabolism of volatile agents and increased F^- ion production

13. Obesity hypoventilation syndrome (Pickwickian syndrome)

  (a) Distinguished by the presence of CO_2 retention, that is, loss of CO_2 drive

  (b) Associated features

    (1) Severe hypoxemia

        (2) Somnolence 2° to obstructive sleep apnea → awakening → resumption of breathing; frequent cycles → sleep deprivation → daytime somnolence

        (3) Periodic breathing

        (4) Pulmonary hypertension

        (5) Systemic hypertension

        (6) Biventricular enlargement, especially R side

        (7) Polycythemia

        (8) Dependent edema

        (9) Pulmonary edema

14. Management preoperative

    (a) Psychology

        (1) Go to see the patient

        (2) Try to gain patient's confidence

        (3) Avoid stereotypical remarks

        (4) Carefully explain procedures and expectations

    (b) History and physical

        (1) Thorough cardiorespiratory evaluation

            [a] Ability to lie flat

        (2) Sleep pattern, narcolepsy, nocturnal sweats, enuresis, snoring

        (3) Exercise tolerance, mobility, SOB, chest pain

        (4) History of hypertension, failure

        (5) Drug history, use + abuse

        (6) Lines, access IV and arterial

        (7) Airway evaluation, mouth opening, neck flexion/extension, thyromental distance

15. Preoperative investigation

    (a) Routine

        (1) Full blood count

        (2) Electrolytes

        (3) Liver function tests

        (4) Glucose

        (5) Arterial blood gas (sitting and supine)

        (6) 12-lead electrocardiogram (ECG)

        (7) Complete x-ray

        (8) Urinalysis

    (b) Additional

        (1) Pulmonary function tests

        (2) MUGA ± dipyridamole thallium stress test

16. Premedication

    (a) H_2 receptor antagonist (ranitidine preferred) night before and on morning of surgery to increase gastric pH

    (b) Gastrokinetic agent (metoclopramide or cisapride) on morning of surgery to decrease gastric volume

    (c) Nonparticulate oral antacid prior to starting rapid-sequence induction

    (d) Avoid sedation, if possible; explain why to the nervous patient and use reassurance as the primary means to allay anxiety

    (e) No intramuscular (IM) drugs

17. Intraoperative management

    (a) Anesthesiologist must have clear plan on how to proceed

    (b) Now is not the time to be vacillating with options

    (c) Operating room table positioning

      (1) May need to join two tables together

      (2) Table adjustment is difficult if two tables are used

      (3) Carefully position patient's arms and protect pressure area

   (d) Monitoring

      (1) Five-lead ECG

   (e) Venous access—may be very difficult, may need to be cut down

   (f) Arterial access—for invasive blood pressure and arterial blood gas (ABG) samples

   (g) Central line—for monitoring volume status

   (h) Plus pulmonary artery flotation catheter—if in heart failure, need to measure PAOP, or right ventricular failure with pulmonary hypertension in patient with obesity hypoventilation syndrome

   (i) Neuromuscular junction monitoring—may require percutaneous needle electrodes

   (j) Temperature: maintain temperature intraoperative to avoid shivering with its concomitant increase in O_2 consumption in the immediate postoperative period

   (k) Pulse oximetry, end tidal CO_2

18. Induction

   (a) Choice will depend on

      (1) Size of patient

      (2) Anticipated ease or difficulty in securing airway

      (3) Presence of other modifying factors

   (b) Options

      (1) Topical anesthetic to base of tongue and pharynx, then do awake look

      (2) If epiglottis and cords visualized, may proceed to rapid-sequence induction with preoxygenation and cricoid pressure

      (3) If any doubts about ability to secure the airway, then

        [a] Do fiberoptic awake nasotracheal intubation

      (4) Remember, breath sounds may be faint or inaudible; therefore, must be able to demonstrate ET_{CO_2} trace to confirm successful intubation

19. Use of regional anesthesia

   (a) Advantages

      (1) May not need to put patient to sleep

      (2) Good abdominal muscle relaxation

      (3) Airway remains protected

      (4) Ventilation may not be compromised

      (5) Avoidance of opiate-induced respiratory depression

      (6) Provision of postoperative pain relief

   (b) Difficulties

      (1) Technical—may have no landmarks to identify

      (2) Patient may be unable to tolerate supine position

      (3) Delayed onset—level may continue to rise over a 30-minute period

      (4) If it goes wrong, may need to do emergency intubation

      (5) Dosing—use a lower dose, 75–80% of estimated dose for age and height

   (c) Advantages of combined general and regional

      (1) Smaller dose of volatile agent

      (2) Less need for neuromuscular blockade

      (3) Postoperative analgesia without respiratory depression from systemic opiates

      (4) Earlier mobilization

      (5) Fewer pulmonary complications in postoperative period

20. Postoperative management

   (a) All obese patients at higher risk for postoperative hypoxemia

      (1) Admit to ICU for aggressive pulmonary therapy

          (2) Provide supplemental oxygen up to 4 days postoperatively

          (3) Adopt semirecumbent position rather than supine

          (4) Provide effective postoperative pain management—whether opiates or regional techniques to allow effective breathing exercises plus clearance of secretions

      (b) Subcutaneous heparin to decrease risk of thrombophlebitis

---

m. Hyperbaric and diving medicine

    1. "Hyper" = high; "baro" = barometric pressure

      (a) Hyperbaric oxygen therapy is a treatment in which the patient breathes 100% oxygen intermittently while the entire body is enclosed in a pressure vessel at greater than sea-level atmospheric pressure

    2. Rationale

      (a) Increased oxygen-carrying capacity

          (1) O_2 carried two ways in body

             [a] Chemically bound to hemoglobin (HbO_2)

             [b] Physically dissolved in plasma

          (2) Hb-bound oxygen

             [a] Each gram of oxygenated Hb carries 1.34 ml of O_2 (four O_2 molecules on each Hb molecule)

             [b] Assuming 15 g/dl Hb concentration, 20 ml of O_2 can be carried per 100 ml blood (i.e., 20 vol%); this is a normal O_2 carrying capacity

          (3) Plasma-dissolved O_2

             [a] At a Pao_2 of 100 mm Hg, only 0.31 ml of O_2 is dissolved per 100 ml blood plasma (i.e., 0.31 vol%)

             [b] Once Hb is saturated, raising inspired O_2 concentration can affect only plasma-dissolved O_2

             [c] As Po_2 increases, O_2 physically dissolved in plasma increases linearly

             [d] Plasma-dissolved O_2 increases approximately 2 vol% for each atmosphere (760 mm Hg) increase in pressure, if breathing 100% oxygen (ATA = atmospheres absolute)

                i) Example: If breathing 100% oxygen, amount of oxygen physically dissolved in plasma: at 1 ATA ≈ 2 vol%, 2 ATA ≈ 4 vol%, 3 ATA ≈ 6 vol% physically dissolved O_2 in plasma

             [e] Tissue oxygen extraction is usually 4–6% vol%. It is, therefore, possible to live solely off plasma-dissolved O_2 in the total absence of Hb, if 100% oxygen is breathed at atmospheric pressures two to three times sea level

             [f] Theoretical Pao_2 can be calculated at any atmospheric pressure

                i) Sea level = 760 mm Hg = 1 ATA

                ii) Assume at 1 ATA (sea level)

                    a) 21% of 760 = 160 mm Hg P_{IO_2}

                    b) 79% of 760 = 600 mm Hg P_{IN_2}

                    c) 100% (air) = 760 mm Hg total

                iii) Theoretical inspired P_{IO_2}

                    a) 2 ATA × 760 × 0.21 = 320 mm Hg P_{IO_2} breathing *air*

                    b) 2 ATA × 760 × 1.0 = 1,520 mm Hg = P_{IO_2} breathing 100% O_2

          (4) Increased O_2 carrying capacity may be beneficial in cases where ischemia results from inadequate O_2 carrying capacity (e.g., carbon monoxide poisoning)

      (b) Increased potential diffusion distance of O_2

(1) At normal Pa_{O_2} of 100 mm Hg, oxygen can diffuse about 64 μm from arterial end of capillary at a rate sufficient to maintain adequate intracellular P_{O_2} to support aerobic metabolism

(2) At Pa_{O_2} of 2,000 mm Hg, the effective diffusion distance for O_2 will increase to approximately 247 μm from arterial end of capillary, thus increasing diffusion distance almost four times

(3) Increased O_2 diffusion distance may be beneficial in cases where some capillaries are not function (e.g., crush injury)

(c) Hyperoxic vasoconstriction

   (1) Hyperoxia causes vasoconstriction of both arterial and venous vessels

   (2) Systemic vascular resistance increases with HBO, as does blood pressure (~10 mm Hg)

(d) Other effects

   (1) May decrease release of leukocyte-mediated vasoactive substances in models of ischemia/reperfusion injury

   (2) Tissue P_{CO_2} increases slightly (~0.04 mm Hg increase in P_{CO_2}) due to

      [a] Decreased Hb buffering of CO_2 (venous Hb remains saturated with oxygen)

      [b] Vasoconstriction of venules, decreasing washout of metabolic waste

3. Oxygen toxicity (see below)

4. Compression of gas spaces due to Boyle's law ($P_1V_1 = P_2V_2$) (see section on "altitude")

5. Approved uses of HBO

  (a) Air embolism

    (1) Cerebral arterial gas embolism (CAGE)

      [a] Iatrogenic causes

         i) May be secondary to direct arterial injection/infusion of gas

         ii) May result from arterialization of venous gas via intracardiac shunt (e.g., patent foramen ovale) or breaching of pulmonary filtration mechanism (in massive venous emboli)

    (2) Iatrogenic air embolism causes

      [a] Cardiac surgery

         i) Postoperative aortic valve replacement (AVR)

         ii) Postoperative atrial septal defect (ASD) repair

         iii) Intra-aortic balloon pump (IAPB) balloons

         iv) Cardiopulmonary bypass (CPB)

      [b] Neurosurgery

         i) Sitting procedure

         ii) Burr hole

      [c] Cardiac angiographic procedure

         i) Catheterization

      [d] Dialysis

         i) Loss of continuity of the dialysis membrane

      [e] Jugular venous catheterization

         i) IJ removal

         ii) PA catheter

      [f] Arthroplasties

         i) Cement placed into air-filled femoral shaft

      [g] Percutaneous needle biopsy of lung mass

      [h] Hysterosalpingogram

      [i] Laparoscopy

    (3) Diving mechanisms: pulmonary overpressurization on ascent with closed glottis after breathing compressed air (i.e., scuba [self-contained underwater breathing apparatus] diving)

      [a] Air within alveoli expands, as per Boyle's law, as ambient pressure decreases

      [b] Alveoli may rupture, allowing escape of air into arterial circulation, presumably via pulmonary veins

         i) CAGE results, with symptoms varying from headache to "strokelike" presentation to sudden death

         ii) Systemic embolization of all great vessels and heart with "vapor lock" described; may also embolize spinal cord or coronary arteries

      [c] Can happen in only 4 feet of water if ascent made with closed glottis after breathing compressed air (greatest relative volume change is always closest to the surface)

      [d] Can *only* occur if breathing compressed air (e.g., scuba), not in breath-hold diving

  (4) Rationale for HBO

      [a] Compress bubble (Boyle's law) with increased atmospheric pressure

      [b] Hasten off-gassing of inert gas across blood–bubble interface (breathing pure oxygen unloads nitrogen from body tissue stores)

      [c] Correct tissue hypoxia

         i) Increased O_2 carrying capacity (see above)

         ii) Increased O_2 diffusion distance (see above)

  (5) Treatment protocol (see below)

(b) Decompression sickness

  (1) Etiology

      [a] Potential problem for scuba divers, commercial divers, and others breathing compressed air, and also for astronauts performing extravehicular activities (e.g., space walks), as current pressure-suit technology provides only approximately one fourth atmosphere of pressure

      [b] For every 33 feet of seawater the diver descends, he or she experiences the equivalent of an atmosphere increase in pressure

         i) 1 ATA = sea level = 760 mm Hg

Depth, Feet of Seawater	Total Atmospheric Pressure	
	Atmospheres Absolute (ATA)	mm Hg
33	2	1,520
66	3	2,280
99	4	3,040

         ii) The diver's regulator delivers air at the same atmospheric pressure as the body. The deeper the diver goes, the higher is the inspired nitrogen partial pressure

         iii) Inert gas dissolves in tissues according to Henry's law (see "altitude")

Gas	1 ATA	3 ATA
21% O_2	160 mm Hg P_IO_2	480 mm Hg P_IO_2
79% N_2	600 mm Hg P_IN_2	1,800 mm Hg P_IN_2
Total	760 mm Hg	2,280 mm Hg

(At 3 ATA [66 fsw], e.g., there will be approximately 1,800 mm Hg nitrogen dissolved in tissues.)

      [c] On ascent, bubbles may form as ambient pressure decreases

      [d] Symptoms range from mild joint pain to paralysis

      [e] Recompression of all cases of decompression sickness advised to prevent permanent neurologic injury or long-term aseptic bone necrosis

  (2) Rationale for HBO same as for CAGE

  (3) Treatment protocol (see "vaporizers")

(c) Carbon monoxide poisoning

  (1) Mechanism of injury

    [a] Most common fatal cause of poisoning in the United States

    [b] CO binds to Hb 200 times more tightly than oxygen

      i) Decreased O_2 carrying capacity

      ii) Stereometric change in CO Hb molecule increases affinity for oxygen of remaining active binding sites. This inhibits release of O_2 of tissues ("left shift")

      iii) Net effect is worse than decreased oxygen carrying capacity secondary to anemia of same degree

    [c] Preferentially binds to heme component of myoglobin (skeletal and cardiac), to mixed-function oxidases, and to cytochrome c oxidase (cytochrome a, a3)

      i) Prevents final electron transfer and energy production

      ii) Is directly toxic to heart and brain

  (2) Rationale for HBO

    [a] Normalize O_2 carrying capacity due to *plasma*-dissolved oxygen

    [b] Shorten half-life of CO Hb

CO Hb T½ (hours)	F_1O_2
5	0.21 at 1 ATA
1	1.00 at 1 ATA
0.25	1.00 at 3 ATA

    [c] Reoxidize brain cytochromes. Sea-level O_2 does not effect cytochrome reoxidation in animal models, as does HBO

      i) Outcome studies show decreased incidence of delayed or permanent neurologic sequelae in HBO-treated patients

      ii) Animal data show decreased brain ischemia/reperfusion injury

      iii) Because considerable tissue loading of CO may occur that is not measurable, CO Hb levels may not accurately represent degree of tissue poisoning by CO

      iv) CO Hb levels correlate poorly with either clinical symptoms or outcome. Outcome more clearly related to concentration time product and delay in treatment

  (3) Criteria for HBO in CO poisoning

    [a] Any history of loss of consciousness, even if alert in hospital

    [b] CO Hb greater than 20–25%

    [c] Pregnancy

    [d] Chest pain or ECG evidence of ischemia

  (4) Treatment protocol (see below)

(d) Clostridial myonecrosis (gas gangrene)

  (1) Mechanism of injury

    [a] Usually in compromised host (hypoxic tissue [e.g., diabetes], or decreased immune response)

    [b] Tissue destruction by *Clostridium perfringens*

    [c] Systemic vascular collapse via exotoxin

    [d] Polymorphonuclear leukocyte (PMN) function inhibited by tissue hypoxia

  (2) Rationale for HBO

    [a] HBO bacteriostatic to anaerobic organism

V. Disease States; m. Hyperbaric and diving medicine (continued)

          [b] *CO perfringens* exotoxin production halted at tissue P_{O_2} over 300 mm Hg. HBO may correct shock due to toxin

          [c] PMN function normalized. Energy requirements increase 20-fold on ingestion of bacteria. In hypoxic tissue, ingestion occurs but oxidative burst requires molecular O_2

          [d] Enhanced antibiotic efficacy, especially aminoglycosides, which is dependent on transport across bacterial cell wall (O_2-dependent transport mechanism)

      (3) HBO only *adjunctive* to proper surgical debridement and appropriate antibiotics

      (4) Treatment protocol (see below)

    (e) Other necrotizing soft tissue infections

      (1) Rationale

          [a] Normalizes tissue P_{O_2} (see above)

          [b] Adjunctive to surgery and antibiotics

    (f) Osteomyelitis

      (1) Rationale

          [a] Intramedullary $P_{O_2} \approx 10$ mm Hg in infected bone. HBO raises intramedullary P_{O_2} to normal levels, thus enhancing neutrophil response and antibiotic efficacy

      (2) Adjunctive to proper surgical debridement of all sequestered bone, and appropriately directed antibiotics

    (g) Compromised skin grafts/flaps

      (1) Rationale

          [a] Increase tissue P_{O_2}

          [b] Decrease ischemia reperfusion injury

          [c] Decrease edema

    (h) Selected nonhealing wounds

      (1) Rationale

          [a] Correct hypoxia

          [b] Encourage collagen production. Cross-linking of nascent procollagen chains requires molecular oxygen to produce collagen fibril, thus allowing fibroblast proliferation

          [c] Encourage angiogenesis; fibroblasts migrate in the direction of hypoxia but require a minimum tissue P_{O_2} of 30 mm Hg for replication

          [d] Patients must have reasonable large vessel flow for HBO to be efficacious

          [e] Transcutaneous oximetry may help select patients for whom HBO is likely to be of benefit

    (i) Burns

      (1) Rationale (see above)

      (2) May decrease need for skin grafting

      (3) Efficacy controversial

      (4) Treatment protocol (see below)

    (j) Soft tissue radionecrosis and osteoradionecrosis

      (1) Rationale

          [a] See above. Often used prior to and following extraction of teeth in irradiated fields as incidence of dry sockets is reduced with HBO

          [b] Enhanced angiogenesis may assist with removal of bony sequestrum by osteoclasts and with new bone growth in irradiated mandible

      (2) May be beneficial in treatment of refractory radiation cystitis, proctitis, etc.

      (3) Treatment protocol (see below)

  6. Implementing HBO treatment

(a) Equipment
   (1) Monoplace chambers—acrylic cylinders, usually compressed with 100% oxygen, which hold one patient supine. Maximum pressure is usually 3 ATA
   (2) Multiplace chambers—steel vessels with more than one com- partment, which can be independently operated. Can usually treat two or more patients at a time. Compressed with *air*, patients breathe oxygen off aviator-type face masks or hoods; maximum pressure rating varies, clinical usage to 6 ATA
(b) Treatment profiles
   (1) CAGE and diver's decompression sickness
      [a] Treatment is standardized by U.S. Navy protocols
      [b] Recompression to either 60 feet of seawater (TT5, TT6) or 165 feet of seawater (TT6A) as outlined in the *USN Diving Manual*
   (2) Carbon monoxide poisoning
      [a] Minimum treatment pressure of 2.4 ATA
      [b] Variable duration depending on protocol
      [c] Usually minimum of 90 minutes
      [d] Retreatment occasionally necessary
   (3) Gas gangrene/necrotizing infections
      [a] Protocols vary from maximum pressure of 68 feet of seawater (3.06 ATA) to 2.4 ATA
      [b] Usually three compressions in first 24 hours, then twice a day thereafter for a minimum of seven treatments
   (4) Wound healing, radionecrosis, failing grafts, burns, etc.
      [a] Standard treatment varies from 2 ATA to 2.8 ATA
      [b] Daily treatments given over variable periods of time, usually days to weeks, depending on response

7. Oxygen toxicity
   (a) Pulmonary oxygen toxicity
      (1) Usually not a factor for routine, brief HBO exposures. Most likely to be encountered after treatment for decompression sickness or arterial gas embolism (USN TT6 or TT6A). May have 2–4% decrement in vital capacity acutely
      (2) Also termed Lorraine-Smith effect
      (3) Reversible with time in all routine HBO exposures
      (4) Decreased incidence with intermittent O_2 delivery. During HBO, oxygen usually given 20 minutes at a time with 5-minute air "break." Such breaks can result in tripling of time until pulmonary symptoms develop
   (b) Central nervous system toxicity
      (1) Exposure over 1.6 ATA P_{O_2} can result in various manifestations of CNS O_2 toxicity
         [a] Twitching, hiccups, grand mal seizures are among possible symptoms; in animals, termed the bean effect
      (2) Risk of CNS O_2 toxicity increases with depth. Maximum P_{O_2} allowed clinically is 3.06 ATA (100% O_2 at depth equivalent to 68 feet of seawater)
      (3) Mechanism of CNS O_2 toxicity may include
         [a] Vasoconstriction
         [b] Damage from oxidative free radicals
         [c] Changes in neurotransmitter population
      (4) Incidence of clinical CNS O_2 toxicity estimated at between one in 2,000 and one in 10,000. Contributing factors are
         [a] Anxiety
         [b] Exertion
         [c] Steroids
         [d] Fever
      (5) No long-term sequelae of CNS O_2 toxicity ever reported in humans

            (c) Ocular O_2 toxicity
- [a] Appears in adults after a series of hyperbaric oxygen exposures as increasing myopia
- [b] May be due to change in distensibility of lens
- [c] HBO has not been implicated in any cases of retrolental fibroplasia of newborns, even in 100 pregnant women treated with HBO for carbon monoxide poisoning

8. Special considerations in HBO treatment
    - (a) Remember that all air spaces are subject to Boyle's law
        - (1) Endotracheal tube cuffs should be filled with saline
        - (2) Prophylactic myringotomies suggested for unresponsive patients to prevent otic barotrauma
        - (3) Sinus pain may occur with compression/decompression; may be helped with Afrin or similar nasal spray
    - (b) Patients with seizure disorder should have therapeutic blood levels of antiseizure medications
        - (1) Patients with high fever may benefit from prophylactic loading with phenobarbital to prevent hyperoxic seizure

9. Contraindications to HBO
    - (a) Absolute contraindications
        - (1) Severe chronic obstructive lung disease
            - [a] On decompression of chamber, pulmonary overexpansion with subsequent pneumothorax, tension pneumothorax, or CAGE may result
    - (b) Relative contraindications
        - (1) Risk versus benefit ratio should be assessed for each individual case
        - (2) Moderate COPD (suggest bronchodilators if pulmonary function tests indicate response)
        - (3) Seizure disorder—increases CNS O_2 toxicity risk
        - (4) High fever—increases CNS O_2 toxicity risk
        - (5) Active carcinoma—no evidence that HBO may enhance tumor growth
        - (6) History of spontaneous pneumothorax
        - (7) History of bleomycin or other pulmonary toxic chemotherapy—may predispose to pulmonary O_2 toxicity
        - (8) Eustachian tube dysfunction—tympanostomy tubes may be needed
        - (9) Cataracts—questionable evidence that HBO may hasten cataract formation

---

n. Near-drowning

1. Physiologic mechanisms
    - (a) Asphyxia
        - (1) Laryngospasm—occurs when fresh water or seawater contacts mucosa of lower respiratory tract
            - [a] May protect from significant aspiration
            - [b] May cause ventricular arrhythmia
            - [c] Has not been proven a factor in drowning or near-drowning
        - (2) Mechanical obstruction
            - [a] Due to aspiration of water or gastric contents
            - [b] Small airway obstruction aggravated by
                - i) Bronchoconstriction
                - ii) Mucosal edema
            - [c] "Plugging" by water, debris, stomach contents, etc.

[d] Decreased lung compliance results in low ventilation/perfusion ratio and shunting

[e] Hypoxia and hypercarbia result

2. Hypoxia/hypercarbia

(a) End result of asphyxia

(b) Aggravated by hypoxemia due to lung injury (see below)

(c) May result in hypoxic encephalopathy

3. Diving reflex

(a) Vestigial in humans, most demonstrable in young children on exposure to cold water

(b) Induce by apnea and facial immersion

(c) Vagally medicated

(d) Causes bradycardia

(e) Near-drowning with prompt hypothermia slows cerebral metabolism; may postpone deleterious effects of anoxia

(f) May improve prognosis of near-drowning in children and in cold-water exposures; otherwise usually not protective or helpful in near-drowning

4. Pathophysiology

(a) Lung injury due to water aspiration

(1) General mechanisms

[a] Loss of surfactant or surfactant activity

[b] Damage to alveolar epithelium and capillary endo- thelium (exposes basement membrane, thus allowing leakage of plasma protein into alveolus; this further inactivates surfactant, worsening ventilation/ perfusion)

[c] Alveolar flooding

(2) Seawater aspiration considerations

[a] Hypertonicity of seawater causes influx of water from pulmonary capillaries into alveoli

i) Contributes to progressive hypoxemia

ii) Removes some surfactant as water egresses from alveolus (seawater does not directly inactivate surfactant)

(3) Fresh-water aspiration considerations

[a] Fluid rapidly absorbed from alveoli (rarely leads to severe electrolyte/ fluid imbalance in humans)

[b] Fresh water removes and inactivates surfactant

[c] Atelectasis requires high airway pressures for reinflation

(4) Consequences of lung injury

[a] Progressive hypoxemia due to intrapulmonary shunting (may reach 70% of cardiac output)

[b] May culminate in adult respiratory distress syndrome (ARDS) hours to days after event in approximately 40% of victims. *Note:* ARDS secondary to near-drowning is more likely to be reversible than ARDS of other etiologies

[c] May necessitate treatment with high F_IO_2, predisposing to pulmonary O_2 toxicity

5. Cerebral injury

(a) Similar to that of global anoxia or severe hypoxia of other etiologies

(b) Cerebral edema—may result when severe, diffuse neuronal damage compromises function of blood–brain barrier

(c) Intracranial pressure (ICP) may rise as edema develops

(1) Profound increases infrequent after near-drowning

        (2) Usually becomes manifest more than 24 hours after initial resuscitation and in patients who already have some evidence of neurologic dysfunction

        (3) Further decreases brain perfusion

        (4) Exacerbates intracellular hypoxia

        (5) May lead to herniation

6. Cardiac arrhythmias

    (a) Ventricular fibrillation may be most common ("cardiac arrest" often given as cause of death)

    (b) May be exacerbated by electrolyte imbalances of near-drowning (actually uncommon in humans with notable exceptions, such as the Dead Sea, due to high mineral content of water)

    (c) Most likely secondary to severe hypoxia and severe metabolic and respiratory acidosis

7. Decreased renal function

    (a) Oliguria

        (1) Acute tubular necrosis (ATN) may result from hypoxia and hypotension

        (2) Rhabdomyolysis, hemolysis, and DIC may contribute

        (3) Recovery of adequate renal function occurs in majority of patients

8. Clinical management

    (a) Evaluate for coexisting conditions predisposing to near-drowning

        (1) Chemical intoxication

            [a] Sedatives, other drugs

            [b] Alcohol

        (2) Myocardial infarction

        (3) Seizures

        (4) Subarachnoid hemorrhage

        (5) Arterial gas embolism in scuba diver

        (6) Spine or skull injuries

    (b) Initial testing

        (1) ECG (for ischemia, injury, and dysrhythmia)

        (2) Arterial blood gases (metabolic acidosis secondary to lactate and hypoxemia are common)

        (3) Serum electrolytes

        (4) Blood glucose (hypoglycemia common)

        (5) CBC (hemolysis, if seen, usually occurs early)

        (6) Drug levels (urine, blood)

        (7) Serial cardiac isoenzymes

        (8) Chest x-ray (findings range from patchy infiltrates to diffuse air-space disease; parenchymal infiltrates developing over hours or days are not unusual)

        (9) Cervical spine films, if indicated

       (10) CT or magnetic resonance images (MRI) of brain (if indicated by coma, neurologic deficit, etc.)

    (c) Indications for ICU admission

        (1) Respiratory distress

            [a] Desaturation, hypoxemia

            [b] Symptoms of

                i) Frothy sputum

               ii) Diffuse crackles, wheezing

        (2) Cardiac arrest or arrhythmia

        (3) Altered mental status

        (4) Hypothermia

    (5) Significant metabolic acidosis
(d) Respiratory care
    (1) Intubation and mechanical ventilation may be necessary
    (2) Atelectasis and pulmonary edema make adequate ventilation challenging
    (3) Sedation and/or paralysis may be necessary to decrease peak airway pressures
    (4) PEEP of 5–15 cm H_2O may decrease atelectasis and intrapulmonary shunt
    (5) Bronchodilator therapy may be beneficial for diffuse wheezing (bronchospasm or mechanical airway obstruction is common)
    (6) Bronchoscopy to evaluate for foreign body advisable for
        [a] Patients with localized atelectasis that fails to improve with effective ventilation
        [b] Localized wheezing
    (7) Prophylactic antibiotics do not improve outcome; however, infection due to contaminated water is common, occurring 2 to 7 days after near-drowning. Reported infectious agents in various types of water include:

Bacteria	Type of Water
Klebsiella oxytoca	Fresh water
Herellea sp.	Fresh water
Neiserria meningitides	Fresh water
Pseudomonas aeruginosa	Fresh water
Listeria monocytogenes	Fresh water
Plesiomonas shigelloides	Fresh water
Edwardsiella tarda	Fresh water
Chromobacterium violaceum	Fresh water
Aeromonas hydrophila	Seawater, fresh water
Escherichia coli	Seawater, fresh water
Proteus mirabilis	Seawater, fresh water
Staphylococcus aureus	Seawater, fresh water
Neiserria mucosas	Brackish
Pseudomonas putrefaciens	Seawater
Francisella philomiragia	Seawater
Vibrio parahemolyticus	Seawater
Fungus	
Pseudoallescheria boydii	Fresh water
Aspergillus	Fresh water

    (8) Respiratory insufficiency in absence of sepsis is seldom the cause of death in near-drowning victims in hospitals with modern intensive care capabilities
(e) Brain resuscitation
    (1) Common classification of neurologic status 1 to 2 hours after resuscitation (may help predict outcome)
        [a] Category A: awake, fully conscious
        [b] Category B: blunted consciousness, stuporous but arousable
        [c] Category C: comatose
            i) C.1: Decorticate posturing
            ii) C.2: Decerebrate posturing
            iii) C.3: Flaccid
    (2) Therapeutic measures controversial and do not differ from brain resuscitation protocols for cerebral hypoxia due to other etiologies
        [a] Corticosteroids—no proved efficacy
        [b] Monitoring ICP advisable in severe neurologic injury

[c] Hyperventilation may be useful for cerebral edema
9. Prognosis
   (a) Overall outcome
      (1) 80% of child and adult near-drowning victims recover without sequelae
      (2) 2–9% victims survive with brain damage
      (3) 12% of all near-drowning victims die
   (b) Prognostic indicators
      (1) 90% of categories A and B and 50% of category C survive with full recovery
      (2) 10–23% of category C survive with permanent sequelae
      (3) Absence of spontaneous respiration after resuscitation is ominous sign, uniformly associated with severe neurologic impairment or death
      (4) No other clinical parameters are predictive (electrolytes, ABG, pH, ECG, body temperature, cardiac arrest, duration of submersion, etc., are all nonpredictive)

B. CARDIOVASCULAR

I. ANATOMY
   a. Heart and major vessels
   b. Electrical activity and conduction
   c. Myocardial innervation
   d. Myocardial blood supply
   e. Systemic circulation
   f. Pulmonary circulation, multiple functions

II. PHYSIOLOGY
   a. Microanatomy
   b. Cardiac cycle
   c. Ventricular function
   d. Coronary blood flow
   e. Blood pressure
   f. Organ flow and autoregulation
   g. Chemical control
   h. Hormonal control
   i. Baro-control

III. PHARMACOLOGY
   a. Inotropes
   b. Antidysrhythmics
   c. Vasodilators
   d. Vasoconstrictors
   e. Antianginal agents
   f. Muscarinic antagonist agents

IV. PHYSICS
   a. Flow and resistance
   b. Vascular pressures and transducers
   c. Function, noninvasive techniques
   d. Pacemaker
   e. Electrophysiology
   f. Assist devices

V. CLINICAL PRIORITIES
   a. Arteriosclerosis
   b. Valvular heart disease
   c. Cardiomyopathy
   d. Tamponade, pericarditis
   e. Pulmonary embolus
   f. New York Heart Association functional classification
   g. Cardiopulmonary bypass
   h. Coagulation defects
   i. Disorders of rhythm

        j. Congenital heart disease

        k. Obstetrics

VI. AGING

    a. Chronologic age

    b. Age-related disease

    c. Age-related diseases associated with increased risk

    d. Elective versus emergency surgery

    e. Pathophysiology

        1. Cardiovascular system

        2. Respiratory system

        3. Central nervous system

        4. Renal function

        5. Liver function

        6. Decreased renal and hepatic functions

        7. Basal metabolic rate and temperature regulation

        8. Airway reflexes

        9. Pharmacokinetics and pharmacodynamics

       10. Protein binding

       11. Putative causes

VII. OBESITY

    a. General

    b. Definition

    c. Pathophysiologic changes

    d. Preoperative management

    e. Use of regional anesthesia

    f. Advantages of combined general and regional anesthetic

    g. Postoperative management

VIII. HEAT STROKE

    a. Cause

    b. Effects

    c. Therapy

I. ANATOMY

a. Heart and major vessels

1. Topographic and gross anatomy

   (a) Retrosternal in middle mediastinum
   (b) Four-chambered based on framework of fibrous tissue and interventricular septum
   (c) Base consists of portions of both atria and attachments of great vesssels
   (d) Apex, left border, and two thirds of the diaphragmatic surface formed by left ventricle (LV)
   (e) Right ventricle (RV) makes up major portion of sternocostal surface
   (f) Pericardium attached to the heart only at the base where great vessels enter

2. Right atrium

   (a) Gross anatomy
      (1) Thin-walled right atrium (RA) with widcr part of the cavity toward the right and narrower part toward the left
      (2) Auricle is a thin projection at the top of the anterior surface and posterior surface is the interatrial septum
      (3) Fossa ovalis is remnant of foramen ovalis, and is patent in 20–30% of patients
   (b) Blood entry into RA
      (1) Superior vena cava (SVC), from right and left brachiocephalic veins
      (2) Inferior vena cava
      (3) Air tends to collect at SVC/RA junction
      (4) Coronary sinus, major return site of myocardial blood flow
      (5) Some direct drainage of right ventricular wall into RA
   (c) Blood exit via narrow left portion of RA via tricuspid valve

3. Right ventricle

   (a) Blood entry via tricuspid valve
   (b) Cavity divided into inflow and outflow tracts by muscular supraventricular ridge
      (1) AV orifice is posterior and to the right
      (2) Tricuspid valve projects into cavity with three cusps
         [a] Anterior
         [b] Septal
         [c] Posterior
         [d] Valve area is 8–11 cm^2
      (3) Outflow tract projects superiorly to the left to the pulmonary orifice and pulmonary valve
      (4) Pulmonary valve
         [a] Semilunar
         [b] Valve area is 4 cm^2
      (5) RV musculature is continuous with that of the LV despite the interventricular septum
   (c) Blood exits through pulmonary trunk to the lungs

4. Pulmonary artery

   (a) After 4–5 cm, the pulmonary trunk divides
   (b) Left pulmonary artery attached to aorta by ligamentum arteriosum (remnant of ductus arteriosus)

5. Left atrium

   (a) Gross anatomy
      (1) Quadrilateral-shaped cavity larger than RA
      (2) Left upper corner is left auricle

(3) Mitral valve on front wall
(b) Blood entry via four pulmonary veins
6. Left ventricle
(a) Gross anatomy
(1) LV cavity is longer than RV
(2) Wall is three times the thickness of RV
(b) Mitral valve
(1) Mitral valve is anchored by the chordae tendinae to the anterior and posterior papillary muscles with valve projecting into the LV cavity
(2) Valve has four cusps that function as two leaflets
(3) Normal valve area is 6–8 cm^2
(4) Critical stenosis at less than 1 cm^2
(c) Aortic valve
(1) Aortic orifice anterior to the mitral valve
(2) Made up of three leaflets
[a] Right
[b] Left
[c] Posterior
(3) Normal valve is 3–4 cm^2 and decreases with age
(4) Critical stenosis is less than 1 cm^2
(5) Right and left coronary arteries arise from respective aortic sinuses
7. Aorta
(a) Ascending aorta
(1) Arises from LV at the level of sternocostal joint
(2) Directed up, forward, and to the right
(3) Has pericardial reflection at its commencement
(4) Coronary arteries are only branches
(b) Aortic arch
(1) Extends from right sternal border to the body of T4 on the left
(2) Left pleura, lung, parasympathetic, and sympathetic nerve supply lie anterior and to the left
(3) Trachea and esophagus are behind, to the right
(4) PA trunk lies inferiorly
(5) Left PA is attached to the arch by the ligamentum arteriosum
(6) Main branches
[a] Brachiocephalic trunk (innominate)—this largest branch ascends to the right of the sternum and divides into the right common carotid and subclavian
[b] Left common carotid—longer than the right, it starts anterior to the trachea and moves to the left
[c] Left subclavian—initially directed vertically in contact with the left pleura
(c) Descending aorta
(1) From lower border of T4 to the diaphragm, initially to the left of the vertebral column (in close contact with pleura) moving anteriorly
(2) Main branches
[a] Bronchial—two right and one left supply the lungs
[b] Pericardial—twigs
[c] Esophageal—anastomose with each other and the left gastric branches
[d] Posterior intercostals—along lower border of ribs to anastomose with anterior intercostals

b. Electrical activity and conduction

1. Electrical anatomy
   - (a) Sinoatrial (SA) node
     - (1) Located at junction of right atrium and superior vena cava
     - (2) Three cell types
       - [a] Nodal cells thought to be origin of impulse formation
       - [b] Transitional cells contain myofibrils, and probably provide functional pathway for impulse to right atrial cells
       - [c] Working atrial cells at margin of node
   - (b) Pathways and conduction through right atrium
     - (1) Anterior nodal pathway
     - (2) Anterior interatrial band
     - (3) Anterior internodal tract
     - (4) Middle internodal tract
     - (5) Posterior internodal tract
     - (6) Preferential functional conduction pathways may exist
   - (c) Atrioventricular (AV) junctional area and AV node
     - (1) Transitional cell zone
     - (2) AV node proper or compact node
     - (3) Penetrating AV bundle
     - (4) AV node considerd a trilaminar structure
       - [a] AN region corresponds to transitional cell groups found posteriorly
       - [b] N region where middle nodal cells and transitional cells merge
       - [c] NH region is anterior region of lower nodal zone
   - (d) Bundle of His
   - (e) Right bundle branch
   - (f) Left bundle branch yields
     - (1) Left anterior fascicle
     - (2) Left posterior fascicle
   - (g) Terminal Purkinje fibers to endocardial region
2. Electrical conduction
   - (a) Five phases of cardiac action potential
     - (1) Phase 0: rapid upstroke
       - [a] Excitation
       - [b] Threshold potential must be attained
       - [c] Na channel major contributor
     - (2) Phase 1: early repolarization
       - [a] Inactivation of Na flux
       - [b] Transient outflow of K
       - [c] Cl may participate
     - (3) Phase 2: plateau
       - [a] Conductance of all ions reduced
       - [b] Ca flux providing some current
     - (4) Phase 3: rapid repolarization, primarily outward current of K
     - (5) Phase 4: resting potential, diastolic depolarization due to Na, some contribution by Ca
   - (b) Additional phenomena
     - (1) Early afterdepolarization
       - [a] Ionic basis unclear
       - [b] Initiated by
         - i) Hypokalemia
         - ii) Hypoxia

I. Anatomy; b. Electrical activity and conduction (continued)

        iii) Ischemia
        iv) Beta-adrenergic agonists
        v) Some antiarrhythmic drugs
        vi) Present in "long Q-T syndromes"
    (2) Late afterdepolarization
        [a] Seen in calcium overload
        [b] Associated with digitalis and inotropes
    (3) Spontaneous depolarization, pacemaker potential

c. Myocardial innervation

1. Sympathetic innervation

    (a) Right stellate ganglion
        (1) Coronary sinus
        (2) AV node
    (b) Left stellate ganglion innervates the ventricle

2. Parasympathetic innervation

    (a) Vagus nerve
    (b) Presynaptic inhibition of norepinephrine
    (c) SA node, decreases rate
    (d) AV node, slows conduction
    (e) Ventricle, negative inotropic effect

d. Myocardial blood supply

1. Coronary arteries

    (a) Left coronary artery
        (1) Dominant in 20% of individuals
        (2) Arises from left aortic sinus
        (3) Supplies left ventricle, anterior two thirds of septum, apex, left atrium, portion of right ventricle
        (4) Branches include left anterior descending (LAD), left circumflex
        (5) May be more susceptible to myocardial infarction
    (b) Right coronary artery
        (1) Originates in right aortic sinus
        (2) Dominant in 50% of individuals
        (3) Branches include posterior descending
        (4) Supplies sinus node and AV node
    (c) Coronary flow "balanced" in approximately 30% of individuals

2. Coronary venous drainage

    (a) Left ventricle drains to the coronary sinus
    (b) Right ventricle drains to anterior cardiac veins, which empty into RA above the AV valves
    (c) Thebesian veins drain deep muscle to RA and RV

e. Systemic circulation

1. Cerebral circulation

    (a) Vertebral arteries join to form basilar artery
    (b) Common carotic yields internal and external carotid arteries
    (c) Circle of Willis

(1) Anterior communicating arteries
(2) Internal carotid arteries
(3) Posterior communicating arteries
(4) Basilar artery from vertebral arteries

2. Upper extremity, subclavian artery yields

(a) Axillary artery
(b) Brachial artery
(c) Radial artery
(d) Ulnar artery

3. Intra-abdominal arteries

(a) Superior mesenteric
(b) Inferior mesenteric
(c) Celiac artery

4. Renal arteries supply approximately 20% of cardiac output to kidneys

5. Lower extremity, aorta bifurcates

(a) Iliac arteries
(b) Superficial and deep femoral arteries

6. Spinal cord

(a) Anterior spinal artery accounts for 75% of spinal cord blood flow
(b) Posterior spinal artery accounts for remaining 25% of spinal cord blood flow

7. Three bronchial arteries (two left and one right) supply nutrients to the lung

8. Liver blood flow

(a) Approximately 20% of cardiac output
(b) Hepatic artery, 65–80% of liver blood flow, remainder from portal system

f. Pulmonary circulation, multiple functions

1. Transport of blood for gas exchange
2. Metabolic transport of humoral agents and drugs
3. Filtration of venous drainage
4. Reservoir for left ventricle

II. PHYSIOLOGY

a. Microanatomy

1. Cardiac myocytes are striated mono- or binucleated cells mechanically connected by intercalated disks and function as a syncytium

2. Sarcomere basic functional unit

3. Z-bands connect repeating sarcomere units where F-actin extends off either side of the Z-line to form I-bands

4. Myosin filaments interdigitate with the actin filaments to form A-bands with M-lines in the middle of A-bands

5. Tropomyosin and the troponin complex bind to calcium and release their inhibiting effects on the actin–myosin contraction interactions, allowing myosin to "ratchet" along the actin molecule, providing movement

6. Sarcoplasmic reticulum provides functional connection to sarcolemma

7. Excitation coupling promotes release of calcium from sarcoplasmic reticulum to initiate contraction

8. ATP provides energy to break calcium binding, resulting in relaxation
9. The high energy requirements necessitate large numbers of mitochondria

b. Cardiac cycle

1. Diastole, relaxation phase, approximately two thirds of a cycle
2. Systole, contraction phase
3. Sequential mechanical events
    (a) End of diastole
        (1) Aortic and pulmonary valves closed
        (2) Mitral and tricuspid valves open
    (b) Systole begins
        (1) Mitral and tricuspid valves close
        (2) Isometric contraction of ventricles
    (c) Ejection phase begins
        (1) Aortic and pulmonic valves open
        (2) Isotonic contraction with ejection
        (3) Ejection fraction approximately 65% in the healthy individual
    (d) Ejection phase terminates
        (1) Aortic and pulmonic valves close
        (2) Closure of aortic valve seen as a dicrotic notch
        (3) Isometric relaxation begins
    (e) Diastolic filling begins
        (1) Mitral and tricuspid valves open
        (2) Diastolic filling occurs from atria
        (3) Major filling is passive
        (4) End diastolic volume approximately 120–140 ml
        (5) Atrial contraction accounts for additional 25% filling

4. Pressures, normal
    (a) Inferior vena cava, 0–5, mean 3
    (b) Superior vena cava, 0–5, mean 3
    (c) Right atrial, 0–5, mean 2
    (d) Right ventrical, <6–25, mean 10
    (e) Pulmonary artery, 10–25, mean 15
    (f) Left atrial, 2–10, mean 7
    (g) Left ventricle, <12–120, mean 60
    (h) Aorta, 120/80, mean 95
    (i) CVP measured from catheter within thorax

5. Cardiac output
    (a) Cardiac output a product of stroke volume and heart rate: CO = SV × HR
    (b) Cardiac output determined by three factors
        (1) Preload, the distension of ventricle secondary to filling pressure
        (2) Afterload, the impedance of ejection by ventricular contraction
        (3) Contractility
        (4) Frank-Starling curve relates filling pressure and cardiac output

c. Ventricular function

1. Descriptive terms
    (a) Inotropy: contractility

     (b) Chronotropy: rate

     (c) Dromotropy: conduction

     (d) Lusitropy: relaxation

2. Systolic function

     (a) Described by *dp/dt*

     (b) Reflected by ejection fraction

3. Diastolic function

     (a) Focuses on ventricular compliance

     (b) Early indicator of ischemic and cardiomyopathic changes

d. Coronary blood flow

1. Two coronary arteries supply myocardium from aorta

2. Superficial coronaries supply the subendocardial plexus with blood via intramural arteries

3. Blood flow to ventricle nearly stops during systole, with most occurring during diastole

4. Increasing heart rate decreases diastolic time for myocardial perfusion

5. Right ventricular myocardium has much lower blood-flow requirements

6. Because myocardium has high oxygen extraction (approximately 70%), increased requirements best met by increasing flow

e. Blood pressure

1. Blood pressure described by three components

     (a) Systolic pressure

     (b) Diastolic pressure

     (c) Mean blood pressure

2. Perfusion pressure described by difference between mean pressure and venous pressure

3. Blood pressure control

     (a) Reflexes, rapid response

          (1) Baroreceptors, stimulated by elevated pressure, inhibits sympathetics

          (2) Elevated CO_2 increases activity of sympathetic activity

          (3) Decreased cerebral perfusion results in elevated pressure

     (b) Renal—slow response, via renin-angiotensin system

     (c) Hormonal—variable response time

f. Organ flow and autoregulation

1. Most organ systems adjust blood flow to metabolic requirements

2. Autoregulation occurs through range beyond which flow is pressure dependent

3. Myogenic theory suggests that vascular smooth muscle contracts in response to stretch resulting from increased distending blood pressure

4. Metabolic products may be basis of autoregulation

     (a) Metabolic products, such as K, CO_2, adenosine, lactate, acidosis, prostaglandin

     (b) Endothelium-derived relaxing factor postulated

g. Chemical control

1. Locally acting metabolites, such as K, Ca, Mg, Na
2. Arachidonic acid derivatives; prostaglandin may have local and distant effects

h. Hormonal control

1. Autonomic nervous system transmitters
   (a) Parasympathetic
       (1) Slows heart
       (2) Decreases contractility
       (3) Dilates vasculature including coronaries
   (b) Sympathetic
       (1) Epinephrine and norepinephrine transmitters
       (2) Increased heart rate
       (3) Increased contractility
       (4) Some vascular beds show vasodilation
2. Atrial natriuretic factor (ANF)
   (a) Released in response to stimulation of stretch receptors in atrial wall
   (b) Increases excretion of Na in the urine; indirectly reduces blood volume
3. Renin-angiotensin system
   (a) Responds to reduced renal blood flow
   (b) Long-term effect is to elevate blood pressure
4. ADH promotes water retention and expansion of blood volume
5. Aldosterone and cortisol both result in elevation of blood pressure
6. Thyroid hormone sensitizes to circulating catechol

i. Baro-control

1. Receptors located in carotid sinus and aortic arch
2. Increased discharge results in reduced sympathetic activity
3. Fall in blood pressure passively results in increased sympathetic activity
4. Is a rapidly responding system
5. Readily adapts and does not function greatly for long-term blood pressure control

III. PHARMACOLOGY

a. Inotropes

1. Adrenergic receptor activities
   (a) Alpha$_1$ postsynaptic adrenoreceptors
       (1) Activation inceases intracellular calcium
       (2) Smooth muscle contraction
       (3) Peripheral vasoconstriction
       (4) Bronchoconstriction
       (5) Inhibits insulin secretion
       (6) Stimulates glycogenolysis and gluconeogenesis
   (b) Alpha$_2$, chiefly presynaptic, receptors

        (1) Inhibits adenyl cyclase activity
        (2) Decreases entry of calcium into cell
        (3) Limits release of norepinephrine
        (4) In CNS
            [a] Sedation
            [b] Decreased sympathetic outflow
            [c] Decreased blood pressure
    (c) $Beta_1$ postsynaptic receptor
        (1) Increases adenyl cyclase activity
        (2) Increased heart rate
        (3) Increased conduction velocity
        (4) Increased myocardial contractility
    (d) $Beta_2$ postsynaptic receptor
        (1) Stimulation leads to smooth muscle relaxation
        (2) Peripheral vasodilation
        (3) Decreased blood pressure
        (4) Increased insulin secretion
        (5) Increased glycogenolysis and gluconeogenesis
        (6) Decreases GI mobility

2. Isoproterenol

    (a) Both $beta_1$ and $beta_2$ actions
    (b) Both an inotrope and a chronotrope
    (c) Vasodilates coronary, renal, and mesenteric beds
    (d) Possible to induce hypotension
    (e) Dose, 0.15 µg/kg/min to effect

3. Norepinephrine

    (a) $Alpha_1$ and $alpha_2 > beta_1$
    (b) Increases systolic, diastolic, and mean blood pressure
    (c) Venoconstriction also occurs
    (d) Reduced blood flow to
        (1) Liver
        (2) Kidneys
        (3) Brain under some conditions
    (e) Some coronary vasoconstriction can occur
    (f) Dose: 0.1–0.4 µg/kg/min

4. Epinephrine, alpha predominates with increasing dose

    (a) Cardiac effects
        (1) Inotrope
        (2) Chronotrope
        (3) Increased flow in normal coronaries
    (b) Peripheral effects dependent on dose
        (1) Renal flow may decrease
        (2) Pulmonary vasoconstriction may occur
    (c) Respiratory effect
        (1) Efficient bronchodilator
        (2) May increase vital capacity by relieving mucosal congestion
    (d) Indications
        (1) Common in cardiac arrest
        (2) Pressor support, bronchodilation, or anaphylaxis
    (e) Dose: 1–4 µg/min

5. Dopamine

    (a) Immediate precursor to norepinephrine
    (b) Receptors: dopamine, beta, and alpha

III. Pharmacology; a. Inotropes (continued)

        (1) Visceral vasodilation with 0.5–5 μg/kg/min
        (2) Beta onset at 5 μg/kg/min
        (3) Alpha onset at 10 μg/kg/min
        (4) May elevate pulmonary artery pressure at higher doses
    (c) Renal effects
        (1) Increases renal blood flow at low doses
        (2) Increases GFR
        (3) Sodium excretion secondary to effect on renal vasculature

6. Dobutamine

    (a) Synthetic derivative of isoproterenol
    (b) Potent inotrope
    (c) May decrease afterload by $beta_2$ effect
    (d) Increases automaticity
    (e) Positive chronotropic effect
    (f) Positive dromotropic effect
    (g) Inhibits hypoxic pulmonary vasoconstriction
    (h) Dose: 2.5–15 μg/kg/min

7. Amrinone

    (a) Phosphodiesterase inhibitor
    (b) Strong inotrope
    (c) Weak vasodilator
    (d) Dose
        (1) 0.75 mg/kg loading
        (2) 5–10 μg/kg/min infusion
    (e) Side effects
        (1) Hypotension
        (2) Thrombocytopenia
        (3) GI effects when given orally

8. Milrinone

    (a) Derivative of amrinone
    (b) Twenty times as potent as amrinone
    (c) Does not reduce thrombocytopenia or GI effects

---

b. Antidysrhythmics

1. Class I

    (a) Class IA
        (1) Sodium channel block + +
        (2) Prolongs repolarization time
        (3) Lengthens effective refractory period
        (4) Prolongs action potential (mild class III effect)
        (5) Proarrhythmic effects
            [a] Prolongs QT
            [b] Torsades de pointes
        (6) Examples
            [a] Quinidine, prototype of class I
                i) Slows conduction and increases refractoriness in retrograde limb of AV nodal tachycardias
                ii) Similarly in both retrograde and antegrade conduction of Wolff-Parkinson-White syndrome
                iii) Effective in ventricular ectopic and tachyarrhythmias

iv) Often used for conversion in atrial flutter and fibrillation
[b] Disopyramide
    i) Similar effects as quinidine
    ii) Stronger anticholinergic effect
    iii) Marked cardiac depressant effect (may be masked by sympathetics)
    iv) In the United States, used only for ventricular dysrhythmias
[c] Procainamide
    i) Often used for lidocaine failure
    ii) Less QT prolongation than quinidine
    iii) Dose
        a) Initial intravenous, 100 mg over 2 minutes, then 25 mg/min up to 1 gram
        b) Maintenence, 2–6 mg/min

(b) Class IB
  (1) Sodium channel block +
  (2) Shortens repolarization time
  (3) Shortcns action potential duration
  (4) Acts preferentially on diseased or ischemic tissue
  (5) Ineffective in atrial dysrhythmias
  (6) Examples
    [a] Lidocaine
      i) Dose
        a) Intravenous only
        b) Initial, 100–200 mg
        c) Maintenance, 2–4 mg/min
      ii) Toxicity
        a) CNS, seizures
        b) Cardiac depression with high doses
        c) Toxicity enhanced by reduced liver clearance
    [b] Phenytoin
      i) Has specific advantages and efficacy
        a) Digitalis toxicity
          • Maintains and/or enhances conduction
          • In presence of hypokalemia, suppresses delayed afterdepolarizations
        b) Effective against ventricular arrhythmias after congenital heart surgery
        c) Congenital prolonged QT syndrome when beta blockade alone fails
        d) Useful when epilepsy present with dysrhythmias
      ii) Dose
        a) Initial IV dose, 10–15 mg/kg over 1 hour
        b) Maintenance dose, 400–600 mg/day (oral)
        c) Hepatic enzyme induction
    [c] Mexiletine
      i) Little toxicity
      ii) Little hemodynamic effect
      iii) Does not prolong QT
      iv) No vagolytic effect
      v) Oral agent, parenteral form not available in the United States
      vi) Effective blood level, 1–2 μg/ml
      vii) Toxicity
        a) Narrow therapeutic–toxic interval
        b) Because of fat solubility, CNS symptoms most common
    [d] Tocainide
      i) Oral analogue of lidocaine

III. Pharmacology; b. Antidysrhythmics (continued)

        ii) Little cardiac depression
        iii) Toxicity
           a) CNS effects similar to those of lidocaine
           b) Polyarthritis and blood dyscrasias
    [e] Ethmozine (also has class IC properties)
        i) A phenothiazine derivative
        ii) Class IB effects, QT unchanged
        iii) Class IC effects, prolongs PR and QRS
        iv) May affect arrhythmias via CNS effect
        v) Effective in both ventricular and supraventricular arrhythmias
        vi) Dose, 600–900 mg in three divided doses at 8-hour intervals
  (c) Class IC
    (1) Sodium channel block + + +
    (2) Marked inhibitory effect on His-Purkinje, QRS widening
    (3) Shortens action potential of Purkinje fibers, leaves surrounding myocardium unchanged
    (4) Promotes nonhomogeneous action potential duration
    (5) Significant proarrhythmic effects
    (6) Used to control ventricular tachyarrhythmias resistant to other agents
    (7) Examples
      [a] Flecainide
        i) Distinctly negative inotrope not used in ischemic heart disease of cardiomyopathy
        ii) Prolongs PR and QRS
        iii) Markedly proarrhythmic, should only be started in hospital setting
        iv) Contraindicated in the absence of life-threatening VT
        v) Aggravates ventricular arrhythmias 5–12%, significant threat of sudden death
        vi) May initiate atrial arrhythmias
      [b] Encainide
        i) Similar action and electrophysiologic effect as flecainide
        ii) Little negative inotropic effect
        iii) Metabolites ODE and MODE are active
      [c] Propafenone
        i) Resembles other class IC agents
        ii) Usually well tolerated
        iii) For life-threatening ventricular arrhythmias
        iv) AV nodal, bundle branch block, and depressed LV function relative contraindications
        v) Asthma relative contraindication
      [d] Ethmozine (also has class IB properties)
2. Class II (beta-blockers)
  (a) Phase IV (depolarizing current); calcium channel
  (b) Repolarization time unchanged
  (c) Beta-blockers
    (1) Nonselective (beta$_1$- and beta$_2$-blockers)
      [a] Reduce heart rate, conduction, and contractility
      [b] May cause bronchoconstriction
      [c] Propranolol is prototype
      [d] Nadolol
      [e] Sotalol, also a class III agent
    (2) Cardioselective (beta$_1$ selectivity)
      [a] Atenolol, most selective

        [b] Esmolol

        [c] Metoprolol

        [d] Cardioselectivity declines or is lost in high doses

    (3) Vasodilatory (partial agonist activity, intrinsic sympathomimetic activity [ISA])

        [a] Pindolol has most ISA

        [b] Acebutolol has sufficiently low ISA; it cannot be destinguished from metoprolol

    (4) Beta- and alpha-blocking activity

        [a] Labetalol

        [b] More active as a beta-blocker than as an alpha-blocker

3. Class III

  (a) Repolarizing K^+ currents affected function

  (b) Repolarization time markedly prolonged

  (c) To be effective, must prolong QT

  (d) May predispose to torsades de pointes, particularly with low potassium

  (e) Promotes more uniform action potential, reduces heterogeneity, which opposes reentry

  (f) Little or no negative inotropic effect (except sotalol)

  (g) Examples

    (1) Amiodarone

        [a] Multiple effects

            i) Lengthens effective refractory period

            ii) Inhibits inactivated sodium channels at high stimulation frequencies

            iii) Blocks alpha and beta receptors

            iv) Possible calcium channel block effect

            v) Low incidence of torsades de pointes

        [b] Slow onset, even when given IV

            i) IV, 5 mg/kg over 20 minutes

            ii) Continue, 1,000 mg over 24 hours

        [c] Serious side effects

            i) Pneumonitis

            ii) Torsades de pointes with QT prolongation with low potassium

            iii) May result in hypothyroidism

            iv) Initiate use in hospital setting

    (2) Sotalol

        [a] Used in lieu of amiodarone when toxicity of latter feared

        [b] Chief hazard is that of torsades de pointes

    (3) Bretylium

        [a] Most often used for VF and VT when lidocaine with DC cardioversion fail, particularly after AMI

        [b] Part of effect is chemical sympathectomy

        [c] Sympathetic activation may occur upon initiation of therapy

        [d] Major side effect is postural hypotension

        [e] Dose, 5–10 mg/kg over 10–30 minutes

4. Class IV

  (a) Calcium channel blockade + +

    (1) L-channel, which is responsible for the plateau to transport calcium to the interior of the cell

    (2) T-channel appears only at more negative potentials

    (3) Both beta-blockers and calcium-blockers have negative inotropic action; only calcium-blockers have vasodilator effect

  (b) K^+ channel openers (hyperpolarization) are indirect calcium antagonists

  (c) Repolarization time unchanged

(d) Specific agents
    (1) Verapamil
        [a] Inhibits slow channel-dependent conduction through AV node
        [b] Increased AV block and effective refractory period reduce ventricular rate in atrial flutter and fibrillation
        [c] Dose: 5–10 mg, repeat after 10 minutes, infusion of 1 mg/min
        [d] Indicated for paroxysmal supraventricular tachycardia
        [e] Indicated for atrial flutter/fibrillation
        [f] With broad complex tachycardia, which is either VT or SVT with aberrant conduction, verapamil *may be fatal if VT*
    (2) Diltiazem
        [a] Inhibits slow channel-dependent conduction through AV node
        [b] Used similarly as verapamil
        [c] Angina and hypertension primary use
    (3) Nifedipine
        [a] Little effect on AV node
        [b] Primarily an arterial vasodilator
    (4) Adenosine
        [a] Opens K^+ channels
        [b] Chief use is paroxysmal supraventricular tachycardia
            i) AV nodal reentrant tachycardia
            ii) AV tachycardia in WPW
            iii) Safer than verapamil with broad complex tachy- cardia, since it is fleeting in nature in its effect in VT
    (5) ATP, probably works by conversion to adenosine

c. Vasodilators

1. Sodium nitroprusside

    (a) Vasodilation by direct action on vascular muscle
    (b) Reduces mean arterial and pulmonary pressures
    (c) Decreases left atrial and ventricular filling pressure
    (d) Decreases afterload and promotes increased forward flow in mitral and aortic regurgitation
    (e) May directly vasodilate coronary arteries
    (f) Does not produce direct myocardial depression
    (g) Metabolism
        (1) Nitroprusside may receive an electron transfer from the iron of hemoglobin and an unstable nitroprusside radical, which breaks down into five cyanide moieties
        (2) Cyanide can react with methemoglobin to form caynomethemoglobin and be converted to thiocyanate in the liver or kidneys
        (3) Leads to release of cyanide, which is converted to thiocyanate by rhodanese in the mitochondria
        (4) Cyanide may combine to inactivate cytochrome oxidase as terminal toxic event
        (5) Toxicity is indicated by evidence of tachyphylaxis, acidosis, increasing venous content, with cardiac dysrhythmias
    (h) Dose
        (1) Precise dosages that avoid toxicity not firmly established
        (2) Recommended doses less than 0.5 mg/kg/hr
    (i) Side effects

(1) Headache, nausea, vomiting, palpitations, and abdominal pain

(2) Worsening intrapulmonary shunting

(3) Thiocyanate inhibits uptake and binding of iodine and may cause hypothyroidism with chronic use

(4) Aqueous form photosensitive and should be protected from light

2. Nitroglycerine

(a) Nonspecific smooth muscle relaxation; preload affected more than afterload

(b) Cardiac vasculature

    (1) Dilates collateral coronary circulation

    (2) Relaxes normal coronary vessels and relieves coronary spasm

    (3) Reduces preload, myocardial wall tension during diastole, and, therefore, reduces myocardial oxygen consumption

    (4) Increases endocardial to epicardial comparative blood flow

(c) Noncardiac vasculature

    (1) Dilates meningeal vessels and may increase intracranial pressure

    (2) Renal blood flow decreases in relation to systemic pressure

    (3) Dilates pulmonary vessels

(d) Metabolism

    (1) Metabolized in the liver by glutathione nitrate reductase

    (2) Nitrate ion oxidizes hemoglobin to methemoglobin

    (3) Chronic administration of long-acting forms may lead to tolerance in arterial vessels but not in the venous vessels

(e) Indications

    (1) Ventricular failure, hypertension

    (2) Ischemic heart disease

(f) Dose

    (1) Initial dose, 0.5 μg/kg/min

    (2) Increase dose to obtain hemodynamic response

(g) Adverse effects

    (1) Postural hypotension

    (2) Tachycardia

    (3) Headache

    (4) Dizziness

    (5) Weakness

    (6) Methemoglobinemia

3. Trimethaphan

(a) Ganglionic blockade, stabilizes postsynaptic nerve membrane

(b) Provides

    (1) Arterial vasodilation

    (2) Decreased peripheral resistance

    (3) Hypotension

(c) Dilates venous system to decrease preload and myocardial wall tension

(d) Causes direct vasodilation in addition to its ganglionic action

(e) Increases cerebral blood flow

(f) Increases intracranial pressure

(g) Adverse effects

    (1) Excessive hypotension and angina

    (2) Mydriasis

    (3) Histamine release

    (4) Noncompetitive inhibitor of pseudocholinesterase

    (5) Development of tachyphylaxis

4. Phentolamine

(a) Alpha-adrenergic blockade and direct-acting dilator

(b) Greater arterial vasodilator effect than venodilator

   (c) Decreases afterload and preload
   (d) Promotes greater ejection fraction and cardiac output
   (e) Decreases pulmonary vascular resistance
   (f) Dose, usually 1–2 µg/kg/min

5. Hydralazine

   (a) Direct-acting vasodilator
   (b) Increases cardiac output
   (c) Causes reflex tachycardia
   (d) Tachyphylaxis may occur
   (e) Dose, 5–10 mg IV may be used intraoperatively and repeated

6. Clonidine

   (a) Central alpha agonist leads to inhibition of sympathetic outflow
   (b) Decreases release of neurotransmitters
   (c) Decreases heart rate, blood pressure, cardiac output, and peripheral vascular resistance
   (d) Abrupt cessation of drug may lead to rebound hypertension
   (e) Adverse effects
       (1) Sedation
       (2) Postural hypotension
       (3) Dry mouth

d. Vasoconstrictors

1. Phenylephrine

   (a) Direct alpha agonist
   (b) Increases peripheral vascular resistance
   (c) Increases systolic and diastolic blood pressure
   (d) Causes reflex bradycardia
   (e) Renal and splanchnic blood flow decreased
   (f) Increases pulmonary artery resistance
   (g) Increases pulmonary artery pressure
   (h) Dose, 50–100-µg bolus to desired response

2. Ephedrine

   (a) Direct-acting agent on alpha and beta receptors
   (b) Also acts indirectly by stimulating the release of norepinephrine
   (c) Increases systolic and diastolic blood pressure
   (d) Increases myocardial contractility
   (e) Increases cardiac output
   (f) Tachyphylaxis, probably related to depletion of norepinephrine stores
   (g) Pressor of choice in obstetrics because of increased uterine blood flow with increased blood pressure
   (h) Bronchial smooth muscle relaxation
   (i) Dose, 5–10 mg IV

3. Metaraminol

   (a) Direct alpha agonist
   (b) Also causes the release of endogenous norepinephrine
   (c) Increases blood pressure
   (d) Increases cardiac output
   (e) Reflex bradycardia occurs

e. Antianginal agents

1. Sources of angina and associated signs of ischemia
   (a) Due to increased oxygen demand
       (1) Increased heart rate
       (2) Increased blood pressure with rise of wall tension
       (3) Increased contractility secondary to sympathetic stimulation or adrenergic agents
   (b) Due to relative decreased oxygen delivery
       (1) Increased heart rate with decreased filling time
       (2) Transient coronary vasoconstriction
       (3) Decreased perfusion pressure
           [a] Decreased systolic and mean arterial pressure
           [b] Increased end diastolic pressure, may be due to increased preload
   (c) ECG changes variable
       (1) ST-T wave changes
       (2) QRS changes with left bundle branch block and left anterior fascicular block
       (3) Ventricular premature beats may be present but not specific for CAD; ventricular tachycardia multiform ventricular ectopy more significant

2. Therapy
   (a) Nitrates
       (1) Decrease afterload
       (2) Decrease preload
       (3) Provide coronary dilation
   (b) Calcium-blockers
   (c) Beta-blockers
   (d) Vasodilators

f. Muscarinic antagonist agents

1. Inhibit salivary, bronchial, pancreatic, and gastric secretions
2. Do not inhibit muscarinic actions uniformly
3. Belladonna alkaloids
   (a) Atropine
   (b) Scopolamine
   (c) Have CNS effects, particularly scopolamine
       (1) Sedation
       (2) Antiemetic
   (d) Inhibit sweating
   (e) Bronchodilation
   (f) Produce paradoxic bradycardia at low doses, secondary to CNS penetration
4. Glycopyrrolate
   (a) More potent antisialogogue
   (b) Less vagolytic effect

IV. PHYSICS

a. Flow and resistance

1. Flow through a tube, defined as a pathway with length greater than its diameter
   (a) Laminar versus turbulent flow
       (1) Laminar
           [a] Pathway of a component is parallel to the wall of the tube
           [b] Laminar flow occurs at low flow rates
       (2) Turbulent
           [a] Pathway of a component is irregular and/or disordered relative to the wall of the tube
           [b] Turbulent flow occurs at high flow rates
       (3) Conversion of laminar flow to turbulent flow occurs at the critical velocity
           [a] Proportional to viscosity
           [b] Inversely proportional to density
           [c] Inversely proportional to tube radius
       (4) Reynold's number relates viscosity, density, and tube diameter where

$$K = \frac{V_c pR}{n}$$

K = Reynold's number
V_c = critical velocity
p = density
R = *radius of tube*
n = viscosity

       (5) Reynold's number close to 1,000 for blood
   (b) Resistance to flow
       (1) Resistance defined in units of pressure change per unit of flow (e.g., mm Hg/L/min)
       (2) Disproportionate and/or dramatic resistance increase with turbulent flow
       (3) Resistance increased by irregularies of tube, sharp bends, changes in diameter
       (4) Resistance proportional to tube length
       (5) Resistance defined by Poiseuille-Hagen law where

$$Res = \frac{8nl}{\pi R^4}$$

Res = resistance
n = viscosity
l = length
π = pi
R = radius

2. Flow through an orifice, defined as a pathway whose diameter exceeds its length
   (a) Flow through an orifice depends on
       (1) Cross-sectional area, diameter squared
       (2) Pressure gradient across the orifice
   (b) Flow through an orifice always contains a turbulent element
       (1) During turbulent flow, density of fluid dominates flow rate
       (2) During laminar flow, viscosity of fluid dominates flow rate
   (c) Examples of flow through an orifice
       (1) Partially obstructed airway, helium mixtures with lower density aids flow, although viscosity is relatively unchanged from oxygen alone
       (2) Gas rotameter flowmeter composed of a bobbin in a tapered tube behaves as a tube at low flow rates (length greater than diameter) and as an orifice (diameter greater than length) at high flow rates. Thus, viscosity is

dominating at low flows, and density at high flows, therefore, helium could be measured in an oxygen flowmeter at low flows (similar viscosities)

b. Vascular pressures and transducers

1. Pressure
   (a) Pressure is defined as force exerted per unit area
      (1) Common units of measurement include
         [a] Pounds per square inch, psi
         [b] Newtons per square meter, pascals or Pa
      (2) Pressure can be expressed as the equivalent of a column of fluid (usually air, water, or mercury) in the earth's gravitational field, thus, atmospheres, cm H_2O, mm Hg
   (b) Gauge versus absolute pressure
      (1) Pressure monitors may be calibrated to read absolute (comparing with vacuum) or gauge pressure (comparing with atmospheric pressure)
      (2) All clinically used transducers and gauges read "gauge" pressure (relate to atmosphere)
      (3) Gauge pressure may be converted to absolute by adding 1 atmosphere of pressure (14.7 psi, 101 kPa, 760 mm Hg)
2. Measurement of pressure
   (a) Devices
      (1) A manometer balances the weight of a column of liquid against the pressure of interest, for example, mercury sphygmomanometer, water-filled CVP or CSF pressure manometers
      (2) Bourdon gauges use elastic properties of metal, measure progressive straightening of curved metal tube as it is pressurized
      (3) Anaeroid gauges and diaphragm gauges measure force resulting from pressure changes acting through a sealed chamber or membrane to move an indicator needle; most high-pressure devices are of this type
   (b) Transducers
      (1) Defined: devices that convert pressure into electrical signals suitable for display and monitoring
      (2) Types
         [a] Resistive or capacative transducers change electrical properties proportionately to applied pressure
         [b] Magnetic or optical transducers provide electromagnetic signals proportionately to mechanical displacement of membrane or diaphragm resulting from applied pressure
      (3) Calibration of transducers includes
         [a] Establishment of a baseline signal relating to ambient pressure, "zero set"
         [b] Range setting of output against known pressure difference, "span"
         [c] Assumes linearity of electrical signal as relative to pressure changes
      (4) Sources of error
         [a] Errors in calibration
         [b] Changes of calibration over time, "drift"
         [c] Lack of linear response to signals
         [d] Resonance and damping phenomena due to the response of tubing to high-frequency signals and/or the presence of air–fluid interfaces (bubbles)

c. Function, noninvasive techniques

1. ECHO
   (a) Provides anatomic and functional information
   (b) Depends on differences of acoustic impedance (tissue density $\times$ speed of sound propagation)
   (c) Generation of image
       (1) A mode: current spikes, proportional to signal
       (2) B mode: modulation of A mode spikes to series of dots, brightness, or density, proportional to height of spikes
       (3) M mode: time display of B mode, which provides image of motion
       (4) Two-dimensional M mode provided by motion of crystal to scan an arc, provides virtual two dimensions

2. Doppler
   (a) Provides indirect measurement of intracardiac flow velocities by detecting changes of carrier frequency reflected to transducer. Governed by the equation

   $$V = \frac{(C \times F_d)}{(2F_0 \times \cos I)}$$

   where

   V = velocity
   C = velocity of sound
   F_d = frequency shift
   F_0 = carrier frequency
   I = angle of interrogation

   (b) Used as a combination of pulsed wave and continuous wave
       (1) Pulsed wave
           [a] Examines limited flow region and localizes flow distribution
           [b] Limited by characteristic of measuring flows at normal velocities (less than 2 meters per second in the adult)
           [c] Rapid velocities result in aliasing, distorts directional characteristics
           [d] Limits defined by Nyquist limit, as defined by flow theorems
           [e] Flow mapping, or color Doppler, provides real-time imaging throughout an entire sector
       (2) Continuous wave
           [a] Avoids aliasing and measures high velocity
           [b] Does not discretely sample along beam

3. Scintigraphic imaging
   (a) Radionuclide method, most commonly employs technetium, thallium, cesium
   (b) Employs sodium iodide crystal detector with a photomultiplier
   (c) Myocardial perfusion scintigraphy
       (1) Assesses myocardial viability, perfusion, and functional reversibility
       (2) Identification of myocardium at significant risk and poor prognosis, reversible perfusion defects
       (3) Dipyridamole perfusion scintigraphy
           [a] Dipyridamole inhibits degradation of adenosine and normally increases coronary flow threefold to fivefold
           [b] Failure of increased flow indicates stenosis or fixed coronary resistance
       (4) Errors secondary to
           [a] Soft tissue attenuation, most frequently in females
           [b] Decreased target-to-background ratio, secondary to prolonged pulmonary transit time and lung uptake
       (5) Defect interpretation: fixed versus reversible, infarction versus ischemia

  (6) Useful for diagnosis, prognosis, and evaluation of treatment
 (d) Invasive scintigraphic methods employ
  (1) Biodegradable microspheres or microaggregated albumin (MAA)
  (2) Xenon washout
  (3) Requires injection into coronary artery
4. Magnetic resonance imaging
 (a) ECG-gated spin-echo technique to obtain anatomic detail, high signal-to-noise ratio
 (b) Cine MRI used for assessment of contractile function
5. Computed tomography (CAT scan)
 (a) Generally requires enhancement by use of
  (1) ECG gating
  (2) Contrast media
  (3) Fast scanning, each exposure approximately 50 milliseconds
 (b) Can assess wall thickening and dynamics
 (c) May be more sensitive than ECHO for assessing pericarditis
 (d) Effectively defines major vascular abnormalities
 (e) Can effectively assess function, single beat imaging
6. Positron emission tomography (PET) scan
 (a) Indicators include $^{13}NH_3$ measures blood flow
 (b) ^{18}F-fluorodeoxyglucose measures glucose uptake by viable tissue
7. Magnetic resonance spectroscopy currently a research technique, but may indicate changes of metabolism
8. Cardiac output, dilution techniques
 (a) Fick principle described by equation

$$Q = \frac{m}{\int c(t)\, dt}$$

where

$$
\begin{aligned}
Q &= \text{flow} \\
\int &= \text{integral symbol} \\
c(t) &= \text{concentration curve} \\
dt &= \text{incremental time} \\
m &= \text{mass of indicator}
\end{aligned}
$$

The equation assumes *constant* flow. To adjust for pulsatile flow

$$Q = A\, f(t)$$

where

$$
\begin{aligned}
Q &= \text{flow} \\
A &= \text{constant} \\
f(t) &= \text{a profile function of time, e.g., a sine curve}
\end{aligned}
$$

d. Pacemaker

1. Modalities
 (a) A = atrium
 (b) V = ventricle
 (c) D = dual (A and V)
 (d) I = inhibited
 (e) T = triggered
 (f) 0 = none
 (g) S = used to indicate single-chamber device suitable for either chamber pacing
 (h) R = rate-adaptive pulse generator
 (i) M = multiprogrammable
 (j) Position of letters indicates type of pacer
  (1) First, denotes chamber paced
  (2) Second, denotes chamber sensed

IV. Physics (continued)

              (3) Third, indicates response to sensing
              (4) Fourth and fifth positions rarely used, except for R

    2. Temporary

       (a) Transvenous, esophageal, transcutaneous, epicardial, and coronary artery
       (b) Indications
          (1) Prophylaxis for new bifaxicular block, complete heart block, Mobitz II block
          (2) Asymptomatic patients with bifascicular do not need temporary pacemaker for surgery and general anesthesia
          (3) AMI

    3. Permanent

       (a) Indications, classification
          (1) Class I, general agreement that permanent pacemaker should be implanted
          (2) Class II, divergent opinion
          (3) Class III, general agreement that pacemaker probably of no benefit
       (b) Pacemaker should be evaluated before and after surgery where electrocautery is used; determine default function, use of magnet
       (c) MRI contraindicated for all patients with permanent pacemaker

e. Electrophysiology

    1. Defibrillation

       (a) Internal, 25–50 joules
       (b) External, 200, 300, and 360 joules
       (c) Ancillary drugs, lidocaine, epinephrine

    2. Cardioversion

       (a) Synchronized shock used for all except ventricular flutter or fibrillation
       (b) Initial shock 50 to 100 joules, except stable ventricular tachycardia, 25 to 50 joules
       (c) Favorable candidates
          (1) Symptomatic AF less than 12 months' duration
          (2) Embolic episodes
          (3) Continue AF after inciting disorder corrected, i.e., thyrotoxicosis
          (4) Rapid ventricular rate that is difficult to control
       (d) Unfavorable candidates
          (1) Digitalis toxicity
          (2) No symptoms, with a well-controlled ventricular response
          (3) Sinus node dysfunction and unstable supraventricular tachyarrhythmias
          (4) Patients who promptly revert despite adequate drug therapy
          (5) Large atrium and long-standing atrial fibrillation
          (6) AF with history of spontaneous reversion to SR
          (7) No mechanical atrial systole after conversion
          (8) AF with advanced heart block
          (9) Cardiac surgery planned in near future
         (10) Antiarrhythmic drug intolerance
       (e) Results
          (1) 70 to 95% favorable
          (2) Less than 50% persist beyond 12 months
       (f) Complications
          (1) Arrhythmias induced by nonsynchronous shock
          (2) Embolic phenomena

    3. Ablation

       (a) Destruction of conduction tissue by current, laser, surgical interruption

    (b) Creation of AV block in patients with flutter/fibrillation
    (c) AV nodal modification for AV nodal reentry
    (d) Ablation of accessory pathway for WPW syndrome
    (e) Ablation of pathway for ventricular tachycardia
    (f) Requires electrophysiologic mapping and provocative maneuvers

f. Assist devices

  1. Intra-aortic balloon counterpulsation

    (a) Counterpulsation requires balloon inflation during diastole and deflation during isometric contraction or early systole
    (b) Placement just distal to the left subclavian artery
    (c) Provides improvement in endocardial viability ratio

$$EVR = DPTI/TTI$$

    where

        EVR = endocardial viability ratio
        DPTI = diastolic pressure time index
        TTI = time tension index

    (d) Improves diastolic coronary perfusion
    (e) Reduces afterload
    (f) May slow heart rate via baroreflex activity changes
    (g) Indications include
        (1) Unstable angina
        (2) Acute myocardial infarction
        (3) Angina
        (4) Postcardiotomy cardiac support
    (h) Contraindications include
        (1) Presence of thoracic or abdominal aneurysm
        (2) Aortic insufficiency
        (3) Severe preexisting peripheral vascular disease
        (4) Lack of definitive therapy for underlying disease processes
    (i) Complications include
        (1) Pulse loss, limb ischemia
        (2) Thromboembolism
        (3) Compartment syndrome
        (4) Aortic dissection
        (5) Local injury and/or infection

  2. Mechanical circulatory assist devices

    (a) Duration of use
        (1) Short term considered, less than 180 days
        (2) Permanent or long term, over 180 days
    (b) Types of devices
        (1) Extracorporeal membrane oxygenation (ECMO) does little to support the left ventricle
        (2) External centrifugal pumps can provide biventricular or left ventricular support, require anticoagulation
        (3) External pulsatile assist devices—cannulae may be placed to either ventricular chamber, and connect to pulmonary vein or aorta; may provide uni- or biventricular support
        (4) Electrical left ventricular assist system designed to provide left ventricular support

  3. Total artificial hearts employed thus far have been pneumatic orthotopic biventricular replacement devices that are sutured directly to the atria

V. CLINICAL PRIORITIES

a. Arteriosclerosis

1. Generic term, characterized by thickened arterial wall and loss of elasticity
   (a) Pathology
       (1) Media hypertrophy
       (2) Subintimal fibrosis
       (3) Atherosclerotic plaques
2. Major risk factors
   (a) Hypertension
   (b) Elevated serum lipids (elevated LDL, low HDL)
   (c) Cigarette smoking
   (d) Diabetes mellitus
   (e) Obesity
   (f) Males
   (g) Family history of premature arteriosclerosis
3. Ischemic heart disease
   (a) Similar risk factors as arteriosclerosis
   (b) Hypercholesterolemia
       (1) Cholesterol should be less than 200 mg/dl
       (2) 15–20% of general population exceed recommended maximum
       (3) Dietary fat a major modifier
       (4) Drug therapy
           [a] Gemifibrozil
           [b] Lovastatin
           [c] Clofibrate
   (c) Hypertension
       (1) Enhances effects of other risk factors
       (2) For each 1 mm Hg, risk of MI decreases 2–3%
   (d) Cigarette smoking
       (1) Smoking equivalent to raising cholesterol by 50–100 mg/dl
       (2) Smoking effects
           [a] Enhances platelet aggregation
           [b] Induces coronary vasoconstriction
           [c] Promotes hypoxemia via carbon monoxide
   (e) Exercise and lifestyle
   (f) Diabetes mellitus, particularly in presence of hypertension
   (g) Currently, 500,000 deaths annually
4. Hypertension
   (a) General
       (1) Definition arbitrary
           [a] Systolic pressure over 160 mm Hg and/or
           [b] Diastolic pressure over 90 mm Hg
       (2) Affects approximately 60 million Americans
       (3) Occurs increasingly with age, two thirds over age 65 afflicted
       (4) Morbidity and mortality increase linearly with either systolic or diastolic pressure
   (b) Etiology
       (1) Essential hypertension accounts for over 90%
       (2) Secondary causes, contributors
           [a] Renal disease most common secondary cause
           [b] Atherosclerosis and peripheral vascular disease
               i) Peripheral arterial occlusive disease

        a) Usually involves coronary and cerebral vessels

        b) Most common form is occlusive disease of femoral arteries

      ii) Acute peripheral vascular disease from emboli

  (c) Antihypertensive drug therapy

    (1) Diuretics

    (2) ACE inhibitors

    (3) Beta-blockers

    (4) Calcium channel blockers

    (5) Vasodilators

  (d) Anesthetic management of hypertensive patient

    (1) Continue antihypertensive control

      [a] Generally, diastolic pressure less than 110 mm Hg acceptable

      [b] Hypokalemia common with diuretics, but incidence of hypokalemia-associated arrhythmias not increased

      [c] Patients receiving potassium and ACE inhibitors may be hyperkalemic

    (2) Patients may have exaggerated response, hypotension upon induction or hypertension with stimulation

    (3) Useful characteristic of volatile agents (particularly insoluble agents) is that of rapid adjustment of dose

    (4) Regional anesthetic may be of advantage

      [a] Fluid state may be more divergent from normal

      [b] Sympathomimetics may be required in addition to fluid therapy

    (5) Postoperative hypertension a frequent occurrence

    (6) Antihypertensive therapy should be resumed as promptly as practical postoperatively

b. Valvular heart disease

  1. Aortic stenosis

    (a) Etiology

      (1) Congenital with unicuspid, bicuspid, or tricuspid valve

      (2) Acquired

        [a] Rheumatic

        [b] Degenerative (senile) calcific

    (b) Symptomatology

      (1) Symptoms typically late in disease

      (2) Angina, average survival 2–3 years

      (3) Syncope, average survival 2–3 years

      (4) CHF, average survival 1½ years

      (5) Sudden death rare in asymptomatic patients, approximately 4%

    (c) Indications for valve replacement

      (1) Onset of symptoms

      (2) Transvalvular pressure gradient over 50 mm Hg

      (3) Valvular cross-sectional area less than 0.75 cm^2/m^2 BSA

    (d) Pathophysiology

      (1) Outflow obstruction

      (2) Early, cardiac output maintained with ability to adjust

      (3) Ventricular contraction progressively more isometric

      (4) Myocardial hypertrophy

      (5) Myocardial stiffness

      (6) Myocardial ischemia

    (e) Anesthetic considerations

      (1) Maintain preload to assure filling of noncompliant ventricle

      (2) Avoid reductions of afterload since heart does not readily adjust stroke volume; anesthetics resulting in sympathectomy somewhat hazardous

V. Clinical Priorities; b. Valvular heart disease (continued)

      (3) Maintain contractility

      (4) Maintain heart rate; ventricle does not readily increase stroke volume in response to bradycardia

      (5) Maintain sinus rhythm to provide "atrial kick" to assure ventricular filling

2. Aortic regurgitation (AR)

  (a) Etiology

      (1) Rheumatic heart disease

      (2) Bacterial endocarditis

      (3) Aortitis with aortic root distortion

          [a] Rheumatoid disease

          [b] Syphilis

          [c] Fallot-type VSD

      (4) Aortitis and aortic root dilation

          [a] Marfan's syndrome

          [b] Syphilis

      (5) Loss of commissural support, dissection tears of aorta

  (b) Symptomatology

      (1) Acute with sudden catastrophic change in hemodynamics versus chronic with evolving disease

      (2) Mild disease, asymptomatic

      (3) Moderate disease

          [a] Dyspnea

          [b] Fatigue

          [c] Palpitations

      (4) Severe with angina (rare)

      (5) Mortality with

          [a] Pulmonary edema

          [b] Dysrhythmias

  (c) Indications for valve replacement

      (1) Emergency replacement of valve for acute aortic regurgitation

      (2) Medical management

          [a] Mortality

              i) 75% survival for 5 years

             ii) 50% survival for 10 years

          [b] Onset of symptoms

              i) Angina, death by 4 years

             ii) CHF, death by 2 years

  (d) Pathophysiology

      (1) Acute aortic regurgitation, with rapid and substantial rise of

          [a] Preload

          [b] Wall tension

          [c] Myocardial oxygen consumption increased

          [d] Coronary perfusion reduced

      (2) Chronic aortic regurgitation

          [a] Ventricular dilation

          [b] Eccentric hypertrophy

          [c] Ratio of ventricular wall thickness of cavity radius (h/R) remains normal

          [d] Largest end-diastolic volumes of any cardiac disease, cor bovinum

          [e] Survival

              i) Poor if end-systolic volume is less than 30 ml/m^2

             ii) Good if end-systolic volume is over 90 ml/m^2

  (e) Anesthetic considerations

      (1) Maintain high preload

  (2) Maintain low afterload
  (3) Maintain good contractility
  (4) Avoid tachycardia
  (5) Maintain sinus rhythm

3. Mitral stenosis
 (a) Etiology
  (1) Rheumatic fever predominant cause
  (2) Rarely congenital
  (3) Rarely carcinoid, systemic lupus erythematosus (SLE), rheumatoid arthritis
 (b) Symptomatology
  (1) Late development of symptoms
   [a] Minimum of 2 years after rheumatic fever
   [b] Up to 20 years for onset, most commonly in third or fourth decade
   [c] Approximately 5 years from onset to severe disability
   [d] Symptoms precipitated by high output states, such as fever, pregnancy
  (2) Dyspnea principal symptom
  (3) Hemoptysis
  (4) Chest pain
  (5) Thromboembolism
  (6) Infective endocarditis, more common with mild multiple sclerosis
  (7) Mortality
   [a] Asymptomatic patients managed medically, 40% worsen or die within 10 years
 (c) Operation should be done for orifice less than 1.0 cm^2/m^2 BSA, surgical or balloon valvuloplasty
 (d) Pathophysiology
  (1) Orifice
   [a] Normal, 4–6 cm^2
   [b] Mild, over 2 cm^2
   [c] Moderate, $\approx$2 cm^2
   [d] Severe, less than 2 cm^2
  (2) Pulmonary hypertension
  (3) Decreased pulmonary compliance
  (4) Dilated left atrium
  (5) Atrial fibrillation, onset decreases cardiac output approximately 20%
 (e) Anesthetic considerations
  (1) Preload, requires accurate monitoring of filling pressure
  (2) Afterload
   [a] Elevation may precipitate acute failure
   [b] Stroke volume relatively fixed, fall in SVR will result in hypotension
  (3) Rate
   [a] Tachycardia impairs LA emptying and precipitates acute failure
   [b] Cannot compensate for severe bradycardia
  (4) Contractility, avoid impairment
  (5) Ventricular response rate more significant than presence or absence of sinus rhythm
  (6) Pulmonary artery pressure elevated, hypoxia, hypercarbia, acidosis, hypothermia, increased airway pressures accentuate

4. Mitral regurgitation
 (a) Etiology
  (1) Acute
   [a] Bacterial endocarditis
   [b] Chordae tendinae rupture
   [c] AMI with papillary muscle dysfunction

V. Clinical Priorities; b. Valvular heart disease (continued)

         (2) Chronic
            [a] Rheumatic heart disease
            [b] Papillary muscle fibrosis secondary to MI
            [c] LV dilation
            [d] MV prolapse
            [e] Mitral annulus calcification
    (b) Symptomatology
         (1) Acute, sudden onset of symptoms of pulmonary edema
         (2) Chronic
            [a] Fatigue
            [b] Dyspnea
            [c] Orthopnea
            [d] Right heart failure
            [e] Mortality
               i) Medical management if severe, 45% survival to 5 years
              ii) Survival predictors
                  a) AV oxygen difference (inverse)
                  b) End-diastolic volume (inverse)
    (c) Pathophysiology
         (1) Mild
            [a] Decreased EF
            [b] Increased LVEDV with normal LVEDP
            [c] Increased stroke volume with decreased forward stroke volume
            [d] Increased LAP
            [e] Frequently atrial fibrillation
         (2) Moderate
            [a] Increased regurgitant fraction
            [b] Markedly reduced forward ejection fraction
            [c] Pulmonary hypertension
            [d] CHF
            [e] Symptomatology
         (3) Severe
            [a] Irreversible myocardial damage, even with valve replacement
            [b] Death
    (d) Anesthetic considerations
         (1) Maintain preload without inducing pulmonary edema, serves as impedance to retrograde flow
         (2) Reduce afterload to promote forward flow
         (3) Maintain higher rates, which promote smaller ventricular size, smaller mitral orifice, and less regurgitation
         (4) Enhanced contractility promotes forward flow

5. Mitral valve prolapse
    (a) Etiology
         (1) Strong hereditary component
         (2) Multiple associations
         (3) May occur with ischemic heart disease or MI
    (b) Symptomatology
         (1) Generally asymptomatic
         (2) Palpitations, chest discomfort
    (c) Pathophysiology
         (1) Generally no functional disturbance unless hypovolemia occurs
         (2) Decreased LVEDV may cause regurgitation because redundant valve leaflets become incompetent

          (3) Increased LVEDV stretches mitral annulus and allows the redundant leaflets to close

     (d) Anesthetic implication, maintain high preload

6. Hypertrophic obstructive cardiomyopathy

     (a) Pathophysiology

          (1) Myocardial hypertrophy of LV outflow obstructs outflow from LV

          (2) Reduced LVEDV accentuates effect of outflow pathway

          (3) Increased LV contractility enhances obstructive influence on outflow tract

     (b) Anesthetic implications

          (1) Maintain high LVEDV

          (2) Avoid use of beta agonists

          (3) Maintain systemic vascular resistance

          (4) Sinus rhythm supports adequacy of diastolic filling and distension

7. IV SBE prophylaxis

     (a) For all prosthetic and abnormal valves associated with turbulent flow

     (b) For mitral valve prolapse if associated with mitral regurgitation

     (c) Ampicillin, 2 g, and gentamicin, 1.5 mg/kg, or

     (d) Vancomycin, 1 g, $\pm$ gentamicin, 1.5 mg/kg, if allergic to penicillin

c. Cardiomyopathy

1. Categories

     (a) Dilated cardiomyopathy (no longer congestive), over 90%

     (b) Hypertrophic

     (c) Restrictive

2. Dilated cardiomyopathy

     (a) Defined

          (1) Syndrome

              [a] Low cardiac output

              [b] Congestive heart failure

              [c] Ventricular dilatation in the absence of

                  i) Pressure overload

                  ii) Volume overload

                  iii) Coronary artery disease

          (2) Key: systolic dysfunction

     (b) Etiology

          (1) Idiopathic

          (2) Inflammatory, initial viral myocarditis leading to autoimmune mediated damage

          (3) Toxins

              [a] Ethanol

              [b] Heavy metals

              [c] Chemotherapeutic agents, e.g., doxorubicin

              [d] Endocrinologic

                  i) Hyper/hypothyroidism

                  ii) Acromegaly

              [e] Metabolic, e.g., thiamine deficiency

              [f] Peripartum, less than 5 months

              [g] Others

                  i) Neuromuscular, e.g., Friedreich's ataxia

                  ii) Hematologic, e.g., sickle cell disease

     (c) Pathophysiology

          (1) Decreased contractility

        (2) Ventricular dilation without increased wall thickness
        (3) Progressive mitral and tricuspid incompetence
        (4) Intracavitary thrombi and systemic emboli
   (d) Clinical
        (1) Initially, paucity of findings due to compensation
        (2) Symptoms of CHF with signs
   (e) Diagnosis
        (1) Cardiomegaly with pulmonary venous congestion on chest x-ray
        (2) ECG shows decreased QRS voltage, conduction defects
        (3) ECHO shows globally impaired ventricular function
   (f) Therapy
        (1) Increase contractility, digoxin
        (2) Reduce preload, salt restriction, diuretics
        (3) Reduce afterload with vasodilators, particularly ACE inhibitors
        (4) Anticoagulation for emboli
   (g) Anesthetic considerations
        (1) Consider pulmonary artery catheter for fluid management
        (2) Avoid myocardial depression, consider inotropes
        (3) Maintain preload in narrow range
        (4) Reduce afterload, consider vasodilators

3. Hypertrophic cardiomyopathy
   (a) Definition
        (1) Excess hypertrophy of the interventricular septum with anterior motion of the mitral valve leaflet causing dynamic LV outflow obstruction
        (2) Also known as
            [a] Asymmetric septal hypertrophy
            [b] Idiopathic hypertrophic subaortic stenosis
   (b) Etiology: autosomal dominant inheritance
   (c) Pathophysiology
        (1) Increased connective tissue and hypertrophied, disorganized myocytes cause primary LVH
        (2) Supranormal systolic function, 80% of SV ejected in first half of systole
        (3) Decreased LV compliance, with impaired diastolic filling and increased filling pressures
        (4) Increased reliance on atrial contribution to filling, up to 75%
        (5) Dynamic subaortic valve obstruction due to acceleration of blood through narrowed area between IVS and anterior leaflet of mitral valve, which causes apposition of MV to IVS by Venturi effect. Worsened by
            [a] Decreased preload
            [b] Decreased afterload
            [c] Increased contractility
   (d) Clinical
        (1) Often silent until third decade
        (2) Symptoms
            [a] Dyspnea, 90%
            [b] Atypical chest pain
            [c] Palpitations
            [d] Syncope, particularly postexercise
        (3) Signs
            [a] May be absent without fixed gradient
            [b] Arrhythmia
            [c] Systolic murmer on left sternal border, increased by Valsalva

   (e) Diagnosis
- (1) Chest x-ray, left atrial enlargement
- (2) ECG: increased QRS voltage, ST/T changes
- (3) ECHO (key)
    - [a] Disproportional septal thickening greater than ventricular free wall
    - [b] Anterior displacement of mitral valve

   (f) Therapy
- (1) Medical
    - [a] Beta-blockers, do not improve survival
    - [b] Calcium channel blockers improve diastolic function and survival
    - [c] Antiarrhythmics: amiodarone
    - [d] Anticoagulation if AF present
- (2) Surgical: myomectomy, mitral valve replacement

   (g) Anesthetic considerations
- (1) Must continue beta-blockers and calcium channel blockers
- (2) Maintain sinus rhythm
- (3) Maintain preload
- (4) Maintain afterload
- (5) Avoid increased inotropy
- (6) Generally neuraxia anesthesia best avoided except opioid epidural for labor

4. Restrictive cardiomyopathy
- (a) Definition: decreased ventricular compliance causing restricted diastolic filling and increased LV filling pressures
- (b) Etiology
    - (1) Idiopathic: "eosinophilic" endocardial fibrosis
    - (2) Infiltrative
        - [a] Amyloid
        - [b] Glycogen storage disease
        - [c] Hemochromatosis
- (c) Pathophysiology
    - (1) Normal systolic function (EF over 40%) but may not be able to increase contractility
    - (2) Severe decrease in ventricular compliance
    - (3) Thromboembolism
- (d) Clinical assessment
    - (1) Pulmonary congestion and edema
    - (2) Right-sided obstruction with ascites, pedal edema
    - (3) Difficult to differentiate from pericardial constriction
- (e) Diagnosis
    - (1) ECG: low QRS voltage
    - (2) Chest x-ray, absence of pericardial calcification
    - (3) ECHO: increased LV thickness with ECG changes
    - (4) Cardiac catheterization with biopsy
- (f) Treatment
    - (1) Treat cause
    - (2) Transplantation
    - (3) Treat symptoms
- (g) Anesthetic considerations
    - (1) Avoid sympatholysis; tachycardia and vasoconstriction are appropriate
    - (2) Maintain preload
    - (3) Avoid bradycardia
    - (4) Maintain inotropy
    - (5) Neuraxial blockade relatively undesired because of fixed stroke volume and increased filling pressures

V. Clinical Priorities (continued)

d. Tamponade, pericarditis

1. Pericardial anatomy
   (a) Closed sac attaches to arch of aorta, branch points of pulmonary veins
   (b) Double layered with up to 50 ml clear fluid, which is an ultrafiltrate of plasma
2. Pericardial function
   (a) Provides relatively fixed position
   (b) Intrapericardial pressure, 0 to 2 mm Hg negative compared with atmosphere
   (c) Limits acute dilation of the heart
   (d) Contributes to ventricular interdependence and diastolic coupling
3. Pericarditis
   (a) Etiologies: idiopathic, infectious, AMI, uremia, neoplasia, radiation, autoimmunity, drug reaction (such as to hydralazine and doxorubicin), trauma
   (b) History and symptoms: chest pain, dyspnea
   (c) Diagnosis
       (1) Pericardial friction rub
       (2) ECG: occurs within hours to days of onset, ST- and T-wave changes occur in approximately 90%
           [a] Stage I accompanies chest pain, ST elevation in all leads but V_r and V_1
           [b] Stage II in several days with ST returning to baseline and flattening of T wave
           [c] Stage III, inversion of T wave with vector opposite of ST, T changes in most leads
           [d] Stage IV, T waves return to normal
       (3) Chest x-ray may show enlargement of the heart shadow
       (4) Management dependent on diagnosis, e.g., antibiotics, anti-inflammatory agents
4. Pericardial effusion
   (a) Enlargement occurs with 250 ml
   (b) ECG shows decreased QRS voltage and T-wave flattening
   (c) Echocardiogram most efficacious and accurate in assessing
5. Tamponade, pericardial effusion with cardiac compression
   (a) Tamponade occurs when right atrial and ventricular diastolic pressures equalize with pericardial pressure
   (b) Pathophysiology
       (1) Cardiac output falls as effective transmural distending pressure gradient is reduced
       (2) Systemic vascular resistance rises as venous pressure rises
       (3) Pulsus paradoxus is an exaggerated fall of arterial pressure during inspiration, over 10%
           [a] Pulsus paradoxus in cardiac tamponade is critically dependent on the inspiratory augmentation of systemic venous return and right ventricular filling
           [b] Transient fall in the pulmonary venous to left heart gradient may occur during inspiration, further accentuates pulsus paradoxus
   (c) Etiology: malignancy, idiopathic pericarditis, uremia, AMI, infection, radiation, immune disorders, iatrogenic dissection, aortic aneurism
   (d) Triad
       (1) Decline in arterial pressure
       (2) Elevation of systemic venous pressure
       (3) Small, quiet heart

(e) Diagnosis
    (1) Chest x-ray not unique
    (2) ECG similar to pericarditis and pericardial effusion
    (3) Echocardiogram very useful

e. Pulmonary embolus

1. Third most common cardiovascular disease after ischemic syndromes and stroke
2. Hypercoagulable states
    (a) Primary
        (1) Antithrombin III deficiency
        (2) Protein C deficiency
        (3) Protein S deficiency
        (4) Lupus anticoagulant
    (b) Secondary
        (1) Abnormalities of coagulation
            [a] Cancer
            [b] Pregnancy
            [c] Oral contraceptives
            [d] Nephrotic syndrome
        (2) Abnormalities of platelets
            [a] Heparin-associated thrombocytopenia
            [b] Myeloproliferative disorders
            [c] Paroxysmal nocturnal hemoglobinuria
        (3) Abnormalities of blood vessels and rheology
            [a] Conditions promoting venous stasis (immobilization, postoperative state, obesity, advanced age)
            [b] Central venous and long-term indwelling catheters
            [c] Hyperviscosity (polycythemia, leukemia, sickle cell disease, leukoagglutination)
3. Deep venous thrombosis, up to 50% risk of pulmonary embolus with DVT of upper leg, less so in the calf
4. Pulmonary embolus (PE) syndrome
    (a) Massive pulmonary embolus
        (1) Sudden increase in right ventricular afterload and pulmonary artery pressure
        (2) Sudden death or long-term pulmonary hypertension
        (3) Syncope, profound dyspnea, cor pulmonale, cardiogenic shock or arrest, tachycardia
    (b) Submassive pulmonary embolus
        (1) Major segments of pulmonary artery involved
        (2) Does not result in pulmonary hypertension
        (3) Unlysed emboli may lead to chronic pulmonary hypertension
    (c) Pulmonary infarction
        (1) Small branch arterioles
        (2) Differential with pneumonia
        (3) Signs and symptoms develop 3 to 7 days following embolism
5. Symptoms of pulmonary embolus
    (a) Chest pain, 88%
    (b) Pleuritic chest pain, 74%
    (c) Dyspnea, 84%
    (d) Apprehension, 59%
    (e) Cough, 53%
    (f) Hemoptysis, 30%
6. Signs of pulmonary embolus
    (a) Tachypnea (RR over 16/min), 92%

    (b) Rales, 48%
    (c) Accentuated second heart sound, 53%
    (d) Tachycardia (HR over 100/min), 44%
    (e) Fever (temperature over 37.8°C), 43%
    (f) Phlebitis, 32%
    (g) Cyanosis, 19%

7. Differential diagnosis of pulmonary embolus

    (a) Myocardial infarction
    (b) Pneumonia
    (c) Congestive heart failure
    (d) Asthma
    (e) Chronic obstructive pulmonary disease
    (f) Intrathoracic cancer
    (g) Pneumothorax
    (h) "Musculoskeletal pain"

8. Diagnostic methods for pulmonary embolus

    (a) Chest x-ray
    (b) Lung scan
    (c) Pulmonary angiography
    (d) Echocardiography

9. Therapy for pulmonary embolus

    (a) Heparin
    (b) Warfarin, coumadin
    (c) Thrombolytic therapy
    (d) Inferior vena cava interruption
        (1) Ligation
        (2) Transvenous devices
    (e) Pulmonary embolectomy

10. Prevention of pulmonary embolus

    (a) Low-dose heparin, 5,000 units preoperatively and every 8 hours
    (b) Warfarin
    (c) Dextran
    (d) Compression stockings
    (e) Intermittent pneumatic compression
    (f) IVC interruption

f. New York Heart Association functional classification

1. Functional Class I: Patients with cardiac disease but *without limitations* of physical activity. Ordinary physical activity does not cause undue fatigue, palpitations, dyspnea, or angina pain

2. Functional Class II: Patients with cardiac disease resulting in *slight limitations* of physical activity. Comfortable at rest. Ordinary activity results in fatigue, palpitations, dyspnea, or anginal pain

3. Functional Class III: Patients with cardiac disease resulting in *marked limitation* of physical activity. They are comfortable at rest. Less than ordinary physical activity causes fatigue, palpitations, dyspnea, or anginal pain

4. Functional Class IV: Patients with cardiac disease resulting in an *inability to carry out any physical activity* without discomfort. *Symptoms* of cardiac insufficiency or of the anginal syndrome *may be present at rest*. If any physical activity is undertaken, discomfort is increased.

g. Cardiopulmonary bypass (CPB)

1. Basic circuit consists of five main components
   (a) Venous reservoir, blood leaves the patient via a venous cannula (usually placed in right atrium) and flows to the venous reservoir by gravity
   (b) Oxygenator
      (1) Bubble
         [a] Tiny oxygen bubbles enter through bottom of a blood column
         [b] Bubbles removed by passing blood past a defoaming agent (a charged silicone polymer)
         [c] Oxygenation depends on
            i) Bubble size
            ii) Number of bubbles
            iii) Oxygen fraction of bubbles
            iv) Transit time of blood in the blood column
            v) Carbon dioxide elimination, which is directly proportional to gas flow
      (2) Membrane
         [a] Thin, gas-permeable silicone membrane, which provides the blood–gas interface
         [b] Oxygenation determined by
            i) Oxygen fraction of bubbles
            ii) Area of interface
         [c] Carbon dioxide elimination is determined by gas flow
   (c) Heat exchanger, blood may be heated or cooled
   (d) Pump provides blood flow back to the patient through the arterial cannula, which is usually placed in the aorta; flow is nonpulsatile
      (1) Roller pumps
      (2) Centrifugal pumps, less hemolysis than roller pumps
   (e) Arterial filter to remove thrombi, tissue debris, and fat globules
2. Management of cardiopulmonary bypass
   (a) Preoperative period
      (1) Work-up dictated by patient's disease and proposed procedure
      (2) Premedications often include opiates with antianxiolytics
   (b) Monitoring
      (1) Usual ASA recommended monitors
      (2) ECG
         [a] Lead V5 is preferred to monitor for ischemia
         [b] Lead II is preferred to monitor rhythm
      (3) Invasive arterial monitor, may be placed preinduction to monitor beat to beat
      (4) CVP
      (5) Pulmonary artery catheter, indications vary widely among individuals and institutions
         [a] Ejection fraction less than 40%
         [b] History of pulmonary hypertension
         [c] Some valvular lesions
      (6) Core temperature
      (7) Urine output
   (c) Induction, specific agent less significant than skill with which it is used
   (d) Maintenance
      (1) IV agents
      (2) Volatile agents via oxygenator
   (e) Prebypass
      (1) Midline sternotomy usual for most CPB procedures
      (2) Pericardium dissected, opened

        (3) Aortic cannula usually placed in ascending aorta. Blood pressure should be reduced to 100 mm Hg systolic to decrease chance of aortic dissection during insertion

        (4) Venous cannula usually placed last because its placement often leads to substantial hemodynamic disturbance. One or two cannulae used

        (5) Anticoagulation
            [a] Heparin, 300 units/kg
            [b] Activated clotting time (ACT), may be used to determine dose, ACT over 400 seconds considered adequate for CPB

(f) Bypass

    (1) Initiation
        [a] Clamps are removed from venous and arterial cannulae, respectively
        [b] As blood drains from the patient by gravity, the reservoir level rises. The CPB pump flow is then gradually increased to approximately 2–2.5 L/min/m^2

    (2) Maintenance
        [a] The reservoir should become constant. A sudden decrease in the reservoir level indicates decreased venous return; cannulae positions should be checked immediately. Pump flow must also be decreased in order to keep the reservoir from completely emptying, which would allow air into the system
        [b] Blood pressure is generally kept between 40 and 70 mm Hg during CPB. Since flow is determined by the pump, blood pressure is manipulated by changing the systemic vascular resistance (SVR). Phenylephrine is typically used to treat hypotension. A vasodilator may be used for hypertension. Since light anesthesia can be a cause of hypertension, adequacy of anesthesia must be determined prior to administration of a vasodilator
        [c] In addition to IV agents for anesthesia during CPB, inhalation agents may be administered via most modern CPB machines

    (3) Arresting the heart
        [a] Cross-clamping and cardioplegia. Once CPB has been established, most cardiac procedures require arresting the heart. A clamp is placed across the aorta proximal to the aortic cannula and cold cardioplegia is administered, usually through a small catheter proximal to the aortic clamp. Cardioplegia is generally a K$^+$-rich crystalloid solution, which will quickly arrest the heart
        [b] Hypothermia used routinely for most procedures. Typically, patients are cooled to 20–25°C. Effective for myocardial preservation and cerebral protection

    (4) Restarting the heart
        [a] Aortic cross-clamp is removed. Blood flow is thus restored to the coronary arteries, washing out cardioplegia
        [b] Rewarming to 37°C is accomplished by heat exchanger
        [c] Most hearts will spontaneously enter a normal sinus rhythm with return of normothermia and perfusion of the coronaries. Ventricular fibrillation should be immediately treated with cardioversion to avoid excessive oxygen consumption

    (5) Termination of bypass
        [a] Checklist for attempting termination of bypass
            i) Core temperature up to 37°C
           ii) Stable rhythm, may require pacing
          iii) Correction of electrolyte abnormalities
          iv) Correction of acidosis
           v) Resumption of ventilation with 100% oxygen

[b] Weaning
    i) The venous cannula is progressively clamped, diverting blood flow to the heart
    ii) As the heart fills, contractility is evaluated and inotropes are added as needed
    iii) Pump flow is gradually decreased as arterial pressure rises
    iv) Visual evaluation of ventricular volume and contractility generally is adequate to dictate administration of volume and inotropes.
    v) If CPB weaning is unsuccessful with inotropes, an intra-aortic balloon pump or other assist device may be employed

(g) Postbypass
  (1) Bypass cannulae are removed
  (2) Heparin is reversed with protamine
  (3) Continued anticoagulation most likely due to hypothermia or platelet dysfunction
  (4) Blood remaining in the CPB circuit may be processed in the cell saver unit and returned to the patient
  (5) Postbypass patients require very careful monitoring in the operating room, during transportation, and in the ICU. The ability to resume CPB quickly should be maintained at all times

h. Coagulation defects

1. Physiology
  (a) Coagulation system incapable of stasis alone in a severed vessel
  (b) Hemostasis requires coagulation factors, platelet function, endothelium, and fibrinolysis
  (c) Initiation of cascade, attachment of von Willebrand factor to exposed subendothelial collagen
  (d) Platelet adhesion from platelet glycoprotein 1b binding on von Willebrand factor, of critical importance in surgical coagulopathies
  (e) Platelets degranulate and deform
  (f) Platelet aggregation, platelet plug formed, solidification with fibrin plug
  (g) Contact phase of coagulation also activated by stimuli leading to platelet adhesion
  (h) Factor XII activation converts prekallikrein to kallikrein, activates intrinsic pathway
  (i) Positive feedback of kallikrein amplifies the activation of factor XII and converts plasminogen to plasmin
  (j) Simultaneously with procoagulation actions, anticoagulation mechanisms are activated, which limit the coagulation. Antithrombin, extrinisic inhibitor, and plasminogen pathways

2. Pathophysiology
  (a) Von Willebrand factor–GP1b binding failure
    (1) Thrombocytopenia, counts over $50,000/mm^3$ result in critical impairment of hemostatic response
    (2) Decrease in platelets in periphery of flowing blood, change in flow characteristics if hematocrits less than 20%
    (3) Lack of platelet GP1b receptor following CPB, platelets stored more than 3 days
    (4) Occupied and/or inert GP1b receptor, following dextran infusion, idiopathic thrombocytopenic purpura
  (b) Poor platelet plug formation
    (1) Thrombocytopenia, thrombocytopathy
    (2) Prior platelet activation, CPB, aspirin exposure, uremia, alcohol ingestion
  (c) Clotting factor dysfunction and/or deficiency
    (1) Anticoagulant therapy, vitamin K deficiency
    (2) Disseminated intravascular coagulopathy (DIC)

V. Clinical Priorities; h. Coagulation defects (continued)

         (3) Massive resuscitation

     (d) Excess fibrinolysis

         (1) DIC

         (2) Resulting from therapy, streptokinase, tPA

  3. Evaluation of hemostasis

     (a) History and examination

         (1) History of excessive blood loss with prior surgeries, spontaneous bleeding, bruising

         (2) Renal, hepatic, and hematologic disease should be excluded

         (3) Note drugs taken, anticoagulants, heparin, aspirin

         (4) Signs of bleeding and/or bruising

     (b) Laboratory evaluation, must be evaluated in light of clinical events

         (1) Activated partial thromboplastin time (aPTT) to assess the intrinsic and common pathways

         (2) Prothrombin time (PT) to assess the extrinsic

         (3) Thrombin time (TT) to assess the amount and quality of fibrinogen present

         (4) Bleeding time a *poor* screening test, a good indicator of platelet functionality in a patient with established coagulopathy

         (5) Platelet count

         (6) Fibrin degradation products (FDPs) assess plasmin activity

     (c) Intraoperative assessment of hemostasis, can be done in the operating room without services of laboratory

         (1) Activated clotting time (ACT). Celite added to whole blood in cuvette, formation of clot sensed by device, time displayed

         (2) Thromboelastography (TEG). Blood placed in rotating cuvette with piston suspended in sample. Energy change or rotation detected as clotting occurs. Trace displayed shows characteristics of clotting and lysis

  4. Specific coagulopathies in cardiovascular procedures

     (a) Cardiopulmonary bypass

         (1) Pathogenesis

            [a] Major injury is on the platelet

            [b] Prolongation of bleeding time directly related to CPB time, hypothermia

            [c] Platelet injuries include loss of GP1b and granules

            [d] Activated platelets cannot contribute to normal platelet aggregation

            [e] Stimulation of fibrinolysis

            [f] CPB may also promote plasmin activation

         (2) Management

            [a] Minimize CPB time

            [b] Platelet transfusions

            [c] Synthetic antifibrinolytics

               i) Epsilon-aminocaproic acid (EACA)

               ii) Tranexamic acid (TA)

               iii) *p*-Aminomethylbenzoic acid (PAMBA)

            [d] Possible increased risk of thrombotic tendency with treatment with antifibrinolytics

            [e] Aprotynin is a naturally occurring antifibrinolytic. May reduce blood loss and coagulopathy. May cause hypersensitivity

     (b) Abdominal aortic aneurism rupture

         (1) Pathogenesis

            [a] Strong association of mortality with coagulopathies and hemorrhage

            [b] Coagulopathy due to

               i) Dilution of platelets and soluble clotting factors

               ii) Consumption of platelets and clotting factor due to activation

[c] Diffuse oozing from trauma and incisions, insertion of cannulae sites
[d] Diagnosis primarily on clinical grounds, laboratory for subsidiary information
[e] With replacement of one blood volume, clinical coagulopathy will occur by dilutional thrombocytopenia
[f] With replacement of two blood volumes, a critical dilution of soluble clotting factors is approached

(2) Management
[a] Platelet count, prothrombin time (PT), and fibrinogen to assess extent of coagulation, not presence. Poor predictors of likelihood of onset of abnormal bleeding
[b] Platelet transfusion initially
[c] If laboratory indicates presence of hypofibrinogenemia or dilutional or consumptive coagulopathy or in the lack of time for confirmation, then cryoprecipitate and fresh frozen plasma
   i) Plasma fibrinogen less than 0.8 g/L
   ii) PT is more than 1.8 times normal and fibrinogen is more than 0.8 g/L, then fresh frozen plasma
[d] Prophylactic infusion of platelets and/or fresh frozen plasma not justified

i. Disorders of rhythm

1. Pathogenesis
   (a) Reentry
       (1) Responsible for most dysrhythmias
       (2) Requires two pathways
       (3) Anterograde pathway conducts impulse forward
       (4) Retrograde pathway conducts impulse backward
       (5) Pharmacologic and/or physiologic conditions may promote heterogeneous conduction with varying refractoriness and permit reentry
   (b) Automaticity changes
       (1) May occur at ectopic focus
       (2) Results from pharmacologic influence and/or physiologic changes
   (c) Should treat those dysrhythmias that compromise cardiac output or threaten to do so, rather than the dysrhythmia per se

2. Diagnosis
   (a) ECG main tool of diagnosis
   (b) Identify P wave for every QRS
   (c) Upright P wave in lead II indicates normal origin of impulse from SA node
   (d) Normal values
       (1) PR, 0.12–0.2 second
       (2) QRS, less than 0.13 second

3. Antidysrhythmic agents (see also "Pharmacology," "Antiarrhythmics" above)
   (a) Should restore normal physiology before initiating drug therapy, e.g., pH, oxygenation, electrolyte balance
   (b) Most generally significant side effect of antidysrhythmics is myocardial depression

4. Electrical cardioversion
   (a) Most useful for
       (1) Atrial flutter
       (2) Atrial fibrillation
       (3) Ventricular tachycardia
       (4) Other ectopic dysrhythmias not responsive to drug therapy

V. Clinical Priorities; i. Disorders of rhythm (continued)

        (5) Note well

           [a] Requires good skin contact

           [b] Higher intensity (e.g., 200 joules) better than repeated attempts at lower intensities

           [c] In the presence of QRS, synchronized shock should be used, otherwise ventricular fibrillation may be provoked

  5. Disturbances of cardiac impulse conduction

    (a) First-degree atrioventricular heart block

      (1) Defined as PR over 0.2 second at heart rate of 70 beats per minute (bpm)

      (2) Pathogenesis

        [a] Usually accompanying aging

        [b] Digitalis

        [c] Ischemia

        [d] May accompany diaphragmatic myocardial infarction

      (3) Usually asymptomatic, requires no intervention

    (b) Second-degree heart block

      (1) Mobitz type I (Wenkebach)

        [a] Progressive increase in PR to complete heart block

        [b] Followed by resumption of AV conduction and cycle repeated

      (2) Mobitz type II

        [a] Sudden interruption of conduction without prolongation of PR

        [b] Disease of His-Purkinje system

        [c] More serious than Mobitz I

        [d] May progress to complete block

      (3) Elective pacemaker for Mobitz II

      (4) External pacemaker if foregoing not done

      (5) No specific therapy for Mobitz I

    (c) Unifascicular heart block

      (1) Left bundle divides into two fascicles, anterior and posterior

      (2) Left anterior hemiblock more common than anterior

      (3) Usually QRS is normal or only minimally prolonged

    (d) Right bundle branch block

      (1) RBBB is present in 1% of adults

      (2) QRS over 0.1 second with a broad RSR in right-sided chest leads

      (3) RBBB often of no clinical significance. May be associated with increased right ventricular pressure

    (e) Left bundle branch block

      (1) Often reflects ischemic heart disease and/or left ventricular hypertrophy

      (2) LBBB has QRS over 0.12 second and wide notched R waves in all leads. Further interpretation of configuration or waves difficult

      (3) Incomplete LBBB, 0.1 less than QRS less than 0.12 second

      (4) Acute appearance of LBBB may indicate occurrence of acute myocardial infarct

      (5) With LBBB, and 5% chance of inducing RBBB with PA catheter, a trifascicular or complete heart block could occur

    (f) Bifascicular heart block

      (1) RBBB with either left anterior or left posterior fascicle blocked; RBBB with left anterior block most common; present in 1% of all ECGs

      (2) Progression to complete heart block in 1% of cases

      (3) RBBB and left posterior block are rare, more frequently progress to complete; insert pacemaker with symptomatic bradycardia

      (4) No evidence that anesthesia or surgery predisposes to development of complete heart block

(g) Third-degree heart block
    (1) Complete heart block with ectopic pacemaker for ventricle beyond block
    (2) Stokes-Adams associated with acute onset
    (3) Etiology
        [a] Most common is fibrous degeneration of conduction system with aging, Lenegre's disease
        [b] Degenerative changes in tissues adjacent to mitral annulus, Lev's disease
        [c] Congenital block usually occurs at level of AV node
        [d] Ischemic heart disease, AMI
        [e] Cardiomyopathy
        [f] Myocarditis
        [g] Ankylosing spondylitis
        [h] Electrolyte derangements, hyperkalemia
        [i] Drugs
           i) Digitalis
           ii) Quinidine
           iii) Beta agonists

6. Disturbances of cardiac rhythm

(a) Sinus tachycardia
    (1) Heart rate over 120 bpm, arising from SA node
    (2) Multiple causes
        [a] Fever
        [b] Thyrotoxicosis
        [c] Hypovolemia
        [d] Pain
        [e] Light anesthesia
        [f] CHF
    (3) Treat *underlying* cause
    (4) Beta-blockers when correctable causes addressed

(b) Sinus bradycardia
    (1) Heart rate less than 60 bpm secondary to slowing of SA node
    (2) May be *normal* in fit patients
    (3) Causes
        [a] Severe pain
        [b] Diaphragmatic myocardial infarct
        [c] Halothane
        [d] Beta antagonists
        [e] Hypothermia
        [f] Hypothyroidism
        [g] Reflex, e.g., ocular reflex
    (4) Therapy when symptomatic

(c) Sick sinus syndrome, bradycardia–tachycardia syndrome
    (1) Bradycardia with episodes of supraventricular tachycardia, most commonly in the elderly
    (2) Usually asymptomatic, may experience syncope and palpitations
    (3) Systemic embolism occurs in up to 20% of patients
    (4) Pacemaker for bradycardia
    (5) If tachycardia incapacitating, surgical ablation of common bundle with pacemaker placed

(d) Atrial premature and junctional premature beats
    (1) Ectopic atrial pacemakers
    (2) Distorted P waves
    (3) QRS normal if conduction through AV node, altered QRS for abnormal conduction pathway
    (4) Acceleration of sinus rate can abolish

        (5) Quinidine occasionally needed
- (e) Paroxysmal supraventricular tachycardia
  - (1) Regular beat of 130–220 bpm, usually sudden onset
  - (2) Usually well tolerated, but may precipitate hypotension or CHF
  - (3) Therapy
    - [a] Initially increase vagal tone, carotid massage, Valsalva, stimulate posterior pharynx
    - [b] Cardioversion
    - [c] Drug conversion
      - i) Adenosine, 3–12 mg
      - ii) Verapamil, 75–100 μg/kg
      - iii) Esmolol, 1–2 mg/kg
- (f) Atrial flutter
  - (1) Regular ECG, rate 250–320 bpm, may have 1:2 AV block
  - (2) Carotid massage ineffective
  - (3) Therapy
    - [a] Digoxin, 0.25–0.75 mg
    - [b] With or without beta-blocker or verapamil
    - [c] Cardioversion
- (g) Atrial fibrillation
  - (1) Most common sustained dysrhythmia, 0.4% of all individuals, 10% of those over 60 years of age
  - (2) Irregular atrial rate, 350–500 per minute with variable slower ventricular response rate
  - (3) Increased incidence of systemic embolization
  - (4) Therapy
    - [a] Digitalis
    - [b] Calcium channel blockers
    - [c] Beta-blockers
    - [d] Electrical cardioversion recommended
- (h) Junctional rhythm
  - (1) Ectopic pacemaker around AV node
  - (2) P wave may precede, follow, or be obscured by QRS
  - (3) Treatment only for falling cardiac output, vagolytic agents
- (i) Ventricular premature beats
  - (1) May arise from a single (unifocal) or multiple (multifocal) ectopic pacemaker sites
  - (2) Diagnosed by
    - [a] Premature occurrence
    - [b] Absence of P wave preceding the QRS
    - [c] Wide and bizarre-appearing QRS
    - [d] ST segment in a direction opposite to the QRS
    - [e] Inverted T wave
    - [f] Compensatory pause after premature beat
  - (3) During relative refractory period (middle third of T wave), heart is vulnerable to initiation of ventricular tachycardia or fibrillation
  - (4) Occurrence
    - [a] Most commonly associated with myocardial disease
    - [b] Electrolyte disturbance
    - [c] Aging
    - [d] Drugs, e.g., digitalis
  - (5) Treatment
    - [a] Suggested when six or more per minute
    - [b] Multifocal origin

       [c] Correct underlying cause preferably
       [d] Drug
          i) Lidocaine first choice
          ii) Long term
             a) Quinidine
             b) Procainamide
             c) Disopyramide
             d) Amiodarone
          iii) See above, "Pharmacology," "Antiarrhythmics"
  (j) Ventricular tachycardia
     (1) Three or more VPBs with a rate greater than 120 per minute
     (2) Requires good ECG to distinguish from supraventricular tachycardia
     (3) Clinical setting aids diagnosis, e.g., following acute myocardial infarction
     (4) Drugs
        [a] Lidocaine
        [b] Procainamide
        [c] Bretylium
  (k) Ventricular fibrillation
     (1) Chaotic asynchronous contraction without discernible QRS, no effective stroke volume
     (2) Electrical cardioversion
     (3) Resuscitation

7. Preexcitation syndromes
  (a) General characteristics
     (1) Anomalous or accessory pathway that bypasses the AV node
     (2) In absence of AV nodal delay, activation of ventricles occurs earlier than normal
     (3) Accessory tracts present in 0.1–0.3% of the population
     (4) Most common dysrhythmia is paroxysmal supraventricular tachycardia; atrial flutter or fibrillation also occurs
  (b) Wolff-Parkinson-White syndrome
     (1) Most common of preexcitation syndromes
     (2) Kent's bundle from atrium to ventricle
     (3) Short PR, less than 0.12 second
     (4) Wide QRS, more than 0.12 second
     (5) Delta wave
     (6) Sudden death in Wolff-Parkinson-White syndrome of 1 in 700–1,000, with first manifestation of syndrome as cardiac arrest in 12% of patients
  (c) Lown-Ganong-Levine syndrome
     (1) James fibers with bypass AV node and insert directly into the bundle of His
     (2) Short PR
     (3) Normal QRS
     (4) No delta wave
     (5) Most common dysrhythmia is atrial flutter or fibrillation
     (6) Often asymptomatic
     (7) Treated as WPW
  (d) Mahaim pathway
     (1) Accessory pathways arising below AV node and inserting directly on ventricular muscle
     (2) Normal or slightly shortened PR
     (3) Wide QRS
     (4) Delta wave
     (5) Treated as WPW

8. Prolonged QT syndrome
  (a) Congenital

        (1) Jervell and Lange-Nielsen syndrome associated with deafness
        (2) Romano-Ward syndrome, without deafness
        (3) Thought to be asymmetrical sympathetic innervation of the heart
        (4) Delayed repolarization renders ventricle susceptible to dysrhythmias

(b) Acquired prolonged QT syndrome
        (1) Drugs
               [a] Quinidine
               [b] Disopyramide
               [c] Tricyclic depressants
        (2) Subarachnoid hemorrhage
        (3) Hypokalemia
        (4) Hypomagnesemia

(c) QT over 0.44 second

(d) Syncope, may be related because of sympathetic effect

(e) Treatment empirical, decrease cardiac sympathetic nervous system activity

(f) Beta-blockers

(g) Stellate ganglion block considered a prophylactic procedure

---

j. Congenital heart disease

1. General considerations

  (a) Occurrence, 6 to 8 in 1,000 births

  (b) Of occurrence, incidence
      (1) Ventricular septal defect (VSD), 25.0%
      (2) Patent ductus arteriosus (PDA), 12.5%
      (3) Pulmonary stenosis (PS), 8.7%
      (4) Tetrology of Fallot (TOF), 7.9%
      (5) Coarctation of aorta (CoA), 6.6%
      (6) Aortic stenosis (AS), 6.3%
      (7) Atrial septal defect (ASD), 5.8%
      (8) Transposition of great arteries (TGA), 5.1%

  (c) Congenital heart disease commonly found in association with other congenital defects

  (d) Anesthetic management in response to four general considerations
      (1) Pulmonary flow increased or decreased
      (2) Outflow obstruction associated with valvular-related abnormality
      (3) Shunts, intracardiac, extracardiac, combined
      (4) Presence of airway obstruction

2. Increased pulmonary blood flow

  (a) Work of breathing increased because of increased pulmonary blood flow

  (b) Cardiac failure secondary to volume overload

  (c) Presence of cyanosis
      (1) No cyanosis
          [a] VSD
          [b] PDA
          [c] ASD
          [d] Endocardial cushion defect, AV canal abnormality
          [e] Anomalous origin of left coronary arteries, ALCA (from pulmonary artery)
      (2) Cyanosis
          [a] TGA
          [b] TA, truncus arteriosus
          [c] Single ventricle
          [d] Total or partial anomalous pulmonary venous drainage, TAPVD or PAPVD

(d) Eisenmenger's complex
  (1) Untreated, develops pulmonary occlusive disease
  (2) Right ventricular failure can occur with closure of defect because of high pulmonary vascular resistance
  (3) Occurs with reversal of left-to-right shunt to right-to-left shunt because of elevated pulmonary vascular resistance

3. Reduced pulmonary flow

  (a) Severe cyanosis, polycythemia, acidosis, and hypoxia with right-to-left shunt exacerbated with reduction of systemic vascular resistance
  (b) Occurs with
    (1) TOF
    (2) Pulmonary atresia with VSD
    (3) Tricuspid atresia
    (4) Ebstein's anomaly, downward displacement of dysplastic tricuspid valve with functionally small right ventricle
    (5) TGA
    (6) Truncus arteriosus
    (7) Single ventricle

4. Obstruction of blood flow

  (a) AS
  (b) PS
  (c) CoA
  (d) Asymmetric septal hypertrophy

5. Obstruction of airway

  (a) Double aortic arch
  (b) Anomalous pulmonary artery

6. Anesthetic considerations in preoperative evaluation

  (a) The neonatal heart is part of series circuit with a high-pressure right ventricle ejecting blood into the main pulmonary artery that ultimately joins the aorta through the PDA. Expansion of the lungs at birth produces a precipitous fall in PVR, with lowering of right-sided pressures. The left side assumes the role of perfusing the systemic circulation
  (b) Some changes require time to fully mature, but under some conditions, may revert to fetal values. Elevations of PVR result in persistent right-to-left shunt, "persistent fetal circulation," or, more accurately, "transitional circulation." Other conditions may promote fetal circulation
    (1) Respiratory obstruction
    (2) Prostaglandin E_1 and E_2
    (3) Acidosis
    (4) Hypercapnea
    (5) Hypoxia
  (c) Neonatal heart is characterized by a poorly compliant right heart and relatively undeveloped left heart. Preload responses are fewer and sensitivity to afterload is increased. Cardiac output is *more dependent on rate*. Neonatal heart less responsive to calcium, beta-induced chronotropy, and inotropy, but very sensitive to beta blockade.
  (d) Multidisciplinary approach for perioperative management is imperative
  (e) History
    (1) Chronologic beginning in prenatal period
    (2) Recurrence of congenital heart disease in sibling is 3%
    (3) History of poor feeding, low weight gain, or delayed development
    (4) Evidence of pallor, syncope, or easy fatigue
    (5) Hypercyanotic episodes (Tet spells) can occur in 20–70% of TOFs

(6) Children who "spell" increase systemic vascular resistance and limit right-to-left shunt. A Tet spell during induction of anesthesia can result in death

(f) Respiratory
   (1) Distress, tachypnea, intercostal recession, grunting, and wheezing may suggest decreased compliance due to large left-to-right shunt
   (2) Infections or bronchial compression by vascular rings can also produce wheezing

(g) Cyanosis due to
   (1) Reduced blood flow to the lungs
   (2) Right-to-left shunt
   (3) Mixing in a common mixing chamber, e.g., TGA, TAPVD, PAPVD, TA, single ventricle

(h) Polycythemia
   (1) Mediated via increased renal
   (2) Perioperative phlebotomy only indicated in symptomatic hyperviscosity with hematocrit over 65%
   (3) Exclude iron deficiency and dehydration
   (4) Long-standing cyanosis may be accompanied by clubbing of the fingers and toes

(i) Hemostasis
   (1) Abnormal in 20% of all congenital heart disease patients
   (2) PT or PPT may be prolonged
   (3) Platelet counts may be decreased and function depressed
   (4) Platelets should be available if counts are less than 120,000

(j) Laboratory
   (1) Hypoglycemia and hypocalcemia significant risk in presence of CHF
   (2) Diuretic therapy may reduce K^+
   (3) PaO_2 of 30–40 mm Hg and saturation less than 70% indicate impaired respiratory reserve and imminent metabolic acidosis

(k) Cardiac investigation
   (1) CXR for size, shape, and position of heart, e.g.,
      [a] TOF, boot-shaped heart
      [b] TGA, "egg on its side"
      [c] TAPVD, "snowman" or "figure-of-eight"
   (2) ECG for evidence of increasing right ventricular hypertrophy
   (3) Echocardiography has decreased need for catheterization
   (4) Cardiac catheterization for identification of specific lesions

(l) Medications
   (1) Diuretics for CHF
   (2) Digitalis for CHF and arrhythmias, consider stopping for CPB
   (3) Beta-blockers to limit functional effects of subvalvular hypertrophy and stenosis
   (4) Prostaglandin E_1 or E_2 to maintain an open PDA
   (5) Oral sodium bicarbonate with acidosis in cyanotic heart disease

7. Anesthetic management
   (a) Antibiotics
   (b) Premedication and preoperative visit
      (1) Unless very ill
         [a] Sedative-hypnotic
         [b] Antisialagogue
         [c] Narcotic
      (2) All preoperative agents continued except digitalis, the latter particularly for CPB

        (3) Oxygen supplementation
  (c) Feeding has been liberalized, consider intravenous hydration
  (d) Monitoring
        (1) Routine or usual
            [a] ECG
            [b] Noninvasive blood pressure
            [c] Precordial stethoscope
        (2) Following induction
            [a] Central or core temperature
            [b] Capnography
            [c] Urine output
            [d] Invasive arterial blood pressure
            [e] CVP
            [f] Left atrial line placed by surgeon
        (3) Oximetry from two sites may be needed
  (e) *Air must be excluded from venous lines*
  (f) Cautious and gentle induction
        (1) Left-to-right shunts, more rapid inhalation induction but slower IV induction
        (2) Right-to-left shunts, slower inhalation induction but more rapid IV induction
  (g) Maintenance
        (1) Note influence of ventilation pressures in presence of low pulmonary flows
        (2) Hypercyanotic spells in TOF can be treated by increasing systemic vascular resistance
        (3) Beta-blocker to relieve infundibular obstruction
  (h) Bypass
        (1) Initiation and continuance
            [a] Heparin, 300–400 μm/kg or 9,000 μm/m^2, whichever is larger, to obtain ACT over 400 seconds
            [b] Circulatory arrest with deep hypothermia usually about 45–90 minutes
            [c] Surface cooling increases margin of safety
        (2) Termination
            [a] Reversal of heparin
            [b] Blood-clotting products may be needed
            [c] Antifibrinolytics may be useful for those undergoing deep hypothermia

k. Obstetrics

1. Cardiovascular changes of pregnancy

  (a) Blood volume increases 35%
  (b) Plasma volume increases 45%
  (c) Red cell volume increases 20%
  (d) Relative anemia from (b) and (c)
  (e) Cardiac output increases 40%
  (f) Stroke volume increases 30%
  (g) Heart rate increases 15%
  (h) Systemic vascular resistance declines 15%
  (i) Both systolic and diastolic pressures decline
  (j) CVP remains unchanged
  (k) Contractility unchanged

2. Induction of pregnant patient must balance following

  (a) Hemodynamics of mother and fetus
  (b) For general anesthesia, rapid induction to avoid aspiration
  (c) Avoid sedation or depression of fetus
  (d) Uterine vasculature maximally dilated and dependent on maternal blood pressure for flow

      (e) Assure adequate hydration

      (f) Avoid aortocaval compression

      (g) Contractions may "autotransfuse" up to 300–500 ml from uterus to effective general circulation

      (h) During labor

          (1) Further increases in cardiac output

          (2) Both heart rate and stroke volume increase

3. Cardiac disease in pregnancy

      (a) More hemodynamically significant lesions

          (1) Primary pulmonary hypertension

          (2) Lesions with right-to-left shunt

          (3) Severe aortic stenosis and coarctation of aorta

          (4) Mitral valve disease

      (b) Severity of disease, New York Heart Association

      (c) Incidence of heart disease in pregnancy, 1.6–2%

          (1) Rheumatic heart disease, decreasing incidence

             [a] Mitral stenosis, 90%

             [b] Mitral regurgitation

             [c] Aortic disease, less than 4%

          (2) Congenital disease, more reaching childbearing age

          (3) Coronary artery disease, increasing

             [a] Smoking

             [b] Overall population with increasing coronary disease

             [c] Postponement of childbearing

      (d) Symptoms of heart disease in pregnancy, may be difficult to distinguish from normal pregnancy or noncardiac origin problems

          (1) Normal

             [a] Decreased exercise tolerance

             [b] Orthopnea

             [c] Dyspnea

             [d] Jugular vein distension, peripheral edema

             [e] Bibasilar rales, secondary to atelectasis from gravid uterus

             [f] Systolic murmur in 96% of patients

             [g] ECG changes

                i) QRS axis deviation

                ii) Q wave in lead III

                iii) ST segment depression

             [h] Syncope

             [i] Arrhythmias more common

                i) Supraventricular tachycardia

                ii) Wandering atrial pacemaker

                iii) PACs

                iv) PVCs

          (2) Abnormal symptoms of pregnancy

             [a] Systolic murmur of intensity greater than 3/6

             [b] Any diastolic murmur

4. Cardiac drugs in pregnancy

      (a) Ephedrine

          (1) Increased SVR

          (2) Decreased venous capacitance

          (3) Increased heart rate

          (4) Increased contractility

      (5) Pro: uterine perfusion generally maintained

      (6) Con: may be hazardous in cardiac disease where chronotropy is undesirable

(b) Phenylephrine

      (1) Increased SVR

      (2) Low dose may decrease venous capacitance without appreciably affecting SVR

      (3) Low doses, 40–100 μg divided, maximum 400 μg, probably safe

(c) Inotropic agents

      (1) Epinephrine, decreases uterine blood flow even in low doses

      (2) Dopamine, decreases uterine blood flow

      (3) Dobutamine, decreases uterine blood flow, although not as much as dopamine

      (4) Norepinephrine, decreases uterine blood flow

      (5) Isoproterenol

          [a] No direct effect on uterine blood flow

          [b] May reduce uterine blood flow secondarily by reducing mean blood pressure

(d) Vasodilators

      (1) Fetal heart rate should be monitored when manipulating maternal blood pressure

      (2) Hydralazine, may increase uterine blood flow

      (3) Nitroglycerin, control of blood flow restores uterine blood flow

      (4) Nitroprusside

          [a] Safe for short-term use

          [b] High dose may be associated with fetal cyanide toxicity

      (5) Trimethaphan

          [a] Limited placental transfer

          [b] No direct fetal adverse effects

(e) Digitalis

      (1) Increased bioavailability in pregnancy

      (2) Crosses placenta

(f) Anticoagulants

      (1) Used in presence of prosthetic heart valves, atrial fibrillation, dilated cardiomyopathy, Eisenmenger's complex

      (2) Coumarin

          [a] Increased spontaneous abortion rate

          [b] Increased malformations

          [c] Increased risk of intracranial hemorrhage

      (3) Heparin

          [a] Does not cross placenta

          [b] No apparent effect on fetal mortality or morbidity

          [c] Anticoagulant of choice in pregnancy

          [d] Discontinue with onset of labor

(g) Antiarrhythmics, see above, "Pharmacology," "Antiarrhythmics"

      (1) Drugs that appear to have no fetal effects at therapeutic doses

          [a] Procainamide

          [b] Verapamil

          [c] Bretylium, may be drug of choice for bupivicaine-induced VF

      (2) Quinidine

          [a] No adverse effects on fetus

          [b] Rarely produces preterm labor

      (3) Dispyramide, oxytocinlike effect

      (4) Phenytoin

          [a] Multiple congenital anomalies from exposure in first trimester

          [b] Use only for refractory digitalis-induced arrhythmias

        (5) Beta-blockers
- [a] Controversial because of potential for fetal bradycardia and adrenergic responses of myometrium
- [b] Myometrium
  - i) Alpha agonist, increases uterine activity
  - ii) Beta agonist, decreases uterine activity
  - iii) Beta blockade, theoretically could
    - a) Increase uterine tone
    - b) Decrease uteroplacental blood flow
    - c) Stimulate preterm labor
- [c] Fetus
  - i) May decrease heart rate
  - ii) Increases umbilical vascular tone
  - iii) All beta-blockers have been used in pregnant women as required with variable fetal results but no clear adverse effects
- [d] Labetalol, alpha-, and beta-blocker
  - i) Effective for severe hypertension
  - ii) Appears safe for chronic or acute use
- [e] Esmolol, purely beta-blocker
  - i) Controversial, animal studies have shown severe bradycardia with hypoxia and acidemia
  - ii) Fetal heart rate should be monitored

5. Valvular cardiac lesions
   - (a) Mitral stenosis
     - (1) Most common valvular lesion
     - (2) Physiologic changes of pregnancy poorly tolerated
     - (3) Frequently pulmonary congestion after 30th week
     - (4) May worsen with labor and delivery
     - (5) Mortality
       - [a] NYHA III, 4–5%
       - [b] With superimposed atrial fibrillation, 14–17%
     - (6) Symptoms
       - [a] Fatigue
       - [b] Dyspnea at rest
       - [c] Orthopnea
       - [d] Paroxysmal nocturnal dyspnea
       - [e] Prone to atrial fibrillation, 33%
       - [f] Severe stenosis may lead to pulmonary edema
     - (7) Physical examination
       - [a] Presystolic or end-diastolic murmur
       - [b] Intensity of murmur does not correlate with severity of lesion
     - (8) Pathophysiology
       - [a] LV underloading
       - [b] Decreased cardiac output
       - [c] Increased left atrial pressure
       - [d] Increased pulmonary vascular pressures
       - [e] Decreased lung compliance, transudation of fluid
       - [f] Dyspnea and orthopnea
       - [g] Eventual right heart failure
     - (9) Factors precipitating cardiac decompensation
       - [a] Tachycardia, shortens LV filling time
       - [b] Decreased SVR, hypotension because of fixed CO
       - [c] Fluid overload

        [d] Worsening pulmonary hypertension
           i) Hypoxia
           ii) Hypercapnea
           iii) Acidosis
           iv) Increased airway pressure
    (10) Anesthetic management
        [a] Monitoring
           i) Pulmonary artery catheter
           ii) Invasive arterial pressue
        [b] Labor and vaginal delivery, epidural
           i) Decreased sympathetic activity
           ii) Close management of fluid
           iii) Avoid epinephrine-containing anesthetics
           iv) Phenylephrine for hypotension
        [c] Cesarean section
           i) Epidural
           ii) Spinal best avoided
           iii) General endotracheal
        [d] Major problems
           i) Atrial fibrillation, treat aggressively
              a) Synchronized cardioversion
              b) Beta blockade
              c) Digitalis
              d) Verapamil
           ii) Pulmonary hypertension
              a) Avoid hypoxia, hypercapnea, acidosis
              b) Vasodilation with nitroglycerin
              c) Inotropic support with dobutamine or dopamine
        [e] Monitor from onset of labor to 24–48 hours postpartum
  (b) Mitral regurgitation
    (1) Second most common valvular lesion
    (2) Pregnancy generally well tolerated
    (3) Pathophysiology
        [a] Chronic LV overload
        [b] Ejection fraction very sensitive to afterload
        [c] Contactile abnormalities may exist
        [d] Pulmonary circulation protected by left atrial compliance until late in disease course
    (4) Factors promoting decompensation
        [a] Increased SVR
        [b] Bradycardia
           i) CO rate dependent with a fixed stroke volume
           ii) Myocardial depressants poorly tolerated
        [c] Pain and anxiety during labor may cause decompensation by increased SVR
        [d] Increased PVR in those patients with pulmonary hypertension
    (5) Anesthetic management
        [a] Labor and vaginal delivery
           i) Epidural to block sympathetic stimulation and increased SVR with contractions
           ii) Invasive monitoring recommended
           iii) Treat hypotension with ephedrine
        [b] Cesarean section
           i) Epidural preferred, decreased SVR facilitates forward CO
           ii) General endotracheal acceptable

V. Clinical Priorities; k. Obstetrics (continued)

        a) Rapid sequence with attempt to attenuate sympathetic
        b) Maintenance with nitrous narcotic or nitrous inhalation agent if LV function maintained

(c) Mitral valve prolapse
  (1) General
    [a] Most common structural lesion
    [b] 5–10% of general population, 17% of women of childbearing age
    [c] Pregnancy usually well tolerated
  (2) Pathologic protrusion of mitral valve tissue into the atrium during systole
  (3) Anesthetic management
    [a] Avoid decreased LVEDV, which increases regurgitation
    [b] Asymptomatic patients require no special therapy, although antibiotic prophylaxis recommended by some
    [c] Symptomatic patients, beta-blockers
    [d] Maintain volume
    [e] Avoid drugs that promote tachycardia
    [f] Epidural reasonable for vaginal and cesarean section
    [g] Spinal blockade may be associated with hypotension
    [h] Hypotension should be aggressively treated with volume, uterine displacement, phenylephrine

(d) Aortic insufficiency
  (1) General
    [a] Uncommon in women of childbearing age
    [b] Generally well tolerated in pregnancy
  (2) Pathophysiology
    [a] LV overload
    [b] Eccentric hypertrophy
    [c] Contractile abnormalities
    [d] Heart failure typically in fourth or fifth decade of life
  (3) Anesthetic management
    [a] Adequate preload will maintain stroke volume
    [b] Avoid increased SVR (with pain) or bradycardia
    [c] Invasive monitoring not required in asymptomatic patient

(e) Aortic stenosis
  (1) General
    [a] Least common valvular disease in pregnancy
    [b] Maternal mortality 17%, fetal mortality 32%
  (2) Pathophysiology
    [a] Concentric hypertrophy
    [b] Contractility well maintained
    [c] Decreased ventricular compliance, dependent on atrial kick for filling
    [d] Increased myocardial oxygen demand with decreased supply
  (3) Hemodynamic decompensation
    [a] Tachycardia, reduced filling time
    [b] Hypovolemia
    [c] Decreased SVR, relatively fixed stroke volume
  (4) Anesthetic management
    [a] Monitoring
      i) Pulmonary artery catheter
      ii) Invasive arterial pressure
      iii) ECG, particularly V5
    [b] Maintenance
      i) Sinus rhythm

          ii) Elevated LVEDV
- [c] Regional anesthesia controversial, but may be used with close monitoring and maintenance of volume
- [d] Treat hypotension with volume, left uterine displacement, phenylephrine
- [e] Cesarean section, general anesthesia recommended
  - i) Mild aortic stenosis may tolerate usual rapid sequence
  - ii) Severe aortic stenosis, recommend high-dose narcotic, prepare for neonatal respiratory depression

6. Congenital heart disease
   - (a) Atrial septal defect
     - (1) Most common congenital heart lesion, adults usually asymptomatic until fourth to fifth decade, pregnancy generally well tolerated
     - (2) Pathophysiology, left-to-right shunt
       - [a] Increased right ventricular volume work
       - [b] Increased pulmonary blood flow
       - [c] Pulmonary hypertension may develop late
     - (3) Avoid
       - [a] Increased systemic vascular resistance
       - [b] Air in IV lines or epidural space
       - [c] Tachycardia
     - (4) Anesthetic management
       - [a] Antibiotic prophylaxis
       - [b] Epidural
         - i) Prevents increased systemic vascular resistance with contractions and laryngoscopy
         - ii) May be used for labor or surgical delivery
         - iii) A precipitous drop in SVR may cause shunt reversal
         - iv) Treat hypotension with phenylephrine
     - (5) General anesthesia may also be used for cesarean section
     - (6) Invasive monitoring rarely required
   - (b) Ventricular septal defect
     - (1) Common congenital defect
     - (2) Pathophysiology dependent on size of lesion
       - [a] Small, minimal effect
       - [b] Moderate
         - i) Increased pulmonary blood flow
         - ii) Right ventricular and pulmonary arterial pressures remain below systemic levels
       - [c] Large
         - i) Right and left ventricular pressure equalize
         - ii) Pulmonary vascular resistance increases
         - iii) Shunt reversal (Eisenmenger's complex)
     - (3) Pregnancy
       - [a] Small VSD, pregnancy well tolerated
       - [b] As severity of disease progresses, maternal mortality increases
     - (4) Avoid
       - [a] Air in IV lines or epidural space
       - [b] Increased systemic vascular resistance
       - [c] Increased heart rate
     - (5) Anesthetic management
       - [a] Antibiotic prophylaxis
       - [b] Epidural
         - i) Prevents inceased SVR, increased HR
         - ii) Titrate slowly to prevent precipitous drop in SVR

    iii) Treat hypotension or desaturation with phenylephrine

    iv) Invasive monitoring not required for small lesions, may be useful to follow PA pressure in more significant lesions

    v) Always remember potential for shunt reversal

    vi) Cesarean section, either epidural or general, high-dose narcotic if LV dysfunction present

(c) Eisenmenger's syndrome

 (1) General

  [a] Pulmonary hypertension at systemic level, due to high pulmonary vascular resistance, with reversed or bidirectional shunt through a large VSD

  [b] Also reported with ASD, PDA, aorticpulmonary window

  [c] Pregnancy poorly tolerated

   i) Maternal mortality, 30%

   ii) Neonatal mortality, 30–50%

    a) Increased prematurity

    b) Intrauterine growth retardation common

 (2) Pathophysiology

  [a] Left-to-right shunt

  [b] Changes in pulmonary circulation, leading to fixed increased pulmonary resistance

  [c] Increased right ventricular pressure

  [d] Increased pulmonary vascular resistance (acidosis, hypercarbia, positive pressure ventilation) will cause increased right-to-left shunting and cyanosis

 (3) Avoid

  [a] Decreased systemic vascular resistance, associated with regional anesthetic

  [b] Increased pulmonary vascular resistance, decreased P_{O_2}, increased P_{CO_2}, decreased pH, high ventilatory pressures

 (4) Monitoring

  [a] ECG

  [b] Pulse oximetry

  [c] Invasive arterial

  [d] CVP

  [e] PA catheter, controversial value, may be difficult to place with increased PVR

 (5) Anesthetic management

  [a] Antibiotic prophylaxis

  [b] Maintain filling pressures

   i) Labor, epidural slowly titrated

   ii) No epinephrine-containing solutions

   iii) Consider subarachnoid or epidural narcotics to minimize local anesthetic use

   iv) Cesarean section epidural reported

   v) General anesthesia preferred

    a) High-dose narcotic or narcotic ketamine induction

    b) Aspiration prophylaxis

    c) May require prolonged ventilation

    d) No nitrous oxide, increased PVR

    e) Extreme caution with inhalation agents, cardiac depression

    f) Intensive monitoring for 48 hours postpartum

(d) Tetrology of Fallot

      (1) TOF lesions
        [a] VSD
        [b] Biventricular origin of aorta, overriding aorta
        [c] RVH
      (2) Pregnancy poorly tolerated, maternal mortality 12%
      (3) Pathophysiology, right-to-left shunt
        [a] Corrected with normal right ventricular function, usual anesthetic management, no invasive monitoring
        [b] Corrected with right ventricular dysfunction
           i) Maintain filling pressures
           ii) Prevent further increased PVR
           iii) Avoid myocardial depressants
        [c] Uncorrected
           i) Monitoring
               a) Invasive arterial pressure
               b) Central venous pressure
               c) Pulse oximetry
           ii) Avoid worsening of right-to-left shunt
               a) Maintain volume
               b) Avoid decrease of SVR
               c) Avoid increase of PVR
           iii) Maintain contractility, excess increase may worsen infundibular obstruction
      (4) Anesthetic management
        [a] Labor, vaginal delivery
           i) Systemic narcotics
           ii) Paracervical and pudendal blocks
           iii) Epidural
               a) Use extreme caution
               b) Low concentrations of local anesthetics and no epinephrine
        [b] Cesarean section
           i) General anesthesia preferred
           ii) Good right ventricular function or minor infundibular stenosis
               a) Ketamine induction
               b) Low-dose inhalational/narcotic maintenance
           iii) Cortical infundibular stenosis
               a) High-dose narcotic
               b) Narcotic/low dose inhalational as tolerated by RV function
        [c] Avoid
           i) Increased heart rate
           ii) Increased contractility
           iii) Cyanosis indicates increased right-to-left shunt, treat with
               a) Volume
               b) Increase SVR with phenylephrine
               c) Beta-blockers if HR increased

7. Cardiomyopathies, peripartum cardiomyopathy
  (a) Primary heart failure
  (b) No previous disease
  (c) Risk factors
    (1) Multiparity
    (2) Multiple gestation
    (3) Age over 30
    (4) Pregnancy-induced hypertension
    (5) Obesity
  (d) Symptoms

V. Clinical Priorities; k. Obstetrics (continued)

          (1) Fatigue
          (2) Dyspnea
          (3) Orthopnea
          (4) Paroxysmal nocturnal dyspnea
          (5) Edema
          (6) Jugular venous distension
          (7) Pulmonary and systemic thromboembolism common, frequently maintained on anticoagulant

       (e) Anesthetic management
          (1) Invasive monitoring generally required for fluid management
          (2) Discontinue anticoagulant and normalize clotting parameters
          (3) Epidural, labor and cesarean delivery, prevents increases in afterload
          (4) Spinal best avoided because of possibility of precipitous drop of blood pressure
          (5) General may be used for cesarean
             [a] Caution with myocardial depressants
             [b] May require high-dose narcotics
             [c] Prolonged intubation may be required for mother and neonate
             [d] Prevent large increase in afterload

  8. Coronary artery disease
       (a) Myocardial infarction during pregnancy, 1 in 10,000; mortality, 30–40%
       (b) Risk factors of coronary artery disease
          (1) Age
          (2) Smoking
          (3) Oral contraceptives
          (4) Cocaine
          (5) Hypertension
          (6) Diabetes mellitus
          (7) Familial
       (c) Testing and medication to optimize maternal condition as per routine management of coronary artery disease
       (d) Anesthetic management
          (1) Invasive monitoring usual
          (2) Epidural minimizes hemodynamic stress and changes
          (3) Epidural/subarachnoid opioids minimize local anesthetic requirements
          (4) Titrate fluids to PCWP to prevent hypotension without fluid overload
          (5) Prevent tachycardia
          (6) Avoid epinephrine-containing local anesthetics
          (7) Single-shot spinal blockade may result in precipitous fall of blood pressure
       (e) General
          (1) Blunt sympathetic stimulation
          (2) Avoid myocardial depressants if ventricular function is compromised
          (3) High-dose narcotic or narcotic/etomidate induction
          (4) Prolonged ventilation may be required

  9. Primary pulmonary hypertension
       (a) Defined
          (1) Pulmonary artery pressure over 30/15 mm Hg
          (2) Mean pulmonary artery pressure over 25 mm Hg
          (3) Etiology unkown, possible autoimmune
          (4) Frequency worsens with pregnancy
          (5) Pregnancy poorly tolerated, maternal mortality 50%
       (b) Pathophysiology

        (1) Increased PVR, eventually irreversible changes in vasculature
        (2) Increased RV afterload
        (3) Right heart failure
        (4) Right ventricular dilation with tricuspid insufficiency
        (5) Decreased LV filling
        (6) Decreased cardiac output

(c) Symptoms
        (1) Dyspnea
        (2) Fatigue
        (3) Chest pain
        (4) Palpitations
        (5) Hemoptysis
        (6) Cyanosis

(d) Anesthetic/medical management of labor and delivery
        (1) Invasive monitoring
            [a] Arterial
            [b] PA catheter may be difficult to pass, discrepancy between PCWP and LVEDP
        (2) Maintain RV functions, avoid negative inotropes
        (3) Avoid increasing pulmonary resistance
            [a] Decreased P_{O_2}
            [b] Increased P_{CO_2}
            [c] Decreased pH
            [d] Pain, hyperinflation
        (4) Maintain volume, failing ventricle may need elevated filling pressures
        (5) Maintain left uterine displacement, maximize volume return
        (6) Maintain systemic vascular resistance, CO limited by fixed right ventricular output

(e) Choice of anesthetic
        (1) General
            [a] Minimize hemodynamic changes
            [b] IV narcotics
        (2) Paracervical block
        (3) Epidural
            [a] Extreme caution
            [b] Narcotics minimize local anesthetic dose
            [c] Cautious hydration
            [d] Slow titration
        (4) Subarachnoid
            [a] Narcotics alone may be helpful for labor
            [b] Single-shot subarachnoid block contraindicated
        (5) Cesarean section
            [a] General anesthetic preferred
            [b] Etomidate/narcotic or high-dose narcotic
            [c] Neonatal depression likely
            [d] Maintenance with narcotic and low-dose inhalational agent if tolerated
        (6) Therapy of rising pulmonary artery pressure
            [a] Correct
                i) Hypoxia
                ii) Hypercapnea
                iii) Acidosis
            [b] Support right ventricular function
                i) Isoproterenol
                ii) Dopamine
            [c] Vasodilate

                i) Nitroglycerine

               ii) Phentolamine

              iii) Prostaglandins

      (7) Monitoring and intensive care must continue postpartum

VI. AGING

a. Chronologic age

1. Chronologic age by itself is not considered a major risk factor for anesthesia, but
2. Increased prevalence of age-related disease
3. Age-related reduction in end-organ function, decreased organ system reserve

b. Age-related disease

1. Rheumatoid arthritis, osteoarthritis
2. Cerebrovascular disease
3. Cardiovascular disease
4. Diabetes mellitus
5. Respiratory disease, COPD
6. Others

c. Age-related diseases associated with increased risk

1. Associated with 10–30-fold greater risk than without concurrent illness
2. Angina, hypertension
3. Cerebrovascular disease
4. Impaired renal function
5. Also, increased number of coexisting medical disorders associated with increased incidence of perioperative mortality

d. Elective versus emergency surgery: perioperative morbidity and mortality increased threefold if surgery performed on emergency basis

e. Pathophysiology

1. Cardiovascular system
   - (a) Heart
     - (1) Increased amounts of fibrous tissue and amyloid
     - (2) Heart is more rigid, progressively less compliant
     - (3) Left ventricular hypertrophy
     - (4) Decreased maximum heart rate
     - (5) Decreased maximum coronary blood flow
   - (b) Vasculature
     - (1) Also becomes less compliant, stiffening of arterial tree
     - (2) Increased impedance to cardiac ejection, increased systolic blood pressure
   - (c) Heart rate

          (1) Resting rate unchanged
          (2) Maximum heart rate decreased, maximum heart rate =
               200 − age in years
    (d) Cardiac output decreased by 1% per year above age 30
    (e) Coronary artery disease
          (1) Increased incidence with age, but may remain occult until critical narrowing
               of vessel occurs
          (2) Lack of symptoms does not equate to lack of disease
    (f) Plasma norepinephrine levels
          (1) Increased resting levels in old as compared with young
          (2) Possibly reflects down-regulation of adrenergic receptors
    (g) Blood pressure regulation
          (1) Systolic hypertension
          (2) Essential hypertension
          (3) Orthostatic hypotension
          (4) Carotid sinus hypersensitivity
    (h) Baroreceptors
          (1) Respond to distension
          (2) Vascular wall rigidity increases with age
          (3) Dampened baroreceptor response
          (4) Clinically significant
               [a] Decreased ability to maintain pressure
               [b] Decreased ability to maintain perfusion
               [c] In face of decreased volume or sudden change in position, PEEP, IPPV

2. Respiratory system

    (a) Decreased ventilatory volumes, VC, TLC, MMV
    (b) Decreased efficiency of gas exchange
    (c) Decreased TLC results from
          (1) Intervertebral disk collapse
          (2) Calcification of cartilages
          (3) Kyposis and scoliosis
    (d) Decreased muscle mass, wastage of diaphragm and intercostal muscles
    (e) Parenchymal changes similar to emphysema, decreased number of alveolae,
        decreased pulmonary capillary density
    (f) Increased closing volume leads to V/Q mismatch
    (g) Resting Pao_2 decreases with age, $Pao_2 = 100 (0.4 \times$ age [years]) mm Hg
    (h) Decreased response to hypoxia and hypercarbia postanesthesia
    (i) All lead to decreased respiratory reserve; thus, elderly patients at much greater
        risk for ventilatory failure in perioperative period

3. Central nervous system

    (a) Daily loss of 50,000 neurons, decreased neuronal density with increasing age
        followed by parallel decrease in CBF and $CMRO_2$
    (b) Age-related decrease in anesthetic requirements
          (1) Decrease MAC for inhalation agents
          (2) Decreased requirement for most drugs, e.g., local anesthetics, narcotics,
               sedatives, IV induction agents
    (c) Increased incidence of delirium and confusional state after general anesthesia,
        anticholinergic agents

4. Renal function

    (a) Decreased number of functional glomeruli
    (b) Decreased GFR, 1–1.5% reduction per year, affects renal clearance of drugs and
        metabolites
    (c) Decreased ability to excrete abnormal solute or volume loads, e.g., excess
        sodium, dehydration, congestive failure

    (d) Renal protection
        (1) Maintain mean arterial pressure
        (2) Maintain urine output, 0.5–1.0 ml/kg/hr intraoperatively

5. Liver function

    (a) Significant decrease in hepatic size with aging, 40–50% hepatic tissue can be lost by age 80
    (b) Decreased hepatic blood flow, important for drugs with high first-pass metabolism, e.g., propranolol
    (c) Isolated reports of decreased microsomal enzyme system activity

6. Decreased renal and hepatic functions combine to give slower decline in plasma concentration of anesthetic drugs and longer duration of action

7. Basal metabolic rate and temperature regulation

    (a) BMR decreased 1% per year over age 30
    (b) Expect decreased metabolism and excretion of drugs
    (c) Exaggerated decrease of temperature intraoperatively
    (d) Decreased autonomic peripheral vascular control leads to decreased ability to vasoconstrict in cold environment
    (e) Intraoperative hypothermia leads to shivering postoperatively, leads to increased metabolic rate and oxygen consumption
        (1) Cardiac and respiratory stress
        (2) Can lead to
            [a] Angina
            [b] Respiratory failure
        (3) Intraoperative hypothermia leads to increased protein catabolism
        (4) Prevention: thermoneutral environment, warm room, warm fluids, warmed air

8. Airway reflexes are decreased with aging

    (a) Patient less able to protect airway
    (b) Imperative that endotracheal tube not be pulled early, patient must have ability to cough
    (c) Coughing
        (1) Decreased volume
        (2) Decreased force
        (3) Decreased flow rate
    (d) More likely to retain secretions

9. Pharmacokinetics (distribution of drug) and pharmacodynamics (effects of drug), changes in

    (a) Plasma protein binding
    (b) Body fat content
    (c) Renal- and hepatic-related changes in metabolism and excretion
    (d) Changing sensitivity to drug changes

10. Protein binding

    (a) It is the "free" or unbound drug that is responsible for drug effects
    (b) With aging, protein binding decreases, leads to increased free drug concentration and increased pharmacologic effect

11. Putative causes

    (a) Decreased serum protein, particularly albumin
    (b) Decreased binding effectiveness of available protein
    (c) Drug displacement by coadministered drugs
    (d) Certain disease states that can inhibit plasma protein binding of drugs

(e) Exaggerated effects will be seen from anesthetic agents that are normally highly protein bound
   (1) Changes in body compartments
      [a] Loss of lean muscle mass, more exaggerated in females
      [b] Increased percent of body fat
         i) Increased availability of lipid storage sites and increased reservoir for lipid-soluble drugs
         ii) Prolonged elimination half-life
      [c] Decreased blood volume, 20–30% by age 75–80
      [d] Leads to increased initial plasma-free drug concentrations
(f) Intravenous drugs
   (1) Barbiturates
      [a] Decreased induction dose required, secondary to decreased plasma volume
      [b] Onset of action delayed, related to decreased cardiac output, slow circulation time
   (2) Benzodiazepines
      [a] Increased sensitivity in elderly
      [b] Prolonged half-life
      [c] Midazolam
         i) Increased sensitivity
         ii) Prolonged half-life
   (3) Opioids
      [a] Increased sensitivity, may require 50% reduction
      [b] Respiratory depression
   (4) Propofol, should reduce dose and administer slowly
   (5) Inhalation agents
      [a] MAC decreases with increased age
      [b] All produce cardiac and respiratory depression
   (6) Muscle relaxants
      [a] Decreased muscle mass
      [b] Decreased volume of distribution
      [c] No decreased initial dose requirements
      [d] Increased duration of action secondary to decreased clearance
(g) Regional versus general anesthesia
   (1) No best techniques
   (2) Regional advantages
      [a] Decreased stress response, nitrogen loss, and blood loss
      [b] Decreased incidence of thromboembolic events
      [c] Decreased mortality in first 4 weeks
   (3) No difference at 6-month to 2-year follow-up
(h) Postoperatively, aged require close attention
   (1) Increased incidence of confusion
   (2) Increased postoperative hypoxemia
   (3) Pulse oximetry
   (4) Clear airway, manage secretions
   (5) Temperature monitoring
   (6) Pain, judicious use of opiates
(i) Summary of practical management
   (1) Preoperative assessment
   (2) History
   (3) Examination
   (4) Investigation
   (5) Premedication
   (6) Anesthetic technique
   (7) Monitoring

VII. OBESITY

a. General

1. Affects 25–45% of population
2. Morbidly obese, 5–7% of obese population
3. Increased risk of surgery and anesthesia
4. Increased risk of system impairment

   (a) Cardiovascular
   (b) Pulmonary
   (c) GI and metabolic

5. Increased incidence of

   (a) Hypertension
   (b) Diabetes mellitus
   (c) Coronary artery disease, AMI, sudden death
   (d) Cancer
   (e) Cholelithiasis
       (1) All may be compounded by psychosocial problems

b. Definition

1. Body mass index (BMI)

$$BMI = weight\ (kg)/height\ (m^2)$$

   (a) Normal = 22–28
   (b) Overweight = 25–30
   (c) Obese = over 30
   (d) Morbidly obese = over 40

2. IBW, ideal body weight for age and gender

   (a) Overweight = less than 20% above IBW
   (b) Obese = more than 20% above IBW
   (c) Morbidly obese = IBW $\times$ 2 or 100 pounds above IBW

c. Pathophysiologic changes

1. Pulmonary

   (a) Metabolic influence
       (1) Increased testing metabolic demand secondary to increased tissue mass
       (2) Increased oxygen consumption
       (3) Increased carbon dioxide production
       (4) Increased minute ventilation
       (5) Increased work and energy cost of breathing
       (6) Decreased wall compliance
       (7) Decreased FRC, ERV, and TCC secondary to decreased compliance
   (b) Closure of small airways
   (c) V/Q mismatch during normal resting ventilation
   (d) Increased shunting
   (e) Closing capacity unchanged
   (f) Supine position, following effects exaggerated
       (1) Further decreased FRC with shift of diaphragm and intra-abdominal pressure
       (2) Closure of more basal alveoli
       (3) Further decrease in compliance
       (4) Clinically significant increased shunting and oxygen consumption

      (g) End result

         (1) Chronic hypoxemia

         (2) With or without hypercapnea

2. Cardiovascular

    (a) Systemic hypertension

    (b) Increased circulating blood volume leads to increased preload leads to increased plasma and red cell mass

    (c) Increased resting cardiac output

    (d) Chronic preload increase leads to LVH and ventricular dilation

    (e) Decreased left ventricular compliance

    (f) Increased LVEDP

    (g) High incidence of pulmonary hypertension

    (h) Increased incidence of sudden death

    (i) Tenfold increase in incidence of PVCs

    (j) Supine position

       (1) Significant increase in PA pressure and cardiac output

       (2) Increased oxygen consumption because of increased work of breathing

3. Gastrointestinal

    (a) Increased gastric volume in fasting state, over 25 cc

    (b) Decreased gastric pH, less than 2.5

    (c) Increased risk of pulmonary aspiration

    (d) Increased incidence of hiatal hernia

    (e) Increased intra-abdominal pressure

    (f) Increased incidence of hepatic fatty infiltration

4. Endocrine

    (a) Glucose intolerance

    (b) Diabetes mellitus

    (c) Abnormal serum lipid profiles

5. Airway

    (a) Decreased flexion of cervical spine

    (b) Decreased mouth opening

    (c) Narrowed airway

    (d) High, anterior larynx

6. Psychologic

    (a) Increased incidence of psychopathology in morbid obesity

    (b) Questionable influence of heredity

    (c) May be demanding emotionally as well as physically

7. Pharmacokinetic, pharmacodynamic

    (a) Obese patients have larger fat compartment

    (b) Biotransformation of drugs may be altered secondary to hepatic disease, or changes in hepatic blood flow

    (c) Renal drug elimination may be affected by changes in glomerular filtration rate

    (d) Biliary excretion may be altered by presence of cholelithiasis

    (e) High incidence of lipoproteinemia may affect drug binding

    (f) Lipophilic drugs will have increased volume of distribution and increased elimination half-life

    (g) Fentanyl pharmocokinetics unchanged, drug should be given on basis of lean body weight

    (h) Hydrophilic drugs have similar volume of distribution if dose adjusted for BSA

    (i) Increased doses of succinyl choline required secondary to increased serum pseudocholinesterase

    (j) Increased metabolism of volatile agents and increased fluoride ion release

8. Obesity hypoventilation syndrome, OHS, pickwickian syndrome
    (a) Distinguished by the presence of CO_2 retention, i.e., loss of CO_2 drive
    (b) Associated features
        (1) Severe hypoxemia
        (2) Somnolence
        (3) Obstructive sleep apnea
        (4) Periodic breathing
        (5) Pulmonary hypertension
        (6) Polycythemia
        (7) Dependent edema
        (8) Pulmonary edema

d. Preoperative management

1. Psychology
2. History and physical
    (a) Cardiorespiratory evaluation
    (b) Ability to lie flat
    (c) Sleep pattern, narcolepsy, nocturnal sweats, enuresis, snoring
    (d) Exercise tolerance, mobility, SOB, chest pain
    (e) History of hypertension, cardiac failure
    (f) Drug history, use and abuse
    (g) Lines, access for IV and arterial
    (h) Airway evaluation
3. Preop investigation
    (a) Usual
        (1) CBC
        (2) Electrolytes
        (3) Liver function test
        (4) Glucose
        (5) Arterial blood gases, sitting and supine
        (6) 12-lead ECG
        (7) Chest x-ray
        (8) Urinalysis
        (9) Pulmonary function tests
        (10) MUGA and dipyridamole thallium stress test
4. Premedication
    (a) H_2 receptor antagonist evening and morning preoperatively to increase pH
    (b) Gastrokinetic agent on morning of surgery to decrease gastric volume
    (c) Nonparticulate oral antacid prior to a rapid-sequence induction
    (d) Avoid sedation
    (e) No IM medications
5. Intraoperative management, clear plan
6. Operating room table positioning
    (a) May require two tables
    (b) Adjustment may be difficult
    (c) Attention to positioning and protection
7. Monitoring
    (a) ECG, five-lead
    (b) Venous access, may require cutdown

        (c) Arterial access for invasive BP and ABG

        (d) CVP for volume status

        (e) Pulmonary catheter, CVP may be inadequate

        (f) Neuromuscular junction monitor

        (g) Temperature

        (h) Pulse oximetry

        (i) End-tidal CO_2

    8. Induction

        (a) Choice

           (1) Size of patient

           (2) Airway assessment, ease of control

           (3) Other factors

        (b) Options

           (1) Topical anesthesia of base of tongue and pharynx

           (2) If epiglottis and cords visualized, proceed with rapid sequence with cricoid pressure

           (3) If doubts, fiberoptic awake intubation

           (4) Demonstrate CO_2 to confirm successful intubation

e. Use of regional anesthesia

    1. Advantages

        (a) May avoid general anesthesia

        (b) Good abdominal muscle relaxation

        (c) Protected airway

        (d) May avoid compromised airway

        (e) Avoidance of opiate-induced respiratory depression

        (f) May provide postoperative pain relief

    2. Difficulties

        (a) Technical

        (b) Patient may not tolerate surgical position

        (c) Delayed onset, may progress for up to 30 minutes

        (d) If inadequate, may require emergency induction

        (e) Dosing, reduce to 75–80% of that estimated for age and height

f. Advantages of combined general and regional anesthetic

    1. Decreased dose of volatile agent

    2. Decreased need for neuromuscular blockade

    3. Postoperative analgesia without respiratory depression

    4. Earlier mobilization

    5. Decreased pulmonary complications in postoperative period

g. Postoperative management

    1. All obese patients at increased risk for postoperative hypoxemia

    2. Admit to ICU for aggressive pulmonary therapy

    3. Provide supplemental oxygen for up to 4 days postoperatively

    4. Adopt semirecumbent position rather than supine

    5. Provide effective postoperative pain management, whether opiates or regional techniques to allow effective breathing exercise and clearance of secretions

    6. Subcutaneous heparin to decrease risk of thrombophlebitis

VIII. HEAT STROKE

a. Cause

1. Occurs as a result of prolonged exposure to excessively high heat loads

    (a) Dry heat up to 130°F may be tolerated with adequate circulation and ventilation
    (b) At 100% humidity, body temperature will rise on exposure to temperatures over 94°F

2. With heavy workload, the critical environmental temperature may be as low as 85–90°F

3. Body has maximum ability to dissipate heat

4. When body heat exceeds 42–43°C, person will likely suffer heat stroke

5. Onset usually rapid and dramatic

b. Effects

1. Hyperpyrexia extremely dangerous with elevated CSF pressure and brain damage

2. General injuries include

    (a) Local hemorrhage
    (b) Parenchymal degeneration of cells

3. Acute circulatory failure may occur

    (a) Hypokalemia
    (b) Acute renal failure
    (c) Acute hepatic failure
    (d) Hemorrhage

c. Therapy

1. Cool as quickly as possible

    (a) Sponge or spray cooling until temperature reduced to 39°C
    (b) Immersion in ice bath, uncontrolled shivering adds to heat production

2. Maintain airway and provide oxygen

    (a) IV hydrocortisone may be lifesaving
    (b) Cold IV fluids to restore salts and water

3. Acclimatization aids in prevention

    (a) May increase maximum rate of sweating
    (b) Reduce loss of salts

C. CENTRAL NERVOUS SYSTEM

I. ANATOMY
  a. **Brain**
  b. **Vertebral column**
  c. **Spinal cord**

II. PHYSIOLOGY
  a. **Electrophysiology**

   1. Electroencephalogram (EEG)
   2. Evoked potentials

  b. **Cerebral blood flow (CBF)**
  c. **Control of other intracranial contents**

   1. Brain volumes
   2. Cerebrospinal fluid (CSF)
   3. Effects of anesthetic agents

  d. **Depth and adequacy of anesthesia**
  e. **Spinal pathways and reflexes**

   1. Anatomy
   2. Spinal reflexes

  f. **Neuronal transmission**
  g. **Neuromuscular transmission**

III. PHARMACOLOGY
  a. **Hypnotics and sedatives**
  b. **Opioids**
  c. **IV anesthetic induction agents**
  d. **Inhaled anesthetics**
  e. **Muscle relaxants**
  f. **Diuretics**
  g. **Vasodilators**
  h. **Vasopressors**
  i. **Miscellaneous**

IV. CLINICAL ENTITIES
  a. **Convulsions**
  b. **Coma**
  c. **Intoxications**
  d. **Spinal cord lesions**
  e. **Air embolism**
  f. **Cerebral protection**
  g. **Vascular lesions**

   1. Intracranial aneurysms
   2. Arteriovenous malformations (AVMs)

  h. **Intracranial hypertension**
  i. **Determination of brain death**

V. PEDIATRICS
  a. Meningomyelocele
  b. Arnold-Chiari malformation (aqueduct stenosis)
  c. Craniosynostosis

I. ANATOMY

a. Brain

1. Morphology
   (a) The brain is the enlarged, convoluted, and highly developed rostral portion of the CNS
   (b) The average adult human brain weighs about 1,400 g, approximately 2% of the total body weight

2. Composition and function
   (a) Brain stem
      (1) Continuous with the spinal cord within the foramen magnum
      (2) Lies on the basioccipital bone in the posterior cranial fossa
      (3) Contains the medulla oblongata and the pons, which regulate bodily functions, such as respiration
      (4) Contains the reticular activating system, which is responsible for maintaining the conscious, alert state
      (5) Lesions in any of these areas may have serious consequences
   (b) Cerebellum
      (1) Extends dorsally from the brain stem and fills the posterior cranial fossa
      (2) Responsible for the coordination of motor activity
   (c) Cerebrum
      (1) Occupies the greater portion of the middle and anterior cranial fossae
      (2) Divided into right and left cerebral hemispheres, which are separated by a deep cleft, the longitudinal cerebral fissure, and connected in the midline by the corpus callosum
      (3) Divided into a number of lobes named by the overlying bone, including frontal, parietal, occipital, temporal, central, and limbic lobes

3. Substructure
   (a) Gray matter
      (1) Covers the surface of the brain
      (2) Consists of cell bodies (neurons) arranged in vertical functional columns with a complex circuitry
      (3) Neurons may die if subjected to damage or ischemia, which may lead to a permanent loss in function
   (b) White matter
      (1) Deeper in the brain
      (2) Consists of tracts or fascicles of axons
   (c) Basal ganglia
      (1) Large ganglia, which lie deep within the base of the cerebral hemispheres
      (2) Comprise the caudate nucleus, the lenticular nucleus (consisting of the putamen and globus pallidus), the subthalamic nucleus, and the substantia nigra (important in motor function)

4. Cerebral vasculature
   (a) Anterior circulation (80% of total cerebral flow is supplied by the paired internal carotid arteries)
   (b) Posterior circulation (20% of the cerebral flow is supplied by the vertebral arteries, which arise from the subclavian arteries)
   (c) Anastomotic circle (of Willis) arises from the carotid and vertebral arteries, which anastomose with each other on the ventral surface of the brain stem
   (d) The cerebral arteries pass dorsally around the sides of the brain within deep fissures; all of the major arteries lie in the subarachnoid space

(e) The cerebral veins consist of deep and superficial groups, which are interconnected by numerous anastomotic channels

---

b. Vertebral column

1. Vertebrae (33 bones)
   - (a) Cervical (seven)
     - (1) The atlas is the first vertebra, which differs in that it lacks a body and spinous process
     - (2) The axis is the second vertebra, which has a superior projection, the dens (odontoid process), that represents the body of the atlas
     - (3) Typical cervical vertebrae contain an extra foramen within their transverse processes for passage of the vertebral artery and they have horizontal spinous processes. The midline approach is possible with a needle in performing central blockade
   - (b) Thoracic (12)
     - (1) Identified by their rib articulations on the transverse process
     - (2) Facet joints are nearly horizontal
     - (3) Spinous processes are very long and oriented caudally
     - (4) Paramedian approach (not midline) is the preferred approach to the interlaminar space since it avoids the oblique spinous processes
   - (c) Lumbar (five)
     - (1) Spinous processes are stubby and project posteriorly
     - (2) Midline approach is easiest with a slight cephalad direction of the needle
   - (d) Sacral (five)
     - (1) Fuse to form the sacrum
     - (2) Sacral hiatus forms from a defect in the roof on the dorsal aspect at the caudal end
     - (3) Administration of local anesthetic into the epidural space of the sacral hiatus results in caudal blockade
   - (e) Coccygeal (four)
     - (1) Formed from fusion of three or four rudimentary vertebrae
     - (2) No anesthetic significance
2. Structure of typical vertebra
   - (a) Body
     - (1) Forms the major supportive portion of the vertebrae
     - (2) Consists of two pedicles anteriorly and two laminae posteriorly
   - (b) Vertebral (neural) arch
   - (c) Vertebral processes
     - (1) Transverse processes are formed by junction of pedicles and laminae
     - (2) Spinous processes are formed by joining each lamina
   - (d) Foramina
     - (1) Contain the spinal cord, its coverings, and its vascular supply
     - (2) Allow spinal nerves to exit
3. Intervertebral disks
   - (a) Form symphyses between the vertebral bodies that permit a limited amount of movement between adjacent vertebrae
   - (b) Composed of
     - (1) Annulus fibrosus (outer portion)
     - (2) Nucleus pulposus (central portion)
   - (c) Clinical considerations include disk degeneration and disk herniation

4. Intervertebral ligaments
   (a) Supraspinous ligament
       (1) Most superficial ligament
       (2) Joins adjacent spinous processes dorsally at their tips from C7 to the sacrum
       (3) Forms the ligamentum nuchae in the cervical region
   (b) Interspinous ligaments
       (1) Run between spinous processes on their horizontal surfaces
       (2) Limit the range of motion of the vertebrae
   (c) Ligamentum flavum (yellow ligament)
       (1) Stretches between adjacent laminae
       (2) Composed of elastic tissue, unlike other ligaments
       (3) Passage through this firm ligament conveys a "gritty" sensation, followed by a distinct "pop" and "loss of resistance" as the dense ligament is exited
   (d) Anterior longitudinal ligament
       (1) Connects the vertebral bodies and intervertebral disks anteriorly
       (2) Runs from the sacrum to the occipital bone
   (e) Posterior longitudinal ligament
       (1) Connects the vertebral bodies and intervertebral disks posteriorly
       (2) Denticulate in shape
5. Spinal curvatures (four)
   (a) Double "C" curve
   (b) Cervical and lumbar curves are convex in a ventral direction, whereas the thoracic and sacral curves are convex dorsally
   (c) Influences the spread of local anesthetic during spinal anesthesia

c. Spinal cord

1. Morphology
   (a) Located in the upper two thirds of the vertebral canal of the bony vertebral column
   (b) Continuation of the brain stem, which is the neural structure anesthetized for central blockade
   (c) Extends from the foramen magnum at the base of the skull to its termination as the conus medullaris
   (d) Enlarged in those segments that innervate the extremities
       (1) Cervical (brachial) enlargement, C5–T1, innervates the upper extremities
       (2) Lumbosacral enlargement, L3–S2, innervates the lower extremities
   (e) Shorter in length than the vertebral column
       (1) Adult: usually ends at level of L1 vertebra
       (2) Infant: usually ends at level of L3 vertebra
   (f) Spinal nerves
       (1) Emerge from the vertebral column *lower* than the spinal cord segments from which the corresponding rootlets originate
       (2) Cauda equina is formed by long roots from the lumbar and sacral nerves
2. Spinal meninges are three individual membranes that surround the spinal cord and are fundamentally similar to those of the brain
   (a) Pia mater
       (1) Highly vascular membrane that closely approximates the spinal cord
       (2) Continues beyond the termination of the spinal cord as the filum terminale, which attaches to the coccyx
       (3) Denticulate ligaments are lateral extensions of the pia mater that help support the spinal cord by binding to the dura
       (4) Contains the blood supply to the spinal cord

I. Anatomy; c. Spinal cord (continued)

   (h) Arachnoid
      (1) Thin, avascular, membranous layer external to the pia mater and connected to it by weblike trabeculations
      (2) Supports the large distribution vessels
      (3) Delimits the subarachnoid space, which is located between the arachnoid and pia mater, and contains the spinal nerves and cerebrospinal fluid (CSF). It extends caudally to the level of S2. Spinal anesthesia is accomplished by infusing the anesthetic about the nerve roots (usually every site between L1–S2 since a needle can be inserted here with relatively little risk of damaging the CNS)
   (c) Dura mater
      (1) Tough, fibrous, single-layered membrane external to the arachnoid that extends from the foramen magnum superiorly to the lower border of S2 anteriorly
      (2) Delimits the subdural space, which is a potential space located between the arachnoid and dura that does *not* contain CSF
      (3) Defines the epidural space, which is unlike the cranial epidural space in that it is an *actual* space. It lies between the dura mater and the periosteum of the vertebral column and contains profuse venous plexuses, along with fat. Epidural anesthesia is accomplished by perfusing the anesthetic agent about the spinal nerves
3. Blood supply
   (a) Anterior spinal artery
      (1) Lies in the anterior median sulcus
      (2) Formed at the level of the foramen by magnum on the union of the two vertebral arteries
      (3) Supplies the anterior two thirds of the spinal cord
      (4) Segmental blood supply with contributions from the two vertebral arteries as well as three radicular branches, including cervical, thoracic, and the radicularis magna of the thoracolumbar region (also known as the artery of Adamkiewicz, which has a variable origin along the cord but arises on the left 80% of the time)
      (5) Anterior spinal artery syndrome results when injury to this artery occurs rendering anterior–central cord ischemia (see "Clinical entities: spinal cord lesions")
   (b) Posterior spinal arteries (two)
      (1) Arise from the vertebral or posterior inferior cerebellar arteries and descend as two branches, one anterior and the other posterior to the dorsal nerve root
      (2) Supplies the posterior one third of the spinal cord
      (3) *Nonsegmental* because of its rich collateral contributions from the subclavian, intercostal, lumbar, and sacral arteries. Thus, segmental arterial injury is an unlikely cause of cord ischemia in the posterior spinal artery distribution

II. PHYSIOLOGY

a. Electrophysiology

1. Electroencephalogram (EEG)
   (a) The scalp EEG is a recording of micropotentials (voltages) produced by the superficial layer (top 1 mm) of pyramidal cells in the cerebral cortex, amplified, and displayed as a time-varying intensity

(b) Techniques
  (1) Numerous schemes of electrode placement can be used and the voltage difference between any two electrodes can be measured
  (2) Diagnostic EEG (raw EEG) uses 10–20 electrodes but processed EEG uses as few as 3–5. Processed EEG monitoring is most commonly used in the operating room setting as a continuous monitor of cerebral function when deemed necessary
  (3) Electrodes must be securely attached and be of *low* resistance
  (4) Regardless of the technique employed, recordings should be bilateral (for comparison) and correlated with intraoperative events
(c) Waveforms are characterized by frequency and amplitude as well as by pattern (regular, spikes, bursts)
  (1) Alpha (8–13 Hz): resting, alert
  (2) Beta (> 14 Hz): awake, central brain pattern
  (3) Theta (4–8 Hz): drowsy, sedated
  (4) Delta (0.5–3 Hz): depressed, injured
  (5) Burst suppression: bursts of waves interspersed with electrical silence
(d) Abnormal patterns
  (1) Electroencephalographic *activation*
    [a] Shift to predominantly high-frequency and low-voltage activity
    [b] Occurs with light anesthesia and surgical stimulation
  (2) Electroencephalographic *depression*
    [a] Shift to predominantly low-frequency and high-voltage activity
    [b] Occurs with deep anesthesia or cerebral compromise
    [c] Detects hemispheric or global ischemia rather than focal ischemia
(e) Anesthetic uses
  (1) Carotid or other cerebrovascular surgery: detects hemispheric ischemia and the need for alteration in surgical technique (shunting)
  (2) Open heart surgery: detects massive embolism or ischemia and allows titration of barbiturates (for cerebral protection) during bypass
  (3) Craniotomy for seizure localization: mapping seizure foci for surgical resection
(f) Intraoperative monitoring
  (1) Ideal system for global monitoring uses four channels (two primary and two backup), for left and right frontal areas
  (2) Spectral analysis is preferable for ease of use
    [a] Compressed spectral array (CSA)
    [b] Density spectral array (DSA)
    [c] Spectral edge frequency
(g) Artifacts and interference
  (1) Muscle movement, from shivering or inadequate relaxation, will result in high-frequency, irregular signals
  (2) ECG artifact
  (3) 60-cycle noise results from equipment (usually blood warmers), or inadequate electrical shielding

2. Evoked potentials
  (a) Small, consistent variations in the EEG that occur at a fixed time after a stimulus
    (1) Allow assessment of the electrical physiologic function of specific pathways; afferent pathways are easier to test than are efferent pathways
    (2) General anesthesia tends to prolong latency and decrease amplitude
  (b) Stimuli
    (1) Peripheral nerve electrical
    (2) Auditory
    (3) Visual
    (4) Motor

    (c) Somatosensory evoked potentials (SSEP)
        (1) Peripheral sensory nerve (most often median) is stimulated and the response over the somatosensory cortex is monitored
        (2) Useful intraoperatively in order to detect dysfunction of the spinal cord during vascular or direct surgical manipulation. Most commonly used during thoracic aortic surgery or spinal instrumentation, such as Harrington or CD rods
        (3) Detect disruption of dorsal *sensory* pathways (not motor) and thus are less useful than intraoperative clinical exam (wake-up test)
        (4) Ischemia is seen as increased latency (delay) or decreased amplitude of waveforms
        (5) Volatile anesthetics (dose related) decrease overall EEG, as well as SSEP waveforms, making detection of ischemia more difficult, and thus nitrous/narcotic/relaxant techniques are preferred
    (d) Brain-stem auditory evoked potentials (BAEP)
        (1) Short-latency responses by the eighth nerve, brain stem, and cortex to auditory stimuli
        (2) Useful in surgery of the temporal bone or the eighth nerve (acoustic neuroma resection), as well as in diagnostic procedures performed on children
        (3) Anesthetic agents have little affect on subcortical responses
    (e) Visual evoked potentials (VEP)
        (1) Cortical electrical responses to visual stimulation (light flashes or regularly shifting patterns)
        (2) Useful for diagnosis of occipital cortical or other visual pathway lesions, although not frequently used in the operating room
        (3) They are applicable to optic chiasm and pituitary surgery
        (4) Most affected by anesthetics (similar in fashion to SSEP)
    (f) Motor evoked potentials (MEP)
        (1) Relatively new technique to assess integrity of motor pathways in the spinal cord
        (2) Stimulation of the motor cortex is done noninvasively via a magnetic coil
        (3) Responses are recorded at cervical, peripheral nerve, and muscle levels

---

b. Cerebral blood flow (CBF)

1. In almost all circumstances, CBF is coupled with metabolism ($CMRO_2$), referred to as activity metabolism flow coupling

    (a) Conditions and drugs that cause reduced cerebral activity also reduce CBF
    (b) Opposite also applies when activity is increased

2. Cerebral blood volume (CBV) is similarly related to flow

    (a) CBV is usually 60–100 ml, depending on
        (1) Temperature
        (2) Wakefulness
        (3) Gravity
        (4) Blood pressure
        (5) Carbon dioxide tension
    (b) CBV is the total of all venous and arterial structures in cranial vault
    (c) Delivered to brain via internal carotid arteries (80%) and vertebrobasilar arteries (20%)

3. CBF versus function

    (a) Normal CBF, 45–50 ml/100 g tissue/min

     (b) Normal function, 20–45 ml/100 g tissue/min

     (c) EEG slowing, 20 ml

     (d) SSEP failure, 15 ml

     (e) No function; survival, 6–20 ml

     (f) Irreversible cell death, 6 ml

  4. Control of CBF

     (a) Autoregulation

        (1) Normally between mean arterial pressure (MAP) of 50 and 150 mm Hg

        (2) Higher limits if untreated hypertension (curve shifted to right)

        (3) Mechanism is poorly understood (H^+ ions)

        (4) Absent in areas of injury or ischemia (maximally dilated)

     (b) Carbon dioxide tension (P_{CO_2})

        (1) Linear relationship between CO_2 and CBF

        (2) CBF increases 1 ml for every 2 mm Hg rise in P_{CO_2}

        (3) Changes cerebral vascular resistance (CVR)

        (4) Affected to a varying degree by inhalation agents

     (c) Oxygen tension (P_{O_2})

        (1) No change when Pa_{O_2} is over 50 mm Hg

        (2) When Pa_{O_2} is less than 50, there is a rapid linear increase in CBF to compensate for reduced O_2 delivery

        (3) There is possibly a 10% reduction in CBF if Pa_{O_2} is over 500 mm Hg

     (d) Temperature

        (1) Directly related to activity; as the brain gets colder, activity is reduced

        (2) As activity is reduced, CBF changes proportionately

c. Control of other intracranial contents

  1. Brain volumes

     (a) Total volume, 1,200–1,600 ml

     (b) Decreases volume

        (1) Atrophy

        (2) Dehydration (extreme)

        (3) Resection

        (4) Diuretics

     (c) Increases volume

        (1) Tumor

        (2) Edema

  2. Cerebrospinal fluid (CSF)

     (a) Normal volume, 120–150 ml

     (b) Produced in the choroid plexus of all ventricles

     (c) Rate of production is 0.35 ml/min (i.e., 450 ml/day); turnover is three times a day

     (d) Absorption takes place in the arachnoid villi and spinal venous plexi

     (e) Normally, rate of formation equals rate of absorption (vf = Ra). If rate of formation increases faster than rate of absorption (Vf greater than Ra) or absorption is obstructed (Ra less than Vf), an increase in CSF volume will occur

     (f) Increases CSF production

        (1) Hyperthermia

        (2) Cervical sympathectomy

        (3) Low serum osmolarity

        (4) Enflurane

        (5) Halothane

        (6) Functioning tumors

     (g) Decreases CSF production

        (1) Hypothermia

II. Physiology; c. Control of other intracranial contents (continued)

   (2) Acetazolamide
   (3) High osmolarity
   (4) Raised ICP
   (5) Steroids
   (6) Ouabain

3. Effects of anesthetic agents on intracranial volume
   (a) Effects on CBF (see table)
       (1) In general, anesthetics reduce cerebral activity and metabolism
       (2) Inhalation agents all produce some direct cerebral vasodilatation causing increases in CBF, CBV, and ICP
       (3) On the other hand, IV agents tend to reduce CBF, CBV, and ICP
       (4) Reactivity to CO_2 is not abolished by inhalation agents
   (b) Effects on CSF
       (1) Volume of CSF is determined by the balance between rate of formation (Vf) and resistance to reabsorption (Ra)
       (2) Only enflurane increases the rate of formation; all others either have no effect on production or produce slight reductions in the rate of formation
       (3) Halothane, enflurane, and sevoflurane probably increase Ra (increase CSF volume)
       (4) Isoflurane, and possibly desflurane, decreases Ra (reduce CSF volume)
       (5) Effects of IV agents are variable, but probably do not have a great impact on intracranial volume

Agent	Metabolism	CBV	CSF	ICP
Halothane	−	+	+	+
Enflurane	−	+	+	+
Isoflurane	−	+	−	+
Desflurane	−	+	?	+
Sevoflurane	−	+	?	+
Nitrous oxide	−	+	0	+
Barbiturates	−	−	0	−
Etomidate	−	−	−	−
Diprivan	−	−	?	−
Benzodiazepines	−	−	−	−
Narcotics	−	−	−	−
Lidocaine	−	−	?	−
Ketamine	+	+	+	+

d. Depth and adequacy of anesthesia

1. Management of general anesthesia is the art of continuously balancing the amount of anesthetic drug in the CNS against the changing intensity of the surgical stimulus
   (a) Surgical stimulus (or pain) is not directly measurable, therefore, reliance must be placed on subjective reporting or, in the case of the unconscious patient, on indirect signs (usually of sympathetic activity)
   (b) Monitoring of anesthetic depth is done to prevent drug overdose or recall of intraoperative events
2. History
   (a) Arthur Guedel published his observations on the "stages" of ether anesthesia, defining the rough categorizations of anesthetic depth still used today

(b) These observations were made with diethyl ether, and are not as applicable to modern agents or to balanced anesthetic techniques

3. Monitoring
    (a) The most reliable measure of anesthetic depth is the absence of movement in response to surgical stimulus in the anesthetized, unparalyzed patient
    (b) The depth and frequency of respiration are valuable monitors in the spontaneously breathing patient
    (c) Autonomic signs of sympathetic activation are commonly used as hallmarks of "light" anesthesia, but these may be confused by autonomically active drugs (atropine, beta blockade) that are often incorporated into anesthetic techniques
    (d) Measurements of spontaneous smooth muscle activity, processed EEG monitoring, and other sophisticated techniques have been proposed to measure anesthetic depth, but none has proved effective for routine use

4. Awareness
    (a) Recall of intraoperative events may be psychologically devastating to patients
        (1) Explicit awareness is conscious recall of intraoperative events, usually auditory or somatosensory
        (2) Implicit awareness has been defined as subconscious recall, usually evidenced as sleep disturbances, nightmares, and other symptoms of posttraumatic stress disorder
    (b) Awareness results from inadequate hypnotic/amnestic effects of anesthetic drugs
        (1) Most common in open heart surgery, cesarean section, and trauma cases (where light anesthesia is often medically necessary)
        (2) Underreported to anesthesiologists; the exact incidence is unknown
    (c) Adequate doses of inhalation agents (0.8 MAC or more) and liberal use of benzodiazepine drugs may reduce the incidence of awareness
        (1) Patients may require psychologic evaluation and counseling
        (2) A significant fraction of liability claims (10%) involve awareness

e. Spinal pathways and reflexes

1. Anatomy
    (a) Afferent pain pathways
        (1) Originate in peripheral receptors and are organized in the dorsal horn of the spinal cord according to fiber size (large medially and small laterally)
        (2) Spinothalamic tract is the primary spinal afferent pathway for nocioception (pain perception)
            [a] Spinothalamic tract is divided into the neospinothalamic tract laterally and the paleospinothalamic tract medially
            [b] Neospinothalamic tract projects into the posterior thalamus and is associated with the location, duration, and intensity of pain
            [c] Paleospinothalamic tract projects into the medial thalamus and is associated with the autonomic and emotional aspects of pain and denervation dysesthesia
        (3) Other afferent pathways include
            [a] Spinoreticular (pain-associated arousal)
            [b] Spinomesencephalic (to reticular formation)
            [c] Spinocervical (to contralateral thalamus)
    (b) Descending inhibitory pathways
        (1) Midbrain periaqueductal gray matter can control analgesia via descending spinal pathways
            [a] Periaqueductal gray matter is rich in endogenous opiates and in opiate receptors
            [b] It projects fibers via the nucleus raphe magnus to the dorsal horn through the dorsolateral funiculus

(2) Adrenergic fibers found in the dorsolateral funiculus are also inhibitory at the spinal cord level

(c) Motor pathways

(1) Primary motor pathway for voluntary movement is the pyramidal or corticospinal tract

[a] Travels from the cerebral cortex, via the pons and medulla (crossing the midline in the lower medulla), and becomes the lateral funiculus of the spinal cord

[b] In the intermediate zone of the spinal cord gray matter, these upper motor neurons synapse with interneurons or directly with lower motor neurons in the anterior horn

(2) Other indirect motor pathways include

[a] Corticorubrospinal

[b] Corticoreticulo-spinal

2. Spinal reflexes

(a) Tendon reflexes (myotactic reflexes)

(1) Afferent pathway arises from muscle spindles (kept tonically active at rest via gamma efferent fibers) in the dorsal horn

(2) Efferent pathway arises from alpha motor neurons in the anterior horn

(3) Activity of the tonic gamma efferent fibers determines resting muscle tone, as well as tone under anesthesia

[a] Gamma efferent tone is inhibited by corticospinal and other supranuclear fibers

[b] Skeletal muscles are not flaccid under general anesthesia in the absence of neuromuscular blocking drugs

(b) Pathologic reflexes

(1) Autonomic hyperreflexia

[a] Presents in cases of upper motor neuron destruction (paraplegia) with an intact sympathetic chain

[b] Usually characterized by sympathetic hyperactivity (hypertension, bradycardia, dysrhythmias) in response to somatic or visceral stimulus *below* the cord injury level

[c] A lesion at or above midthoracic (T5) segments may be associated with this condition

[d] May be treated by drugs that block the sympathetic system at either the central, ganglionic, or peripheral level

[e] Adequate spinal or general anesthesia usually prevents occurrence of this syndrome

(2) Reflex sympathetic dystrophy

[a] Syndrome of sympathetically mediated pain following trauma, surgery, or illness

[b] Characterized by pain, hyperalgesia, autonomic dysfunction, and dystrophic changes, usually in an extremity

[c] Possibly related to dysfunction of skin and muscle efferent vasoconstrictors and heightened sympathetic activity

[d] Treatment may involve surgical lumbar symphathectomy, neurolytic lumbar sympathetic block, or even local anesthetic sympathetic blockade

f. Neuronal transmission

1. Neuron structure

(a) Each neuron is composed of

(1) Nucleus (karyon)

   (2) Cell body (perikaryon)

   (3) Axon and dendritic processes

  (b) Neurons are supplied by glial tissue and classified by

   (1) Morphology

    [a] Unipolar

    [b] Bipolar

    [c] Multipolar

   (2) Function

    [a] Sensory; receive impulses and transmit them

    [b] Motor; deliver efferent impulses through PNS

    [c] Interneurons; form circuits in CNS

   (3) Diameter (see table)

 2. Synapses

  (a) Definition

   (1) Site of functional contact between the axonal membrane of one neuron and the membrane of another, or with effector cell next in line

   (2) Anatomic basis of intercellular communication

  (b) Classification

   (1) Axon dendritic; between axon and dendrite of two neurons

   (2) Axon somatic; between axon and axon of perikaryon of another neuron

   (3) Dendrodendritic synapses; interdendritic synapses (uncommon)

  (c) Morphology

   (1) Presynaptic membrane (axonal terminal)

   (2) Synaptic cleft

   (3) Postsynaptic membrane

  (d) Function

   (1) Electrical impulse travels to the presynaptic membrane

   (2) Stored chemicals, neurotransmitters, are released into the synaptic cleft and combine with chemical receptors on the postsynaptic membrane to produce an electromechanical change

 3. Neurotransmitters

  (a) Classification

   (1) Excitatory (e.g., norepineprine)

   (2) Inhibitory (e.g., glycine, GABA)

   (3) Each neuron receives thousands of excitatory and inhibitory synapses. The final response arises from summation of neurotransmitters at any given time

 4. Neuronal transmission

  (a) The flow of transmission is usually unidirectional from axon to dendrite, called neuronal polarization

   (1) In certain peripheral neuropathies of the axon, or in experimental stimulation, the wave of depolarization may become bidirectional

   (2) It may spread distally toward the axonal tip (orthodromic conduction) or peripherally toward the cell body (antidromic conduction)

    [a] Axonal transmission

     i) Ionic changes run continuously along the nerve fibers (axon)

     ii) Unmyelinated type C fibers

    [b] Saltatory conduction

     i) Ionic changes/action potential occur at the nodes of Ranvier, allowing faster transmission

     ii) Myelinated type A fibers

II. Physiology; f. Neuronal transmission (continued)

	Myelinated	Fiber Diameter (μm)	Conduction Velocity (m·sec^{-1})	Function	Sensitivity to Local Anesthetic (Subarachnoid, Procaine) (%)
A					
A-alpha	Yes	12–20	70–120	Innervation of skeletal muscles Proprioception	1
A-beta	Yes	5–12	30–70	Touch Pressure	1
A-gamma	Yes	3–6	15–30	Skeletal muscle tone	1
A-delta	Yes	2–5	12–30	Fast pain Touch Temperature	9.5
B	Yes	3	3–15	Preganglionic autonomic fibers	0.25
C	No	0.4–1.2	0.5–2	Slow pain Touch Temperature Postganglionic sympathetic fibers	0.5

g. Neuromuscular transmission

1. Quantal theory

   (a) Acetylcholine (ACh), formed from choline and acetate, is stored in vesicles and in the cytoplasm

   (b) Nerve action potential causes voltage-dependent Ca^{+2} channels to open and Ca^{+2} ions to enter the nerve ending

   (c) Ca^{+2} ions combine with calmodulin to form calmodulin–Ca^{+2} complex

   (d) Complex activates vesicular discharge (quanta of ACh) into the synaptic cleft

2. Depolarization

   (a) Resting transmembrane potential is -90 mV, which is maintained by unequal distribution (ratio) of Na^+ and K^+ ions across cell membrane

   (b) ACh binds to specific receptors (nicotine cholinergic) on the postsynaptic membrane, leading to influx of Na^+ ions and efflux of K^+ ions

   (c) Transmembrane (end-plate) potential changes from -90 mV to -45 mV (depolarization)

   (d) This action potential will spread over the surfaces of skeletal muscle fibers and lead to a contraction

   (e) Released ACh is hydrolyzed to choline and acetate by acetylcholinesterase in the region of motor end plate; restimulation requires new ACh release

3. ACh receptors

   (a) Glycoproteins, consisting of five subunits

      (1) Alpha (two)

      (2) Beta

      (3) Delta

      (4) Epsilon

   (b) Location

      (1) Postjunctional

         [a] Densely located in junctional folds

         [b] ACh and some nondepolarizing muscle relaxants (NDMRs) bind to alpha subunits competitively

[c] Depolarizing muscle relaxants (DMRs) combine with one alpha unit, whereas ACh binds to both alpha units, in order to produce an effect

(2) Extrajunctional

[a] Located outside the end plate

[b] Normally present in small amounts due to synthesis suppression by neuronal stimulation

[c] Proliferate whenever stimulation is less active (e.g., posttrauma, denervation)

[d] Suxamethonium stimulation of these receptors in pathologic conditions can lead to exaggerated K^+ efflux from muscle

(3) Prejunctional

[a] Differ from postjunctional receptors in their binding characteristics

[b] Control Na^+ and Ca^{+2} ions, which can affect presynaptic ACh release

[c] Blocked by aminoglycosides and some NDMRs, leading to muscle weakness

[d] Can be partially reversed by calcium chloride infusion

III. PHARMACOLOGY

a. Hypnotics and sedatives

1. Depress the CNS in a dose-dependent, relatively nonselective manner, with the exception of benzodiazepines

2. Benzodiazepines

   (a) Cause a moderate parallel reduction in CBF and $CMRO_2$

   (b) Safe to administer to patients with intracranial HTN, provided that respiratory depression and hypercapnia do not occur

3. Flumazenil

   (a) Has no effect on CBF in unanesthetized normal human volunteers. However, in two dog studies, when used to reverse the effects of midazolam, there was an overshoot in CBF and ICP

   (b) Used with caution in the reversal of benzodiazepine-induced sedation in patients with raised ICP, until further human data become available

b. Opioids

1. In general, there is little effect on CBF or ICP with small doses of an opioid drug, unless there is a rise in arterial partial pressure of carbon dioxide (Pa_{CO_2}) due to respiratory depression

2. Morphine and meperidine

   (a) Minimal effect on CBF and $CMRO_2$

   (b) If normocapnia and normotension are maintained, ICP, CBF autoregulation, and CO_2 responsiveness are not affected

3. Fentanyl causes a moderate reduction in CBF, $CMRO_2$, and ICP

4. Alfentanil (similar to fentanyl)

5. Sufentanil

   (a) Conflicting reports of cerebral vasodilation

   (b) Although not contraindicated in neuroanesthesia, it should be used in conjunction with hypocapnia

c. IV anesthetic induction agents

1. General
   (a) With the exception of ketamine, their use results in a parallel reduction in CMR and CBF
   (b) Ketamine causes an increase in CBF and $CMRO_2$
   (c) Autoregulation and CO_2 responsiveness are preserved
2. Barbiturates
   (a) Cause a dose-dependent reduction in CBF and $CMRO_2$ throughout the brain
   (b) May be used to induce coma in the intensive-care setting
3. Etomidate
   (a) Decreases CBF less than it decreases $CMRO_2$
   (b) Results in regionally variable reductions in $CMRO_2$
4. Propofol
   (a) Decreases CBF and $CMRO_2$ to a similar degree
   (b) Cerebral function recovers faster

d. Inhaled anesthetics

1. Volatile anesthetic agents
   (a) Cause cerebral vasodilation, resulting in an increase in CBF and CBV, as well as in ICP; (halothane $\gg$ enflurane $>$ isoflurane)
   (b) Cerebral vasodilation can be restricted if reduced MAC (Minimum Alveolar Concentration) of an agent is combined with hyperventilation
   (c) Desflurane and sevoflurane behave like isoflurane
   (d) Cause a dose-dependent reduction in $CMRO_2$
2. Nitrous oxide
   (a) Elevates CBF and ICP, but there is no consensus on its effect on $CMRO_2$
   (b) Cerebral vasodilation can be blunted by the simultaneous administration of fixed anesthetics
   (c) Safely used in neurosurgery, but should be discontinued if ICP is consistently elevated, or if the brain is "tight"

e. Muscle relaxants

1. Succinylcholine
   (a) Increases ICP secondary to increased CBF and $CMRO_2$, which is due to an increase in cerebral activity caused by afferent input from muscle spindles
   (b) Poor correlation between increase in ICP and muscle fasciculations
   (c) Not contraindicated if there is a need for rapid onset of paralysis (e.g., full stomach, possible difficult intubation)
2. Nondepolarizing muscle relaxants
   (a) No direct effect on CBF and $CMRO_2$, as they do not cross the blood–brain barrier (BBB)
   (b) Histamine release (atracurium) may increase ICP (cerebral vasodilation) and decrease MAP, thereby decreasing CPP, although the effect is clinically insignificant
   (c) May elevate ICP if there is an abrupt increase in MAP

f. Diuretics

1. Mannitol

   (a) Osmotherapeutic agent of choice in reducing ICP; dose 0.25–1 g/kg
   (b) Removes water from normal (not edematous) brain
   (c) Serum electrolytes and volume status should be monitored
   (d) Caution its use in patients with congestive heart failure
   (e) Rebound intracranial HTN may occur
   (f) Large doses or rapid infusion (less than 10 minutes) may result in hyperosmolarity-induced dilation of vascular smooth muscle, resulting in transient increase in ICP and a decrease in MAP
   (g) Administration of mannitol should be used with care in surgery for vascular pathologies before opening the cranium

2. Furosemide (loop diuretic)

   (a) Lowers ICP without increasing intravascular volume or blood osmolality
   (b) Decreases CSF formation, increases water loss, and resolves cerebral edema
   (c) Slower onset of action when compared with mannitol (40 minutes compared with 15 minutes)
   (d) Potentiates the action of mannitol, but their combination results in rapid water and electrolyte loss

g. Vasodilators

1. Systemic vasodilators (sodium nitroprusside, nitroglycerine, hydralazine)

   (a) Cause cerebral vasodilation, and thus may increase CBF and ICP
   (b) ICP effects are less pronounced if hypotension is induced slowly

2. Ganglion blocking agents (trimethaphan)

   (a) Produce less of an increase in CBF and ICP
   (b) Postoperative neurologic assessment may be difficult due to drug-induced mydriasis and cycloplegia

3. Beta-adrenergic receptor blockers

   (a) Minimal effects on CBF and ICP if cerebral perfusion pressure is not decreased
   (b) Often drug of choice for neurosurgical procedures

h. Vasopressors

1. General

   (a) Minimal effect on undamaged cerebral vasculature, as they do not normally cross the BBB
   (b) CBF may rise as an indirect effect of increased sympathetic tone

2. Alpha-1 agonists (phenylephrine)

   (a) May decrease CBF; no effect on $CMRO_2$
   (b) Norepinephrine may cause vasodilation if the BBB is damaged

3. Epinephrine

   (a) With normal cerebral vasculature, there is little effect on CBF and $CMRO_2$, unless CPP is raised
   (b) If the BBB is damaged, increases CBF and $CMRO_2$

4. Dopamine

   (a) With normal cerebral vasculature, vasodilation occurs with minimal change in $CMRO_2$
   (b) May produce alpha-mediated vasoconstriction in large doses

III. Pharmacology (continued)

i. Miscellaneous

1. Analeptics

   (a) Low dose results in carotid body stimulation
   (b) Higher doses stimulate the respiratory centers of the medulla, causing a concomitant increase in blood pressure
   (c) Overdose may result in seizures

2. Antipsychotics

   (a) Have antidopaminergic, antihistaminic, anti-alpha-1, and anticholinergic effects, resulting in changes in affect, cognition, and motor performance
   (b) The EEG is slowed, with increases in theta activity and voltage
   (c) May lower the seizure threshold
   (d) Alpha-1 blockade may result in postural hypotension and heat loss due to peripheral vasodilation

3. Antidepressants

   (a) Tricyclic antidepressants
       (1) May produce confusional states, especially in elderly patients
       (2) Cardiac dysrhythmias have been reported, especially in patients anesthetized with halothane and undergoing dental procedures
   (b) Monoamine oxidase inhibitors (MAOIs)
       (1) Commonly cause orthostatic hypotension, especially in elderly patients
       (2) Hypertensive crises may occur if tyramine-containing substances are administered concurrently with MAOIs
       (3) Potentiate the action of some sympathomimetics, possibly resulting in a hypertensive crisis
       (4) Potentiate the effects of opioids, barbiturates, and alcohol
       (5) Two potential interactions with concurrent opioid administration
           [a] Depressive form, in which CNS depression occurs
           [b] Excitatory form, in which hypertension, hyperthermia, and convulsions occur

4. Antiparkinsonian medications (levodopa)

   (a) May cause cardiac dysrhythmias and postural hypotension
   (b) Hypotensive as well as hypertensive reactions have been reported when used with inhalational agents

IV. CLINICAL ENTITIES

a. Convulsions

1. Classification

   (a) Localization-related epilepsies and syndromes
   (b) Generalized epilepsies and syndromes
   (c) Undetermined epilepsies and syndromes
   (d) Special syndromes

2. Diagnosis

   (a) Partial (temporal lobe epilepsy)
       (1) Motor
       (2) Sensory
       (3) Automatic behaviors
       (4) Psychic manifestations

   (b) Complex partial
      (1) Altered consciousness
      (2) Often automatism
      (3) Typical EEG discharge, most frequently from temporal or frontal lobes
   (c) Generalized seizures—involve both cerebral hemispheres simultaneously; always impair consciousness
      (1) Absence
         [a] 20 years old or younger
         [b] Brief duration
         [c] Usually tonic clonic, automatic behaviors
         [d] Can be precipitated by hyperventilation
         [e] EEG shows generalized 3-Hz spike and wave discharge
      (2) Myoclonic
         [a] Symmetric, involving extremities or facial musculature
         [b] EEG shows "fast" 4–6-Hz spike and wave discharge
      (3) Atonic (drop attacks)
         [a] Loss of muscle tone without impaired consciousness
         [b] EEG shows generalized polyspikes, flattening, or low-voltage fast activity
      (4) Clonic
         [a] Generalized jerking movements
         [b] EEG shows fast activity with generalized spike/polyspike and wave discharge
      (5) Tonic
         [a] Muscle stiffness and rigidity
         [b] EEG similar to clonic
      (6) Tonic–clonic (grand mal)
         [a] Combination of clonic and tonic
         [b] EEG similar to clonic and tonic
   (d) Treatment
      (1) Guided by diagnosis of seizure type
      (2) Do not overtreat isolated seizures; e.g., IV diazepam following a seizure may cause dangerous central depression and is ineffective
      (3) Phenobarbital
         [a] Popular in the pediatric population for all forms of neonatal, generalized, partial, or febrile seizures, as well as status epilepticus
         [b] May aggravate absence seizures
         [c] Reduce dosage in renal and hepatic disease
         [d] Therapeutic level 10–30 µg/ml
      (4) Phenytoin
         [a] Partial and secondary generalized tonic/clonic seizures
         [b] Also effective in status epilepticus
         [c] Ineffective against absence seizures and febrile convulsions
         [d] Therapeutic range 10–20 µg/ml
      (5) Primidone
         [a] Partial seizures or refractory myoclonic seizures
         [b] Metabolized to phenobarbital in liver, therefore, phenobarbital levels should be monitored
         [c] Phenytoinlike action
         [d] Therapeutic level 5–12 µg/ml
      (6) Ethosuxamide
         [a] Absence seizures
         [b] Therapeutic range 40–100 µg/ml
      (7) Carbamazepine
         [a] All types of partial seizures

        [b] Induces own metabolism requiring increased dosage over time

        [c] Therapeutic range 4–12 µg/ml

    (8) Valproic acid

        [a] All forms of primary generalized and refractory partial seizures

        [b] Therapeutic levels 50–100 µg/ml

        [c] Most serious adverse effect is hepatic failure in children older than 2 years of age, which usually occurs if receiving multiple antiepileptic drugs

(e) Status epilepticus

    (1) An epileptic seizure that is sufficiently prolonged or repeated at sufficiently brief intervals so as to produce an unvarying and enduring epileptic condition

    (2) Life-threatening medical emergency; mortality 10%

    (3) Precipitated by inadequate anticonvulsant Rx in epileptics, severe hypoxic brain injury, cerebrovascular disease or ischemic event, tumors, metabolic derangement, alcohol withdrawal

(f) Management of status epilepticus

    (1) Aim is to control seizures within 60 minutes

    (2) Evaluate patient and provide basic cardiopulmonary support

    (3) Use benzodiazepine, e.g., diazepam or lorazepam and phenytoin together to treat seizure. If ineffective, consider introducing secondary antiepileptic medication

    (4) General anesthesia may be necessary

    (5) Ensure that appropriate chronic therapy is instituted once status epilepticus resolved

(g) Nonconvulsive status epilepticus

    (1) Diagnosis is difficult

    (2) Manifests as absence attacks, aphasia, confusional states, stupor, behavioral disturbances

(h) Anesthetic considerations for patients with seizure disorder

    (1) Patient will not convulse under general anesthesia

    (2) Regional anesthesia does not increase the risk of seizures

    (3) Knowledge of anticonvulsant medications is essential to assess potential cardiopulmonary effects and interactions with anesthetic agents

    (4) Patients taking phenytoin or carbamazepine have increased requirements for NDMRs, therefore, monitor their administration using a peripheral nerve stimulator

    (5) Rapid infusion of IV phenytoin can cause respiratory arrest, hypotension, or death

(i) Anesthetic agents and seizures

    (1) Enflurane

        [a] Most epileptogenic of the inhalational agents

        [b] In doses of 1–5–2 MAC, seizure patterns (spike and wave activity) appear on the EEG, particularly during hypocapnia

        [c] May induce seizures in patients with no previous history on emergence, and for up to 1 week postanesthesia

    (2) Methohexital and etomidate

        [a] Induce epileptiform activity in temporal lobe epilepsy and generalized epilepsy

        [b] Inhibit the progress of ongoing seizures

    (3) Propofol

        [a] Anticonvulsant activity

        [b] More effective than barbiturates in limiting ECT-induced seizures

[c] Effective in status epilepticus refractory to thiopental
(4) Meperidine
[a] Avoid
[b] Primary metabolite, normeperidine, is a convulsant
[c] Other opioids are safe

b. Coma

1. Pathophysiology

   (a) Supratentorial and subtentorial lesions
   (b) Metabolic processes
   (c) Psychiatric disorders

2. Assessment

   (a) Level of consciousness
       (1) Arousal (ability to awaken or open eyes)
       (2) Awareness
           [a] Ability to interact meaningfully with the environment
           [b] Normal awareness includes orientation to person, place, and time
       (3) It is important to distinguish between arousal and awareness
   (b) History
       (1) Reveals cause of neurologic dysfunction
       (2) Past medical problems, such as diabetes, recent injury, access to drugs, and psychiatric history, should be elicited
   (c) Neurologic examination
       (1) Glasgow coma scale
           [a] Simple, reliable, and reproducible scale that has been widely accepted
           [b] Obtained by scoring the response of three aspects (motor, eye opening, and verbal response) of the clinical examination
           [c] The sum can be used to describe the severity of altered responsiveness, with a score of less than 8 considered coma
       (2) Focal neurologic exam
           [a] Eye exam (cranial nerves)
           [b] Motor exam
           [c] Sensory testing
           [d] Reflex testing

3. Immediate stabilization is necessary

   (a) First priority is to prevent potentially irreversible injury due to
       (1) Hypotension
       (2) Hypoxemia
       (3) Hyperglycemia
       (4) Thiamine deficiency (Wernicke's encephalopathy)
       (5) Status epilepticus
       (6) Intracranial hypertension
       (7) Profound hyper- or hypothermia

4. Monitors and tests

   (a) Lumbar puncture
   (b) Computed tomography
   (c) Cervical spine films—15% of head-injured patients have concomitant vertebral injury
   (d) Magnetic resonance imaging
   (e) Cerebral angiography
   (f) Cerebral radionuclide scan
   (g) Skull films—little use

IV. Clinical Entities (continued)

c. Intoxications

1. Exogenous toxins
   (a) Drugs
      (1) Such agents as phenobarbital, ether, and chloroform produce depression of respiratory centers and cause death without organic neural damage
      (2) Some drugs (e.g., morphine) produce nerve cell degeneration, especially if taken chronically
      (3) Acetaminophen
         [a] Clinical symptoms may include pallor, lethargy, N/V, and diaphoresis
         [b] Hepatotoxicity may occur when normal metabolic pathways become saturated
         [c] Initial treatment involves induction of emesis or gastric lavage followed by administration of activated charcoal
         [d] *N*-acetylcystine significantly reduces the incidence of hepatotoxicity
   (b) Alcohol
      (1) Ethanol
         [a] Depresses ventilation, decreases myocardial contractility, predisposes to hypothermia, and causes hypoglycemia, especially in children
         [b] There is no antidote and no method of hastening its metabolism
         [c] Treatment may include hemodialysis and critical-care support with assisted ventilation of the lungs, in addition to the treatment of associated illnesses
      (2) Methanol and ethylene glycol
         [a] Methanol is present in windshield washer antifreeze, solvents, and organic synthetic processes
         [b] Ethylene glycol is the major automotive antifreeze
         [c] Metabolites are potent poisons and may lead to irreversible toxicity if they go undetected
         [d] Treatment is systemic alkalinization to decrease ocular and renal toxicity, followed by hemodialysis to accelerate elimination of the alcohols and their metabolites
   (c) Carbon monoxide (CO)
      (1) Colorless, odorless, tasteless, nonirritating gas produced by the incomplete combustion of carbonaceous material
      (2) The major cause of death in patients exposed to smoke inhalation from fires
      (3) Exerts its toxic effects through tissue hypoxia by combining with hemoglobin at oxygen-binding sites, displacing oxygen, and shifting the saturation curve to the left (hemoglobin molecule has an affinity for CO that is over 200 times greater than for oxygen)
      (4) Symptomatology depends on
         [a] Patient's activity level
         [b] Tissue oxygen demands
         [c] Amount of CO present
         [d] Hemoglobin concentration
      (5) Clinical symptoms include headache, visual disturbances, N/V, convulsions, coma, and respiratory paralysis
      (6) Skin and mucous membranes exhibit classic cherry-red color
      (7) Treatment is to remove the offending agent and provide a highly oxygen-enriched environment
      (8) Treatment modalities may include hyperventilation with 100% oxygen, hyperbaric oxygen, and transfusion therapy, as well as diuretics and steroids for the treatment of complicating cerebral edema

2. Bacterial toxins
   (a) Tetanus
       (1) Chiefly affects motor neurons of the spinal cord and brain stem since the neurotoxin irreversibly binds to the motor neurons of the spinal cord, as well as to the neuromuscular junction
       (2) Early signs include spasms of the jaw, face, and neck muscles; even minor sensory stimulation may produce intense muscle spasms and respiratory arrest
       (3) Other manifestations include sympathetic hyperactivity, such as HTN, tachyarrythmias, sweating, pallor, and cyanosis
       (4) Treatment may include tracheostomy, although the best treatment is prophylaxis
   (b) Botulism
       (1) Toxin inhibits the presynaptic release of acetylcholine at the neuromuscular junction
       (2) GI irritability usually occurs before or shortly after onset of neurologic symptoms (affects brain-stem nuclei)
       (3) The bulbar musculature is affected initially, particularly the extraocular muscles, producing diplopia, ptosis, or both
       (4) Further signs of cranial dysfunction include vertigo, dysphagia, hoarseness, and/or breathy nasal speech
       (5) Trivalent (ABE) antitoxin should be given initially and type-specific antitoxin administered after the type of toxin has been identified
       (6) Treatment effectiveness depends on early diagnosis; mortality has decreased with improved respiratory intensive care

d. Spinal cord lesions

1. Myelopathy
   (a) May impair motor, sensory, or autonomic function, which will vary in severity
   (b) If partial or incomplete, it will present as one of several major spinal-cord syndromes, each having a certain propensity for recovery
   (c) Etiology may include congenital, degenerative, traumatic, infectious, or neoplastic disease processes
2. Anterior cord syndrome
   (a) May result from
       (1) Damage to the anterior two thirds of the spinal cord
       (2) Sustained hypoperfusion, such as prolonged anesthesia-related hypotension
       (3) Obstruction of the feeder vessels to the anterior spinal artery
   (b) Occurs more commonly in the cervical region
   (c) Characterized by LMN paralysis of the arms and UMN paralysis of the legs
   (d) There is motor paralysis with complete deficits of pain (sharp/dull), temperature, and light-touch sensory modalities below the level of injury
   (e) A partial myelopathy is often due to ventral compression from retropulsed bone or disk, a flexion injury, or interruption of anterior spinal artery blood flow
   (f) Variable sparing of the posterior columns accounts for residual tactile, vibration, and position sense in the lower extremities
   (g) Treatment is aimed at relieving any existing contributory pathology and providing general support
3. Central cord syndrome
   (a) Common myelopathy
   (b) Acute central cord syndrome can be caused by trauma to the central cord, such as contusion or hematoma

IV. Clinical Entities; d. Spinal cord lesions (continued)

    (c) Acute syndromes are characterized by sacral sparing of pain and temperature sensory modalities and by a dense motor weakness in the arms versus the legs

    (d) Motor, sensory, and bladder functions have good prospects for recovery, with earlier improvements noted in the legs

    (e) Chronic central cord syndrome can be caused by cysts, such as syringomyelia, or by intrinsic cord tumors

    (f) Chronic syndromes are characterized by a dissociated sensory disorder, LMN-type flaccid paralysis, and muscle atrophy of the upper extremities

    (g) Progressive disruption of the dorsal horns accounts for the trophic disorders that may involve the arms and fingers

4. Syringomyelia

    (a) Disease of the central part of the spinal cord in which a tubelike enlargement of the central canal develops, typically at lower cervical or upper thoracic levels

    (b) May present as an incomplete myelopathy and may extend rostrally to the medulla (syringobulbia) to impair various lower cranial nerve functions

    (c) Patient loses pain and temperature sensation

    (d) Can be caused by abnormalities at the foramen magnum level, such as congenital Chiari malformation, as well as cord trauma, tumor, arachnoiditis, and compressive spondylosis

5. Complete transection of the spinal cord

    (a) Most commonly caused by trauma. Other causes include neoplasms, vascular occlusion, multiple sclerosis, or even malposition (e.g., excessive neck flexion)

    (b) Quadriplegia results if the insult or injury occurs above the arm level and paraplegia if below this level

    (c) Caudal to the level of the lesion, the patient shows

        (1) Paralysis of all voluntary movements

        (2) Anesthesia

        (3) Loss of bladder and bowel control

        (4) Anhidrosis and loss of vasomotor tone

        (5) Paralysis of volitional and automatic breathing if the lesion is in the rostral part of the cervical cord

    (d) Anesthetic considerations

        (1) Acute injury

            [a] Associated injuries may be problematic

            [b] Spinal shock

                i) Unopposed parasympathetic tone, manifested by peripheral pooling of blood and bradycardia

                ii) Heart cannot increase its chronotropic or inotropic state

                iii) Associated with acute pulmonary edema

        (2) Chronic injury (see "Spinal reflexes: pathologic reflexes")

            [a] Autonomic hyperreflexia (follows spinal shock)

            [b] Osteoporosis

            [c] Impaired renal function secondary to recurrent urinary tract infections

        (3) Choice of technique

            [a] General

                i) Moderate depth required to ensure that hyperreflexia is blocked

                ii) Risk of hypotension

            [b] Regional

                i) Excellent for blocking reflex

                ii) Difficult to assess level of anesthesia

        (4) Pharmacologic considerations

            [a] Atropine may be administered before intubation to prevent bradycardia

          [b] Titrate all drugs slowly

          [c] Avoid succinylcholine for 24 hours after injury

          [d] Pancuronium for muscle relaxation

     (5) Monitoring

          [a] Standard monitoring, including temperature, since thermoregulation is impaired

          [b] Invasive monitoring, including Foley, CVP, or Swan-Ganz catheter, may be necessary

     (6) General care

          [a] Position carefully to prevent pressure sores and damage to osteoporotic bones

          [b] Deep venous thrombosis precautions should be taken

     (7) Postoperative

          [a] If lesion is high and patient unable to cough, leave intubated

          [b] Treat pain above sensory level

6. Brown-Séquard syndrome (spinal cord hemisection)

  (a) Impairment of one half of the spinal cord while sparing the opposite half

  (b) Clinical findings (caudal to level of lesion)

     (1) Contralateral effects

          [a] Loss of pain and temperature sensation

     (2) Ipsilateral effects

          [a] Paralysis of voluntary movements

          [b] Hyperreflexia, spasticity, and extensor toe sign

          [c] Loss of vibration, position sense, form perception, and two-point discrimination

          [d] Segmental weakness, atrophy, and anesthesia

          [e] Loss of sweating

          [f] Horner's syndrome if lesion is cervical

  (c) The prognosis for motor recovery is better than that of other incomplete myelopathies but remains influenced by the nature of the insult, rapidity of diagnosis, and, when appropriate, expeditious decompression

  (d) Can be caused by unilateral encroachment of epidural tumor through the neural foramina or intradural tumor from the nerve root, as well as trauma that impairs one lateral half of the cervical or thoracic cord

7. Posteriorcord syndrome

  (a) Rare presentation of an incomplete myelopathy

  (b) Results in ipsilateral loss of discriminatory touch and vibration sense, as well as loss of position sense below the level of the lesion with preservation of motor function

  (c) Most commonly caused by multiple sclerosis, vitamin B_{12} deficiency, Friedreich's ataxia, tabes dorsalis, or pure sensory neuropathies

  (d) Rarely, it may be caused by a dorsal extramedullary tumor

8. Conus medullaris syndrome

  (a) Results from injury to the conus medullaris

  (b) Produces impotence, loss of bowel and bladder control, anesthesia of the saddle region, reduced anal sphincter tone, and variable sparing of the lower extremities

  (c) Prognosis for recovery of bowel and bladder control is poor

9. Cauda equina syndrome

  (a) Typical physical findings include variable LMN sensory and motor loss to the lower extremities and sphincter disturbances

  (b) Prognosis for motor recovery is excellent

e. Air embolism

1. History and definition
   (a) Defined as bubbles of air (gas) in the venous or arterial circulations
   (b) Clinically recognized since the middle of the 19th century
2. Mechanism
   (a) Venous
       (1) Entrained into veins when a gradient of over 5 cm exists between open venous structures and the right atrium
       (2) Increased potential for entrainment when venous structure is rigid (spongy bone, bony venous sinuses) or supported by rigid structures (bridging veins)
       (3) Can also be driven in under pressure; e.g., injected through a syringe, infused through an IV under pressure, driven in by air-powered surgical instruments, forced in during radioimaging studies, forced in during reaming for total hip arthroplasty
       (4) Important to be aware of mechanism because of varying clinical picture, depending on volume and rate of air entrainment
   (b) Arterial
       (1) Can be directly injected into arterial tree; e.g., cardioplegia followed by air, direct chest trauma to bronchial veins, etc.
       (2) Can be paradoxic; i.e., crossing over from venous side unexpectedly
       (3) Routes of potential crossover include
           [a] Intracardiac defects; e.g., patent foramen ovale (PFO)
           [b] AV shunts in pulmonary circulation
           [c] Forced across alveolar microcirculation by raised pulmonary arteriolar driving pressure
       (4) Can be formed during decompression, e.g., divers, astronauts, etc.
3. Procedures with reported incidence of air embolism
   (a) Neurosurgery
       (1) Incidence is approximately 40–50% in sitting position
       (2) Other positions have smaller incidences but no guarantee that it will not occur; has even occurred during prone lumbar laminectomy
   (b) Obstetrics and gynecology
       (1) Patients in Trendelenberg position have a gradient to the right atrium (RA)
       (2) Large exposed venous channels during cesarean section or dilation and curettage procedures
       (3) Injection may occur through epidural catheters for anesthesia and labor
   (c) Head and neck surgery
       (1) Large vascular areas and organs
       (2) Frequently operate in head-up position for better venous drainage (gradient)
   (d) Central venous pressure lines
       (1) During insertion
       (2) Access to large vessels
       (3) Noncollapsible catheter with direct route to right atrium
   (e) Miscellaneous
       (1) Dental air drills
       (2) Lithotripsy
       (3) Irrigation of wounds with hydrogen peroxide
       (4) Chest trauma
       (5) Total hip replacement
       (6) Liver transplantation

(7) GI endoscopy

(8) Hip arthrography

4. Pathophysiology

(a) Venous

(1) Slow infusion

[a] Air vortex at junction of superior vena cava and right atrium

[b] Gradual obstruction of pulmonary outflow tract with air bubbles

[c] Raised pulmonary artery pressure (PAP)

[d] Right ventricular strain

[e] Acute cor pulmonale

[f] Cardiovascular collapse

(2) Rapid injection

[a] Rapid accumulation of air into right ventricle

[b] Foaming of blood and air

[c] No forward output from right ventricle

[d] Acute right ventricular air lock

[e] Sudden cardiovascular collapse

(b) Arterial

(1) Usually from venous side

(2) Small bubbles cross over through unidentified AV connection

(3) Obstruction of nutrient arteries to heart (coronary), brain (carotid, circle), spinal cord (arterial spinal artery)

(4) Ischemia, infarction, stroke, heart failure, paralysis, failure to waken, and sudden death may occur

(c) Paradoxical

(1) No obvious point of crossover from venous side

(2) Sitting position can change left atrial to right atrial pressure gradient

(3) Some 25–30% of asymptomatic, healthy adults have probe patent foramen ovale (PPFO); therefore, possible incidence of paradoxical air embolism (10%)

5. Monitoring

(a) Aims

(1) Early detection of air entry

(2) Prevention of early air entry once detected

(3) Removal of as much air as possible

(4) Preservation of normal hemodynamics

(5) Treatment of cardiovascular collapse, dysrhythmias, or pulmonary edema

(b) History

(1) Until late 1970s, no reliable method of detection; waited for clinical signs to change

(2) First clinical sign was gasp during spontaneous respiration at 0.38 ml air/kg/min

(3) Changes in CVP, PAP, heart rate, cardiac output, ECG, blood pressure, and rhythm may follow

(4) "Mill-wheel" murmur is a late sign on auscultation

(c) Current clinical practice

(1) Echocardiography (most sensitive)

[a] Very expensive, dynamic monitoring tool

[b] Demands some expertise and experience

[c] Not generally available in operating room setting

[d] Very fast recognition of gas embolism in the right atrium

[e] Able to monitor right-to-left shunting

[f] Able to detect venous, arterial, and paradoxical air embolism

[g] Able to monitor success of therapy

IV. Clinical Entities; e. Air embolism (continued)

    (2) Mass spectrometry
       [a] Detection of decreased end-tidal carbon dioxide
       [b] Detection of nitrogen in expired gas
       [c] Available in operating room sampling devices
       [d] Relatively fast and specific, although some false positives if end-tidal CO_2 is used and there may be a delay if multiple operating rooms using same system
    (3) Doppler
       [a] Inexpensive device that detects very small volumes of air
       [b] Readily available in operating room setting
       [c] Reliable, although gives some false positives
       [d] Sometimes difficult to locate the probe accurately
       [e] Bovie interference
       [f] Fast enough to prevent serious intraoperative problems
    (4) Capnography
       [a] Reliable method
       [b] Faster than multiple operating room mass spectrometry
       [c] False positives
       [d] Old-fashioned
       [e] Best used in conjunction with other methods
    (5) Transcutaneous CO_2 detection
       [a] Nonspecific
       [b] Slow
    (6) Pulmonary artery pressure (PAP)
       [a] Mirrors end-tidal CO_2 changes
       [b] Increases with air obstruction of catheter
       [c] Auto monitor left-to-right gradient by monitoring wedge pressure and CVP
       [d] Regular Swan-Ganz does not allow fast enough aspiration of air from right atrium
       [e] Limited infusion rate for resuscitation
    (7) Central venous pressure line
       [a] Often a routine monitor for neurosurgical cases
       [b] Multiorifice catheter placed for maximal air aspiration
       [c] Important for right-to-left atrial shunt monitoring
       [d] Location of catheter important (see below)
       [e] Also useful for proper location of Doppler
    (8) Hemodynamics
       [a] Changes in blood pressure, heart rate, or the occurrence of cardiac dysrhythmias are late changes
       [b] Treat hemodynamics appropriately
    (9) Murmur
       [a] Classic "mill-wheel" murmur
       [b] Very late sign

6. Clinical practice
  (a) Patient position (sitting versus prone)
    (1) Lower incidence of air embolism in prone position, although blood loss is greater
    (2) Better exposure in sitting position
  (b) Nitrous oxide
    (1) Expands intravascular bubbles
    (2) Allows earlier detection
    (3) More hemodynamic disturbance since increased pulmonary artery obstruction

        (4) Use is controversial

        (5) Can be used as a test of whether or not bubbles are still present in pulmonary vasculature

    (c) Positioning right arterial catheter

        (1) Air vortex at junction of SVC and RA

        (2) Location of orifice of catheter at precise air vortex difficult

        (3) Methods of location

            [a] ECG—monitoring P wave (biphasic)

            [b] Chest x-ray

            [c] Pressure-wave transduction

    (d) Monitoring

        (1) Doppler and CVP routine

        (2) Use of mass spectrometry, echocardiography on the rise

        (3) Dedicated gas monitoring units now available at bedside for pulse oximetry, transcutaneous CO_2, and anesthetic/respiratory gases

    (e) Anesthetic technique

        (1) Mainly IV narcotics with low-dose isoflurane

        (2) Nitrous oxide controversial

        (3) Paralyzed with controlled ventilation

7. Treatment

    (a) Good communication with surgeon, call for help

    (b) Turn off N_2O; 100% Fio_2

    (c) Aspirate CVP catheter if present

    (d) Treat hemodynamics as needed

    (e) Change position if air entrainment continues

    (f) CPR if necessary

    (g) Obstruct venous drainage through neck manually if necessary (compression of ipsilateral internal jugular vein)

    (h) Consider hyperbaric oxygen if paradoxical air bubbles to cerebral, spinal cord, and/or coronary circulations

8. Future

    (a) Less sitting, more prone positioning

    (b) More sophisticated monitoring—echocardiography, mass spectrometry

    (c) Neurophysiologic monitoring—EEG, SSEP, and motor-evoked responses

    (d) Increased use of IV anesthetic techniques

f. Cerebral protection

1. General

    (a) Protection of the brain against ischemic or hypoxic insults is the focus of cerebral protective strategies

    (b) Most significant in neurosurgical and cardiovascular procedures involving transient ischemia

    (c) Protection can be prospective, in anticipation of an insult, or retrospective, to minimize the loss of cerebral function after an event

    (d) Most protective strategies involve metabolic suppression, in an effort to minimize the demand for metabolic substrate in situations of reduced supply

2. Cerebral metabolic requirements

    (a) The brain is an obligate aerobe, intolerant of reduction of O_2 delivery below 2 ml/min/100 g

    (b) Anaerobic metabolism

        (1) Less efficient, producing 2 ATP/glucose molecules versus 38 ATP/glucose in aerobic metabolism

IV. Clinical Entities; f. Cerebral protection (continued)

        (2) Productive of intracellular acidosis via pyruvate-lactate pathway
    (c) Cerebral metabolism, like other cellular metabolism, is primarily (60%) concerned with maintenance of transmembrane gradients of ions
        (1) ATP-dependent processes (such as Na^+/K^+ ATPases) maintain chemical and electrical dysequilibrium across cell membranes at high energetic cost
        (2) Failure of ATP-driven pumps causes
            [a] Unopposed leak of Na^+ (into) and K^+ (out of the cell) (depolarization)
            [b] Ca^{++} leaks into the cell and there is a subsequent release of sequestered intracellular Ca^{++}
            [c] Intracellular pH decreases and phospholipases, triggered by Ca^{++}, increase, start to break down cell structures

  3. Excitatory amino acids (glutamate)
    (a) May cause secondary ischemic damage
    (b) Produce excess activity in damaged brain
  4. Protective strategies
    (a) Hypothermia
        (1) Most reliable and safe method of reducing metabolic demand
            [a] $CMRO_2$ is reduced 50% by a 10°C decrease in brain temperature
            [b] Circulatory arrest is tolerated for 30–60 minutes at 12–15°C
            [c] Metabolic demand is reduced and membranes are stabilized by even mild (33–35°C) hypothermia
        (2) Complications
            [a] Cardiac complications (primarily dysrhythmias) become a problem below 32°C unless circulation is supported (bypass)
            [b] Research is ongoing toward minimizing the complications of deep hypothermia, which should allow this strategy to be applied more often in difficult cases
    (b) Pharmacologic strategies
        (1) Barbiturates
            [a] Titrated to EEG burst suppression or electrical silence in order to provide suppression of electrical activity
            [b] Effects of barbiturates in focal ischemia may also be linked to vasoconstriction of normal vessels and shunting to ischemic areas
        (2) Propofol
            [a] May be protective, although it is still under investigation
            [b] Faster emergence times are attractive for neurosurgery
        (3) Ion channel blockers
            [a] Ca^{++} blockers include nimodipine and nicardipine
            [b] Na^+ channel blockers reduce the load on ATP-driven pumps
        (4) Lidocaine and its derivatives
            [a] Membrane stabilizers
            [b] Promising agents
        (5) Dizocilipine
            [a] Glutamate blocker
            [b] Has shown some mild protective effects in experimental models
        (6) Dexmedetomidine and dextromethorphan
            [a] NMDA antagonists
            [b] Possibly useful in focal ischemia
        (7) Anesthetic agents
            [a] Inhaled anesthetics reduce CMR, increase CBF, and may show some mild protective effect

[b] The risk of increasing ICP through increases in CBF must be weighed against the benefits derived from using these agents

5. Summary
    (a) Only hypothermia is of undisputed benefit as a cerebral protective agent
    (b) Anesthetic drugs may provide a limited benefit in focal ischemia
    (c) New membrane-stabilizing drugs show promise in reducing the energetic demands of ionic pumping across intrinsically leaky membranes

g. Vascular lesions

1. Intracranial aneurysms
    (a) Incidence
        (1) Symptomatic (SAH): 15–20 per 100,000
        (2) Asymptomatic: 4–6% found at autopsy
        (3) Peak age range for rupture is 55 to 60 years
        (4) Before age 40, aneurysms occur predominantly in men; after age 40, more women are afflicted
        (5) Varies according to country and racial group
        (6) Aneurysm rupture during pregnancy most often occurs during the 30th and 40th weeks of gestation or in the postpartum period, in contrast to AVM bleeds, which occur most commonly at delivery
    (b) Outcome
        (1) Of the 30,000 new cases of SAH secondary to aneurysm rupture each year, roughly 3,000 die immediately, and another 8,000 die from recurrent hemorrhage
        (2) Only 17,000 to 18,000 patients are admitted to the hospital, of which 70% come to the operating room, with a surgical mortality of less than 10%
    (c) Classification
        (1) Classified according to location and size
        (2) Patients are also assigned a clinical grade, depending on the presence of signs of meningeal reaction, level of conscious- ness, and evidence of focal neurologic dysfunction
        (3) Either Bottrell's original classification or the modification proposed by Hunt is used by neurosurgeons to provide a means of estimating surgical risk and outcome
    (d) Signs and symptoms of SAH
        (1) Result from the abrupt, marked increase in ICP
        (2) Most common symptom is "worst headache of my life"
        (3) Other symptoms may include neck stiffness, photophobia, N/V, loss of consciousness, or major neurologic deficit
        (4) A small bleed or "warning leak" precedes a major aneurysmal rupture in about 50% of patients
    (e) Diagnosis
        (1) Definitive diagnosis is made by lumbar puncture
        (2) CT scan may confirm subarachnoid blood, as well as provide information about the site and source of bleeding
        (3) Angiography will localize the source of the bleed and rule out other causes of SAH, such as arteriovenous malforma- tion or neoplasm
    (f) Preoperative care
        (1) Goals are to help the brain recover from the effects of SAH and to prevent recurrent hemorrhage
        (2) Bed rest, sedation, and analgesics are recommended to minimize stress
        (3) Anticonvulsants are prescribed for seizure prophylaxis
        (4) Blood pressure is controlled and stabilized

      (5) Fluid balance and nutrition are maintained

      (6) The use of antifibrinolytic agents to prevent recurrent hemorrhage is controversial

(g) Complications

    (1) Rebleeding

      [a] The most devastating complication (high morbidity and mortality)

      [b] Results when the bursting pressure within exceeds the tensile strength of either the clot or the wall of the sac

      [c] Antifibrinolytic agents are often used for prevention

      [d] If it occurs, control ICP

    (2) Vasospasm

      [a] Occurs in approximately 30% of patients

      [b] Associated with neurologic deterioration in 50% of these patients

      [c] Results in diminished cerebral perfusion and loss of cerebral autoregulation

      [d] Cerebral ischemia and infarction may result

      [e] Treatment is usually "triple H therapy": HTN, hemodilution, and hypervolemia; calcium channel blocking drugs are used for prevention

    (3) Hydrocephalus

      [a] Occurs in 15–20% of patients

      [b] Results from blood and cellular exudate blocking the basal cisterns and CSF efflux

      [c] Results in a gradual decrease in the level of consciousness

      [d] Treatment may include temporary ventricular CSF diversion or shunt

    (4) Brain edema and swelling

      [a] Results from irritation of the parenchyma by the subarachnoid clot, edema around an intracerebral hematoma, or ischemia from vasospasm

      [b] Treatment may include steroid therapy and/or mannitol (osmotic diuretic)

    (5) Other complications include deep venous thrombosis, pulmonary embolism, sepsis, and metabolic abnormalities, such as hyperglycemia or hyponatremia

(h) Surgical management

    (1) Involves isolation of the aneurysmal sac from the remainder of the cerebral circulation in order to prevent rebleeding

    (2) The aneurysm may be clipped at its neck or wrapped, depending on its size and location

    (3) Temporary occlusion of the parent vessel proximal to the aneurysm is now often performed

    (4) Early surgery (24–48 hours) is usually preferred

      [a] Reduces incidence of rebleeding and vasospasm

      [b] Facilitates the treatment of vasospasm should it occur (triple H therapy)

      [c] Allows earlier ambulation and shorter hospitalization

(i) Induction

    (1) A smooth induction is critical to avoid large increases in the transmural pressure gradient and aneurysm rupture

    (2) Preoperative sedation is continued as appropriate

    (3) In addition to standard monitoring, an arterial line and possibly a CVP line are placed

    (4) The patient should be deeply anesthetized during periods of stimulation, including intubation and head pinning

    (5) Administration of lidocaine, esmolol, opioids, or an additional dose of the induction agent will help blunt the cardiovascular response to intubation

(6) Succinylcholine has been reported to cause serious dysrythmias as a result of an increase in serum potassium, and thus its use is often avoided

(j) Maintenance

(1) Any technique (narcotics, volatile agents, barbiturates) may be used for maintenance as long as it allows for prompt awakening and early neurologic examination

(2) Techniques to "shrink" the brain and provide better surgical exposure include

[a] Hyperventilation to a Pa_{CO_2} 28–32 mm Hg

[b] Adequate oxygenation

[c] CSF drainage via a spinal catheter or ventriculostomy

[d] Optimal venous drainage

[e] Administration of barbiturates or mannitol (steroid use is controversial)

[f] Discontinuing N_2O if pneumocephalus develops

[g] Discontinuing or reducing volatile agent

(3) Maintain normovolemia in order to support an adequate blood pressure and CO by using isotonic or hypertonic IV fluids

(4) Avoid hyperglycemia as it may worsen any neurologic insult that occurs

(k) Special techniques

(1) Controlled hypotension

[a] Decreases tension across the wall of an aneurysm and reduces arterial hemorrhage in the event of aneurysm rupture

[b] Although once a mainstay of the intraoperative management of aneurysm clipping, its value has diminished with the use of temporary occlusion

[c] Maintenance of an adequate cerebral perfusion pressure (mean of 50–60 mm Hg) determines a "safe" level of hypotension

[d] Can be achieved with the use of various vasoactive drugs and inhalational agents

[e] Instituted as the surgeon approaches the aneurysm and continues until the aneurysm is clipped

[f] Complications are primarily related to end-organ hypoperfusion

(2) Induced hypertension

[a] Augments cerebral perfusion via collateral circulation during temporary occlusion of parent artery

[b] Augmenting systemic blood pressure increases cerebral perfusion pressure (CPP = MAP − ICP)

[c] Phenylephrine is the drug of choice since it does not cause direct cerebral vasoconstriction, although norepinephrine and dopamine have also been used safely

[d] Complications include an increased risk of cerebral edema and intracranial hemorrhage

(3) Hypothermia

[a] Prolongs safely tolerated periods of cerebral ischemia as cerebral oxygen demand is reduced by 7–8% per 1°C

[b] The relationship between "brain protection" and hypothermia is not linear

[c] Although mild hypothermia (34°C) is protective, profound hypothermia (less than 20°C) and circulatory arrest may be used for giant aneurysms that would be otherwise inoperable

[d] Potential complications include cardiac dysrhythmias and ischemia, postoperative shivering, increased blood viscosity, coagulopathy, prolonged drug clearance, and increased rates of infection

(4) Pharmacologic protective therapy (see "Cerebral protection")

IV. Clinical Entities; g. Vascular lesions (continued)

- (l) Emergence
    - (1) Rapid emergence is desirable to allow early neurologic assessment
    - (2) The sympathetic response to noxious stimuli (HTN and tachycardia) may be controlled by the use of labetalol, esmolol, hydralazine, propofol, or SNP
    - (3) Extubation should be planned for patients who were neurologically intact before surgery and whose operative course was uneventful
2. Arteriovenous malformations (AVMs)
    - (a) Vascular malformations in which there are direct communications between arteries and veins without an intervening capillary network
    - (b) Incidence
        - (1) One seventh as prevalent as cerebral aneurysms (approximately 280,000 in the United States)
        - (2) Males more than females, 1–1.5 to 1
        - (3) No familial influence
        - (4) Majority present by age 40
        - (5) Supratentorial and superficial compose 90% of AVMs compared with infratentorial and deep (10%)
        - (6) Lesions may be multiple or associated with cerebral aneurysms
    - (c) Classification
        - (1) Classified according to location, size of AVM midus (core), number and distribution of feeding arteries, pattern of venous drainage, amount of flow, and the amount of steal from the adjacent normal brain
        - (2) Grading systems are intended to predict the risk of neurologic impairment resulting from treatment, especially surgery
        - (3) Most commonly used grading system is that by Spetzler and Martin
    - (d) Treatment
        - (1) Surgical removal
        - (2) Embolization
        - (3) Radiation therapy
    - (e) Unique problems
        - (1) Impaired autoregulation
        - (2) Abnormalities in regional cerebral blood flow
        - (3) Abrupt fluctuations in hemodynamics
        - (4) Changes in ICP
        - (5) Fragility of cerebral vessels
    - (f) Preoperative case
        - (1) Very similar to aneurysms
        - (2) Early recurrent hemorrhage and cerebral vasospasm are not major concerns
    - (g) Anesthetic management
        - (1) Same general considerations as for aneurysm surgery
        - (2) Induced hypotension is not employed unless there are episodes of cerebral engorgement
        - (3) Intraoperative arteriograms are often obtained to assess proper resection
    - (h) Pediatric AVMs
        - (1) Tend to be larger and to bleed more easily
        - (2) Usually involve enlargement of the vein of Galen
        - (3) Often have impaired cardiac function
            - [a] Neonate: high output CHF
            - [b] Infant/child: hydrocephalus, mild cardiac dysfunction
        - (4) Other symptoms include seizures, cerebral steal, and bruits

h. Intracranial hypertension

1. Cranial vault

    (a) Functions as a rigid box

    (b) Contains
        (1) Brain, 85%
        (2) Cerebrospinal fluid, 5–10%
        (3) Blood, 4–8%

    (c) Normal intracranial pressure (ICP) is 0–10 mm Hg

    (d) When contents increase in volume rapidly, ICP rises

    (e) When contents increase gradually, there is time for compensation and ICP does not rise; once compensation is maximal, pressure rises steeply, even with small increments in volume

2. Pathophysiology

    (a) Defined as ICP over 20 mm Hg

    (b) Dangerous because of the potential for ischemia to develop when cerebral perfusion pressure (CPP) falls below 50 mm Hg

    (c) Normal CPP is 90 mm Hg (CPP = MAP − ICP)

    (d) Herniation may occur, especially in the posterior cranial fossa (coning)

    (e) Changes in ICP can be mediated by very small changes in intracranial volume (blood and CSF)
        (1) Increase elastance (decrease compliance)
            [a] Hypercapnia
            [b] Hypoxia
            [c] REM sleep
            [d] Ketamine
            [e] Inhalation agents (increased flow)
        (2) Decrease elastance (increase compliance)
            [a] Hypocapnia
            [b] Hypothermia
            [c] IV anesthetics (reduced metabolism)

3. Causes of elevated ICP

    (a) Acute
        (1) Hematoma
            [a] Extradural
            [b] Subdural
            [c] Subarachnoid (aneurysm, AVM)
        (2) Edema
            [a] Diffuse
            [b] Focal

    (b) Chronic
        (1) Hematoma
            [a] History of trauma
            [b] Senile atrophy
            [c] Recurrence of drained hematoma
        (2) Tumors
            [a] Supratentorial
            [b] Infratentorial
        (3) Infective processes
            [a] Abscess
            [b] Encephalitis
            [c] Pseudotumor cerebri
            [d] Meningitis

    (4) Mechanical
       [a] Hydrocephalus
       [b] Congenital malformations

4. Signs and symptoms of elevated ICP
  (a) Mildly elevated ICP
    (1) Headache
    (2) Irritability
    (3) Nausea and vomiting
    (4) Papilledema
    (5) Confusion
  (b) Moderately elevated ICP
    (1) Disturbed level of consciousness
    (2) Hypertension
    (3) Bradycardia
    (4) Irregular respiration
  (c) Severely increased ICP
    (1) Cardiovascular collapse
    (2) Coma
    (3) Respiratory depression
    (4) Dilated pupils
    (5) Respiratory arrest (brain-stem compression)

5. Clinical management of anesthesia
  (a) Preoperative care
    (1) All preoperative medications depress CNS; therefore, do not use unless very anxious (small doses of benzodiazepines are usually well tolerated)
    (2) Continue steroids
    (3) Anticonvulsants
  (b) Induction of anesthesia
    (1) Avoid agents that increase CBF, CBV, CSF, and ICP
    (2) Thiopental, etomidate, and diprivan, all decrease ICP by decreasing CBF (activity-flow coupling)
    (3) Important to preserve arterial pressure and CPP, while decreasing cerebral metabolic activity
    (4) HTN and tachycardia may already be present to compensate for elevated ICP
    (5) Avoid hemodynamic exacerbations
      [a] Avoid pancuronium
      [b] Muscle relaxant for rapid-sequence induction is controversial (high-dose rocuronium versus succcinylcholine)
      [c] Succinylcholine is the drug of choice for the difficult airway
      [d] Esmolol, lidocaine, or narcotics should be available to control blood pressure
  (c) Maintenance
    (1) Maintain paralysis
      [a] Use vecuronium, rocuronium
      [b] Caution concerning use of pancuronium or atracurium
    (2) IV narcotics
      [a] Fentanyl
      [b] Alfentanil (may drop blood pressure)
      [c] Sufentanil (may cause cerebral vasodilation)
    (3) Low-dose isoflurane and possibly N_2O
    (4) Control Pa_{CO_2} between 28 and 32 mm Hg

(5) Use positioning to help venous, CSF drainage

(6) Remain intubated if brain-stem compression or edematous brain

(7) Control blood pressure once cranial vault decompressed

(8) Monitor arterial blood gases, dynamic blood pressure, blood volume, and even ICP, if possible

(9) Control brain swelling with mannitol, furosemide, and by monitoring osmolarity and possibly brain oxygen consumption

i. Determination of brain death

1. Clinical diagnosis

    (a) The patient should have no signs of brain-stem function and have no other reversible cause for these findings

    (b) Clinical findings include

       (1) Normothermia and absence of hypotension

       (2) Absence of CNS depressants and muscle relaxants

       (3) No doll's eyes and absence of oculovestibular reflexes

       (4) No response to noxious stimulus applied to the trunk

       (5) No evidence of spontaneous ventilatory movement. An apnea test is conducted in which the patient is placed on FiO_2 1.0, monitored with a pulse oximeter, and is not ventilated for 10 minutes, at which time an ABG is drawn, and ventilation resumed. The $PaCO_2$ should rise to near 60 mm Hg without respiratory movement

       (6) Spinal reflexes may still be present (withdrawal of extremity that is stimulated)

2. Confirmatory tests may be done at the clinician's discretion, although they are not required. a-c should demonstrate absence of cerebral blood flow

    (a) Four-vessel carotid angiogram

    (b) Radionuclide cerebral blood flow study

    (c) Transcranial Doppler

    (d) EEG should be isoelectric at highest sensitivity

V. PEDIATRICS

a. Meningomyelocele

1. Congenital herniation of part of the meninges, spinal cord, and nerve roots through a defect in the lumbar vertebral column (spina bifida)

2. Incidence

    (a) 0.2–4 per 1,000 live births

    (b) Females more than males

    (c) Whites more than blacks

3. Etiology

    (a) Uncertain

    (b) Presumed polygenic inheritance with environmental influences, especially poor maternal diet

4. Prevention

    (a) Folic acid, 4 mg/day, plus multivitamins from conception until 7 weeks' gestation

    (b) Overall incidence has decreased by 40% in the last 10 years

5. Diagnosis (antenatal)

    (a) 75% have elevated alpha-fetoprotein levels in serum and amniotic fluid at 14–20 weeks' gestation

V. Pediatrics; a. Meningomyelocele (continued)

    (b) 90% lesions seen on fetal ultrasound sonography (USS) with or without ventriculomegaly after 20 weeks' gestation

    (c) Together, 96–100% diagnoses made by 24–28 weeks' gestation

6. Overall survival (1990)

    (a) 5-year survival 83%

    (b) 6–12-year survival 79%

7. Clinical abnormalities

    (a) Protective integument often absent over the lesion, allowing CSF to leak and increasing the risk of infection

    (b) Nerve roots below lesion nonfunctional, causing muscle paralysis, neurogenic bladder and bowel, and orthopedic deformities

    (c) Hydrocephalus, 65–85%, of which 73% are secondary to an Arnold-Chiari malformation

    (d) Altered ventilatory pattern secondary to diminished central response to hypercapnia compared with normal individuals

    (e) Short trachea

    (f) Strabismus (30–50%)

8. Surgical intervention

    (a) Urgent: within 72 hours of birth

    (b) Indications for early closure

        (1) Maximizes function of the dysplastic spinal cord within the lesion and the structures it innervates

        (2) Prevents infection

        (3) Reduces large evaporative fluid losses

        (4) Reduces risk of hypothermia

    (c) Operative procedure involves primary closure or staged closure with insertion of tissue expanders and synthetic coverings

9. Anesthetic considerations

    (a) Follow general management of anesthesia in neonates

    (b) Preoperative

        (1) Ensure adequate preoperative hydration

        (2) Physiologic saline to replace evaporative losses from defect

        (3) Cross-matched blood should be available

    (c) Perioperative

        (1) Suxamethonium is safe to use because it does not cause exaggerated hyperkalemia; however, it is not always indicated

        (2) Posture for induction

            [a] Large lesions: induce and intubate in the left lateral position

            [b] Small/medium lesions: place supine with padding around the lesion to prevent trauma

            [c] Hydrocephalus: airway management may be awkward, therefore, consider best posture, supine/lateral

        (3) Prone for surgery: care with positioning with respect to ETT, IPPV, and pressure points

        (4) Blood and fluid losses

            [a] May be high

            [b] Are related to size of lesion and area of skin undermined to create flaps for closure

            [c] Require a minimum of two peripheral IV lines and an arterial line

        (5) Prevention of hypothermia

            [a] Warm IV fluids

[b] Warm and humidify inspired gases

[c] K thermic blanket

[d] Space blanket and warmed covers or heated air cover, e.g., Bair hugger

(6) Avoid exposure to latex since minimizing exposure may prevent or delay sensitization

(d) Postoperative

(1) Increased risk of apnea and/or hypoventilation, especially in the presence of hydrocephalus; therefore, ICU setting appropriate

(2) Monitor by pulse oximetry

(3) If there is any doubt about the adequacy of spontaneous ventilation, leave the patient intubated. Have a low threshold for reintubating extubated patients

10. Outlook when defect corrected within 24 hours (1991)

(a) 75% of survivors have normal intelligence

(b) 90% of survivors have achieved bladder/bowel control by school age

(c) Greater than 80% of survivors are ambulant by school age with or without walking aids; 10–15% of survivors are not socially competitive

11. Additional information

(a) If a patient with previous meningomyelocele repair presents for surgery, he or she may have latex sensitivity

(1) Take full latex precautions to avoid allergen exposure

(2) Give pharmacologic prophylaxis as premedication or at induction

[a] H_1 antagonist

[b] H_2 antagonist

[c] Corticosteroid

b. Arnold-Chiari malformation (aqueduct stenosis)

1. Description

(a) Complex developmental anomaly associated with meningomyelocele and other neural tube defects

(b) Involves a bony abnormality of the posterior fossa and upper cervical spine with downward displacement of the cerebellar tonsils into the upper cervical spinal canal, as well as elongation of the medulla oblongata and fourth ventricle, resulting in obstructive hydrocephalus and brain-stem dysfunction

(c) Abnormal vascular architecture of the brain stem is also present

2. Incidence

(a) Most common anomaly involving cerebellum

(b) Cause of 73% of hydrocephalus in patients who also have meningomyelocele

3. Clinical manifestations

(a) Frequently asymptomatic, although 20% of patients with meningomyelocele are symptomatic

(b) Clinical signs arise from cranial nerve and brain-stem dysfunction

(1) Large head associated with raised ICP

(2) Apnea: abnormal ventilatory pattern secondary to decreased response to hypoxia and hypercapnia

(3) Stridor/upper airway obstruction: one or both vocal cords may be paretic or paralyzed

(4) Dysphagia

[a] Feeding difficulties

[b] Pooling of oral secretions

(5) Aspiration secondary to diminished or absent gag reflex

   (6) Arm weakness

   (7) Opisthotonos

  (c) Extreme neck flexion and extension may cause brain-stem compression in otherwise asymptomatic patients

  4. Survival

  (a) Rapid progression of vocal cord paralysis and arm weakness is associated with increased mortality

  (b) Death can occur within 2 weeks of presentation

  5. Surgical intervention

  (a) Usually within the first 3 months of life but after meningomyelocele repair

  (b) Often in two stages

   (1) Hydrocephalus decompression by VP shunt or ventriculostomy

   (2) Posterior fossa decompression with upper cervical laminectomy and opening of dura to release cerebellar tonsils and relieve brain-stem compression

  (c) Usual position for surgery is prone with slight neck flexion

  6. Anesthetic considerations

  (a) Preoperative

   (1) Airway

    [a] Presence of hydrocephalus may make intubation difficult

    [b] Chronic respiratory compromise is associated with repeated aspiration

    [c] May need intubation before surgery

    [d] Consider best posture and technique for securing airway, e.g., supine versus left lateral, awake versus asleep

    [e] May be intubated already if presented with stridor/apnea/aspiration

   (2) ICP precautions should be taken in patients with hydrocephalus that has not been decompressed

   (3) Cardiovascular stability

    [a] Perioperative dysrythmias are common during manipulation of the floor of the fourth ventricle

    [b] Dysrhythmias include bradycardia, junctional rhythm, and premature ventricular contractions

   (4) Air embolism

   (5) Latex allergy if associated with meningomyelocele

  (b) Intraoperative

   (1) IV access

    [a] Two peripheral IVs

    [b] CVP in right atrium

   (2) Monitors

    [a] Standard

    [b] Precordial Doppler

    [c] Arterial line, CVP

   (3) Position carefully in order to prevent injury to patient and displacement or kinking of endotracheal tube

  (c) Postoperative

   (1) Immediate

    [a] Intensive-care setting

    [b] Protective reflexes and vocal cord function may still be diminished or absent; if in doubt, leave intubated

    [c] Ventilation abnormalities may persist

   (2) Late

    [a] Vocal cord function and gag reflex may not return

[b] A tracheostomy and/or gastrostomy feeding tube may be needed to secure and protect the airway

c. Craniosynostosis

1. Congenital, premature fusion of one or more cranial sutures, occurring alone or as part of a syndrome
2. Incidence
   (a) One in 2,000 live births
   (b) Males more than females
   (c) Location
      (1) Sagittal (56%)
      (2) Single coronal (11%)
      (3) Bilateral coronal (11%)
      (4) Metopic (7%)
      (5) Lambdoid (1%)
      (6) Three or more sutures (14%)
3. Etiology
   (a) Genetic
      (1) Most common
      (2) Approximately 39% of cases have a positive family history
   (b) Metabolic
      (1) Elevated thyroxine (T_4) secondary to hyperthyroidism or excessive exogenous intake
      (2) Hypercalcemia
      (3) Hypophosphatasia
      (4) Rickets
   (c) Teratogens
      (1) Phenytoin
      (2) Methotrexate
      (3) Retinoic acid
   (d) Compression of fetal head in utero
4. Diagnosis
   (a) Clinical observation
   (b) Radiology
      (1) X-ray
      (2) CT scan
5. Clinical manifestations
   (a) Physical deformity of the skull
   (b) Chronic intracranial hypertension with brain compression may result in decreased intelligence if uncorrected
   (c) Psychologic disturbances may arise from the combination of deformity and raised intracranial pressure
6. Surgical intervention
   (a) Elective; age 4 to 6 weeks old
   (b) Allows brain growth and normal development
   (c) Allows better remodeling of bone
7. Procedure
   (a) Extradural, not intracranial
   (b) Strip craniectomy or reconstruction of sutures
   (c) Up to 20% require VP shunt for hydrocephalus; more likely if the synostosis is associated with other abnormalities

8. Anesthetic considerations
    (a) Same general considerations regarding anesthesia in infants
    (b) Preoperative
        (1) Airway
            [a] Intubation may be difficult due to facial dysmorphia
            [b] Use reinforced ETT if movement of the head is anticipated during surgery
        (2) Anticipate large blood loss
            [a] Can be up to 400% of blood volume
            [b] Significant losses from scalp and cranium with possible sudden, catastrophic bleeding if venous sinus opened
            [c] Cross-matched blood, coagulation factors, and platelets should be immediately available
        (3) Intracranial HTN
            [a] May or may not be present, depending on severity of craniosynostosis
            [b] IV induction is best
            [c] If inhalation induction is necessary, isoflurane is the preferred agent as it causes a smaller rise in ICP
            [d] Hyperventilate slightly once airway is secured
        (4) Air embolism
    (c) Intraoperative
        (1) Prevention of hypothermia (see "Meningomyelocele")
        (2) Monitoring and IV access similar to Arnold-Chiari management if multiple-suture synostosis or cranial reconstruction
        (3) Prone position is most common
        (4) Often difficult to keep up with blood loss
            [a] Administer 10% of estimated blood volume as whole blood or 5% albumin prior to incision in patients with normal cardiovascular status
            [b] Transfuse 10% more than estimated blood loss during the procedure
            [c] Tachycardia means hypovolemia until proved otherwise, therefore, give blood and/or colloid
        (5) Avoid deliberate hypotension to reduce bleeding as this can cause decreased brain perfusion in association with retraction
        (6) Normovolemic hemodilution techniques have been used to limit the total volume of blood transfused
            [a] Requires frequent measurements of hematocrit and blood gases to ensure that the oxygenation remains adequate
            [b] Diuretics may be given at the end of the procedure to aid excretion of excess crystalloid
        (7) Aim for rapid awakening and extubation if the airway is not compromised; if airway patency is in doubt, leave the patient intubated
    (d) Postoperative
        (1) Intensive-care setting
        (2) Postoperative ventilation is often necessary (24–48 hours)
            [a] Allows fluid shifts to normalize
            [b] Controls ICP
            [c] Allows resolution of upper airway edema
        (3) Review dressings, cardiovascular status, general condition, and hematocrit often and regularly since bleeding is common
        (4) Monitor consciousness level; if there is intracranial hemorrhage, LOC will decrease

9. Additional conditions
   (a) Apert's syndrome
       (1) Described: 1906
       (2) Incidence: 1 in 160,000 live births
           Males equal females
       (3) Inheritance—autosomal dominant
       (4) Clinical features
           [a] Acrobradycephaly
           [b] Wide forehead
           [c] Prominent supraorbital ridge in infancy
           [d] Syndactyly
       (5) Possible clinical features
           [a] Hypertelorism
           [b] Proptosis
           [c] Downward slanting of palpebral fissures
           [d] Splenoethmoidmaxillary hypoplasia or hypoplastic midface
           [e] Cleft palate (30%)
           [f] Mental retardation
           [g] Normal life span
   (b) Crouzon's disease
       (1) Described in 1912
       (2) Incidence: males equal females
       (3) Inheritance is autosomal dominant with complete penetrance but variable
           expressivity
       (4) Clinical features
           [a] Craniosynostosis—commences after birth; commonly lambdoid ±
               others (variable)
           [b] Hypertelorism
           [c] Proptosis
       (5) Possible clinical features
           [a] Strabismus
           [b] Nystagmus
           [c] Hypoplastic maxilla
           [d] Palate high arched, short, ± with or without cleft malocclusion
           [e] Rarely, may be elevated intracranial pressure
           [f] Normal intelligence, unless increased ICP or craniosynostosis is
               untreated
           [g] Normal life span
   (c) Anesthetic considerations for craniofacial reconstruction are similar to those for
       craniosynostosis. In addition
       (1) Blood loss at least 100–200% of blood volume
       (2) Greater likelihood of intraoperative death or neurologic sequelae
       (3) Perioperative extubation risk if midface moved forward, e.g., 3 cm. May
           need to reintubate nasal → oral, or vice versa, during procedure

D. UROLOGIC SYSTEM

I. ANATOMY
   a. Kidney

   b. Drainage system

   c. Anatomic imaging

II. PHYSIOLOGY
   a. Renal blood flow (RBF), renal plasma flow (RPF)

   b. Glomerular filtration rate (GFR)

   c. Tubular transport

   d. Tubular transport and permeability

   e. Regulation of tubular function

   f. Metabolic or endocrine functions of the kidney

   g. Acid-base balance

   h. Sodium balance (MW = 23)

   i. Potassium balance (MW = 39)

   j. Calcium balance (MW = 40)

   k. Chloride balance (MW = 35.5)

   l. Phosphate balance (PiMW = 31)

   m. Magnesium balance (MW = 24)

   n. Glucose (MW = 180)

   o. Amino acids

   p. Water balance

III. DIAGNOSTIC EVALUATION
   a. Urine flow rate (V)

   b. Urinalysis

   c. Measurement of RBF

   d. Measurement of GFR

   e. Tests of tubular function

   f. Tests of concentration

   g. Tests of tubular injury

   h. Erythropoietin

IV. PHARMACOLOGY
   a. Diuretics

   b. Anesthetic effects

V. CLINICAL DISEASE STATES
   a. Kidney failure

   b. Kidney trauma

   c. Polyuria

   d. Oliguria

VI. PERIOPERATIVE CONSIDERATIONS

    a. Fluid management with preexisting renal insufficiency

    b. Fluid management with functional anephric state

    c. Nephrectomy

    d. Transurethral surgery

    e. Effects of mechanical ventilation

    f. Induced hypotension

    g. Aortic cross-clamping

    h. Cardiopulmonary bypass

    i. Preoperative evaluation

I. ANATOMY

a. Kidney

1. Location
   (a) Retroperitoneal
   (b) Extends from L1–L4 when upright and from T12–L3 when supine, move 1–7 cm during ventilation
       (1) Right slightly lower than left
   (c) Partially covered by 11th to 12th ribs
2. Size
   (a) Neonate: 50 g
   (b) Adult kidneys are approximately 13 by 6 cm
   (c) Normal adult weight is 250–300 g, declining with age by about 30% to 175–200 g by the 80s
3. Gross anatomy
   (a) Cortex
       (1) Superficial nephrons (85% of nephrons) have short loops of Henle
       (2) Juxtamedullary nephrons (15%) have long loops of Henle
       (3) Most of loss with aging is from cortex, mostly capillary tufts
   (b) Medulla
       (1) Outer medulla
           [a] Outer stripe
               i) Contains third segment of proximal tubule
           [b] Inner stripe
               i) Contains thick ascending limbs
       (2) Inner medulla
           [a] Contains descending and ascending limbs of the loops of Henle and vasa recta
4. Microscopic anatomy
   (a) Glomerular filtration barriers
       (1) Capillary endothelium diaphragmed fenestrated pores 50–100 nm in diameter
       (2) Basement membrane is 350 nm thick, with fixed negative charges that retard passage of negatively charged molecules
       (3) Visceral epithelium (Bowman's capsule) is lined by podocytes separated by slits 25–60 nm wide
       (4) Parietal epithelium
       (5) Mesangium, which contains contractile cells that decrease the ultrafiltration coefficient (Kf) by decreasing the surface area
   (b) Proximal tubule divided into S1, S2, and S3 segments
       (1) Epithelial cells are joined by tight junctions
           [a] Spaces between cells (paracellular spaces) are in continuity with the interstitial space
           [b] Numerous microvilli form the brush border, which increases the absorptive surface area
       (2) High metabolic activity with numerous mitochondria
   (c) Loop of Henle
       (1) Descending limb and thin ascending limb are lined by a relatively simple, flat epithelium
       (2) Thick ascending limb is lined by tall epithelial cells, with numerous mitochondria reflecting its high metabolic rate
   (d) Distal tubule is lined by tall epithelial cells with numerous basolateral infoldings

(e) Connecting segment (collecting tubule)
(f) Innervation is derived from the celiac plexus and from thoracic and lumbar nerves
5. Vasculature
   (a) Renal artery
      (1) Arises from aorta just below superior mesenteric artery at L1–2 disk space and progressively subdivides into interlobar arteries, arcuate arteries, interlobular arteries, afferent arterioles (major resistance to flow), glomerular capillaries, efferent arterioles, peritubular capillary, descending vasa recta, and capillaries of inner stripe
      (2) Ascending vasa recta drain between vascular bundles
         [a] Ascending vasa recta of inner medulla join vascular bundle to form countercurrent relationship with descending vasa recta from inner stripe
      (3) Interlobular veins, arcuate veins, renal vein
   (b) Juxtaglomerular apparatus (JGA) components
      (1) Macula densa of the thick ascending limb
      (2) Glomerulus
      (3) Modified smooth muscle cells of the afferent and efferent arterioles that produce renin
   (c) Lymphatics
6. Developmental—aging
   (a) Vascular
      (1) Radiologically increased tortuosity, rapid tapering of diameter
      (2) Hyaline afferent arteriolosclerosis
      (3) Atherosclerosis of large renal arteries found in 70% of elderly
      (4) Hypertension causes myointimal hyperplasia of arterioles and arteries and accelerates atherosclerosis of larger arteries
   (b) Glomeruli
      (1) Nephrogenesis is complete at 34 weeks' postconception
      (2) Healthy individuals lose glomeruli with age
         [a] Hyaline deposition, smooth muscle atrophy, luminal obliteration
      (3) Decreased size of glomerular tuft
      (4) Increased mesangial tissue
      (5) Loss is greatest in superficial cortex
         [a] Entire nephron is lost
      (6) Juxtamedullary region
         [a] Glomeruli are lost
         [b] Afferent to efferent arteriolar connection continues, explaining better preservation of juxtamedullary than cortical circulation in elderly
         [c] Preferential loss of glomerular and proximal tubular volume
   (c) Tubules
      (1) Reduced number with aging
      (2) Length and volume of tubules decline
      (3) Tubular diverticula appear

b. Drainage system

1. Renal pelvis accepts urine from papillae
2. Ureters arise from the renal pelvis
   (a) Right ureter starts behind the duodenum, passes in front of the psoas, crosses the common iliac artery as it enters the pelvis
   (b) The left ureter follows a similar route into the pelvis, and then passes behind the sigmoid colon
3. Bladder
4. Urethra passes through prostate in male

c. Anatomic imaging

1. Ultrasound detects
   - (a) Size, shape, uniformity of parenchyma
   - (b) Dimensions of renal pelvis, ureters
   - (c) Stones
2. Intravenous pyelogram (IVP) detects
   - (a) Size, shape, uniformity of parenchyma
   - (b) Dilation and course of renal pelvis, ureters
   - (c) Stones
   - (d) Estimate of arterial inflow, glomerular function, and comparison of right versus left
3. Arteriogram
   - (a) Vascular anatomy
   - (b) Glomerular function
4. Nuclear medicine scan
   - (a) Semiquantitative flow, comparisons of right with left
   - (b) Semiquantitative assessment of renal size
   - (c) Depending on the particular agent, filtration and/or tubular function may be assessed
5. CT with contrast
   - (a) Visualize kidney parenchyma
   - (b) Trace course of ureters to bladder

II. PHYSIOLOGY

a. Renal blood flow (RBF), renal plasma flow (RPF)

1. 1,000–1,200 ml/min; 20% of cardiac output for 0.5% of body mass
   - (a) Low O_2 extraction, $(a-v)O_2$ difference of only 1.5 ml/100 ml
   - (b) RBF falls about 1% a year
     - (1) RBF/CI fraction and RBF/gram fall slightly with aging
     - (2) PAH clearance (estimated renal plasma flow) fell from 649 in 30–40 age range to 289 ml/min in 80s
       - [a] Cortical component falls more than medullary
     - (3) Vasoconstriction in response to angiotensin II similar in old and young
2. Distribution
   - (a) Cortex: 90% of RPF
     - (1) 2.0–5.0 ml/g/min
     - (2) Cortical $O_2ER = 0.18$
   - (b) Medulla
     - (1) Outer medulla receives about 1.0 ml/g/min
     - (2) Inner medulla flow is about 1% of total RBF
     - (3) Medullary $O_2ER = 0.79$, Pao_2 8–15 mm Hg
3. Regulation of RBF
   - (a) Renal perfusion pressure (RPP)
     - (1) $RPP = (MAP - RVP)/RVR$
       - [a] Where MAP is mean systemic arterial pressure, RVP is renal venous pressure, RVR is total renal vascular resistance

(2) RVP is slightly higher than inferior vena caval pressure, which is higher than central venous pressure. RVP is also higher than intra-abdominal pressure, which is approximated by bladder pressure

4. Renal vascular resistance is determined by
   (a) Autoregulation
      (1) Constancy of blood flow in the face of changes in renal perfusion pressure ranging from 70 to 180 mm Hg
   (b) Endothelial derived relaxing factor (EDRF)
      (1) Major regulator of vascular tone
      (2) Is nitric oxide (NO) or closely related substance
      (3) Half-life 1–2 seconds
         [a] Inactivated by hemoglobin, myoglobin, superoxide anions
      (4) Mediates vasodilation of many drugs and hormones
      (5) Production is impaired if endothelium is damaged, e.g., ischemia
   (c) Adrenergic system
      (1) Alpha agonists vasoconstrict with some preference for afferent arteriole
      (2) Beta agonists
         [a] Mild vasodilation
         [b] Release renin
         [c] Beta-antagonist agents
            i) Usually decrease RBF, GFR; increase RVR
            ii) Labetalol has no effect on RBF or GFR
            iii) Nadolol and teratolol actually increase RBF, decrease RVR, and at least do not decrease GFR
      (3) Dopamine
         [a] Dopaminergic$_1$ receptor (DA$_1$) mediate vasodilation
         [b] DA$_2$ receptors inhibit norepinephrine release
         [c] Dopexamine
            i) Beta$_2$ selective agonist and weak DA$_1$ and DA$_2$ agonist
            ii) Increase RBF
            iii) Increase urine flow rate
            iv) Inhibit catecholamine uptake
            v) Increase creatinine clearance in patients with CHF, but not after cardiopulmonary bypass
         [d] Fenoldopam is a selective DA1 agonist
   (d) Renin controls the generation of angiotensin II. Renin release from the macula densa is
      (1) Stimulated by
         [a] Hypotension via intrarenal baroreceptors
         [b] Beta-adrenergic agonists
         [c] Decreased delivery of sodium to the distal nephron JGA
         [d] Prostaglandin E$_2$ (PGE$_2$)
      (2) Depressed by
         [a] Angiotensin II
         [b] ANP
         [c] High rate of Na or Cl transport in distal nephron at the JGA
      (3) Angiotensinogen is produced in the liver
      (4) Angiotensin I is produced by the action of renin on angiotensinogen
      (5) Angiotensin converting enzyme (ACE) catalyzes the conversion of angiotensin I to angiotensin II
      (6) Angiotensin II
         [a] Receptors
            i) Distribution similar to that for ANP
         [b] Angiotensin II effects
            i) Vasoconstriction

II. Physiology; a. Renal blood flow (RBF), renal plasma flow (RPF) (continued)

        ii) Constricts the efferent arteriole more than the afferent arteriole

        iii) Efferent arteriole constricts in response to angiotensin II at 1/1000th the concentration required for afferent arteriolar constriction

        iv) Inhibits renin release

        v) Potentiates norepinephrine release

        vi) Reduces GFR by glomerular constriction

        vii) Releases aldosterone

        viii) Stimulates drinking

        ix) Stimulates proximal tubular sodium absorption

        x) Stimulates proximal tubular H^+ absorption

(7) Developmental

  [a] Aging

    i) Renin substrate concentration does not change with age

    ii) Lower baseline plasma renin activity (PRA)

    iii) Active renin falls with age, but PRA does not, suggesting a defect in conversion of inactive to active renin

    iv) Response to Na restriction blunted

    v) Response to upright posture blunted

(8) Interactions

  [a] Physiologic

    i) Head-down tilt during abdominal surgery had no effect on PRA

    ii) Positive fluid balance suppressed PRA

    iii) PRA is higher during general than epidural anesthesia

    iv) Cardiopulmonary bypass activates RAA

(e) Endothelial-derived-hyperpolarizing factor (EDHF)

  (1) Vasodilator

(f) Endothelin

  (1) Production stimulated by

    [a] Shear stress

    [b] Endothelial injury

    [c] Thrombin

    [d] Angiotensin II

    [e] Interleukin-1

    [f] Arginine vasopressin (AVP)

    [g] Epinephrine

    [h] Transforming growth factor beta

    [i] Endotoxin

    [j] Hypoxia

  (2) Metabolism

    [a] Half-life less than 2 minutes

    [b] Removed by lungs, kidneys, liver

    [c] Degraded by neutral endopeptidase 24.11

  (3) Three subtypes

  (4) Receptors

    [a] Belong to G protein–coupled superfamily of receptors

    [b] Found throughout kidney with higher concentrations in glomerular mesangial and epithelial cells, inner medulla, vasa recta

  (5) Actions inhibited by ANP, PGE_2, PGI_2, and calcium channel blockade

  (6) ET_1 and ET_2 are potent vasoconstrictors

    [a] Increase RVR, decrease RBF

      i) Efferent constriction greater than afferent

      ii) Greater effect in medulla than cortex

iii) Renal response much greater than most other vascular beds

iv) Antibodies to ET improve renal function after experimental renal artery occlusion

(7) Release EDRF, PGI_2, ANP, aldosterone, renin

(8) Renal effects

    [a] Decreases GFR

    [b] Decreases Na excretion

    [c] Releases PGE_2, PGI_2

    [d] Inhibits Na-K-ATPase

(9) Increases renin release after high dose, slightly decreases it after low dose

    [a] Increase may be due to renal ischemia

    [b] Renin release is inhibited in vitro

(10) Stimulates aldosterone production in zona glomerulosa and enhances release

(g) Tubuloglomerular feedback (TGF)

  (1) Increased delivery of NaCl to the macula densa causes afferent arteriolar constriction and renin-mediated angiotension II generation, thereby decreasing GFR

    [a] Protects against unregulated Na and H_2O loss when proximal tubule is damaged

  (2) Accounts for about 25% of resting RVR

  (3) DA_1 agonists in the lumen inhibit TGF

  (4) Adenosine-1 agonists inhibit TGF

  (5) Blunted by volume expansion

  (6) Enhanced by volume depletion

(h) Prostaglandins of the E series

  (1) Predominant renal eicosanoid

  (2) Act as vasodilators

  (3) No basal vasodilator action

  (4) When vasoconstriction occurs, PGE_2 is released and blunts the increase in arteriolar tone

  (5) When cyclooxygenase is inhibited (e.g., NSAID), excessive and prolonged vasoconstriction may result

  (6) Cyclosporine A, FK 506 inhibit synthesis

(i) Adenosine

  (1) Kinetics

    [a] Production increases during hypoxia as high-energy phosphates decline

    [b] Metabolized to uric acid

  (2) Effects

    [a] Receptors

      i) Adenosine-1

        a) Decreases cardiac output

        b) Inhibits renin release

        c) Decreases NE release

        d) Antagonizes adrenergic agonist effects on vasculature

      ii) Adenosine-2

        a) Direct active vasodilation in nearly all vascular beds

    [b] Renal

      i) Blood flow

        a) Afferent arteriolar vasoconstriction

        b) May tonically control RBF, because antagonism increases RBF

      ii) Filtration

        a) Reduces GFR

      iii) Transport

        a) Decreases urine output, UNaV (sodium excretion)

II. Physiology; a. Renal blood flow (RBF), renal plasma flow (RPF) (continued)

                b) May have basal inhibitory effect on Na excretion, because antagonists increase UNaV

(j) Vasopressin
- (1) Potent vasoconstrictor
  - [a] Appears to divert blood from the superficial cortex to juxtamedullary nephrons
- (2) Produced in the hypothalamus, transported to the posterior pituitary, where it is stored
- (3) Released when action potentials initiated in the hypothalamus depolarize the cell membrane
- (4) Release is initiated by
  - [a] Increasing osmolality of the interstitial fluid
    - i) Normal threshold for release is 285–290 mOsm/kg H_2O with maximal release at 290–295 mOsm/kg H_2O
    - ii) Full suppression occurs at osmolalities less than 280–285 mOsm/kg H_2O
  - [b] Hypovolemia, with a threshold value of about 10%
  - [c] Hypotension via afferents in the aorta and carotids
  - [d] Other
    - i) Stimuli associated with stress, including pain, nausea, anxiety. These appear to be mediated via dopaminergic central neurons
- (5) Effects of AVP are mediated by V_1 and V_2 receptors
  - [a] V_1 receptors mediate vasoconstriction
  - [b] V_2 receptors mediate changes in collecting tubule permeability to water

(k) Atrial natriuretic peptide (ANP)
- (1) Renal vasodilation when it is preconstricted, especially by angiotensin
- (2) ANP tends to oppose angiotensin II
- (3) Reduce afferent tone in relation to efferent tone

(l) Parathyroid hormone (PTH)
- (1) Increases RBF

(m) Miscellaneous factors of unknown physiologic significance that affect RBF
- (1) Acetylcholine: vasodilation
- (2) Bradykinin: vasodilation
- (3) Serotonin
- (4) Thromboxane: vasoconstriction

5. Interactions affecting RBF

(a) Diseases affecting RBF
- (1) Hypoxia increases RVR
- (2) Hypertension
  - [a] Increased RVR
  - [b] Decreased renal plasma flow (RPF)
  - [c] Increased glomerular capillary pressure
    - i) May lead to progressive glomerular sclerosis
    - ii) Seen only with MAP over 107 mm Hg
  - [d] Reducing BP slows the rate of loss of GFR
  - [e] Autoregulation curve shifted to right
- (3) Sepsis, septic shock
  - [a] PGE_1 reduces ratio of RBF/CO
- (4) Hypovolemic shock
  - [a] Inhibition of NO (EDRF) with L-NMMA raised MAP, RVR, RPF in hypovolemic rats

(b) Drug effects on RBF
- (1) Adrenergic

[a] Epinephrine infusion raises BP, SVR
  i) During the first 30 minutes, RVR increases, then returns toward control, resulting in a transient reduction, followed by a sustained elevation above baseline of RBF
(c) Surgery, anesthesia
  (1) Patients undergoing aortic surgery while anesthetized with halothane had lower RPF and GFR as compared with isoflurane

b. Glomerular filtration rate (GFR)

1. 140 ml/min/1.73 m^2 at 25–34 years
2. Filtration rate is determined by forces described in the modified Starling equation
   (a) GFR = Kf{(Pgc − Pt) − r(πgc − πt)}
      (1) Kf is the ultrafiltration coefficient, which is a function of area and conductivity
         [a] Kf is proportional to hydraulic conductivity
            i) Capillary pores filter out cells
            ii) Basement membrane filters out proteins
            iii) Negative charges retard passage of negatively charged substances
            iv) Allows passage of molecules smaller than proteins
            v) Filtration slits between negatively charged foot processes filter smaller molecules
            vi) Molecules less than 18–20Å are freely filtered
            vii) Molecules 18–36Å are filtered selectively depending somewhat on charge
            viii) Molecules larger than 36Å are not normally filtered
         [b] Kf is proportional to glomerular surface area
            i) Number of glomeruli
            ii) Area of individual glomerulus is regulated by contractile mesangial cells
            iii) Endothelin-1, AVP, angiotensin II, sympathetic nerve stimulation, norepinephrine, and thromboxane cause contraction
            iv) Dopamine, alpha-$_2$ agonists, and PGE$_2$ increase intracellular cAMP and relax mesangial cells
      (2) Pgc is determined by MAP, afferent arteriolar resistance, and efferent arteriolar resistance
      (3) Pt (the pressure in Bowman's space and the proximal tubule) is relatively constant ($\sim$10 mm Hg) in the absence of obstruction
      (4) r is the reflection coefficient, which is a term describing the relative ability of a semipermeable membrane to prevent the passage of molecules of a defined size and/or charge
         [a] r is 1.0 if the molecule is completely prevented from passing, and is 0 if the molecule passes as freely as water
      (5) πgc − πt are the oncotic (colloid osmotic) pressures in the glomerular capillary (20–25 mm Hg) and proximal tubule (0 mm Hg), respectively
   (b) Filtration fraction is GFR/RPF
      (1) Normally 0.20 (roughly 10–12% of RBF)
      (2) Increased if ratio of efferent/afferent resistance increases, e.g., angiotensin II
3. Regulation of GFR
   (a) Autoregulation similar to RBF autoregulation
   (b) Tubuloglomerular feedback
      (1) GFR falls when NaCl delivery to the distal nephron is increased
      (2) TGF is mediated in part by the renin-angiotensin system

    (c) Atrial natriuretic peptide (ANP) increases GFR
    (d) Glucocorticoids increase GFR
    (e) Protein intake increases GFR
       (1) A measure of renal functional reserve capacity

4. Age
    (a) Perinatal
       (1) Premature infants have low GFR due to incomplete nephrogenesis and high-renin-induced renal vasoconstriction
    (b) Elderly
       (1) GFR declines about 1% per year after age 30
          [a] 140 ml/min/1.73 m^2 at 25–34 years to 97 at 75–84 years
          [b] A reduction of 8 ml/min/1.73 m^2 per decade
          [c] At age 85 to 90 years, GFR is reduced about 50% of normal
          [d] Decline is variable and one third have no decline at all
          [e] Rate of decline increases with increased age
          [f] Intercurrent diseases of the elderly that result in progressive deterioration include hypertension, diabetes, atherosclerosis, infections, drugs, excess protein intake
       (2) Cockcroft equation quantitates loss with age

$$GFR = \frac{(140 - Age\ [in\ years]) \cdot Weight\ (kg)}{72 \cdot Creatinine\ (mg/dl)}$$
$$(multiply\ by\ 0.85\ for\ females)$$

          [a] Use ideal body weight (IBW) if very obese, edematous. IBW = 50 kg + 2.3 kg × (height in inches − 60) for men. Substitute a baseline weight of 45 kg for women
       (3) Kf and r appear to be normal in the elderly

---

c. Tubular transport

1. Active (energy-dependent) transport by Na-K-ATPase creates concentration gradients for sodium between the interstitial fluid and cell interior

    (a) Na-K-ATPase is located mostly in basolateral membranes
    (b) Na-K-ATPase has low activity at birth but increases rapidly postnatally due to increased enzyme synthesis
    (c) Na pumping accounts for most of the O_2 consumption of kidney

2. Passive diffusion down electrochemical gradients accounts for transport of most substances in the kidney; the electrochemical gradients are produced by sodium pumps

3. Carrier-mediated transport
    (a) Secondarily active transport (cotransport and countertransport)
       (1) Active transport produces concentration gradients that then drive other carrier proteins
    (b) Cotransport (symporters)
       (1) Carrier molecule in the membrane has a receptor for a molecule that exists in differing concentrations inside as compared with outside the cell, the driving molecule, which is usually sodium
          [a] Gradient for the driving molecule is produced by energy-consuming primary transport
          [b] The carrier also binds with another type of molecule being transported, for example, glucose
          [c] When both the sodium and glucose are bound, the carrier transports

both the sodium and glucose from the lumen into the cell, releasing them into the interior when the sodium dissociates from the carrier

    [d] The maximal rate of glucose transport declines about 1% per year

        i) Associated with fewer mitochondria, lower enzyme concentration, lower Na-K-ATPase concentration, lower Na pumping, and decreased O_2 consumption

  (c) Countertransport (antiporters) is similar to cotransport, except that the molecule being transported (e.g., PAH) moves in the direction opposite to that of the driving molecule (sodium)

    (1) Maximal rate of PAH secretion declines about 1% per year

d. Tubular transport and permeability vary significantly among the different nephron segments

1. Proximal convoluted tubule
   (a) Freely permeable to water via paracellular route
   (b) High level of primary and secondarily active transport
       (1) Sodium absorption
       (2) Phosphate absorption
       (3) Amino acids absorption
       (4) Small proteins absorbed
       (5) Glucose absorbed
       (6) Organic acids absorbed and secreted
       (7) Organic bases absorbed and secreted

2. Descending limb
   (a) Little or no active or mediated transport
   (b) Highly permeable to water, which moves into interstitium
   (c) Impermeable to solute

3. Thin ascending limb
   (a) Little or no activity or mediated transport
   (b) Impermeable to water
   (c) Permeable to solute

4. Thick ascending limb
   (a) Impermeable to water
   (b) High level of active transport
       (1) Sodium
       (2) Calcium
       (3) Magnesium

5. Distal convoluted tubule
   (a) Water permeability low
   (b) Active transport
       (1) Sodium absorption
       (2) Potassium secretion

6. Connecting tubule
   (a) Water permeability low
   (b) Active transport
       (1) Sodium absorption
       (2) H^+, K secretion

7. Collecting duct
   (a) Permeability to water regulated primarily by vasopressin acting via V_2 vasopressin receptors

e. Regulation of tubular function

1. Aldosterone
    (a) Produced from cholesterol in zona glomerulosa of adrenal cortex
    (b) Release
        (1) Stimulated by
            [a] Angiotensin II
            [b] Hyperkalemia
            [c] ACTH
                i) Effect lasts less than 24 hours
            [d] Negative Na balance
            [e] Endothelin
        (2) Inhibited by
            [a] Chronic heparin therapy
            [b] Dopamine
                i) Metoclopramide blocks dopamine, thus stimulating aldosterone
                   release
            [c] ANP
    (c) Effects of aldosterone
        (1) Receptors are intracellular
            [a] Binds to DNA to induce production of Na channels, K channels,
                Na-K-ATPase
            [b] Neonates have blunted response
        (2) Renal
            [a] Transport
                i) Stimulates the reabsorption of sodium
                    a) Increases either the percentage of time that apical sodium
                       channels are open or the number of channels or both
                    b) Increases Na-K-ATPase activity in the basolateral membrane of
                       the distal tubule and collecting duct, particularly the cortical
                       collecting duct
                    c) Effect takes 3 to 6 hours to develop
                ii) Stimulates secretion of potassium
                    a) Increases potassium conductance in the basolateral membrane
                       of the distal tubule and collecting duct
                    b) Increased cellular entry of sodium creates a negative luminal
                       electrical potential
                    c) Potassium and protons move down their electrical gradients
                       from the cell to the lumen, causing kaliuresis, hypokalemia and
                       proton excretion, and alkalosis
                iii) Redistributes K to intracellular space
    (d) Aldosterone interactions
        (1) Physiologic
            [a] Dopamine suppresses release
        (2) Diseases
            [a] Plot the aldosterone level (pmol/L) against the aldosterone/PRA ratio
            [b] Hypoaldosteronism is characterized by
                i) Hyponatremia
                ii) Volume depletion
                iii) Hyperkalemia
                iv) Etiology
                    a) Tuberculosis
                    b) Metastatic neoplasms

                c) Autoimmune diseases
                d) Cytomegalovirus (CMV)
                e) Human immunodeficiency virus (HIV)
                f) Septic shock
            [c] Hyperaldosteronism is characterized by
               i) Hypertension
              ii) Hypokalemia
              iii) Metabolic alkalosis
              iv) Etiology
                  a) Adrenal hyperplasia
                  b) High renin level
                  c) Adrenal adenoma
                  d) Enzyme deficiencies (e.g., licorice ingestion)
        (3) Drug effects on aldosterone
            [a] Dopamine suppresses release
            [b] Metoclopramide blocks dopamine inhibition of release
            [c] Etomidate blocks production
            [d] Ketoconazole blocks production
        (4) Levels lower in elderly

2. Parathyroid hormone (PTH)

    (a) Kinetics
        (1) Produced in four parathyroid glands
        (2) Release stimulated by
            [a] Hypocalcemia
            [b] Mg^{++}
               i) Mild hypomagnesemia stimulates
            [c] Beta- and alpha-adrenergic agonists
            [d] Dopamine
            [e] Volume expansion
            [f] Prostaglandins
            [g] Hyperchloremic acidosis
            [h] 1,25-dihydroxyvitamin D
        (3) Release inhibited by
            [a] Hypercalcemia
            [b] Severe hypomagnesemia
            [c] Hypermagnesemia
            [d] Vitamin D
            [e] Calcitriol suppresses PTH by decreasing set point for PTH release by Ca, decreasing production of PTH precursor, and depressing PT cell proliferation
        (4) Excretion
            [a] Cleared by kidney (accumulates in renal failure)
    (b) Effects
        (1) Renal
            [a] Increases RBF
            [b] Transport
               i) Phosphate, HCO_3^-
              ii) Increases urinary acid excretion resulting in metabolic alkalosis (see "Acid base")
        (2) Stimulates Ca reabsorption by proximal tubule

3. Alpha-adrenergic

    (a) Stimulates proximal sodium reabsorption

4. Angiotensin II

    (a) Effects

II. Physiology; e. Regulation of tubular function (continued)

    (1) Releases aldosterone
    (2) Stimulates drinking
    (3) Renal
        [a] Stimulates proximal tubular sodium absorption
        [b] Stimulates proximal tubular H^+ absorption
    (4) Cardiovascular
        [a] Vasoconstriction
            i) By stimulating Ca influx via voltage-dependent Ca channels, perhaps mediated by G protein
            ii) Stimulates formation of IP3
            iii) Stimulates formation of DAG

5. Dopaminergic

  (a) Concentration of receptors higher in kidney than in most tissues
    (1) Preferential localization to the cortex
    (2) Probably basal dopamine-mediated vasodilation
    (3) Dopamine-$_1$ receptor activation inhibits Na absorption
        [a] Stimulates adenyl cyclase activity
        [b] Inhibits the Na-H antiporter
            i) Reduces proximal NaCl and $NaHCO_3$ absorption
        [c] Inhibits Na-K-ATPase
    (4) May be produced by conversion of filtered dopa by dopadecarboxylase inside the tubular cells
    (5) Catabolized by monoamine oxidase, type A
        [a] Increasing sodium concentrations increase renal dopamine production
    (6) ANP decreases DA formation by the kidney
    (7) Glomerular mesangial relaxation
        [a] Increased Kf
    (8) Increased Pgc
        [a] Due to afferent dilation
    (9) Net effect is diuresis
        [a] Primarily by inhibition of Na absorption
        [b] Secondarily by increasing RBF and GFR

6. Atrial natriuretic peptides (ANP)

  (a) Related compounds
    (1) Urodilatin
    (2) Brain NP (BNP)
    (3) C-type NP
  (b) Receptors
    (1) Prime receptor is termed ANP-Rgc(A) (also known as type B, type I(R1), ANPR-A, guanylate cyclase-A, GC-A)
        [a] Membrane-bound (particulate) guanylate cyclase is an integral part of the receptor
            i) Increases intracellular cGMP, which decreases intracellular calcium levels
            ii) ANP increases cGMP content of cultured smooth muscle cells 20-fold
            iii) Involves an action on the inhibitory G protein
        [b] Also contains protein kinase
        [c] Mediates the physiologic effects of ANP
        [d] Found in the glomerular mesangial cells, descending vasa recta, inner medullary collecting duct, renal medullary interstitial cells, vascular

smooth muscle, endothelial cells, lung tissue, lung fibroblasts, and adrenal zona glomerulosa cells

    i) Receptors and physiologic action demonstrated definitively in the glomerulus and the inner medullary collecting duct

    ii) Indirect evidence that they exist in all parts of the nephron except the thick ascending limb and distal tubule

    iii) The highest concentrations occur in the inner medullary collecting duct

    iv) Low density of receptors in the proximal tubule

(2) ANP-Rgc(B) is activated by C-type NP

    [a] Contains guanylate cyclase and protein kinase

    [b] Found in kidney, cerebellum, pituitary, lung, and adrenal medulla

(3) C receptors (ANP-Rc, ANPR-C)

    [a] Do not contain protein kinase or guanylate cyclase sequences

    [b] Have no known physiologic effects

    [c] Bind the agonist with high affinity

    [d] Mediate destruction of the hormone

    [e] Account for 95% of all ANP receptors

    [f] ANP-Rc receptor density is increased by dehydration

(c) Regulation of ANP

(1) Produced and stored in cardiac atrial myocytes, R > L

(2) Released by atrial stretch

(3) Endothelin releases ANP

(4) ANP levels tend to parallel atrial size

    [a] Elevated in fluid overload, heart failure

    [b] Depressed when cardiac size is diminished (PEEP or cardiac tamponade)

    [c] ANP levels increase by 10–15 pmol/L for each 1 mm Hg rise in atrial pressure

(5) ANP markedly increased in traumatic hypovolemia and falls to normal after resuscitation

(6) Plasma levels correlate directly with sodium balance

(7) Glucocorticoids, testosterone, adrenocorticotrophic hormone, and cardiac hypoxia may increase ANP secretion

(8) Elderly tend to have higher ANP levels

    [a] Correlates with increased exchangeable sodium

    [b] Less depression of ANP levels in the upright posture

    [c] Greater response to infused saline

(9) Urodilatin

    [a] Contains 32 amino acids

        i) Identical to ANP with the addition of four amino acids

    [b] Produced in the distal nephron

    [c] Synthesized and released from the kidney by hypervolemia by a mechanism requiring cardiac innervation

    [d] Released by saline infusion by a more direct intrarenal action, or by an effect of sodium concentration within the brain

(d) Effects of ANP

(1) Renal

    [a] Little change in RBF

    [b] High concentrations increase GFR

        i) Glomerular mesangial cell relaxation

            a) Increases the ultrafiltration coefficient

        ii) Afferent arteriolar dilation and efferent constriction increases glomerular capillary pressure

II. Physiology; e. Regulation of tubular function (continued)

a) Afferent dilation is minimal unless preexisting constriction is present
- Especially if induced by angiotensin II

iii) Delivers an abnormally large volume of filtrate to the proximal tubule, which has limited capacity to increase the fraction of filtrate absorbed

iv) An increased volume reaches the distal nephron

v) ANP also inhibits tubuloglomerular feedback

[c] ANP and urodilatin block apical sodium channels in the inner medullary collecting duct after binding to basolateral receptors coupled to guanylate cyclase

i) Reduces the probability of the apical channel's being open without affecting its conductance or ion selectivity

ii) It is possible that ANP does not normally reach the distal nephron because of degradation by proximal tubular endopeptidase

a) Urodilatin may be the physiologically active hormone in the collecting duct

iii) ANP also increases excretion of calcium, magnesium, and phosphate, suggesting a proximal tubular action

[d] ANP, but not urodilatin, inhibits aldosterone secretion directly and by blunting renin release

i) ANP blunts aldosterone release induced by adrenocorticotrophic hormone (ACTH), angiotensin II, and potassium

(2) Cardiovascular

[a] Reduction in mean arterial blood pressure (MAP)

[b] Reduced plasma volume

i) Decreased cardiac output

[c] More effective in relaxing preexisting vascular tone (e.g., induced by angiotensin II, norepinephrine (probably via alpha-$_1$ receptors), serotonin, histamine)

(3) Brain natriuretic peptide (BNP) when injected into cerebrospinal fluid (CSF) inhibits sodium intake, water intake, AVP, and ACTH release, and raises blood pressure

(e) ANP is rapidly inactivated by endopeptidase

(f) Interactions

(1) Physiologic

[a] Blunts AVP response to hypovolemia

[b] Inhibits aldosterone release response to hypotension

[c] Inhibits sympathetic nervous system (SNS) response to hypotension

[d] ANP is physiologic angiotensin II antagonist

[e] Na depletion blunts diuretic effect of ANP, as does hypotension

[f] ANP levels were not changed by head-down tilt during abdominal surgery

(2) Drugs

[a] Patients anesthetized with narcotics appropriately elevate ANP levels during fluid infusion

[b] Morphine and fentanyl (mu agonists) increase ANP levels, while kappa agonists do not

[c] Fentanyl per se did not change ANP levels or the response to fluid loading

[d] Phenylephrine increases ANP levels and fentanyl appears to blunt this effect

[e] Alpha$_1$- and alpha$_2$-adrenergic stimulation increases ANP secretion

           [f] Halothane increased or failed to change, while pentobarbital decreased, ANP levels. Deep anesthesia with halothane potentiated the rise in ANP induced by volume loading

    (g) Diseases

        (1) Patients with COPD have higher levels than normal, but not affected by level of PA pressure

    (h) Miscellaneous

        (1) Cardiopulmonary bypass does not change ANP levels

7. Arginine vasopressin (AVP)

    (a) Regulation of release controlled by hypothalamus

        (1) Osmolality

           [a] Fully suppressed at osmolality less than 280–285 mOsm/kg H_2O

           [b] Fully activated at osmolality over 290–295 mOsm/kg H_2O

        (2) Hypovolemia

           [a] Overrides osmoregulation

           [b] 10% reduction in plasma volume is threshold

        (3) Hypotension

           [a] Overrides osmolar and volume regulation

           [b] Most drug effects are actually secondary to hemodynamic effects of drug

        (4) Stress

           [a] Nausea, vomiting, pain, hypoxia

           [b] Mediated by dopaminergic neurons

        (5) Alpha$_2$ agonists inhibit secretion

    (b) Effects

        (1) Cardiovascular

           [a] Vasoconstriction by V_1 receptor stimulation

             i) Reduced blood flow

             ii) Minimal effect on blood pressure due to reduction in sympathetic system activation

        (2) Increased permeability of collecting duct to water and urea by V_2 receptor stimulation

           [a] If medullary interstitium is hypertonic, fluid is reabsorbed and urine flow rate falls

           [b] Maximal dilution if AVP less than 1 pmol/L

           [c] Maximal concentration, if AVP is greater than 5 pmol/L

        (3) Platelet aggregation by V_1 receptor

        (4) Release of coagulation factors

    (c) Interactions

        (1) Drugs

           [a] Diuretic effect impaired by PGE_2, alpha$_1$, alpha$_2$, adrenergic stimulation, lithium

             i) Clonidine increased urine output during isoflurane anesthesia

           [b] Kappa agonists inhibit AVP release

           [c] EtOH inhibits release

         (2) Pregnancy resets release threshold to about 275 mOsm/kg H_2O

        (3) Aging

           [a] AVP release and kinetics in the elderly are probably not very different from those in the young adult

           [b] Kidney responsiveness to vasopressin falls with age, resulting in impaired urinary concentrating ability after water deprivation

             i) After an overnight fast, urine osmolality (UOsm) is 400–600 in the healthy 85-year-old, contrasted with a UOsm of 1,000 mOsm/kg H_2O in the 30-year-old

II. Physiology; e. Regulation of tubular function (continued)

        [c] Elderly persons responded normally at low doses of AVP, but did not reach the same maximal UOsm at higher infusion rates, suggesting a failure to develop concentrated interstitium rather than impaired AVP responsiveness

  (4) Miscellaneous

        [a] Head-down tilt during abdominal surgery had no influence on AVP levels

---

f. Metabolic or endocrine functions of the kidney

1. Erythropoietin (EPO)

  (a) Kinetics

     (1) Production

        [a] Abnormal ectopic production can lead to polycythemia in renal cell carcinoma, hepatoma, uterine fibromyoma, cerebellar hemangioblastoma

        [b] Inappropriately low levels

           i) Renal disease

          ii) Inflammatory diseases (anemia of chronic disease)

         iii) Malignancy

          iv) HIV infection

           v) Prematurity

        [c] Functional protein is 165 amino acids

        [d] Produced primarily in liver in fetus, but by the kidney after birth although liver (Kupffer and hepatocytes) may contribute during hypoxic stress; anephric patients produce some EPO

           i) Produced primarily in the inner cortex and outer medulla in a peritubular interstitial cell

     (2) Release

        [a] Regulation of release is primarily related to hypoxia and anemia

           i) Not affected by acute or chronic exercise

          ii) Renal O_2 tension seems to be a primary stimulus

         iii) Cobalt, nickel, manganese may stimulate production

          iv) CO inhibits hypoxia-induced production

             a) May involve a heme protein

     (3) Concentration

        [a] Normal level 4–30 mU/ml plasma

  (b) Effects

     (1) Induces proliferation and differentiation of erythroid precursor cells

  (c) Interactions

     (1) Diseases

        [a] Response to acute anemia blocked in critically ill children compared with those with chronic anemia

        [b] Erythropoietin therapy may worsen hypertension in end-stage renal disease (ESRD) patients

        [c] Erythropoietin therapy requires 12–14 weeks to raise hemoglobin (Hb) from 7.4 to 10 g/dl in ESRD

        [d] EPO is used in conjunction with autologous blood donation to reduce transfusion requirements during elective surgery

2. Vitamin D

  (a) Kinetics

     (1) Uptake and production

        [a] Absorbed from the gut

[b] Produced in skin under influence of ultraviolet light
    i) Reduced efficiency in elderly
[c] Hydroxylated in the liver to 25-hydroxyvitamin D
[d] Kidney hydroxylates to 1,25-dihydroxyvitamin D
    i) Stimulated by PTH
    ii) Stimulated by low inorganic phosphate (Pi)
    iii) Inhibited by high Pi, low pH, 1,25-dihydroxyvitamin D, renal insufficiency, sepsis, rhabdomyolysis, and pancreatitis

(b) Effects
  (1) Renal
    [a] Stimulates Ca reabsorption

(c) Interactions
  (1) Elderly have marked reduction in capacity for hydroxylation of 25-OH-vitamin D to 1,25(OH)2-vitamin D

g. Acid-base balance

1. Kinetics
(a) Net acid load $\approx$ 1 mMol/kg/day
  (1) 40% titratable acid
  (2) 60% ammonium
  (3) Filters and absorbs 65 mEq/kg/day bicarbonate
(b) Proximal tubule pumps protons into lumen
  (1) 65% via Na-H antiporter, driven by Na gradient produced by basolateral Na-K-ATPase
    [a] Activated by intracellular acidosis, increased GFR, angiotensin II, potassium depletion, glucocorticoids, growth hormone, and alpha$_2$-adrenergic agonists
    [b] Inhibited by increased peritubular (blood) bicarbonate or pH, PTH, and cAMP
  (2) 35% via H-ATPase located inside the apical membrane
  (3) Apical membrane Cl^--OH and a Cl^--formate exchanger, which balance the Na^+ uptake
  (4) Protons combine with bicarbonate to produce carbonic acid (H_2CO_3)
  (5) H_2CO_3 forms CO_2 and H_2O under influence of carbonic anhydrase (CA) in the brush border
  (6) CO_2 enters the tubular cell
    [a] Under the influence of CA, CO_2 is hydrated to H_2CO_3, which dissociates into H^+ and HCO_3^- intracellularly
  (7) The bicarbonate exits from the cell via a basolateral membrane $Na^+(HCO_3^-)_3$ symporter activated by sodium and following the electrogenic gradient; cell negative in relation to the interstitium
  (8) The pH of the fluid leaving the proximal convoluted tubule is about 6.7 and the HCO_3^- about 8 mEq/L
  (9) Volume loading increases paracellular back-diffusion of bicarbonate
  (10) Proximal tubule generates two ammonium ions and bicarbonate from glutamine
    [a] Ammonium production accelerated by PTH, metabolic acidosis, acute respiratory acidosis, and potassium depletion
    [b] Metabolic alkalosis and hyperkalemia decrease NH_3 production
  (11) Phosphate is reabsorbed by the proximal tubule via a Na-PO$_4$ cotransporter
    [a] Parathyroid hormone inhibits PO$_4$ absorption
      i) Increases titratable acid excretion

II. Physiology; g. Acid-base balance (continued)

    (c) Thin descending limb
      (1) Selectively removes water, thus causing the HCO_3^- concen- tration to increase from 8 mEq/L to 24 mEq/L at the bend
    (d) Thin ascending limb
      (1) Permeable to NH_4^+, which probably diffuses into the interstitium
      (2) High medullary interstitial concentration of NH_3 facilitates uptake into the medullary collecting duct
    (e) Thick ascending limb (TALH)
      (1) Absorbs 75–80% of delivered HCO_3^-
      (2) Lowers HCO_3^- to about 5 mEq/L
      (3) Absorbs 10–15% of filtered HCO_3^-
      (4) H^+ secretion via Na-H antiporter, HCO_3^- extrusion across basolateral membrane driven by voltage gradient
      (5) Absorbs 50% of the delivered ammonium
         [a] Via a paracellular cation-selective pathway due to a lumen-positive transepithelial gradient
         [b] At least 65% of TALH NH_4^+ absorption occurs by substitution for K^+ in the Na^+-K^+-$2Cl^-$ cotransporter in the apical membrane
            i) Thus, furosemide and hyperkalemia inhibit NH_4^+ uptake
    (f) Collecting duct
      (1) Responsible for the final pH
      (2) pH declines progressively along duct
      (3) Secretes only 10% of the hydrogen ion (low capacity)
      (4) It can generate a 3 pH unit gradient (1,000:1)
      (5) Contains type A (acid-secreting) and type B (bicarbonate-secreting) intercalated cells
         [a] Stimulated by aldosterone
      (6) During acidosis, the luminal membrane proton pump of type A intercalated cells secretes protons into the lumen, resulting in HCO_3^- absorption
      (7) During alkalosis, the proton pump in the basolateral membrane of the type B cells pumps protons into the interstitium, resulting in HCO_3^- excretion
      (8) Collecting duct secretes most of the NH_4^+
         [a] NH_3 accumulated in the medullary interstitium provides a gradient to move into the collecting duct lumen, where it can combine with secreted H^+
      (9) Despite normal pH and HCO_3^-, elderly subjects had reduced ability to excrete an acid load due to reduced ammonia excretion
  2. Regulation of renal acid-base balance
    (a) Aldosterone facilitates proton excretion
      (1) Stimulation of sodium absorption by the principal cells causes the lumen to become more negatively charged, thus facilitating lumenal entry of H^+
      (2) Direct stimulation of the proton pump rate capacity, but not gradient generating capacity
      (3) NH_4^+ secretion into the collecting duct is impaired by aldosterone deficiency, as is proton secretion
    (b) Angiotensin II may stimulate net activity of the Na-H antiporter
      (1) May also stimulate the antiporter by activating protein kinase C directly
    (c) PTH markedly stimulates HCO_3^- absorption in the cortical collecting tubule (CCT), probably due to increased phosphate delivery
    (d) Beta$_2$-agonists increase HCO_3^- absorption
    (e) Alpha$_2$-agonists reduce proximal HCO_3^- absorption
    (f) Dopamine$_1$-receptor activation reduces $NaHCO_3$ absorption
    (g) Chronic severe K depletion stimulates HCO_3^- reabsorption and can produce

alkalosis when combined with Na restriction or hypovolemia; also depresses aldosterone secretion, which leads to metabolic alkalosis

(h) Acute hyperkalemia or K infusion depresses HCO_3^- reabsorption; chronic K loading depresses proton secretion, ammonium excretion, and net acid excretion

(i) AVP-V_2 receptor stimulation stimulates HCO_3^- absorption in the CCT

(j) ANP inhibits angiotensin II–induced volume absorption and Na-H antiporter and Na-PO_4 transporter activity; both effects may be due to dopamine release

(k) Glucagon stimulates net HCO_3^- secretion by type B intercalated cells of the CCT

3. Interactions
(a) Elderly
(1) Normal pH, HCO_3^-
(2) Delayed excretion of an acid load with a smaller percentage as NH_4^+, although amount per GFR was normal

h. Sodium balance (MW = 23)

1. Kinetics
(a) Normal intake 1–2 mEq/(kg × day)
(b) Kidney matches Na output to equal intake minus nonrenal losses
(c) Proximal tubule absorbs 60–80% of filtered load
(d) Thick ascending limb absorbs about 20% of filtered Na
(e) Neonates
(1) Preterm infants have limited ability to excrete Na load due to low GFR, hyperaldosteronism, preferential perfusion of juxtamedullary nephrons, increased clearance of ANP, catecholamine-induced Na absorption, extracellular fluid (ECF) redistribution
(2) Limited ability to tolerate Na restriction due to impaired aldosterone production, impaired distal nephron responsive- ness to aldosterone, decreased proximal Na absorption

2. Regulation
(a) ANP increases excretion
(b) Angiotensin II decreases excretion
(c) Aldosterone decreases excretion

3. Interactions
(a) Elderly fail to reduce Na excretion as quickly as do young subjects when Na intake is restricted
(b) Disease
(1) Hypernatremia
[a] Pathophysiology
i) Usually due to excess water loss
[b] Therapy
i) Severe chronic hypernatremia may be well tolerated
ii) Stop abnormal water loss
iii) Administer hypotonic fluid
(2) Hyponatremia
[a] Pathophysiology
i) Usually due to water retention
ii) Often associated with mild Na depletion
iii) Thiazides are often implicated
iv) Risk factors
a) Females account for most cases, with premenopausal women most at risk

        b) Hypothyroidism, renal disease, pneumonia, dehydration, seizure disorder, EtOH abuse, diabetes, UTI, liver disease, anemia, pulmonary disease, GI disease, heart failure, mental disorders, cancer, hypertension

   [b] Therapy

      i) Myelinolysis, especially in pons, may occur 2–3 days after rapid correction

         a) In animal models, lesion correlates not with hyponatremia, but with rapid elevation of Na

         b) Correlates with magnitude of correction better than with rate of correction

         c) Also seen in rapidly developing hypernatremia

      ii) Rate of correction should be proportional to rate of development

         a) Rapid correction should be slowed as soon as the CNS symptoms begin resolving

         b) An increase of 4–6 mEq/L over 3–4 hours may be reasonable for patients with convulsions

         c) If less than 24 hours in duration, correct by as much as 20 mEq/L per 24 hours (0.6 mEq/L/hr) but only until over 120 mEq/L

         d) If more than 72 hours in duration, correct by no more than 12 mEq/L per 24 hours (0.5 mEq/L/hr) until over 120

      iii) If due to thiazide diuretic, stopping diuretic causes rapid reversal

      iv) Correction of hypokalemia facilitates redistribution of Na from intracellular space

      v) Restoration of plasma volume facilitates production of dilute urine

      vi) Electrolyte-free H_2O should be restricted

      vii) Measurement of urinary Na excretion (UNaV), UOsm, [Na] in GI or other losses will allow calculation of minimal amount of Na to administer

i. Potassium balance (MW = 39)

  1. Kinetics

    (a) Normal intake 1.5–2 mEq/(kg × day)

    (b) Kidney matches K output to equal intake

    (c) Proximal tubule absorbs most filtered K

  2. Regulation

    (a) Aldosterone

      (1) Redistributes K to intracellular space

      (2) Increases urinary K excretion chronically

    (b) Beta-adrenergic agonist

      (1) Redistributes K to intracellular space

    (c) H^+

      (1) Acidosis redistributes K to extracellular space

      (2) Alkalosis redistributes K to intracellular space

    (d) Insulin

      (1) Redistributes K to intracellular space

  3. Hypokalemia

    (a) Pathophysiology

      (1) Renal loss

        [a] Diuretics

        [b] Nephrotoxins

[c] Diabetic ketoacidosis may lead to 5-mEq/kg deficit
(2) Redistribution to intracellular space
[a] Reversal of catabolic state during nutritional support
[b] Beta-adrenergic stimulation
[c] Alkalosis
(3) Diuresis
(4) Gastric suction
(b) Effects
(1) Ventricular arrhythmia with K less than 3.0 mEq/L
(2) Impair response to antiarrhythmic agents
(3) Muscle weakness
(4) Rhabdomyolysis
(5) Vasoconstriction
(6) Renal magnesium wasting
(7) Increased susceptibility to aminoglycoside toxicity
4. Hyperkalemia
(a) Pathophysiology
(1) Redistribution from intracellular space
[a] Tissue damage
[b] Acute acidosis
(2) Reduced excretion
[a] Kidney failure
[b] Trimethoprim inhibits K excretion, by amiloridelike action
[c] K-sparing diuretics

j. Calcium balance (MW = 40)

1. Regulation
(a) PTH raises Ca^{++}
(b) Parathyroid hormone–related protein raises Ca^{++}
(c) Calcitonin lowers Ca^{++}
(d) Vitamin D formed in kidney by hydroxylation of 25-hydroxyvitamin D raises Ca^{++}
(1) Stimulated by PTH
(2) Stimulated by low Pi
(3) Inhibited by high Pi
(4) Inhibited by low pH
(5) Inhibited by 1,25-dihydroxyvitamin D
(6) Inhibited by renal insufficiency
(7) Inhibited by sepsis, rhabdomyolysis, pancreatitis
(8) Stimulates renal reabsorption of Ca
2. Hypocalcemia
(a) Pathophysiology
(1) 67% of critically ill are hypocalcemic, but only 15% have ionized hypocalcemia
(2) Increased binding on protein
(3) Precipitation in tissue
[a] Pancreatitis
[b] Rhabdomyolysis
(b) Effects
(1) Decreases sensitivity to digoxin
(2) Potentiates nephrotoxins
(3) Lowered seizure threshold

k. Chloride balance (MW = 35.5)

1. Kinetics
   (a) Proximal tubule passively absorbs about two thirds of filtered Cl in the later parts of the tubule down its concentration gradient
2. Hypochloremia
   (a) Chloride dose = $(Cl_{desired} - Cl_{measured}) \times 0.2 \times weight$
3. Hyperchloremic metabolic acidosis
   (a) Common in acutely ill patients after saline resuscitation, especially with renal injury

l. Phosphate balance (Pi MW = 31)

1. Kinetics
   (a) 10 mmol/1,000 kcal
   (b) Absorbed in duodenum and jejunum
      (1) Stimulated by vitamin D
      (2) 1 mmol/kg/day
   (c) Filtered at glomerulus
   (d) Proximal tubule absorbs most (80%) of filtered phosphate by Na-Pi symporter, 10% absorbed distally
   (e) Secreted into gut
      (1) May be trapped by angiotensin I antacids, Ca, sucralfate
2. Regulation
   (a) PTH inhibits proximal reabsorption
   (b) Cortisol inhibits proximal reabsorption
   (c) Glucagon inhibits proximal reabsorption

m. Magnesium balance (MW = 24)

1. Kinetics
   (a) Excretion
      (1) Filtered
      (2) 25–30% absorbed proximally
      (3) 60–75% reabsorbed by thick ascending limb
         [a] Inhibited by osmotic and loop diuretics, tubular toxins, hypercalciuria
      (4) 2–5% reabsorbed distally
   (b) Uptake
      (1) Intake 18–20 mmol/day, of which about one third is absorbed, i.e., 0.1 mmol/kg*day of absorbed Mg
      (2) PTH increases gut absorption
2. Regulation
   (a) Aldosterone increases excretion
   (b) PTH decreases excretion, increases gut absorption
   (c) Insulin causes shift to intracellular space
3. Hypomagnesemia
   (a) Cause
      (1) Poor intake
         [a] Alcoholism
         [b] Malabsorption

        (2) Intestinal loss
          [a] Diarrhea
          [b] Gastric suction
        (3) Renal loss
          [a] Loop diuretics
          [b] Digoxin
          [c] Hypokalemia
          [d] Aminoglycosides
          [e] Alcohol abuse
          [f] Hyperaldosteronism
          [g] Cisplatin
          [h] Cyclosporine
          [i] Amphotericin B
          [j] Postobstructive diuresis
     (b) Effects of hypomagnesemia
        (1) Hypokalemia due to renal K wasting
        (2) Hypocalcemia
          [a] Hypomagnesemia impairs PTH secretion
          [b] Hypomagnesemia inhibits mobilization of calcium from bone induced by PTH
        (3) Hyponatremia
        (4) Hypophosphatemia
        (5) Digoxin toxicity
        (6) Arrhythmias
        (7) Increased intracellular Ca
        (8) Heart failure
        (9) Hypertension
        (10) Increased mortality in hospitalized patients
  4. Hypermagnesemia
     (a) Etiology
        (1) Laxatives containing magnesium
        (2) Antacids containing magnesium
        (3) Lithium
        (4) Renal dysfunction
        (5) Adrenal insufficiency
        (6) Hypothyroidism
     (b) Effects
        (1) Hypotension
        (2) Mental status changes (lethargy, confusion, slurred speech)
        (3) Abnormal ECG (prolonged QT)
        (4) Respiratory depression

n. Glucose (MW = 180)

  1. Reabsorbed by the proximal tubule by a saturable mechanism
     (a) When net glucose filtration exceeds tubular maximal reabsorptive capacity (T_{max}), glucose is excreted in the urine
        (1) Glucose filtration rate is equal to the plasma glucose concentration multiplied by the GFR

o. Amino acids

  1. Kinetics
     (a) Fully reabsorbed by the proximal tubule

p. Water balance is maintained by varying urinary concentration to match urinary output with intake minus nonrenal losses and varying thirst to replace deficits

1. Neonate undergoes progressive modification of fluid balance
   (a) Day 1
       (1) ECF volume 415 ml/kg
       (2) Weight 100% (baseline)
   (b) Days 5–20
       (1) ECFV = 375 ml/kg
       (2) Weight day 5 = 87% of baseline
       (3) Weight day 10 = 89% of baseline
       (4) Weight day 15 = 95% of baseline
       (5) Weight day 20 = 100% of baseline
   (c) Dilutional ability is normal, but low GFR precludes elimination of very large water loads
   (d) Concentrating ability impaired
       (1) Preterm max = 550 mOsm/kg H_2O
       (2) Full term max = 700 mOsm/kg H_2O
       (3) Limited urea concentration in medulla due to positive nitrogen balance
       (4) Collecting ducts relatively less responsive to AVP

2. Elderly

Age	Maximal Osmolality
Neonate	500–700
1 week	1,000–1,200
30 years	1,000–1,200
80 years	400–600

   (a) Urine concentration after 12 hours of water deprivation was 1,109, 1,051, 882 mOsm/kg H_2O in young, middle-aged, and elderly normal subjects, respectively. Elderly did not increase UOsm as much as did young adults after 24 hours of water deprivation, although they significantly increased UOsm
   (b) Elderly responded normally at low doses of AVP, but did not reach the same maximal UOsm at higher infusion rates, suggesting a failure to develop concentrated interstitium rather than impaired AVP responsiveness
   (c) AV communications form at site of degenerating glomeruli, which increases medullary flow, washing out hyperosmolality
   (d) Thirst is impaired in elderly after water deprivation and they fail to increase water intake sufficiently to replace deficit
   (e) Required milliliters of H_2O = ([osmolar intake + production]/maximal UOsm)*1,000

III. DIAGNOSTIC EVALUATION

a. Urine flow rate (V)

1. Oliguria is volume of urine too low to maintain osmolar balance, excrete metabolic byproducts, maintain water balance
   (a) Common definition is 0.5 ml/kg/hr
   (b) Normal osmolar intake

           (1) Electrolytes (3–5 mOsm/kg/day)

           (2) Protein breakdown to nitrogen byproducts, especially urea (6–10 mOsm/kg/day)

               [a] Each gram of protein produces about 5.7 mOsm of solute

               [b] Catabolic patients with accelerated protein turnover, or those on high protein or amino acid loads, will have correspondingly increased osmolar loads

        (c) Average osmolar load is 12 mOsm/kg/day

           (1) Each milliliter of maximally concentrated urine can excrete 1 mOsm

           (2) Thus, 0.5 ml/kg/hr (12 mOsm/kg per 24 hours) will excrete this normal load

        (d) Patients with reduced lean body mass, low rates of protein turnover, minimal protein intake (e.g., elderly patients, debilitated patients) will have lower osmolar loads and will maintain osmolar balance with lower urine output

    2. V = GFR − reabsorption

        (a) V = urine flow rate

        (b) V does not correlate with GFR in nonoliguric states due to variable reabsorption

        (c) Oliguria can only occur when GFR is reduced

        (d) Nonoliguria could occur with a normal GFR and normal reabsorption, or with a very low GFR and impaired reabsorption. Examples are

           (1) GFR = 100 ml/min (near normal)

               [a] Fractional reabsorption = 0.99, or 99 ml/min, will lead to V = 1 ml/min

           (2) GFR = 20 ml/min (severely reduced)

               [a] Fractional reabsorption = 0.95, or 19 ml/min, will lead to V = 1 ml/min

        (e) Oliguria (and low GFR) can occur without permanent tubular damage

b. Urinalysis

    1. Microscopic

        (a) Cells

           (1) Red blood cells (may arise anywhere in urinary tract)

           (2) White blood cells (suggest inflammation anywhere in urinary tract)

               [a] Eosinophils (suggest allergic interstitial nephritis)

        (b) Casts

           (1) Hyaline

           (2) Granular

           (3) Cellular

               [a] Red blood cells (glomerular diseases)

               [b] WBC (inflammation of kidney)

               [c] Tubular cells (ATN)

        (c) Crystals

    2. Chemical

        (a) Protein (high levels suggest glomerular disease)

        (b) Glucose (suggests proximal tubular damage, hyperglycemia, hyperfiltration)

        (c) Ketones (secreted, so appear before plasma ketonemia)

        (d) pH (should be directly related to plasma pH)

        (e) Osmolality

        (f) Electrolytes

c. Measurement of RBF

    1. Para-aminohippurate (PAH) clearance is often called effective renal plasma flow (eRPF)

    2.
$$eRPF = \frac{C_{PAH}}{1 - Hct}$$

III. Diagnostic Evaluation; c. Measurement of RBF (continued)

   (a) PAH extraction averages 92% in young and old subjects

   (b) In the presence of tubular injury, the proportion of PAH extracted from the plasma decreases and thus falls variably below true RPF

     (1) $$E_{PAH} = \frac{PAH_a - PAH_v}{PAH_a}$$

     (2) If E_{PAH} is measured, then

$$\text{true RPF} = \frac{C_{PAH}}{E_{PAH}}$$

3. A special thermodilution catheter with a 180-degree bend near the tip is positioned in the renal vein and blood flow can be measured repetitively

4. Duplex Doppler ultrasound can be used to study interlobar artery flow repetitively

5. Inert gas washout

6. Radionuclide flow scan

7. Positron emission tomography

8. Dynamic CT

9. MRI

10. Radioactive or colored microspheres

d. Measurement of GFR

1. An ideal marker of filtration is
   - (a) Eliminated only by the kidney
   - (b) Freely filtered, MW less than 15–20Å, uncharged
   - (c) Nontoxic
   - (d) Not secreted, absorbed, produced, or metabolized by the kidney
   - (e) Easily measured accurately

2. Inulin clearance is the gold standard
   - (a) Problems with inulin
     - (1) Analysis is laborious
     - (2) Induction of diuresis may be clinically unacceptable or impossible
     - (3) Accurate timing of plasma and urine samples in the operating room or ICU may be impractical

3. Creatinine clearance (CCr)
   - (a) CCr = UV/Pt
     where CCr = creatinine clearance, U = urine concentration of creatinine, V = volume of urine, P = plasma creatinine concentration, t = duration of urine collection
   - (b) Creatinine is secreted in addition to being filtered
     - (1) As filtration falls and creatinine rises, the proportion secreted increases
     - (2) Secretion is inhibited by cimetidine, trimethoprim, salicylates

4. Plasma creatinine is proportional to creatinine production and inverse to excretion
   - (a) Production is proportional to muscle mass
     - (1) Creatinine production decreased due to loss of muscle mass (aging, sedentary lifestyle, liver disease, hyperthyroidism, glucocorticoid therapy, muscle wasting, bed rest during illness or injury)
     - (2) Estimated turnover of 1.6–1.7% per day
     - (3) For men, the excretion of creatinine is 28.2 g − 0.172 × age
       - [a] Creatinine excretion in the 80s is 11.7 mg/kg/day ± 4.0 (95% CI 3.7–19.7)
     - (4) For women, 25 g − 0.175 × age

     (5) Creatinine production is increased by muscle damage or ingestion of meat that contains 3.5–5.0 mg of creatinine per gram, with plasma elevations persisting for 8–12 hours

     (6) Total creatinine excretion correlates best with lean body mass

    (b) When the plasma level rises, some (perhaps as much as 65%) is destroyed in the gut, leading to levels of plasma creatinine that are lower than expected for the level of GFR

    (c) When measured colorimetrically by the Jaffe reaction, temperature, pH changes, bilirubin, glucose, protein, ketones, ascorbic acid, pyruvate, acetoacetate, uric acid, barbiturates, cephalosporins, and penicillins cause false elevations; high doses of furosemide produce falsely low values

    (d) Serum creatinine half-life is measured in hours. It takes five half-lives to reach a new steady state after a change in clearance. The lower the clearance, the longer the half-life, and the longer it takes to reach equilibrium

5. Acceptable substitutes for inulin

    (a) Diatrizoate, cyanocobalamin, EDTA, iothalomate, iohexol, and gadolinium-DTPA

6. Plasma clearance of filtration markers

    (a) Give results nearly equivalent to that of urinary clearance

    (b) Marker injected as a bolus

    (c) Samples are drawn after the alpha redistribution phase

    (d) Standard pharmacokinetic models are applied to calculate clearance. For example, the elimination rate constant (Ke) = 0.0024 CCr + 0.01

e. Tests of tubular function

1. Reabsorption of glucose is calculated from GFR and plasma and urine glucose

    (a) Reabsorption = $GFR \times P_{glucose} - U_{glucose} \times vol/time$

    (b) Normal maximal rate is about 300 mg/min

    (c) Upper limit of urine glucose is 15 mg/dl (0.8 mmol/L)

    (d) Normal renal threshold is plasma glucose over 8.9 mmol/L

    (e) 61% incidence of glucosuria in critically ill patients without marked hyperglycemia

2. Secretion of PAH

    (a) Normally 85–90% extraction

    (b) By using a dose that raises delivery to a rate higher than can be secreted, a maximal rate of secretion can be estimated, analogous to the maximal rate of absorption of glucose

3. Fractional excretion of any substance (FeS) is the clearance of any substance as a fraction of the amount filtered, or the rate of clearance divided by the GFR

$$FeS = \frac{\frac{Us*V}{Ps}}{GFR}$$

    (a) FeS = fractional excretion of any substance, S

    (b) Us = urine concentration of S

    (c) V = urine flow rate (ml/min)

    (d) Ps = plasma concentration of S

    (e) The V term appears in the numerator and denominator and cancels; thus, a single sample can be used, rather than a timed specimen

    (f) For FeNa, the percentage of filtered Na that is excreted is

$$FeNa = \frac{\frac{UNa}{PNa}}{\frac{UCr}{PCr}} \times 100$$

     (1) Normal reabsorption of Na is 98–99.5%; that is, FeNa is 2.0–0.5%

(2) In tubular dysfunction, FeNa exceeds 2%

(3) However, FeNa is also increased by any diuretic agent, by vigorous Na, and by volume loading

f. Tests of concentration

1. Osmolality is proportional to the number of particles in solution in a kilogram of pure water, expressed as mOsm/kg H_2O; it is the preferred measure of urine concentration

   (a) Osmolarity is the number of osmoles per liter of solution

2. Each molecular particle contributes to osmolality; thus, a nondissociating molecule, such as glucose, contributes 1 osmole per mole, whereas dissociating molecules, such as NaCl, could theoretically contribute 2 osmoles per mole

   (a) However, at physiologic concentrations, dissociation is not com- plete, so each mole of NaCl contributes about 1.8 osmoles/mole

3. The osmotic pressure increases by 19.3 mm Hg per mOsm/kg H_2O

   (a) Urine and serum or heparinized plasma, but not oxalated plasma, is an acceptable specimen for measurement of osmolality, but must be thoroughly centrifuged to remove any particulate matter

   (b) Increasing solute concentration depresses vapor pressure and freezing point and elevates osmotic pressure and boiling point

      (1) When 1 mole of solute is dissolved in 1 kg of H_2O, the freezing point falls by 1.858°C

         [a] The accuracy and reproducibility of the freezing point depression method are ± 2 mOsm/kg H_2O

         [b] Freezing-point depression method is more accurate and reproducible than the vapor pressure osmometer

      (2) One mole of solute dissolved in 1 kg of H_2O decreases vapor pressure by 0.3 mm Hg

         [a] Reproducibility of the vapor pressure method, ± 3 mOsm/kg H_2O

         [b] Vapor pressure method fails to account for volatile solutes, such as ethanol, methanol, dissolved CO_2, and presumably volatile anesthetics

   (c) Urine/plasma ratio of osmolality indicates whether the kidney is diluting or concentrating the urine in relationship to plasma

   (d) In circumstances in which urine should be concentrated (dehydration, hypovolemia, hypotension, hyperosmolality, oliguria), the ratio should be much greater than 1.0; i.e., 1.5–4.0

   (e) During water loading, the ratio should be 0.2–0.67

4. Specific gravity (SG) is related to the weight of a solute in water

   (a) Physiologic range is 1.000 up to 1.025

   (b) Urine contains multiple solutes, each with its own relationship between molar concentration and specific gravity

   (c) Larger molecules (e.g., protein, glucose, mannitol, radiocontrast agents, dextran, and dextrose) contribute greatly to specific gravity, but because their molar concentration per unit of weight is low, do not contribute proportionally to osmolality

   (d) Thus, the relationship between osmolality and specific gravity in a complex solution, such as urine, is quite variable

   (e) Errors in the measurement of specific gravity

      (1) Poor technique by busy caregivers

      (2) Equipment poorly maintained

         [a] Accuracy depends on true specific gravity and on surface tension,

requiring that the surfaces of the measuring instruments must be completely clean
- (3) The float must not touch the side wall
- (4) No bubbles may be allowed to cling to the stem
- (5) One gram per deciliter of protein adds 0.003 to SG
- (6) One gram per deciliter of glucose adds 0.004 to SG

5. The total solids meter or refractometer estimates specific gravity from the refractive index, which, in turn, estimates osmolality; it should be used only as a very rough guide to actual urine osmolality

(a) Each substance in solution contributes differently to specific gravity and refractive index
- (1) Glucose and protein invalidate the relationship between refractive index and specific gravity

6. Free-water clearance

(a) $C_{H_2O} = V - C_{osm}$ where C_{H_2O} is free-water clearance, V is urine flow rate in ml/min, C_{osm} is osmolar clearance in ml/min. If C_{H_2O} is zero, the urine is isoosmotic to plasma; if negative, it is concentrated
- (1) Zero represents no net concentration
- (2) Positive numbers reflect excretion of dilute urine
- (3) Negative numbers reflect excretion of concentrated urine

g. Tests of tubular injury

1. Cellular casts
2. Granular casts
3. Eosinophiluria is characteristic of allergic interstitial nephritis
   - (a) Detected by Hansel's stain
   - (b) Found in interstitial nephritis but not in acute tubular necrosis (ATN)
   - (c) Postinfectious and rapidly progressive glomerulonephritis
   - (d) Acute prostatitis
   - (e) Atheroembolic disease
4. Brush border enzymes of the proximal tubule include L-alanine aminopeptidase, beta-galactosidase, angiotensin converting enzyme, angiotensinase A, gamma-glutamyltranspeptidase (GGT), dipeptidyl aminopeptidase IV, leucineaminopeptidase (LAP), and alkaline phosphatase (AP)
   - (a) Found in urine after proximal tubular cellular damage
5. Lysosomal enzymes include beta-glucuronidase and *N*-acetyl-beta-*D*-glucosaminidase (NAG)
6. Increased excretion of substances may indicate tubular damage
   - (a) Beta$_2$-microglobulin is filtered and fully reabsorbed proximally; excretion rises with proximal tubular damage
   - (b) Amylase is filtered and normally completely reabsorbed and fractional excretion rises in ATN
   - (c) Retinol binding protein is normally filtered and totally reabsorbed and is stable in urine
   - (d) Adenosine deaminase binding protein is a proximal tubular antigen that is stable in urine and reliably elevated in ATN

h. Erythropoietin

1. Production and release are controlled by O_2
   - (a) Renal O_2 tension
     - (1) Acute anemia

III. Diagnostic Evaluation; h. Erythropoietin (continued)

    (2) Hypoxemia
   2. Therapy
    (a) Evaluate iron stores
     (1) Total iron binding capacity rises with Fe deficiency
     (2) Ferritin falls as Fe stores fall
     (3) Fe falls only after iron depleted
     (4) Fe/TIBC falls as Fe stores fall
     (5) Zn protoporphyrin/heme rises as Fe falls
     (6) RBC VDW is elevated with Fe deficiency
     (7) RBC volume falls as end-stage Fe deficiency anemia occurs
    (b) Check erythropoietin levels
    (c) Check reticulocyte count
    (d) Start 50–100 U/kg three times per week, increasing by 12.5–25 U/kg every 2–6 weeks
    (e) Recheck reticulocyte count in 10–14 days, B_{12}, folate levels, iron studies

IV. PHARMACOLOGY

a. Diuretics

   1. Carbonic anhydrase inhibitors

    (a) Reduce GFR by 10–30% due to TGF
    (b) Proximal tubular HCO_3^- absorption is diminished by 80–90%
     (1) Proximal luminal pH falls due to accumulation of H_2CO_3
     (2) HCO_3^- absorption decreases by 67%
     (3) Collecting duct secretions of HCO_3^- and H^+ are inhibited
      [a] Fractional excretion of HCO_3^- can increase to 20–30%
     (4) NH_4^+ excretion is reduced
     (5) Fractional excretion of Na increases up to about 5%
     (6) Urine pH, potassium (FeK = 50–60%), and phosphate ($FePO_4$ = 20–30%) excretions increase

   2. Loop diuretics

    (a) Furosemide
     (1) Kinetics
      [a] Uptake
       i) PO
        a) Onset less than 60 minutes
        b) Bioavailability 60–65%
       ii) IV
        a) Onset less than 5 minutes
      [b] Distribution
       i) 91–99% protein bound
      [c] Metabolism
       i) Hepatic glucuronidation
      [d] Excretion
       i) Renal filtration
       ii) Renal secretion
       iii) Terminal half-life = 2 hours
     (2) Effects
      [a] Block Na-K-2Cl transporter of thick ascending limb by binding to Cl binding site

[b] Lower urinary pH, increase net acid excretion by increasing NH_4^+ and titratable acid excretion

[c] Upper level of response curve is 160 mg in chronic KF

[d] Continuous infusion is more effective than bolus doses because the longer the exposure of the TALH to drug, the greater the diuresis, natriuresis for the same dose

    i) Without bolus dose, maximal effect occurs by 3 hours

    ii) Up to 4 mg/min (240 mg/hr) or 4 g/day appear to be safe, but usual doses reported are 1–9 mg/hr

    iii) Discolors when exposed to light and should be discarded. Stable for 24 hours if pH greater than 5.5. Refrigeration causes precipitation or crystallization

    iv) Compatibilities (see table)

Drug	Furosemide	Bumetanide
Amikacin	C	C
Aminophylline	C	C
Amrinone	I	U
Atropine	C	C
Chlorpromazine	I	U
Ciprofloxacin	I	U
Dextrose 5%	C	C
Diazepam	I	U
Diphenhydramine	I	U
Dopamine	I	U
Dobutamine	I	I
Epinephrine	C	U
Esmolol	I	U
Fluconazole	I	U
Gentamicin	I	U
Heparin	C	C
Isoproterenol	I	U
Lidocaine	C	U
Meperidine	I	U
Metoclopramide	I	U
Morphine	I	U
Milrinone	I	U
NaCl, 0.9%	C	C
Netilmicin	I	U
Nitroglycerin	C	U
Prochlorperazine	I	U
Quinidine	I	U
Ranitidine	C	U
Ringer's lactate	C	C
Bicarbonate	C	U
Tobramycin	C	U

C = compatible; I = incompatible; U = unknown

[e] Adverse effects

    i) Pancreatitis

    ii) Intrahepatic cholestasis

    iii) Systemic vasculitis

    iv) Interstitial nephritis

    v) Tinnitus, hearing loss

IV. Pharmacology; a. Diuretics (continued)

        vi) Paresthesia
       vii) Thrombocytopenia
      viii) Hypokalemia
       ix) Hyperglycemia
        x) Hyperuricemia
- (3) Interactions
  - [a] Increases ototoxic potential of aminoglycosides
  - [b] Elevates salicylate level by competing for renal secretion
  - [c] Increase risk of renal dysfunction induced by NSAID
  - [d] Antagonizes nondepolarizing neuromuscular block
  - [e] Potentiates depolarizing neuromuscular block
  - [f] Increased risk of lithium toxicity by reducing Li clearance
  - [g] High levels make creatinine unmeasurable by Jaffe method
- (b) Bumetanide
  - (1) Kinetics
    - [a] Uptake
      - i) PO
        - a) Onset 30–60 minutes
        - b) Peak 60–120 minutes
      - ii) IV
        - a) Onset less than 5 minutes
        - b) Peak 15–30 minutes
    - [b] Distribution
      - i) 95% protein bound
    - [c] Metabolism
      - i) Hepatic oxidation of about 55%
    - [d] Excretion
      - i) At least 81% in urine as drug and metabolites
      - ii) Renal filtration
      - iii) Renal secretion
      - iv) Half-life: 1–1.5 hours
  - (2) Effects
    - [a] Blocks ascending limb Na-K-2Cl transporter
    - [b] Proximal tubular action
      - i) Phosphaturia
    - [c] 1 mg approximates 40 mg furosemide
    - [d] Continuous infusions of 0.25–1 mg/hr have been used
    - [e] Adverse effects
      - i) Hyperuricemia by inhibiting renal excretion, hypochloremia, hypokalemia, azotemia, hyponatremia, increased serum creatinine, hyperglycemia, and variations in phosphorus, CO_2 content, bicarbonate, and calcium; deviations in hemoglobin, prothrombin time, hematocrit, LDH, total serum bilirubin, serum proteins, SGOT, SGPT; increases in urinary glucose
      - ii) Ototoxicity
      - iii) Muscle cramps, dizziness, hypotension, headache, nausea, and encephalopathy (in patients with preexisting liver disease)
  - (3) Interactions
    - [a] Enhanced ototoxicity
    - [b] Reduced lithium clearance may lead to toxicity
    - [c] Indomethacin blunts natriuresis of bumetanide
- (c) Metolazone (Zaroxolyn)
  - (1) Kinetics

          [a] Uptake
                i) PO
                    a) Onset: less than 60 minutes
                    b) Peak: 2–4 hours
                    c) Duration: 24 hours
                    d) Bioavailability
          [b] Distribution
                i) Protein bound
          [c] Metabolism
                i) Hepatic: small fraction
          [d] Excretion
                i) Renal: most of drug unchanged
                ii) Terminal half-life: 14 hours
    (2) Effects
          [a] Blocks Na absorption in diluting segment of TALH
          [b] Some proximal Na absorption block
          [c] Increased potassium, phosphate, magnesium excretion
          [d] Adverse effects
                i) Dizziness (lightheadedness); headaches, muscle cramps; fatigue
                    (malaise, lethargy, lassitude); joint pain, swelling, chest pain
                    (precordial discomfort)
    (3) Interactions
          [a] Potentiates furosemide diuresis
    (4) Pharmaceutic
          [a] Similar to thiazides
3. Osmotic
    (a) Mannitol
        (1) Nonreabsorbable solute
        (2) Proximal tubule
              [a] Na is absorbed, but osmolality increases as water is absorbed and
                  mannitol concentration rises. Water absorption is thus impaired. This
                  dilutes the remaining intratubular Na. Because the Na pump in this
                  segment cannot generate large concentration gradients, Na and water
                  reabsorption are diminished
        (3) Thick ascending limb can generate high concentration gradients, but the
            massively increased Na load exceeds the absorptive capacity of the distal
            nephron
        (4) Collecting duct permeability leads to water reabsorption if the medullary
            interstitium is concentrated. However, the increase in fluid flow into the loop
            of Henle dilutes the concentration of the interstitium
        (5) The net result is an increase in Na and water excretion with urine osmolality
            tending to become isoosmotic
    (b) Metabolic
        (1) Hyperglycemia will have the same effects as mannitol when the rate of
            glucose filtration exceeds the rate of tubular reabsorption
        (2) Uremia with a high BUN is associated with an osmotic diuresis; thus, urine
            output in patients in renal failure often decreases during and after dialysis as
            the BUN decreases
4. Thiazide diuretics inhibit distal tubular Na reabsorption
    (a) Increase excretion of HCO_3^-, Na, K, Cl, and PO_4 acutely
5. Aldosterone antagonism with spironolactone will lead to a moderate increase in Na
    absorption distally if aldosterone levels are high
6. Potassium sparing diuretics
    (a) Triamterene

IV. Pharmacology; a. Diuretics (continued)

    (1) Blocks apical Na channels in collecting duct, increasing Na excretion moderately

    (2) Blocked Na absorption lessens the normal electrical gradient (lumen negative in relation to interstitium), which drives K secretion into the lumen; thus, K excretion is not increased as much as with other diuretics

b. Anesthetic effects

1. Regional

    (a) Blockade of T4 through T10 suppresses the sympathoadrenal response to surgery and preserves RBF and GFR

2. General anesthesia

    (a) Inhalation

        (1) Reduced GFR

        (2) Reduced urine flow rate

        (3) Hypotension is the most important contributor to reduced RBF

        (4) Maintenance of BP depends on angiotensin II due to sympathetic suppression

        (5) Desflurane

            [a] No effect on RBF by 2 MAC

            [b] No renal toxicity

                i) Urinary retinol binding protein, NAG, serum, and urine fluoride failed to change after 1.5 hours at 3.6%

        (6) Isoflurane

            [a] Essentially no metabolism to fluoride

        (7) Sevoflurane

            [a] 1 MAC does not change RBF

            [b] No evidence of direct or fluoride-related toxicity despite metabolism to fluoride; this may relate to less intrarenal metabolism in comparison with methoxyflurane

            [c] Degradation by soda lime or baralyme produces a nephrotoxic olefin

    (b) IV narcotics

        (1) Minimal effects on RBF and GFR

    (c) Benzodiazepines

        (1) Minor reductions in RBF and GFR

    (d) Ketamine

        (1) Increases RBF

V. CLINICAL DISEASE STATES

a. Kidney failure

1. Acute kidney failure (AKF), etiology

    (a) Immune

        (1) Glomerulonephritis

        (2) Interstitial nephritis

    (b) Obstructive

        (1) Neoplasms

        (2) Metabolic

            [a] Stones

                i) Calcium

                ii) Uric acid

(c) Ischemic (the most common contributing factor in perioperative period)
   (1) Vascular obstruction
     [a] Arterial
     [b] Venous
   (2) Arterial embolism
   (3) Severe vasoconstriction
   (4) Prolonged hypotension
   (5) Cortical necrosis occurs during extreme and prolonged hypotension, especially in hypercoagulable states; the infarction of the cortex is irreversible
   (6) Acute tubular necrosis results from moderate prolonged hypoperfusion. Although tubular epithelial cells die, the basic nephron structure is preserved, and thus is at least partially recoverable
     [a] Accounts for 90% of perioperative cases
     [b] Complications (see "Chronic kidney failure")
       i) Mortality
         a) Perioperative cases have mortality rates of 40–90%
         b) Increased by coexisting organ dysfunction
         c) Doubled if oliguric
         d) Lower if nephrotoxic in origin
       ii) Cardiovascular
         a) Hypertension is not characteristic of ATN and suggests preexisting hypertension, or AKF due to a glomerular lesion, or large renal vessel stenosis
       iii) Metabolic
         a) Calcium
           • Hypocalcemia may be seen early due to deposition in damaged tissue as in rhabdomyolysis, acute pancreatitis
           • Later hypocalcemia is related to hyperphosphatemia as in chronic failure
           • During resolution, hypercalcemia may occur due to
             —Overzealous Ca, vitamin D therapy
             —Mobilization from bone due to bed rest, from dead tissue reabsorption
       iv) Chronic renal insufficiency may follow. The longer the duration and the more severe the oliguria, the less likely is full recovery
     [c] Pathophysiology of AKF due to ischemic ATN
       i) Ischemia
         a) Prerenal
           • Lowered GFR due to low glomerular capillary pressure due to vasoconstriction and/or hypotension and/or glomerular constriction
           • Maximal tubular reabsorption of electrolyte and water
             —Low urine Na, fractional excretion of Na, and oliguria, high urine osmolality, negative free-water clearance
           • Imbalance between O_2 delivery and utilization leads to widened AV O_2 difference and reduced lactate extraction
         b) Cellular death phase (acute tubular necrosis, ATN)
           • Proximal tubular and thick ascending limb cells die, slough into lumen due to high metabolic rate and marginal perfusion
           • Fail to modify concentration of electrolytes in filtrate
             —Urine Na and FeNa rise, oliguria is common (about 50%), osmolality approaches plasma level, free-water clearance near zero

V. Clinical Disease States; a. Kidney failure (continued)

- Appearance of epithelial cells, cellular and granular, and wide brown casts in urinalysis
  - ii) Intratubular obstruction due to concentration of protein and cellular debris forming obstructive casts raises intratubular pressure until filtration stops
  - iii) Back leak through damaged tubule
- [d] Therapy of AKF
  - i) Stabilize BP, cardiac output, O_2 delivery
  - ii) Maintain blood volume in upper normal range
  - iii) Minimize nephrotoxins
  - iv) Correct fluid and electrolyte problems
  - v) Insulinlike growth factor, epidermal growth factor shorten the course of ATN in animals
  - vi) Control administration of water, electrolytes (Na, K, Ca, PO_4, Mg), drugs to match output
- (7) Sepsis
  - [a] Activated WBCs plus mild renal ischemia potentiate damage
  - [b] PGE_1 infusion decreased the RBF/CO ratio in septic shock model
- (8) Hepatorenal syndrome (HRS)
  - [a] Diagnosis of HRS
    - i) Severe hepatic disease, usually cirrhosis, often with ascites
    - ii) Low urine output
    - iii) Very low urine Na and FeNa
    - iv) Urinalysis with hyaline casts or normal
  - [b] Pathogenesis of HRS
    - i) Severe renal hypoperfusion
      - a) Arterial hypotension
      - b) Increased intra-abdominal pressure
      - c) Intense renal vasoconstriction
        - Elevated endothelin levels
    - ii) Variable aldosterone levels
  - [c] Management of HRS
    - i) Optimize intravascular volume
    - ii) Raise arterial pressure
    - iii) Relieve ascites to lower intra-abdominal pressure
    - iv) Treat underlying liver disease
    - v) Adjust doses of potential nephrotoxins
- (9) Preeclampsia, eclampsia
  - [a] Pathophysiology
    - i) Excessive vasoconstriction (angiotensin, thromboxane), sodium retention, altered coagulation, endothelial damage
    - ii) Hypovolemia
  - [b] Management
    - i) Adequate fluid loading
- (d) Toxic
  - (1) Radiocontrast
    - [a] Acute reduction in RBF
      - i) Crenated RBC may obstruct vasculature
    - [b] Tubular toxicity
    - [c] Hypovolemia due to osmotic diuresis
    - [d] Risk factors
      - i) Preexisting renal disease (most important single factor)
      - ii) Diabetes

iii) Dehydration and hypovolemia
iv) Myeloma
v) Heart failure
[e] Dye exposure potentiates effects of subsequent minor ischemic events
[f] Management
    i) Establish saline diuresis
    ii) Mannitol does not help and may worsen risk
    iii) Furosemide increases risk
(2) Aminoglycoside
    [a] Pathogenesis
        i) Filtered
        ii) Binds to brush border phospholipid
        iii) Taken up by pinocytosis into lysosomes
        iv) Released into cytoplasm
            a) Half-life in cortex is several days
            b) Toxicity usually not seen until 10 days of therapy
        v) Inhibits oxidative phosphorylation
        vi) Cells die
        vii) Proximal tubular transport defects
        viii) Declining GFR with maintained urine flow
        ix) Risk factors
            a) Volume depletion
            b) Hypokalemia
            c) Hypomagnesemia
            d) Obstructive liver disease
            e) Vancomycin
            f) Cephalosporins
            g) Cisplatin, doxorubicin
            h) Corticosteroids
            i) NSAID
            j) Radiocontrast
    [b] Treatment
        i) Prevention
            a) Monitor serum levels daily in critically ill
            b) Avoid peaks over 8 μg/ml
            c) Maintain trough under 1.0 μg/ml
            d) Avoid hypovolemia
            e) Keep K normal
            f) Keep Mg high normal
(3) Vancomycin
    [a] New formulations are minimally toxic alone
    [b] Toxicity increased by coadministration with other nephrotoxins, sepsis, cardiovascular instability
    [c] If CCr is decreased, monitor vancomycin levels daily to guide dosing
(4) Amphotericin B
    [a] Excreted by liver, thus dose not reduced in AKF
    [b] Not dialyzed
    [c] Avoid hypokalemia
(5) Fluoride
    [a] Levels over 50 mg/dl are associated with renal toxicity of methoxyflurane
    [b] Intrarenal metabolism to Fl may be more important than plasma level per se
(6) Sulfonamides
    [a] Crystals deposit, causing obstruction and inflammation
    [b] Alkalinization of urine decreases precipitation

          (7) Nonsteroidal anti-inflammatory drugs (NSAIDs)
              [a] Block generation of vasodilator PGE_2, PGI_2
              [b] Vasoconstrictor agents then cause more intense vasoconstriction, leading to greater and longer ischemia
                  i) May lead to ATN, papillary necrosis
              [c] May also cause interstitial nephritis
          (8) Cisplatin
              [a] Acute and chronic renal failure
              [b] Magnesium wasting
      (e) Metabolic
         (1) Hypercalcemia
         (2) Hyperuricemia
         (3) Heme pigment (hemoglobin, myoglobin)
         (4) Hyperosmotic
      (f) Immune
         (1) Glomerulonephritis
              [a] Poststreptococcal
              [b] Associated with abscess, bacterial endocarditis, V-P shunt infections
         (2) Interstitial nephritis
              [a] Drug related
                  i) Penicillins
                  ii) Cephalosporins
                  iii) Sulfonamides, including furosemide
      (g) Traumatic
         (1) Contusions, lacerations
         (2) Vascular obstruction, avulsion
  2. Pyelonephritis
    (a) Cause of AKF in elderly in absence of fever or symptoms
  3. Chronic kidney failure
    (a) Epidemiology
      (1) 11/100,000 ages 10–40; 470/100,000 over 80 years
    (b) Pathogenesis
      (1) Hypertension
      (2) Diabetes
      (3) Toxic agents
          [a] NSAIDs
          [b] Cisplatin
          [c] BCNU
          [d] CCNU
          [e] Streptozocin
          [f] Mithramycin
      (4) Glomerulonephritis
  4. Complications of kidney failure
    (a) Hematologic
      (1) Anemia
    (b) Neurologic
      (1) Peripheral neuropathy in slow and rapid forms
      (2) Encephalopathy
      (3) Sympathetic hyperactivity reversed by nephrectomy, but not dialysis
    (c) Cardiac
      (1) Accelerated coronary disease
      (2) High output failure due to oversized AV fistula

(d) Vascular
  (1) Hypertension
  (2) Accelerated atherosclerosis
  (3) Loss of venous access due to multiple AV fistulae
(e) Pulmonary
  (1) Edema
(f) Metabolic
  (1) Hyperkalemia
  (2) Hyperphosphatemia
  (3) Hyponatremia due to H_2O retention
  (4) Hypocalcemia due to hyperphosphatemia
  (5) Acidosis due to failure to excrete "fixed acids" (PO_4, SO_4, Cl)
  (6) Hyperuricemia
(g) Endocrine
  (1) Hyperparathyroidism due to prolonged hypocalcemia may lead to hyperplastic parathyroid
  (2) Endothelin levels are elevated in KF during hemodialysis
(h) Bone
  (1) Reabsorption due to hyperparathyroidism
(i) Gastrointestinal
  (1) Bleeding
  (2) Nausea, vomiting
(j) Pharmacologic effects of kidney failure
  (1) General
    [a] Water-soluble drugs will be filtered at reduced rates
    [b] Many lipid-soluble drugs are metabolized to water-soluble metabolites, which are excreted by the kidney
    [c] Total body water (TBW) and extracellular fluid volume (ECFV) are often increased in acute and chronic kidney failure. ECFV is variable during intermittent dialysis. Thus, the volume of distribution of drugs is often increased
    [d] Protein binding of many drugs is decreased
  (2) Acyclovir
    [a] Dose must be reduced
  (3) Allopurinol
    [a] Metabolized to oxipurinol
    [b] Oxipurinol accumulates in KF
    [c] Allopurinol dose should not exceed 300 mg/day
  (4) Amantidine
    [a] Accumulates in failure
      i) Can cause arrhythmias, neuropsychiatric symptoms
  (5) Aminoglycosides
    [a] Filtered, minor reabsorption
    [b] Dosing must be guided by measuring levels in perioperative period and acute illness because both clearance and volume of distribution change rapidly
  (6) Angiotensin converting enzyme inhibitors (ACEI)
    [a] Some renal excretion
      i) Accumulate in KF
  (7) Aztreonam
    [a] Two thirds renal elimination
    [b] Reduce dose
  (8) Barbiturates
    [a] Long-acting drugs have important renal excretion; short-acting agents are metabolized in liver

V. Clinical Disease States; a. Kidney failure (continued)

      [b] Phenobarbital excretion in the urine can be increased by alkaline diuresis
- (9) Benzodiazepine
  - [a] Metabolized in liver to metabolites, which are excreted in urine
  - [b] Metabolites of chlordiazepoxide, diazepam, flurazepam have active metabolites
  - [c] Lorazepam and oxazepam metabolites are not active
- (10) Beta-adrenergic antagonists
  - [a] Highly dependent on renal excretion
    - i) Nadolol, sotalol, atenolol, practolol
  - [b] Little dependence on renal excretion
    - i) Propranolol, pindolol, labetalol, alprenolol, bufuralol, mepindolol, terazosin, timolol, tolamolol
- (11) Bretylium
  - [a] Accumulates in KF
- (12) Cancer chemotherapeutic agents
  - [a] Bleomycin accumulates
  - [b] Cyclophosphamide
    - i) Toxic metabolites accumulate
  - [c] Methotrexate accumulates
- (13) Cephalosporins
  - [a] Filtered and secreted
  - [b] Side chain responsible for coagulopathy accumulates in kidney failure
  - [c] The dose of most cephalosporins should be decreased to 25–30% of normal. Exceptions
    - i) 50% reduction
      - a) Cefachlor, cefixime, cefotaxime, cefuroxime
    - ii) 20% reduction
      - a) Cefoperazone, ceftriaxone, cefaprin
- (14) Clonidine
  - [a] Eliminated predominantly by kidney
  - [b] Reduce dose by 75–50%
- (15) Digoxin
  - [a] Volume of distribution reduced
  - [b] Filtered
  - [c] Accumulates in KF
    - i) Reduce dose by 75% and measure levels
- (16) Diuretics
  - [a] Acetazolamide
    - i) Should be avoided
    - ii) Accumulates in KF
  - [b] Amiloride
    - i) Accumulates in KF
  - [c] Bumetanide
    - i) Minimal accumulation
  - [d] Furosemide
    - i) Accumulates in KF
  - [e] Spironolactone
    - i) Metabolites accumulate
- (17) Histamine antagonists
  - [a] Dosages reduced by about 50%
- (18) Hypoglycemics, oral
  - [a] Require major dose reduction

(19) Lithium
    [a] Filtered and reabsorbed
    [b] Accumulates in KF and is toxic
(20) Metoclopramide
    [a] Accumulates in KF
(21) Narcotics
    [a] Morphine
        i) Glucuronides are active and accumulate in KF
    [b] Meperidine
        i) Normeperidine accumulates and causes delirium and seizures
(22) Neuromuscular blocking agents
    [a] Pancuronium, metocurine, gallamine accumulate in KF
    [b] Increased sensitivity to mivacurium
(23) Nitroprusside
    [a] Metabolized to thiocyanate
    [b] Thiocyanate accumulates in KF
        i) Toxicity causes hypothyroidism, psychosis
(24) Penicillins
    [a] Filtered and secreted
    [b] Penicillin G has 1.7 mEq/million U of potassium
    [c] Synthetic penicillins have Na 5 mEq/g
(25) Pentamidine
    [a] No effect on short-term therapy
(26) Phenothiazines
    [a] No effects on kinetics
    [b] Uremic patients more susceptible to extrapyramidal effects
(27) Phenytoin
    [a] Protein binding is decreased substantially, so half-life decreases but free level rises
    [b] Measure free level, not total, in KF
(28) Procainamide
    [a] Reduce dose by 80%
    [b] N-Acetyl procainamide (NAPA) accumulates to greater extent than parent compound
(29) Tetracyclines
    [a] Aggravate azotemia
(30) Tricyclic antidepressants
    [a] No effect on kinetics of parent drugs, but metabolites accumulate in KF and some are active
(31) Vancomycin
    [a] Filtered
    [b] Dosing must be guided by levels in AKF

5. Therapy of kidney failure
    (a) Nutrition
        (1) Maintain normal caloric intake
        (2) Prior to institution of dialysis, either reduce protein intake or provide a diet rich in essential amino acids
        (3) Normalize protein composition and intake after dialysis begins
        (4) Protein restriction does not seem to affect progression of chronic KF
        (5) Albumin level less than 4 g/dl associated with increased risk of death in dialysis patients
    (b) Electrolytes
        (1) Intake of electrolytes should be minimized

V. Clinical Disease States; a. Kidney failure (continued)

    (2) No K should be administered in maintenance fluids, such as in total parenteral nutrition (TPN) or enteral feeding, until a clear-cut requirement is demonstrated

    (3) Calcium replacement should be guided by measurement of ionized Ca, not total Ca, and kept in the low normal range

  (c) Hemodynamics

    (1) Blood pressure should be normalized

      [a] Keep DBP at under 95 mm Hg in AKF to minimize additional kidney damage, especially in black patients

      [b] In chronic KF, to minimize other end-organ damage, as well as progression of KF

      [c] ACEI may be advantageous, especially in diabetic nephropathy

      [d] ACEI markedly increases incidence of hypotension following induction of anesthesia

  (d) Dialysis

    (1) Peritoneal

    (2) Hemodialysis

      [a] Intermittent (IHD)

        i) Chronic KF

          a) Urea reduction of at least 60% with dialysis associated with better survival

          b) About one third of patients have episodic hypotension associated with reduction in SNS output and hypovolemia

        ii) Cuprophane membranes increase duration and mortality of acute kidney failure

      [b] Continuous

        i) Arteriovenous (CAVH)

          a) With dialysis (CAVHD)

        ii) Veno-venous (CVVH)

          a) With dialysis (CVVHD)

      [c] Hemoperfusion

  (e) Transplantation

    (1) Immune suppression

      [a] Cyclosporine

        i) Hypertension

        ii) Hyperkalemia

      [b] OKT$_3$

      [c] Steroids

      [d] Azathioprine

      [e] Transfusion

    (2) Graft protection

      [a] Calcium channel blockade

      [b] Recipient volume loading to a CVP of 15–18 associated with improved outcome

---

b. Kidney trauma

  1. IVP not needed in adult victims of blunt trauma with stable BP and microscopic hematuria

c. Polyuria

1. Definition

    (a) Urine output greater than required to maintain fluid and electrolyte balance
    (b) Generally greater than 2 ml/kg per hour

2. Pathophysiology

    (a) Failure to reabsorb filtrate
    (b) Low vasopressin level
        (1) Physiologic
            [a] Hypervolemia
            [b] Hyponatremia, hypoosmolality
        (2) Pathologic
            [a] Hypothalamic damage
            [b] Pituitary stalk damage
            [c] Posterior pituitary damage
    (c) Failure of kidney to respond to AVP
        (1) Blood flow redistribution
            [a] Vasodilators, sepsis, sickle cell anemia
        (2) Tubular dysfunction
            [a] Ischemia
            [b] Toxins, such as aminoglycosides
            [c] Drug induced
                i) Diuretics

3. Effects

    (a) Hypovolemia
    (b) Hypernatremia (hypertonic dehydration)

d. Oliguria

1. Definition

    (a) Urine output too low to maintain fluid and electrolyte balance and excretion of metabolic waste products
    (b) Less than 400 ml per day in acute kidney failure defines patients with increased risk of mortality
    (c) Less than 0.5 ml/kg per hour

2. Pathophysiology

    (a) Reduced GFR with maximal tubular reabsorption
    (b) Oliguria as defined is due to low GFR
        (1) Absence of oliguria does not preclude low GFR
        (2) Low GFR does not necessarily imply tubular damage

VI. PERIOPERATIVE CONSIDERATIONS

a. Fluid management with preexisting renal insufficiency

1. Fluid loading prior to induction helps sustain urine flow and GFR

b. Fluid management with functional anephric state

1. Avoid K

2. If nonoliguric, administer enough fluid to sustain urine flow rate

3. If oliguric, maintenance fluids are only 30% of usual

c. Nephrectomy

1. Reduce maintenance fluids to 30% of usual

d. Transurethral surgery

1. Cystoscopy
2. Prostatic resection
    (a) Complications
        (1) Bladder rupture
            [a] Abdominal pain
            [b] Shoulder pain due to diaphragmatic irritation and referral to C4 distribution
        (2) Fluid overload
            [a] Absorption via venous sinuses correlated with duration of resection
            [b] Rising CVP with hypertension
            [c] Nonelectrolyte fluid used for irrigation to prevent current dispersal
                i) Leads to hyponatremia
                    a) Causes CNS dysfunction
                        • Agitation, confusion, seizures, coma
            [d] Glycine commonly used to normalize osmolality with good visual characteristics
                i) Glycine and NH_3 intoxication may occur
            [e] EtOH may be added to irrigant and monitored via exhaled gas
        (3) Hemorrhage
            [a] May be associated with fibrinolysis

e. Effects of mechanical ventilation

1. Decreased cardiac output and blood pressure
    (a) Decreased atrial size causing decreased ANP release, increased AVP release leading to hyponatremia
    (b) Decreased urine flow rate, RBF, GFR, Na excretion

f. Induced hypotension

1. Trimethophan decreases RBF
2. Nitroprusside causes renal vasodilation, so has little impact on RBF until discontinued
3. Nitroglycerin causes little reduction in GFR
4. Adenosine markedly decreases RBF, GFR

g. Aortic cross-clamping

1. Suprarenal
    (a) Acute reduction in GFR lasting at least 24 hours
    (b) Impaired concentrating ability, Na and water absorption, maintains urine flow
    (c) Clamp times over 50 minutes associated with prolonged reductions in GFR
2. Infrarenal clamping associated with short-term reduction in GFR

h. Cardiopulmonary bypass

1. Decreased RBF during bypass
2. Decreased cardiac output and RBF postoperatively
3. Role of nonpulsatile flow probably not important
4. Incidence of AKF about 2%
5. No benefit for prophylactic dopamine infusion
6. Pretreatment with ACEI prevented fall in ERPF and maintained higher UNaV and GFR without influencing blood pressure or fluid requirements

i. Preoperative evaluation

1. History
   (a) Any kidney disease?
   (b) Glomerulonephritis, nephritis?
   (c) Frequency, nocturia, polyuria?
   (d) Hematuria?
   (e) Dysuria?
   (f) Kidney stones, flank pain?
   (g) Kidney, bladder, or urinary tract infections?
   (h) Diseases associated with renal damage?
      (1) Diabetes mellitus
      (2) Hypertension
         [a] ACEI therapy predisposes to hypotension, associated with volume-dependent blood pressure; increases vagal activity; interferes with sympathetic nervous system function
      (3) Atherosclerosis
      (4) Collagen vascular disease or vasculitis
      (5) Obstructive jaundice, cirrhosis
      (6) Cardiac failure
      (7) Treatment with nephrotoxic antibiotics, chemotherapeutic agents
2. Preoperative testing
   (a) Indications for obtaining creatinine, BUN
      (1) Age over 64
      (2) Diabetes
      (3) Hypertension
      (4) Cardiovascular disease or surgery
      (5) History of renal disease
      (6) Vasculitis
      (7) Sepsis
      (8) Acute muscle injury (rhabdomyolysis)
      (9) Therapy with nephrotoxic drugs
         [a] Aminoglycoside
         [b] Radiocontrast media
         [c] NSAIDs
      (10) CNS disease
      (11) Use of diuretics
      (12) Use of digoxin
      (13) Hepatobiliary surgery
      (14) Evidence of hepatic disease
      (15) Conditions associated with hypovolemia or dehydration

E. HEPATIC SYSTEM

I. ANATOMY
a. Gross anatomy

b. Histology

c. General information

d. Dual blood supply

II. PHYSIOLOGY
a. Drug metabolism

b. Synthetic function

c. Coagulation function

d. Tests of coagulation

e. Excretory actions of the liver

f. Cytochrome p450 system

g. Liver function tests

III. PHARMACOLOGY
a. Enzyme induction

b. Pharmacokinetics

c. Drug excretion

IV. CLINICAL PRIORITIES
a. Hepatitis

b. Cholangitis

c. Portal hypertension

d. Ascites

e. Liver failure

f. Liver transplantation

g. Transfusion reaction/hemolysis

I. ANATOMY

a. Gross anatomy

1. Right and left hepatic lobe
2. Caudate and quadrate lobe
3. Gallbladder

b. Histology: three zones of hepatocytes surrounding a terminal afferent blood vessel

1. Zone 1
   - (a) Close proximity to terminal vessels
   - (b) First to regenerate
   - (c) Last to develop necrosis
2. Zone 2
   - (a) Receives blood after flow through zone 1
   - (b) Less oxygen and nutrient content
3. Zone 3
   - (a) Least resistant to hypoxia, hepatotoxins, damaging cellular agents

c. General information: largest visceral organ in the body

1. Total hepatic blood flow averages 100 ml/min/100 g of tissue or 1.5 L/min
2. 25% of cardiac output
3. 20–30 ml of blood per 100 g of liver tissue contained in liver parenchyma
4. 15% of the total blood volume

d. Dual blood supply

1. Portal vein: 65–80% of hepatic blood flow provides 50–60% of the total oxygen delivered and consumed
2. Hepatic artery: 20–35% of hepatic flow and 30–50% of the hepatic oxygen requirements
3. Unusual phenomenon: the venous system provides majority of oxygen to liver

II. PHYSIOLOGY

a. Drug metabolism

1. Phase 1 reactions: functionalization
   - (a) A lipid-soluble molecule has a charge placed on it, making it sticky
   - (b) Oxidation or reduction
   - (c) Susceptible to impairment due to disease
2. Phase 2 reactions: conjugation
   - (a) A polar group is stuck to charged compound, creating a water-soluble substance the kidney can excrete
   - (b) Rugged; functions despite disease

II. Physiology (continued)

b. Synthetic function

1. Carbohydrate metabolism

   (a) Gluconeogenesis
   (b) Glycolysis
   (c) Glucose buffer function

2. Lipid metabolism

   (a) Regulation of lipids, HDL and VLDL cycles

3. Ammonia regulation

4. Hemoglobin metabolism

   (a) Hg biliverdin bilirubin
   (b) Conjugation and excretion of bilirubin

5. Protein metabolism

   (a) Site of protein synthesis
   (b) Deamination of amino acids
   (c) Albumin is responsible for plasma oncotic pressure

6. Electrolyte regulation

c. Coagulation function

1. Liver synthesizes all clotting factors except VIII

2. Diminished vitamin K absorption results in decreased production of vitamin K–dependent factors II, VII, IX, and X

3. Liver disease leads to decreased synthetic function, resulting in coagulopathy

d. Tests of coagulation

1. PT: prothrombin time

   (a) Measures extrinsic coagulation pathway
   (b) Slight change in PT usually reflects profound liver dysfunction
   (c) Affected by coumadin and heparin

2. PTT: partial thrombin time

   (a) Measures intrinsic coagulation pathway
   (b) Affected by heparin

3. Platelet count

   (a) Quantitative measure of platelets
   (b) Normal mean platelet count 150,000–300,000
   (c) Multifactorial etiology of thrombocytopenia, including bone marrow failure, hemodilution, or blood loss
   (d) Dilutional thrombocytopenia is most common platelet abnormality encountered in the operating room

4. Fibrin degradation products (FSP)

   (a) Grossly quantified by bioassay
   (b) Normal value less than 10 mg%
   (c) Elevation signals an ongoing lytic process

5. Bleeding time (BT)

    (a) Provides assessment of initial platelet plug formation

    (b) Measures qualitative defect in platelet function

    (c) Poor predictor of perioperative blood loss

6. Thromboelastograph (TEG)

    (a) Rapid qualitative assessment of coagulation

    (b) Examines whole blood clot dynamics

    (c) Assesses interaction of coagulation cascade and platelets

    (d) Provides a guide to blood component therapy

7. Activated clotting time (ACT)

    (a) Most commonly utilized intraoperative coagulation test for heparin function

    (b) Automated adaptation of a Lee-White whole blood coagulation test

    (c) Affected by severe platelet dysfunction, hypofibrinogenemia, cold or excess protamine

e. Excretory actions of the liver

1. Bilirubin

    (a) Conjugated in the liver to glucuronic acid

    (b) Excreted by active transport into the bile

2. Urobilinogen

f. Cytochrome p450 system

1. Hemoprotein system located in the smooth endoplasmic reticulum of the hepatocyte

2. Responsible for drug metabolism and production of toxic metabolites

3. Over 50 p450 systems have been identified

4. Genetic differences in catalytic activity may determine idiosyncratic untoward drug reactions

g. Liver function tests

1. Aminotransferases

    (a) Aspartate transaminase: AST (SGOT)

        (1) Elevation may assist early diagnosis of hepatocellular disease

        (2) Normal value 5–40 IU/L

    (b) Alanine transaminase: ALT (SGPT)

        (1) Nonspecific

        (2) ALT than AST in alcoholism

        (3) Normal value 5–35 IU/L

    (c) Gamma-glutamyl transpeptidase: GGT

        (1) Elevated with alcohol abuse, also marker for biliary cholestasis

        (2) Normal value 10–48 IU/L

2. Alkaline phosphatase

    (a) Useful for diagnosis of cholestasis, hepatic infiltration, obstruction

    (b) Normal value 35–130 IU/L

3. Albumin

    (a) Best measure of hepatic synthetic function

    (b) Assess severity of liver disease

    (c) $T_{1/2}$ of 20 days, therefore, low only after 3–4 weeks of liver compromise

4. Prothrombin time (PT)
   (a) Normal value 12–16 seconds
5. Bilirubin
   (a) Total
      (1) Increase due to increased production
         [a] Massive transfusion
         [b] Absorption of large hematoma
         [c] Hemolysis
      (2) Increase due to decreased metabolism
         [a] Hereditary abnormalities
   (b) Conjugated
      (1) Increase due to
         [a] Hepatocellular diseases
         [b] Disease of small bile ducts
         [c] Congenital syndromes
         [d] Obstruction of extrahepatic biliary ducts

III. PHARMACOLOGY

a. Enzyme induction

1. Refers to increasing activity of cytochrome p450 enzymes leading to enhanced production of metabolites and altered pharmacologic effect
2. May be accompanied by liver enlargement
3. Drugs that cause enzyme induction
   (a) Barbiturates
   (b) Alcohol
   (c) Anesthetics
   (d) Hypoglycemic and anticonvulsant agents
   (e) Griseofulvin
   (f) Rifampicin
   (g) Glutethimide
   (h) Phenylbutazone
   (i) Meprobamate

b. Pharmacokinetics

1. Influenced by many factors
   (a) Method of drug delivery
   (b) Efficiency of drug metabolizing enzymes
   (c) Intrinsic clearance
      (1) Drugs avidly taken up by the liver have high first-pass metabolism
   (d) Liver blood flow
      (1) Rate-limiting factor in hepatic uptake
   (e) Plasma protein binding
      (1) Limits presentation of drug to hepatic enzymes
2. Pharmacologic effects of drugs vary according to the relative importance of these factors

c. Drug excretion

1. Multiple factors determine whether metabolized drug is excreted in bile or urine
    (a) Polarity
        (1) Highly polar substances are excreted unaltered in bile
        (2) Substances more polar after conjugation are usually excreted in the bile
    (b) Molecular weight
        (1) Substances with molecular weights over 200 tend to be excreted in the bile
        (2) As molecular weight falls, the urinary route of excretion becomes more important

IV. CLINICAL PRIORITIES

a. Hepatitis

1. A nonspecific term referring to inflammatory process of the hepatic parenchyma. If hepatitis persists, fibrosis follows
2. General information
    (a) Signs and symptoms
        (1) Onset may be gradual or sudden
        (2) Dark urine
        (3) Fatigue
        (4) Anorexia, vomiting
        (5) Low-grade fever
        (6) Enlarged, tender liver
    (b) Laboratory tests
        (1) Mild anemia and lymphocytosis
        (2) Elevated aminotransferases
        (3) Hepatitis serology
    (c) Clinical course
        (1) Clinical course usually uneventful
        (2) Dark urine and jaundice usually preceded by symptoms for 1–2 weeks
        (3) As jaundice worsens, symptoms improve
        (4) Aminotransferases usually decrease just before peak jaundice occurs and decrease rapidly thereafter
3. Viral: morbidity and mortality as high as 25% in patients exposed to anesthesia and surgery
    (a) Hepatitis A (infectious)
        (1) Transmission: fecal–oral route
        (2) 20–37-day incubation period
        (3) Does not progress to chronic liver disease
        (4) Prevention: pooled gamma globulin
        (5) Mortality: less than 0.2%
    (b) Hepatitis B (serum or long incubation)
        (1) Transmission: percutaneous or venereal
        (2) 60–110-day incubation period
        (3) Chronic liver disease in 1–10%
        (4) Prevention: hepatitis B vaccine, hepatitis B immunoglobulin
        (5) Mortality: 0.3–1.5%
    (c) Hepatitis C (or non-A, non-B)
        (1) Transmission: percutaneous
        (2) 35–70-day incubation period
        (3) Chronic liver disease develops in over 50%
        (4) Prevention and mortality unknown

III. Clinical properties; a. Hepatitis (continued)

4. Serum
5. Drug induced
    (a) Drugs associated with hepatic dysfunction
        (1) Antibiotics
        (2) Antihypertensives
        (3) Anticonvulsants
        (4) Analgesics
        (5) Tranquilizers
        (6) Anesthetics
    (b) Clinical features
        (1) Idiosyncratic reactions
        (2) Rare, unpredictable, not dose dependent
        (3) Signs of dysfunction usually occur 2–6 weeks after initiation of therapy
    (c) Treatment
        (1) Early recognition of liver dysfunction
        (2) Discontinuation of responsible drug
6. Halothane
    (a) United States National Halothane Study
        (1) Demonstrated that halothane hepatitis is an exceedingly rare complication, less than 0.01%
        (2) One in 35,000 cases
    (b) Increased risk in patients with
        (1) Multiple exposures
        (2) Procedures with higher risk of death
    (c) Risk factors
        (1) Previous exposure to halothane
        (2) Mild hepatic dysfunction
        (3) Other drug allergies
        (4) Obesity
        (5) Advancing age (uncommon in pediatrics)
        (6) Female gender
    (d) Diagnosis
        (1) Diagnosis of exclusion
        (2) No distinctive hepatic pathology or test
    (e) Signs and symptoms
        (1) Broad clinical spectrum
        (2) Asymptomatic elevation in serum transaminase
        (3) Fever of unknown origin
        (4) Clinical jaundice
        (5) Massive hepatic necrosis

b. Cholangitis

1. General information
    (a) Some 15–20 million U.S. adults have biliary tract disease, displayed by presence of gallstones
    (b) Radiolucency
        (1) 90% are radiolucent
        (2) Composed of hydrophobic cholesterol molecules
    (c) Radiopaque
        (1) 10% are radiopaque
        (2) Composed of calcium bilirubinate
        (3) Usually with cirrhosis or hemolytic anemia

2. Acute cholecystitis
   (a) Etiology: almost always due to obstruction of cystic duct by gallstones
   (b) Cardinal symptom: abrupt onset of severe midepigastric pain that radiates to right upper quadrant
   (c) Signs and symptoms
      (1) Murphy sign: pain accentuated by inspiration
      (2) Localized tenderness may indicate perforation with peritonitis
      (3) Fever, mild leukocytosis
      (4) Increased plasma bilirubin, alkaline phosphatase, and amylase
      (5) Jaundice if cystic duct obstructed
   (d) Diagnosis
      (1) Cholescintography: IV injection of labeled material selectively excreted by the gallbladder
      (2) Ultrasonography
   (e) Differential diagnosis
      (1) Acute viral hepatitis
      (2) Alcoholic hepatitis
      (3) Penetrating peptic ulcer
      (4) Appendicitis
      (5) Pyelonephritis
      (6) Right lower lobe pneumonia
      (7) Pancreatitis
      (8) Myocardial infarction
   (f) Treatment
      (1) Initial: IV fluids and gastric suction
      (2) Opiates will relieve intense pain
      (3) If perforation is suggested by free air under diaphragm or peritonitis, an emergency laparotomy is indicated
3. Chronic cholelithiasis and choledocholithiasis
   (a) Occurs after repeated acute attacks
   (b) Gallbladder becomes fibrotic and unable to contract and expel bile; leads to dilated bile ducts
   (c) Percutaneous transhepatic cholangiography allows direct visualization of biliary tree

c. Portal hypertension

1. Complication of chronic cirrhosis
2. Progressive scarring of liver leads to increased resistance to blood flow through the portal vein system
3. Physical examination
   (a) Hepatomegaly
   (b) With or without splenomegaly and ascites

d. Ascites

1. General
   (a) Common with severe parenchymal liver disease
   (b) Generally implies a grave prognosis
   (c) Aggravates poor cardiac function
2. Associated factors
   (a) Portal vein hypertension
   (b) Hypoalbuminemia
   (c) Increased ADH secretion

3. Diagnosis
   (a) Fluid wave on physical examination
   (b) Right-sided pleural effusion

4. Signs and symptoms
   (a) Increased abdominal pressure and girth
   (b) Upward shift of diaphragm
   (c) Decreased functional residual capacity and tidal volume with increased intrathoracic pressure
   (d) Decreased venous return and cardiac output

5. Treatment
   (a) Adequate nutrition
   (b) Diuresis usually with aldosterone antagonist, such as spironolactone
   (c) Paracentesis if respiratory compromise is life-threatening
   (d) LeVeen shunt: routes ascitic fluid subcutaneously from peritoneal cavity to internal jugular vein through a one-way valve

e. Liver failure

1. General
   (a) Liver disease, primarily cirrhosis, is one of top five causes of death in the United States
   (b) High perioperative mortality rates
   (c) Liver parenchyma has large reserve; only severe hepatitis and end-stage liver disease will affect drug metabolism in a clinically significant manner

2. Clinical features of cirrhosis
   (a) Enlarged spleen and liver
   (b) Ascites
   (c) Mild to moderate jaundice
   (d) Weakness
   (e) Anorexia, nausea, vomiting
   (f) Abdominal pain

3. Associated signs and symptoms
   (a) Hepatic encephalopathy
   (b) Pulmonary
      (1) Intrapulmonary shunt
      (2) Arterial oxygen desaturation
      (3) Orthodeoxialess dyspnea in supine position due to improvement in shunt fraction
      (4) Orthopnea and platypnea
      (5) Ventilation perfusion mismatch
   (c) Cardiovascular
      (1) Hyperdynamic circulation with increased CO and SVR
      (2) Resistance to inotropic drugs
      (3) Diminished cardiac reserve
   (d) Ascites
   (e) Palmar erythema, dilated peripheral veins, and spider angiomas
   (f) Prerenal azotemia and acute tubular necrosis
   (g) Hypersplenism—source of thrombocytopenia

f. Liver transplantation

1. Accepted therapeutic option for end-stage liver disease in suitable candidates
2. General indications
    (a) End-stage cirrhosis
        (1) Primary biliary cirrhosis
        (2) Chronic active hepatitis
        (3) Cryptogenic cirrhosis
        (4) Hemochromatosis
        (5) Sclerosing cholangitis
        (6) Budd-Chiari syndrome
    (b) Fulminant hepatic failure
    (c) Metabolic disorders
        (1) Wilson's disease
        (2) Protoporphyria
        (3) Hemochromatosis
        (4) Type IV hyperlipidemia
        (5) Budd-Chiari syndrome
    (d) Hepatocellular carcinoma
3. Contraindications
    (a) Metastatic disease
    (b) Coexisting life-threatening disease
4. Major perioperative complications
    (a) Hemorrhage
    (b) Coagulopathy
        (1) Factor deficiencies
        (2) Thrombocytopenia
        (3) Hypofibrinogenemia
        (4) Fibrinolysis
    (c) Hypothermia
    (d) Metabolic abnormalities
        (1) Metabolic acidosis
        (2) Hypocalcemia
        (3) Hyperkalemia
        (4) Hyperglycemia
    (e) Hypoxia
    (f) Immunosuppression

g. Transfusion reaction/hemolysis

1. Causes of transfusion-associated deaths in order of frequency from 1976 to 1985
    (a) Acute hemolysis
    (b) Non-A, non-B hepatitis
    (c) Acute pulmonary edema
    (d) Hepatitis B
    (e) Delayed hemolysis
2. Potential risks of blood transfusion
    (a) Hemolytic transfusion reaction
        (1) Immediate
        (2) Delayed
    (b) Transfusion-transmitted disease
        (1) Viral hepatitis

          (2) Cytomegalovirus

          (3) Acquired immunodeficiency syndrome (AIDS)

    (c) Recipient alloimmunization

    (d) Allergic reaction

3. Acute hemolytic transfusion reaction

    (a) Mortality rate 17–54%

    (b) Only a minimal amount of blood is necessary (30 ml) to cause lethal reaction

    (c) Occurs when ABO-incompatible red blood cells are transfused

          (1) Ag–Ab reaction occurs

          (2) This complex binds complement

          (3) Intravascular hemolysis results

    (d) Signs and symptoms

          (1) Fever

          (2) Tachycardia

          (3) Hypotension

          (4) Back pain

          (5) Dyspnea

          (6) Chest pain

          (7) Hemoglobinemia

          (8) Diffuse bleeding

          (9) Nausea

         (10) Flushing

         (11) Apprehension

         (12) Chills

    (e) Treatment

          (1) Aimed at preventing renal failure and DIC

          (2) Discontinue transfusion

          (3) Volume loading with crystalloid

          (4) Furosemide: increases renal blood flow and urine output

          (5) Return all units of blood to bank

F. ENDOCRINE SYSTEM

I. ANATOMY

    a. Pituitary

    b. Thyroid

    c. Parathyroid

    d. Adrenal

    e. Pancreas

II. PHYSIOLOGY

    a. Hypopituitarism

    b. Diabetes insipidus

    c. Acromegaly

    d. Hyperthyroidism

    e. Hypothyroidism

    f. Hyperparathyroidism

    g. Hypoparathyroidism

    h. Glucocorticoid excess

    i. Mineralocorticoid excess

    j. Adrenocortical insufficiency

    k. Pheochromocytoma

    l. Carcinoid

    m. Diabetes mellitus

III. PHARMACOLOGY

    a. Hormones

    b. Corticosteroids

I. ANATOMY

a. Pituitary

1. Located in the sella turcica (saddle-shaped cavity in the sphenoid bone)
2. Average glandular size: 10 mm by 13 mm by 6 mm
3. Weight: 0.5–0.7 grams
4. Two lobes

    (a) Anterior (75% of total glandular weight)
    (b) Posterior (neurohypophysis)

b. Thyroid

1. Anatomic proximity

    (a) Trachea/larynx
    (b) Esophagus
    (c) Carotid
    (d) Vagus

2. Weight: 20–25 grams
3. Vascular supply

    (a) Superior thyroidal artery
    (b) Inferior thyroidal artery

4. Innervation

    (a) Superior laryngeal
    (b) Recurrent laryngeal

5. Mediator of metabolism and thermoregulation
6. Control of synthesis and $Na+/K+$ ATPase and membrane channels
7. Tests of thyroid function

    (a) T_3, T_4, rT_3 measure total (bound and free) hormone
    (b) FTI, T_3RU: compensate for increased TBG (pregnancy, oral contraceptives, cirrhosis)
    (c) TSH: most sensitive to mild hypothyroidism
    (d) Functional testing: radionuclide scan

c. Parathyroid

1. Mediator of calcium metabolism in bone, gut, and kidney
2. Usually four but can be anywhere from 1 to 12 yellow glands located posteriolateral to thyroid with some variation in location (but usually symmetric); common blood supply with thyroid
3. Calcium

    (a) GI absorption 0.5–1.0 g/day (duodenum/jejunum)
    (b) Body reservoir of 1,000 grams calcium
    (c) 40% ionized, 40% protein bound, 20% chelated
    (d) Normal renal excretion of 300–400 mg per day (maximum of 500 mg per day)

d. Adrenal

1. General

    (a) Produces 50 types of steroids

    (b) Two glands, each located extraperitoneally at the upper poles of each kidney lateral to the 11th thoracic to first lumbar vertebrae

    (c) Each gland weighs 4 grams

    (d) Is 2–3 cm wide and 4–6 cm long

    (e) Arterial supply

        (1) Abdominal aorta

        (2) Renal arteries

        (3) Phrenic arteries

    (f) Venous drainage

        (1) Left gland: renal vein

        (2) Right gland: inferior vena cava

    (g) Autonomic innervation

    (h) Regulation

        (1) ACTH

        (2) Angiotensin II

        (3) Serum potassium

2. Cortex

    (a) Composes 90% of adrenal gland

    (b) Contains three zones

        (1) Zona glomerulosa

            [a] Outermost portion

            [b] 15% of cortex

            [c] Produces aldosterone

        (2) Zona reticularis

        (3) Zona fasciculata

            [a] 75% of cortex

3. Medulla

    (a) Principal site of catecholamine biosynthesis

    (b) Catecholamines produced

        (1) Epinephrine

        (2) Norepinephrine

        (3) Dopamine

    (c) Synthesized from tyrosine and phenylalanine

    (d) Catecholamines, $T_{1/2}$ is 1–2 minutes

e. Pancreas

1. Endocrine and exocrine organ

2. Anatomy

    (a) Approximately 15 cm in length and weighs 60–140 grams

    (b) Anatomic relationships

        (1) Duodenum

        (2) Ampulla of Vater

        (3) Common bile duct

        (4) Superior mesenteric artery

        (5) Portal vein

        (6) Spleen

        (7) Transverse colon

        (8) Left lobe of the liver

    (c) Composed of two tissue types

        (1) The acini: secrete digestive fluids into the duodenum

        (2) Islets of Langerhans: secrete insulin, glucagon, and somatostatin directly into the blood

            [a] Alpha cells secrete glucagon

I. Anatomy; e. Pancreas (continued)

        [b] Beta cells secrete insulin
        [c] D cells secrete somatostatin
        [d] PP cells secrete pancreatic polypeptide

3. Physiology
   - (a) Endocrine
     - (1) Produces insulin and glucagon
     - (2) Regulates glucose, lipid, and protein metabolism
   - (b) Exocrine
     - (1) 80–85% of the pancreas
     - (2) Secretes 1.5–3.0 liters of isosmotic alkaline fluid per day
     - (3) Contains 20 enzymes and zymogens to aid in digestion
     - (4) Proteolytic enzymes
       - [a] Trypsin
       - [b] Chymotrypsin
       - [c] Carboxypolypeptidase
       - [d] Ribonuclease
       - [e] Deoxyribonuclease
     - (5) Carbohydrate enzymes
       - [a] Amylase
     - (6) Lipid enzymes
       - [a] Lipase
       - [b] Cholesterol esterase
   - (c) Regulation of secretion
     - (1) Cholinergic and beta-adrenergic stimulation increases insulin, glucagon, and pancreatic polypeptide secretion
     - (2) Secretion stimulated by secretin and cholecystokinin

II. PHYSIOLOGY

a. Hypopituitarism

1. Presentation depends on rate of onset and hormonal system affected
2. Etiology
   - (a) Pituitary tumor
     - (1) 30% or more have one or more hormone deficiencies
     - (2) Growth hormone deficiency most common
   - (b) Parasellar tumor (meningioma)
   - (c) Suprasellar tumor (hypothalamic) tumor
   - (d) Postoperative
   - (e) Postirradiation
   - (f) Pituitary apoplexy
     - (1) Abrupt destruction of pituitary tissue resulting from infarction or hemorrhage into the pituitary, usually from an undiagnosed tumor
     - (2) Clinical presentation
       - [a] Sudden onset
       - [b] Severe headache
       - [c] Visual loss
       - [d] Cranial nerve palsies (III, IV, or VI)
       - [e] Variably depressed mental status
   - (g) Infiltrative diseases (hypothalamic or pituitary)
     - (1) Sarcoid
     - (2) Giant-cell granuloma

        (3) Eosinophilic granuloma
        (4) Wegener's granulomatosis
        (5) Lymphocytic hypophysitis
        (6) Hemachromatosis
        (7) Metastatic breast or lung cancer
    (h) Miscellaneous causes
        (1) Empty sella
        (2) Trauma
            [a] May occur without basilar skull fracture
        (3) Internal carotid artery aneurysm

3. Treatment

    (a) Replace the hormones that the target endocrine glands are no longer capable of producing
    (b) Goals of hormone-replacement therapy
        (1) Raise circulating hormone concentrations to levels that are within the normal range
        (2) Attempt to mimic normal diurnal variations
        (3) Ameliorate symptoms of underlying hormone deficiency

4. Anesthetic management

    (a) No special anesthetic considerations
    (b) Continue specific hormone replacement as necessary (i.e., corticosteroids)
    (c) Mineralocorticoid not usually necessary

b. Diabetes insipidus (DI)

1. General

    (a) Clinical manifestations
        (1) Polyuria
            [a] 3–15 liters per day
            [b] Abrupt onset
            [c] Urinary output may exceed 700 ml per hour
        (2) Thirst
        (3) Nocturia
        (4) Intravascular volume depletion
        (5) Hypertonic encephalopathy
    (b) Diagnosis
        (1) Polyuria
        (2) Hypernatremia (essential to the diagnosis)
        (3) Inappropriately dilute urine
            [a] 60–200 mOsm
            [b] Specific gravity less than 1.005
    (c) Management
        (1) Intravascular volume repletion
            [a] Correct hemodynamic instability
            [b] Rapid infusions of hypotonic solutions may induce seizures
            [c] Correct serum sodium to normal over 36–48 hours while matching urinary output
            [d] Reduce serum sodium by 1 mEq/L every 2 hours
        (2) ADH
            [a] 1-desamino-8-*D*-arginine vasopressin (DDAVP), desmopressin
               i) Synthetic analogue of vasopressin
              ii) Limited systemic effects
             iii) 1–2 mg SC or IV
             iv) $T_{1/2}$: 2–6 hours

            [b] Aqueous vasopressin (Pitressin)
               i) 5–10 IU IM or SC
              ii) $T_{1/2}$: 2–6 hours IV, 24–48 hours IM

2. Pituitary DI (central)
   (a) Pathology
       (1) Lack of ADH
       (2) Unable to appropriately concentrate urine or conserve water
       (3) Presents as polyuria: inappropriately dilute urine in the presence of a concentrated serum, and in the absence of a renal concentrating defect
       (4) Urine osmolality increases with supplemental vasopressin
   (b) Etiology
       (1) Trauma to neurohypophysis
           [a] Accidental
           [b] Surgical
       (2) Tumor (primary or metastatic)
       (3) CNS granulomatous diseases
       (4) Vascular lesions
       (5) 30–40% idiopathic
   (c) Triphasic acute DI following hypophysectomy
       (1) Polyuric, hyposthenuric phase of hours to days; inhibition of ADH release
       (2) Decreasing urine volume with increased urine osmolality
       (3) If DI permanent, then recurrent polyuria and hypostheuria

3. Nephrogenic DI
   (a) Pathology
       (1) Renal tubular unresponsiveness to ADH
   (b) Etiology
       (1) Familial
       (2) Acquired
           [a] Drugs
               i) Demeclocycline
               ii) Volatile fluorocarbon anesthetics
               iii) Lithium
           [b] Systemic diseases
               i) Sarcoidosis
               ii) Sjogren's syndrome

4. Differential diagnosis of polyuria
   (a) Pituitary (central) DI
   (b) Nephrogenic DI
   (c) Solute diuresis (i.e., postoperative)
   (d) Renal concentrating defect
   (e) Primary polydipsia

5. Anesthetic management
   (a) Monitor serum electrolytes and urine output
   (b) Treat free-water losses as needed in a patient who is NPO
       (1) Replace urine output
       (2) DDAVP as needed

c. Acromegaly

1. Hypersecretion of growth hormone (GH)

2. Increased GH secondary to pituitary tumor (common) or hyperplasia (rare)

3. Clinical features
    (a) Depend on age of onset
    (b) Pediatric
        (1) Gigantism
        (2) Hypogonadism
    (c) Adult
        (1) Signs and symptoms develop slowly
        (2) Soft-tissue swelling and hypertropy of the extremeties and face
        (3) Increasing ring, glove, and shoe sizes
        (4) Skin thickened, leathery, and oily, and increased sweating
        (5) Prominent skin folds
        (6) Increased hair growth and pigmentation
        (7) Prognathism due to mandibular enlargement (overbite of lower incisors and increased spacing of teeth)
        (8) Bony overgrowth of frontal, malar, and nasal bones
        (9) Vocal cord hypertrophy
        (10) Peripheral entrapment neuropathy (carpal tunnel)
        (11) Visceromegaly (cardiomegaly)
        (12) Mild hypertension
    (d) Laboratory
        (1) Elevated GH levels that do not respond to stimulation or suppression
    (e) Treatment
        (1) Pituitary adenomectomy
        (2) Irradiation
        (3) Pharmacologic
            [a] Dopaminergic agonist: bromocriptine
            [b] Somatostatin analogue: octreotide
4. Anesthetic management
    (a) Airway problems
        (1) Poorly fitting mask
        (2) Enlarged tongue and epiglottis
        (3) Enlarged cords, narrow glottis
        (4) Enlarged turbinates
    (b) Poor collateral circulation
        (1) Perform Allen's test before radial artery cannulation
    (c) Carefully monitor for coexisting disease
        (1) Diabetes mellitus
        (2) Skeletal muscle weakness
    (d) Careful airway evaluation
    (e) Awake fiberoptic intubation may be necessary (prepare ahead of time)
    (f) Small endotracheal tube
    (g) No change necessary in anesthetic drug requirements or usage

d. Hyperthyroidism

1. Fivefold greater incidence in females
2. Pathology
    (a) Most often diffuse hyperplasia
    (b) Graves' disease: autoimmune, systemic disease
    (c) Hyperfunctioning (hot) nodule
    (d) Ectopic thyroid
    (e) Chorionic tissue

II. Physiology; d. Hyperthyroidism (continued)

3. Clinical signs/symptoms
   (a) Nervousness, palpitations, fatigue, weakness, fine tremor, dyspnea on exertion, insomnia, weight loss, increased appetite
   (b) Tachycardia, arrhythmia, edema, pigment changes, organomegaly
   (c) Ocular changes (signs): lid retraction (Dalrymple's), lid lag (Graefe's), infrequent blink (Stellwag's)

4. Thyroid storm
   (a) Hyperpyrexia
   (b) Tachycardia
   (c) Hypotension

5. Systemic effects
   (a) Metabolic
       (1) Increased basal metabolic rate
       (2) Hyperthermia
       (3) Osteopenia
       (4) Osteoporosis
   (b) Renal
       (1) Increased calcium and phosphate excretion
   (c) Hematologic
       (1) Anemia
       (2) Lymphocytosis
   (d) Ocular
       (1) Extraocular muscles enlarged
       (2) Optic nerve compression
   (e) Cardiac
       (1) Increased cardiac output
       (2) Tachycardia
   (f) Neurologic
       (1) Proximal muscle weakness
       (2) Fine hand tremor

6. Anesthetic management
   (a) Remember—patients are hypermetabolic
   (b) Normalize thyroid function prior to surgery, if possible
   (c) Premedicate with barbiturate or benzodiazepine
   (d) Induce with thiopental
       (1) Questionable antithyroid effect due to thiourea structure
       (2) Probably not clinically significant
   (e) Avoid sympathetic stimulants (i.e., ketamine)
   (f) Inhalation induction slowed by increased cardiac output
   (g) Maintenance of anesthesia
       (1) Avoid sympathetic stimulation and vagolytic drugs
       (2) No documented increases in anesthetic requirements have been found
       (3) However, anesthetic requirements are increased with coexisting hyperthermia
       (4) Avoid indirect sympathomimetics (ephedrine) due to unpredictable response
       (5) Monitor temperature carefully
       (6) Treat tachyarrhythmias aggressively with beta blockade
       (7) Consider coexisting myasthenia (more common in hyperthyroid patients)
       (8) Protect eyes due to the presence of exophthalmos

e. Hypothyroidism

1. 0.5–0.8% incidence

2. Tenfold greater incidence in females

3. Pathology

    (a) Mostly iatrogenic (postsurgery, ablation)
    (b) Inadequate hormone replacement
    (c) Dietary: inadequate iodine leading to TSH stimulation leading to hypertrophy and goiter
    (d) Secondary: pituitary hypofunction or tumor

4. Clinical signs/symptoms

    (a) Fatigue, hair loss, constipation
    (b) Hoarseness, cold intolerance, menorrhagia, memory impairment
    (c) Periorbital edema, lateral eyebrow thinning, dry skin, hypothermia, bradycardia, and slow relaxation of deep tendon reflexes

5. Myxedema coma

    (a) Severe hypothyroidism
    (b) Hypothermic
    (c) Hypoventilation (chronic respiratory acidosis)
    (d) Hyponatremic (SIADH)
    (e) Hypoglycemic

6. Basal metabolic rate 55–60% of normal

7. Susceptible to environmental hypothermia

8. Cardiovascular function compromised by both metabolic depression and structural changes

    (a) Pericardial effusions
    (b) Prolonged preejection period and decreased left ventricular ejection time
    (c) Cardiac output may decrease by 40%
        (1) Bradycardia
        (2) Decreased stroke volume
        (3) Systemic vascular resistance increased
    (d) Decreased blood volume (10–24%)
    (e) Increased extracellular water

9. Respiratory changes

    (a) Impaired hypoxic ventilatory response
    (b) Depressed CO_2 response

10. Neurologic changes

    (a) Altered baroreceptor response
    (b) Increased sympathetic tone
    (c) Enhanced adrenal response to hypoglycemia
    (d) Polyneuropathy (peripheral)

11. Renal changes

    (a) Decreased glomerular filtration rate and creatinine clearance
    (b) Decreased free-water excretion

12. Miscellaneous changes

    (a) Decreased factors VIII and IX
    (b) Increased cholesterol
    (c) Concomitant adrenal insufficiency
    (d) Ileus, gastroparesis

II. Physiology; e. Hypothyroidism (continued)

13. Anesthetic management
    (a) Very sensitive to depressant drugs
    (b) Decreased cardiac output and cardiac reserves
    (c) Slowed drug metabolism (especially opiates)
    (d) Minimal baroreceptor reflexes
    (e) Decreased intravascular volume
    (f) Blunted ventilatory drive to hypoxia and hypercarbia
    (g) Delayed gastric emptying
    (h) Decreased free-water clearance (hyponatremia)
    (i) Hypothermia
    (j) Anemia
    (k) Hypoglycemia
    (l) Adrenal insufficiency
    (m) No standard premedication
    (n) Consider the use of perioperative steroids
    (o) Induction with ketamine or *small* doses of other hypnotic
    (p) Consider rapid-sequence induction with aspiration prophylaxis
    (q) Anesthesia maintenance
        (1) Minimize use of volatile anesthetics
        (2) MAC not decreased by hypothyroidism
        (3) Controlled ventilation
        (4) Avoid hypothermia
    (r) Anesthesia recovery
        (1) Postoperative respiratory depression common
        (2) Consider adrenal insufficiency in refractory hypotension

f. Hyperparathyroidism

1. Increased PTH
2. Primary: benign adenoma (90%), carcinoma, or hyperplasia; adenomas associated with MEN I (parathyroid, pituitary, and islet cells) or MEN IIa (thyroid, parathyroid, and pheochromocytoma)
3. Produces bone resorption, osteopenia, and hypercalcemia
4. Symptoms and signs of hypercalcemia
    (a) Generalized weakness most frequent
    (b) Renal: calculi, polyuria, polydipsia
    (c) Cardia: hypertension, short QT, prolonged PR
    (d) Skeletal: pain, pathologic fractures
    (e) Hematologic: anemia
    (f) CNS: somnolence, psychosis, decreased pain
5. Serum ionized calcium over 5.5 mEq/L
6. Serum chloride over 102 mEq/L (renal bicarbonate excretion)
7. Hypophosphatemia
8. Therapy
    (a) Fluids
    (b) Diuretics
    (c) Mithramycin
    (d) Calcitonin
    (e) Dialysis
    (f) Parathyroidectomy

9. Secondary: renal disease (decreased phosphate excretion, decreased hydroxylation of vitamin D, decreased serum calcium, increased PTH)

10. Pseudohyperparathyroidism

    (a) Ectopic PTH or analogue
    (b) Usually produced by tumor (lung, breast, pancreas, kidney, or lymphoproliferative disease)
    (c) Most frequently accompanied by anemia, chloride less than 102 mEq/L, and increased alkaline phosphatase

11. Anesthetic management

    (a) Maintain hydration and urine output
    (b) Possible skeletal muscle weakness and decreased relaxant requirements
    (c) Careful positioning (osteoporosis)

g. Hypoparathyroidism

1. Primary

    (a) Glandular dysfunction
    (b) Surgical removal
    (c) Hypomagnesemia
    (d) Chronic renal failure
    (e) Malabsorption
    (f) Anticonvulsant drugs
    (g) Acute pancreatitis

2. Produces symptomatic hypocalcemia

    (a) Acute hypocalcemia
        (1) Perioral paresthesias
        (2) Restlessness
        (3) Neuromuscular irritability
            [a] Facial nerve (Chvostek's)
            [b] Carpopedal spasm (Trousseau's)
    (b) Chronic hypocalcemia
        (1) Fatigue
        (2) Muscular cramps
    (c) Ionized calcium (Ca^{2+}) less than 4.5 mEq/L
    (d) Prolonged QT with normal PR
    (e) Hyperphosphatemia
    (f) Therapy
        (1) Acutely: calcium infusion
        (2) Chronically
            [a] Oral calcium
            [b] Vitamin D supplements

3. Pseudohypoparathyroidism

    (a) Renal unresponsive to circulating PTH
    (b) Mental retardation
    (c) Short stature
    (d) Calcification of basal ganglia

4. Pseudopseudohypoparathyroidism

    (a) Same as pseudohypoparathyroidism, but with normal Ca^{2+} values

5. Anesthetic management

    (a) Monitor Ca^{2+} and neuromuscular signs
    (b) Postoperative stridor and tetany possible

      (c) Treatment of acute hypocalcemia includes IV calcium and/or use of thiazide diuretics

---

h. Glucocorticoid excess

1. Cushing's syndrome

    (a) Chronic glucocorticoid excess
    (b) Usually supraphysiologic glucocorticoid doses
    (c) Rarely spontaneous
        (1) Adrenal tumors (15% of cases)
        (2) Excessive pituitary (Cushing's disease, 66% of cases) or nonpituitary, ectopic (15% of cases) (50% of cases due to oat-cell carcinoma of the lung) ACTH secretion
        (3) Excessive CRF secretion from hypothalamus
    (d) Cushing's disease
        (1) Spontaneous glucocorticoid excess due to excessive pituitary ACTH
        (2) Females 20–40 years old
        (3) 90% with pituitary adenomas

2. Clinical features

    (a) Classic features seen in Cushing's disease
    (b) Develop insidiously over several years
    (c) In order of incidence: obesity, facial plethora, hirsutism, menstrual disorders, hypertension, muscular weakness, back pain, striae, acne, psychologic disorders, bruising, congestive heart failure, edema, renal calculi, headache, polyuria, polydipsia, and hyperpigmentation

3. Diagnosis

    (a) 24-hour urine for free cortisol
    (b) Low-dose dexamethasone suppression test
    (c) If (a) and (b) normal, then Cushing's excluded
    (d) If (a) and (b) abnormal, then plasma ACTH and high-dose dexamethasone suppression test should be performed
    (e) If Cushing's syndrome confirmed, then an etiologic diagnosis needs to be pursued
    (f) If tumor suspected, then obtain MRI

4. Treatment

    (a) Pituitary microsurgery for Cushing's disease
    (b) Pituitary irradiation
    (c) Bilateral adrenalectomy reserved for patients unresponsive to initial treatments
    (d) Drugs to suppress ACTH secretion
        (1) Reserpine
        (2) Bromocriptine
        (3) Cyproheptadine
        (4) Valproate sodium

5. Anesthetic management

    (a) Increased cortisol release during surgery not preventable
    (b) Skeletal muscle weakness implies
        (1) Relaxant dose may be reduced
        (2) Controlled ventilation preferred
    (c) Hypokalemia may be present
    (d) Supplement cortisol during hypophysectomy or bilateral adrenalectomy

i. Mineralocorticoid excess

1. Primary aldosteronism
   - (a) Clinical manifestations
     - (1) Sodium retention
       - [a] Increased extracellular fluid volume
       - [b] Edema rarely present
     - (2) Hypertension
     - (3) Suppression of plasma renin
     - (4) Urinary excretion of potassium and hydrogen ions
       - [a] Hypokalemia
       - [b] Muscular weakness
       - [c] Cardiac irritability and arrhythmias
     - (5) Nephrogenic DI
     - (6) Carbohydrate intolerance
     - (7) Baroreceptor abnormalities (volume-dependent hypertension)
     - (8) No characteristic physical findings
   - (b) Etiology
     - (1) Adrenocortical adenoma (70% in females)
     - (2) Bilateral adrenocortical hyperplasia
     - (3) Adrenal carcinoma
   - (c) Peak incidence in third and fourth decades
   - (d) Diagnosis
     - (1) Document hypokalemic hypertension (no diuretic therapy)
     - (2) Plasma renin
     - (3) 24-hour urine for aldosterone and plasma aldosterone
     - (4) CT or MRI of the adrenals
   - (e) Treatment
     - (1) Unilateral adrenalectomy for adenomas
     - (2) Antimineralocorticoid therapy
       - [a] Spironolactone
       - [b] Amiloride

2. Secondary aldosteronism: adrenal stimulation by the renin-angiotensin system
   - (a) Physiologic
     - (1) Protective against increased potassium intake
     - (2) Luteal phase of the menstrual cycle
     - (3) Rarely with oral contraceptives
     - (4) Normal pregnancy
   - (b) Pathophysiologic
     - (1) Excessive sodium loss or dietary sodium restriction
     - (2) Congestive heart failure
     - (3) Hypoalbuminemia (nephrotic syndrome)
     - (4) Cirrhosis (usually with ascites)
     - (5) Bartter's syndrome
     - (6) Renal artery stenosis
     - (7) Unilateral renal ischemia
     - (8) Accelerated hypertension
     - (9) Renin-secreting tumors

3. Anesthetic management
   - (a) Correct hypokalemia
   - (b) Treat hypertension
   - (c) Detect and treat hypovolemia (orthostasis)
   - (d) Intraoperatively
     - (1) Avoid hyperventilation (hyperkalemia)

II. Physiology; i. Mineralocorticoid excess (continued)

      (2) Monitor intravascular volume invasively with CVP or pulmonary artery catheter

      (3) Cortisol supplementation unnecessary unless surgery is bilateral

j. Adrenocortical insufficiency

1. General
   (a) Clinical presentation
       (1) Insidious, unmasked during stress
       (2) Catastrophic syndrome: adrenal crisis
       (3) Due to cortisol and aldosterone deficiency
   (b) May require empiric replacement therapy prior to diagnosis

2. Physiology
   (a) Adrenal cortex secretes two hormones
       (1) Glucocorticoid (cortisol)
           [a] Increases gluconeogenesis
           [b] Enhances catabolism
           [c] Increases lipolysis
           [d] Inhibits neutrophil and macrophage migration
           [e] Increases free-water clearance
           [f] Enhances peripheral vascular responses to endogenous vasoconstrictors
           [g] Secretion controlled by adrenocorticotropic hormone (ACTH)
       (2) Aldosterone
           [a] Regulates extracellular fluid volume
           [b] Secretion controlled by reninangiotensin system, serum K^+, and ACTH

3. Primary adrenocortical insufficiency (Addison's disease)
   (a) Rare; equally affects males and females
   (b) More than 90% glandular destruction
   (c) 80% idiopathic, 50% with antiadrenal antibodies
   (d) Other etiologies
       (1) Tuberculosis
       (2) Cryptococcosis
       (3) Cytomegalovirus
       (4) Metastatic neoplasms
       (5) Radiation
       (6) Hemachromatosis
   (e) Clinical signs
       (1) Hyperpigmentation in skin exposed to light, friction, or pressure (primary)
       (2) Postural and supine hypotension (primary and secondary)
   (f) Symptoms (common to both primary and secondary)
       (1) Asthenia
       (2) Muscle weakness
       (3) Malaise
       (4) Anorexia
       (5) Abdominal pain
       (6) Vomiting
       (7) Diarrhea or constipation
       (8) Weight loss
       (9) Salt craving
       (10) Myalgias, arthralgias
       (11) Mental status changes
   (g) Increased sensitivity to CNS depressants, especially opioids

4. Secondary adrenocortical insufficiency
    (a) Etiology
        (1) ACTH deficiency
            [a] Pituitary deficiency
            [b] Hypothalamic deficiency
        (2) Hypothalamic-pituitary-adrenal suppression
            [a] Exogenous corticosteroid
        (3) Pituitary dysfunction (rare)
            [a] Neoplasms
            [b] Infections
            [c] Hemorrhage
            [d] Infarction
            [e] Radiation
            [f] Granulomatous infiltration
5. Acute adrenocortical insufficiency (addisonian crisis)
    (a) Etiology
        (1) Worsening of chronic hypoadrenalism
            [a] Insufficient hormone to respond to stress
        (2) Cessation or too rapid reduction of exogenous steroid
        (3) Exogenous steroid–drug interaction (rifampin, barbiturates, phenytoin)
        (4) Adrenal hemorrhage
            [a] Sepsis
            [b] Anticoagulants
            [c] Burns
            [d] Surgery
            [e] Trauma
            [f] Postpartum
            [g] Pituitary apoplexy
            [h] Drugs that inhibit steroid metabolism
            [i] Etomidate
    (b) Clinical presentation
        (1) Shock unresponsive to volume or vasopressors
        (2) Precipitating event
            [a] Surgery
            [b] Sepsis
        (3) History of exogenous steroids
        (4) Fever
        (5) Malaise, weakness
        (6) Anorexia, nausea, vomiting, abdominal pain
        (7) Altered mental status
    (c) Diagnosis
        (1) High clinical suspicion
        (2) Document functional adrenal insufficiency
            [a] Low baseline serum cortisol with insufficient response to cosyntropin (synthetic ACTH)
        (3) Hypoglycemia
        (4) Metabolic acidosis and respiratory acidosis
        (5) Intravascular volume depletion
        (6) Abdominal CT scan to evaluate adrenals
    (d) Treatment
        (1) Steroid supplementation (may begin prior to ACTH stimulation test) (dexamethasone does not interfere with the cortisol assay)
        (2) Intravascular volume repletion
        (3) Vasopressors as needed
        (4) Treat and monitor hypoglycemia

II. Physiology; j. Adrenocortical insufficiency (continued)

    6. Anesthetic management

      (a) Acute insufficiency very unlikely in normal patients with only a history of recent steroid use

      (b) Exogenous corticosteroid supplementation intra- and postoperatively

      (c) Urgent surgery in untreated hypoadrenocorticism may involve

        (1) Extreme sensitivity to drug-induced myocardial depression

        (2) Glucose and electrolyte disturbances

        (3) Skeletal muscle weakness

k. Pheochromocytoma

    1. General

      (a) Catecholamine-releasing tumors

      (b) Typically present with hypertension, which is curable with tumor resection

      (c) May produce malignant hypertension

      (d) Pheochromocytoma occasionally malignant

      (e) Considered malignant if tumor metastasizes

      (f) May be part of polyglandular syndromes (MEN IIa and IIb)

      (g) 90% arise from the adrenal medulla

      (h) Multiple pheochromocytomas present 10% of the time

    2. Clinical manifestations

      (a) Due to released catecholamines and not tumor mass effect

      (b) Symptoms

        (1) Paroxysmal and associated with increases in blood pressure

        (2) Headache

        (3) Palpitations

        (4) Diaphoresis

        (5) Abdominal/chest pain

        (6) GI: diarrhea

        (7) Weakness

        (8) Visual

        (9) Increased metabolic rate

          [a] Weight loss

          [b] Heat intolerance

      (c) Signs

        (1) Usually intermittent hypertension

      (d) Laboratory

        (1) Elevated plasma catecholamines during symptomatic hypertensive episodes

      (e) Diagnosis

        (1) Clinical suspicion

          [a] Paroxysmal symptoms

          [b] Intermittent/refractory hypertension

          [c] Family history

        (2) Biochemical

          [a] Plasma norepinephrine and epinephrine when supine and when not symptomatic and repeated during symptoms

          [b] Urinary catecholamines or metanephrines

        (3) Tumor localization

          [a] CT scan of adrenals; if negative, then scan the pelvis and thorax

          [b] MRI

          [c] Iodobenzylguanidine scan

3. Anesthetic management
    (a) General principles
        (1) Avoid sympathetic stimulation
        (2) Use invasive monitoring
        (3) Regional anesthesia usually not indicated
    (b) Preoperatively
        (1) Continue alpha blockade
        (2) Premedicate with narcotic/benzodiazepine
        (3) Place arterial line and pulmonary artery catheter
    (c) Anesthesia induction
        (1) Barbiturate or benzodiazepine
        (2) Succinylcholine or nondepolarizing relaxant with minimal cardiovascular effects
        (3) Ensure adequate anesthetic depth before intubation
        (4) Nitroprusside or phentolamine for acute hypertension
    (d) Anesthesia maintenance
        (1) Nitrous oxide/isoflurane
        (2) Avoid droperidol
        (3) After resection, hypotension may require phenylephrine
        (4) Monitor arterial blood gases, electrolytes, glucose, urine output, and temperature frequently
        (5) Hypoglycemia possible following resection
    (e) Postoperatively
        (1) Early extubation
        (2) Continue invasive monitoring for 24–48 hours

l. Carcinoid

1. Overview
    (a) Carcinoid tumors arise from enterochomaffin (Kulchitsky's) cells, located primarily in the gastrointestinal mucosa
    (b) Syndrome due to overproduction of serotonin
    (c) Carcinoid tumors
        (1) Common
        (2) Most commonly found in the appendix or rectum
        (3) Rarely produce carcinoid syndrome
    (d) Carcinoid syndrome
        (1) Rare
        (2) Produced by tumors in the
            [a] Ileum (with metastases to the liver)
            [b] Stomach
            [c] Bile duct
            [d] Duodenum
            [e] Pancreas
            [f] Lung
            [g] Gonads
    (e) Survival usually less than 5 years

2. Serotonin
    (a) 5-Hydroxyindoleacetic acid (5-HIAA) is the major metabolite of serotonin
    (b) Serotonin synthesized from dietary tryptophan
    (c) Normal 5-HIAA excretion less than 10 mg per 24 hours
    (d) Carcinoid syndrome 5-HIAA excretion 50–100 mg per 24 hours

3. Clinical manifestations
    (a) Produced by ileal carcinoid tumor with liver mets
    (b) 90% with cutaneous flushing
        (1) Precipitated by alcohol, food, stress, liver palpation
        (2) Not due to serotonin
    (c) 75% with diarrhea
        (1) Serotonin mediated
    (d) 33% with right-sided endocardial fibrosis
        (1) Possibly chronically high serotonin
    (e) 20% with bronchoconstriction
4. Diagnosis
    (a) High clinical suspicion
    (b) Increased urinary 5-HIAA
    (c) Metastatic hepatomegaly
5. Treatment
    (a) Somatostatin decreases flushing, diarrhea, and bronchoconstriction
    (b) Tumor resection not indicated with metastatic disease
    (c) Nicotinamide to prevent pellagra
    (d) Serotonin antagonists
6. Anesthetic management
    (a) General principles
        (1) Block histamine, serotonin, bradykinin if possible (diphenhydramine, cimetidine, cyproheptadine, aminocaproate)
        (2) Avoid histamine-releasing drugs (morphine, atracurium)
        (3) Minimize catecholamine release
        (4) Avoid hypotension (stimulates tumor secretion)
        (5) Regional anesthesia may be complicated by persistent hypotension
    (b) Intraoperative complications include
        (1) Bronchospasm (sometimes refractory)
        (2) Hypotension
        (3) Tachycardia and hypertension (serotonin release)

m. Diabetes mellitus

1. Perioperative management
    (a) Noninsulin dependent
        (1) NPO
        (2) Omit a.m. hypoglycemic
        (3) Fasting serum glucose measurement
        (4) IV in place prior to any interventions
        (5) Slow dextrose infusion
        (6) Monitor glucose intraoperatively
        (7) Low-dose insulin only if profoundly hyperglycemic
        (8) Resume oral hypoglycemic as soon as patient tolerates PO intake
    (b) Insulin dependent
        (1) NPO
        (2) IV in place prior to insulin administration
        (3) Half of usual a.m. dose of insulin SC (given as regular insulin and not NPH)
        (4) Glucose infusion intraoperatively
        (5) Frequent serum glucose determinations
        (6) IV insulin infusion if serum glucose is labile

2. Hypo/hyperglycemia: general principles

   (a) Symptoms of hypo- and hyperglycemia are masked by general anesthesia
   (b) Frequent monitoring of blood glucose is essential
   (c) Regional anesthesia helpful to monitor mental status

3. Diabetic ketoacidosis

   (a) Overview
      (1) Lack of effective insulin
      (2) Clinical hallmarks
         [a] Metabolic acidosis
         [b] Dehydration
         [c] Electrolyte abnormalities
      (3) Pathophysiology
         [a] Ingested carbohydrate not utilized and resultant hyperglycemia produces an osmotic diuresis and a hyperosmolar state results
         [b] Ketosis and acidosis attributable to lack of an insulin effect on adipose tissue
         [c] With low insulin levels, markedly increased glucagon levels with unchecked lipolysis and fatty acids converted in the liver to ketone bodies
   (b) Precipitating causes
      (1) 25% of patients omit or reduce insulin dose
      (2) 25% present as the initial manifestation of diabetes
      (3) 25% secondary to infection
      (4) 25% others: pulmonary embolism, myocardial infarct, etc.
   (c) Signs and symptoms
      (1) Polyuria
         [a] Osmotic diuresis occurs when renal glucose threshold exceeded (180–200 mg/dl)
      (2) Polydipsia
      (3) Anorexia
      (4) Nausea/vomiting
      (5) Abdominal pain, can mimic an acute abdomen
      (6) Weakness and myalgias
      (7) Headache
      (8) Dyspnea
         [a] Kussmaul's respirations
            i) Long, deep, sighing breaths
            ii) Ventilatory response to metabolic acidosis
            iii) Usually appears when pH is less than 7.20 and/or $[HCO_3^-]$ is less than 12 mEq/L
      (9) Hypothermic
      (10) Acetone breath
      (11) Intravascular volume depletion
      (12) Hyporeflexia
      (13) Altered mental status
         [a] Difficult to relate to degree of ketosis or acidosis
   (d) Differential diagnosis
      (1) Cerebrovascular accident (altered mental status)
      (2) Brain-stem hemorrhage (hyperventilation, glycosuria)
      (3) Symptomatic hypoglycemia
      (4) Elevated anion gap metabolic acidosis

A—alcohol	*S*—salicylates
M—methanol	*U*—uremia
P—paraldehyde	*D*—DKA
L—lactate	*S*—starvation
E—ethylene glycol	

II. Physiology; m. Diabetes mellitus (continued)

    (e) Initial laboratory values
       (1) Glucose
         [a] 300–800 mg/dl
         [b] Not related to severity of DKA
       (2) Ketones
         [a] Usually 1:2 or greater
         [b] Measures acetoacetate but not beta-hydroxybutyrate
       (3) HCO_3^-
         [a] 0–15 mEq/L
       (4) pH
         [a] 6.80–7.30
       (5) Na^+
         [a] Total body depletion
         [b] Measured value normal, high, or low
         [c] Pseudohyponatremia secondary to hyperglycemia
       (6) K^+
         [a] Total body potassium depletion
         [b] Measured value normal, high, or low
         [c] Carefully follow ECG
       (7) PO_4^-
         [a] Total body depletion
         [b] Measured value normal or high
       (8) Creatinine/BUN
         [a] BUN slightly elevated secondary to prerenal azotemia
         [b] Creatinine elevated out of proportion to BUN because acetoacetate interferes with the laboratory measurement of creatinine, giving a falsely elevated value
       (9) Hemoconcentration (volume contraction)
      (10) Leukocytosis
      (11) Hyperuricemia
         [a] Volume contraction
         [b] Increased protein breakdown
      (12) Elevated lactate
    (f) Caveats
       (1) Diagnosis of DKA cannot be made without the presence of ketones
       (2) Glucose concentrations are not a good index of the severity of metabolic derangement (17.5% of patients have glucose less than 300 mg/dl)
       (3) Initially give normal saline (NS) to restore intravascular volume regardless of Na^+ or K^+ values
       (4) Phosphaturia accompanies all forms of metabolic acidosis
    (g) Treatment
       (1) Immediate goals of therapy
         [a] Replete volume
         [b] Treat hyperglycemia
         [c] Correct hyperosmolality
         [d] Reverse ketonemia
         [e] Reverse acidemia
         [f] Correct K^+ depletion
       (2) General principles
         [a] Accurate, up-to-date flow sheets are essential
         [b] Accurate intake and output records
         [c] Careful fluid management
         [d] Anticipate metabolic and fluid changes

        [e] Evaluate for inciting etiology

        [f] Aspiration precautions

        [g] Serial electrolytes

    (3) Fluid resuscitation

        [a] Normal saline, 2–3 liters over first 2 hours

        [b] Thereafter, one half NS at high flow rates

        [c] When serum glucose approaches 250 mg/dl, add D5W

        [d] Discontinue IV fluids when diet is tolerated and anion gap acidosis resolved

    (4) Insulin replacement

        [a] IV bolus of regular insulin at 0.15 units/kg lean body weight, usually safe with 10 units

        [b] Continuous regular insulin IV infusion at 0.15 units/kg per hour

        [c] Cover patient with SC regular insulin 2 hours prior to discontinuation of insulin infusion to prevent rebound DKA

    (5) $NaHCO_3$

        [a] Controversial

        [b] Cardiovascular instability or altered mental status with pH less than 7.10

    (6) K^+

        [a] Profoundly depleted regardless of initial K^+

        [b] Usually have lost 5–10 mEq K^+/kg

        [c] Serum K^+ increases by 0.6 mEq/L for each 0.1 decrease in pH below 7.40

        [d] 20–30 mEq/hr

        [e] Observe for adequate urine output

        [f] Rehydration produces hypokalemia (dilutional and improved renal perfusion increases osmotic diuresis and urinary K^+ losses

        [g] Insulin therapy produces hypokalemia

            i) Stimulates cellular K^+ uptake

            ii) Transported intracellularly with glucose

            iii) Correction of acidosis causes H^+ to leave cells and K^+ to enter cells to maintain electroneutrality

    (7) PO_4^-

        [a] Deficit of 70–100 mmol

        [b] Give IV as potassium phosphate

(h) Complications

    (1) Infection

    (2) Arterial thrombosis

    (3) Shock

    (4) Lactic acidosis

    (5) Hyperchloremic acidosis

    (6) Cerebral edema

        [a] Headache

        [b] Papilledema

        [c] Altered mental status that persists or recurs with treatment

    (7) 5% mortality

    (8) Hypokalemia

    (9) Hypophosphatemia

4. Hyperosmolar nonketotic coma (HNKC)

(a) Overview

    (1) Severe hyperglycemia usually greater than 800 mg/dl

    (2) Severe hyperosmolality usually greater than 350 mOsm/L

    (3) Profound intravascular volume depletion

        [a] More severe than in DKA

        [b] 10–20% of total body weight (9 liters)

II. Physiology; m. Diabetes mellitus (continued)

     (4) Absence of ketoacidosis
     (5) Impaired renal function
    (b) Typical patient profile
     (1) Elderly
     (2) Mild, type II diabetes
     (3) Symptomatic polyuria
     (4) Loss of ability to ingest or retain fluids as a result of illness, drugs, or injury
    (c) Conditions associated with HNKC onset
     (1) Diseases
      [a] This may be the initial manifestation of diabetes
      [b] Infection
       i) Urinary tract
       ii) Pulmonary
       iii) Sinuses
       iv) Biliary tract
      [c] Acute pancreatitis
      [d] Pancreatic carcinoma
      [e] Acromegaly
      [f] Cushing's syndrome
      [g] Thyrotoxicosis
      [h] Subdural hematoma
      [i] Uremia
     (2) Drugs
      [a] Diuretics
      [b] Drugs that inhibit insulin secretion
       i) Diphenylhydantoin
       ii) Diazoxide
      [c] Propranolol (inhibits lipolysis)
      [d] Glucocorticoids (insulin antagonists)
      [e] $NaHCO_3$
     (3) Miscellaneous
      [a] Burns
      [b] Dialysis
      [c] Hypothermia
      [d] Heat syndromes
    (d) Signs and symptoms
     (1) Same symptoms as DKA except for absence of dyspnea (Kussmaul's respirations)
     (2) Signs
      [a] Neurologic
       i) Altered mental status
       ii) Focal or generalized seizures
       iii) Hemiparesis
       iv) Coma
      [b] Hyper- or hypothermia
      [c] Profound volume depletion
       i) Tachycardia
       ii) Orthostatic hypotension
       iii) Dry mucosa
    (e) Concurrent illnesses
     (1) Acute myocardial infarction

(2) Infection
    [a] Dermatologic
    [b] Sinusitis/otitis
    [c] Genitourinary
    [d] CNS
    [e] Pulmonary
(3) Vascular
    [a] Pulmonary embolism
(4) Acute renal failure

(f) Treatment
  (1) General guidelines
    [a] Expand intravascular volume
    [b] Correct hyperglycemia
    [c] Treat associated/concurrent illnesses
    [d] Careful hemodynamic monitoring
       i) Potential for too rapid volume expansion
  (2) Replacement fluids
    [a] Correct 50% of calculated total body water deficit in first 24 hours
    [b] If [Na] is less than 150 mEq/L, replace initially with NS
    [c] If [Na] is more than 150 mEq/L, use one half NS
    [d] Use 1–2 liters in first 1–2 hours
  (3) Insulin
    [a] Same as for DKA
    [b] Do not decrease glucose to less than 250 mg/dl
  (4) K^+
    [a] Same as for DKA except without acidosis; intracellular K^+ shifts do not occur
    [b] Higher incidence of underlying renal disease than with DKA
    [c] Lower urinary K^+ losses

Comparison of DKA and HNKC		
	DKA	HNKC
Age	< 40	> 40
Sx duration	< 2 days	> 5 days
Glucose (mg/dl)	< 800	> 800
Na^+	More likely to be normal or low	More likely to be normal or high
K^+	Anything	Anything
HCO_3^-	Low	Normal
Ketones	Elevated	Usually normal
pH	Low	Normal
Osmolality (mOsm/L)	< 350	> 350
Cerebral edema	Often present	Rare
Mortality	5%	30–50%

  (5) Pancreatic transplant
    [a] Experimental therapy for diabetes mellitus
    [b] Often performed simultaneously with renal transplantation
    [c] Can normalize blood glucose
    [d] Whole organ more successful than islet cell transplantation alone

III. PHARMACOLOGY

a. Hormones

1. Anterior pituitary hormones

   (a) Corticotropin-related peptides
      (1) Corticotropin (ACTH)
      (2) B-LPH
      (3) Endorphins
   (b) Glycoprotein hormones
      (1) Thyroid-stimulating hormone (TSH)
      (2) Luteinizing hormone (LH)
      (3) Follicle-stimulating hormone (FSH)
   (c) Somatomammotropic hormones
      (1) Growth hormone (GH)
      (2) Prolactin

2. Posterior pituitary hormones

   (a) Arginine vasopressin (AVP)
   (b) Oxytocin

3. Thyroid hormone synthetic pathways

   (a) Uptake of iodine (normally 100 μg per day)
      (1) From iodine in the diet
      (2) Active transport into thyroid gland
         [a] Inhibited by perchlorate, thiocyanate (nitroprusside), and high intracellular iodine levels
   (b) Peroxidase-mediated conversion to free radical
   (c) Binding of tyrosine on thyroglobulin
   (d) Combination of iodotyrosine residues
      (1) Oxidative coupling
      (2) Catalyzed by the same peroxidase and inhibited by thioamides (PTU, methimazole, carbimazole)
   (e) Hormone stored extracellularly in follicle
   (f) Hormone release
      (1) Endocytosis, hydrolysis, and secretion
      (2) Inhibited by intrathyroid iodine and lithium
      (3) Daily secretion of T_4 is 90 μg
      (4) Daily secretion of T_3 is 8 μg
   (g) Fate of hormone
      (1) Bound to TBG and TBPA
      (2) Free/bound ratio determines metabolic activity
      (3) Peripheral conversion of T_4 to T_3
      (4) T_3 is principal active hormone
      (5) Some T_4 is conjugated in liver and GI excreted
   (h) Differential activity base on receptors
      (1) Thyroxine responsive: liver, kidney, heart
      (2) Thyroxine unresponsive: spleen, testes, brain

4. Thyroid hormone feedback control

   (a) TRH → TSH → thyroxine
   (b) TRH release from hypothalamus augmented by hypothermia and blocked by atropine and diethyl ether (rat model)
   (c) TSH (pituitary) release stimulated by cAMP, theophylline, epinephrine
   (d) TSH release inhibited by T_3 and T_4

(e) Effects of exogenous iodine
(1) Thyroid organic iodine reserves of 5,000–7,000 μg act as buffer
(2) Increased intake inhibits uptake, synthesis, and release

5. Thyroid hormone reserves
(a) In thyroid: 2 weeks
(b) Extrathyroidal: 900 μg T_4 and 50 μg T_3 evenly divided between plasma and liver/kidney

6. Parathyroid hormone (PTH)
(a) 84 amino acid peptide
(b) Modulated inversely by extracellular ionized calcium (Ca^{2+})
(c) Magnesium (Mg) affects release
(d) Not directly affected by phosphate (PO_4)
(e) Hepatic transformation, renal cleavage, and elimination
(f) Mediates bone catabolism and resorption
(g) Increases renal PO_4 excretion and Ca^{2+} reabsorption
(h) Increases production of 1,25-OH vitamin D (which, in turn, increases gut Ca^{2+} absorption)

7. Calcitonin
(a) 32 amino acid peptide
(b) Mostly produced in thyroid, widely distributed in other tissues
(c) Release triggered by hypermagnesemia
(d) Not affected by acute changes in Ca^{2+}
(e) Increases renal Ca^{2+} and PO_4 excretion
(f) Synthetic form useful for acute treatment of hypercalcemia

8. Adrenal glucocorticoids
(a) General functions
(1) Carbohydrate regulation
(2) Hemodynamic functions
(3) Developmental processes
(b) Cortisol
(c) 90% protein bound
(d) Plasma $T_{1/2}$ 80–120 minutes
(e) Regulation
(1) Hypothalamus: corticotropin-releasing factor (CRF) and arginine vasopressin (AVP) released
(2) Anterior pituitary: CRF and AVP stimulate ACTH release
(3) Adrenal: ACTH increases cortisol production
(f) ACTH
(1) Plasma $T_{1/2}$ 10 minutes
(2) Stimulates cortisol release within 2–3 minutes
(g) Stress increases cortisol production sixfold

9. Adrenal mineralocorticoids
(a) General functions
(1) Sodium regulation
(2) Potassium regulation
(3) Hydrogen balance
(4) Secondarily affect blood pressure
(b) Aldosterone
(1) 60% protein bound
(2) Plasma $T_{1/2}$ 15 minutes

III. Physiology; a. Hormones (continued)

    (3) Regulation

      [a] Renin: produced by juxtaglomerular cells of afferent renal arteriole. $T_{1/2}$ 15 minutes. Stimulated by low blood pressure, erect posture, salt depletion, and beta-adrenergic and CNS stimulation. Acts in plasma to cleave angiotensinogen to yield angiotensin I

      [b] Angiotensin II: converted from angiotensin I by plasma-converting enzyme. Potent vasoconstrictor. Feedback inhibition of renin release.

      [c] Potassium: hyperkalemia stimulates and hypokalemia inhibits aldosterone production

  (c) Androgenic steroids in females

10. Insulin

  (a) Secreted by beta cells of the pancreas

  (b) Polypeptide

  (c) Secretion stimulated by

    (1) Increased blood glucose

    (2) An excess of certain amino acids

    (3) Free fatty acids

    (4) Serum ketones

    (5) $Beta_2$ and cholinergic activity

    (6) Several GI hormones

  (d) Secretion inhibited by

    (1) Low blood glucose

    (2) $Alpha_2$ stimulation

  (e) $T_{1/2}$ about 5–6 minutes

  (f) Function

    (1) Facilitates cellular glucose uptake

    (2) Promotes glycogen storage

    (3) Enhances protein and fatty acid synthesis

    (4) Promotes lipid storage

    (5) Inhibits gluconeogenesis

11. Glucagon

  (a) Secreted by alpha cells of the pancreas

  (b) 29 amino acid polypeptide

  (c) Secretion inhibited by

    (1) Increased blood glucose

    (2) Somatostatin

    (3) Free fatty acids

    (4) Serum ketones

  (d) Secretion stimulated by

    (1) Excess of certain amino acids

    (2) Sympathetic activity

  (e) Function

    (1) Stimulates hepatic glycogenolysis

    (2) Stimulates hepatic gluconeogenesis

    (3) Promotes uptake of amino acids by hepatocytes

    (4) Increases lipolysis

    (5) Increases cardiac contractility

b. Corticosteroids

Drug	Equivalent Dose	Sodium Retaining	$T_{1/2}$ (hours)	Activity (hours)
Hydrocortisone	20	+ +	1.5	8–12
Cortisone	25	+ +	1.5	8–12
Prednisone, prednisolone	5	+	>3	>18
Methylprednisolone	4	−	>3	>18
Betamethasone	0.6	−	>3	>36
Dexamethasone	0.76	−	>3	>36

G. AUTONOMIC SYSTEM

I. ANATOMY

a. Autonomic nervous system (ANS)—major components

b. ANS—nerves and ganglia

c. Bodily functions under ANS control

d. Centers of ANS function

e. Feedback to the ANS

II. SYMPATHETIC NERVOUS SYSTEM (SNS)

a. The fight-or-flight system

b. SNS (fight-or-flight) responses

c. General anatomy of the SNS

d. Organs affected by the SNS

III. PARASYMPATHETIC NERVOUS SYSTEM (PNS)

a. PNS function

b. Energy-conserving/building responses

c. General anatomy of the PNS

d. Organs affected by the PNS

IV. INFORMATION TRANSMISSION IN THE ANS

a. Neurotransmitters

b. Nerves using acetylcholine (Ach) as a neurotransmitter

c. Nerves using norepinephrine (NE)/epinephrine (EPI) as a neurotransmitter

d. ANS receptors

e. Ach receptors

f. Adrenergic receptors

V. ANS PHARMACOLOGY

a. Alpha agonists

b. Alpha antagonists

c. Beta agonists (no pure beta$_1$ agonist)

d. Beta antagonists

e. Cholinergic agonists (parasympathomimetics)

f. Cholinergic antagonists

VI. CLINICAL

a. Induced hypotension

b. Temperature and temperature regulation

c. Malignant hyperthermia

d. Autonomic hyperreflexia

e. Neuroleptic malignant syndrome

I. ANATOMY

a. The autonomic nervous system (ANS) consists of two major components that are separated anatomically and physiologically. Both are active

1. Sympathetic nervous system (SNS)
2. Parasympathetic nervous system (PNS)

b. The ANS consists of nerves and ganglia that provide innervation to the heart, vasculature, glands, visceral muscles, and smooth muscles, and functions below the level of consciousness

c. Bodily functions under ANS control include

1. Respiration
2. Circulation
3. Digestion
4. Body temperature
5. Metabolism
6. Sweating
7. Certain endocrine functions

d. Centers of ANS function

1. Cerebral cortex
2. Hypothalamus
3. Brain stem
4. Spinal cord

e. Feedback to the ANS

1. Afferent neurons from peripheral chemoreceptors, baroreceptors, and pain receptors
2. Afferent fibers carried by vagus, pelvic, splanchnic, and other auto- nomic nerves. About 80% of the fibers in the vagus nerve are afferent
3. For cardiovascular autonomics: pressure receptors in the carotid sinus and aortic arch sense changes in peripheral arterial blood pressure. Afferents from the carotid sinus enter the central nervous system (CNS) via the glossopharyngeal nerve (IX). Afferents from the aortic arch enter the CNS via the vagus (X)

II. SYMPATHETIC NERVOUS SYSTEM (SNS)

a. Commonly called the fight-or-flight system. The term "fight or flight" is indicative of the homeostatic mechanisms that are activated with sympathetic stimulation

II. Sympathetic nervous system (continued)

b. SNS (fight-or-flight) responses

1. Tachycardia
2. Increased contractility
3. Hypertension
4. Mydriasis (pupillary dilation)
5. Bronchodilation
6. Hyperglycemia
7. Piloerection ("goose bumps")

c. General anatomy of the SNS

1. Neurons of the SNS arise from the intermediolateral cell column of the thoracic and lumbar portions of the spinal cord with outflow from segments T1–L3
2. Short myelinated preganglionic SNS axons exit the spinal column via the ventral root with motor fibers and either synapse in sympathetic ganglia, traverse the ganglia, or travel up/down the ganglion chain. Acetylcholine (Ach) is the neurotransmitter of the sympathetic chain ganglia
3. Sympathetic ganglia
   (a) Paravertebral ganglia lie on either side of the vertebral column and form lateral chains
   (b) Significant ganglia include
       (1) Stellate (inferior of three cervical ganglia; blocked with interscalene/supraclavicular brachial plexus blocks)
       (2) Celiac (can be blocked for therapeutic reasons in chronic abdominal pain syndromes)
       (3) Superior mesenteric
       (4) Aorticorenal
       (5) Inferior mesenteric
   (c) Long postganglionic unmyelinated SNS axons innervate end organs except for the adrenal medulla and use norepinephrine (NE) as their neurotransmitter. The postganglionic sympathetic neurons synapse directly on the organs affected (the visceral structures of the thorax, abdomen, head, and neck). This postganglionic organization allows one preganglionic fiber to synapse with many postganglionic fibers, thereby providing for exponential sympathetic output (e.g., mass sympathetic reflexes in the patient with spinal cord injury)
4. Adrenal medulla
   (a) Acts to amplify the sympathetic response
   (b) Homologous to sympathetic ganglia
   (c) Releases primarily epinephrine (EPI) directly into the bloodstream (also releases a smaller quantity of NE)

d. Organs affected by the SNS

1. Heart
   (a) Increased heart rate
   (b) Increased contractility
2. Vascular
   (a) Arteriolar vasoconstriction

    (b) Both venoconstriction and dilation

3. Pulmonary

    (a) Bronchodilation

    (b) Decreases secretions

4. Ocular

    (a) Pupillary dilation (mydriasis)

    (b) Improved far vision

5. Stomach and intestinal tract

    (a) Decreased motility

    (b) Inhibits secretion

6. Kidney

    (a) Increased renin secretion

7. Uterus

    (a) Relaxation

8. Skin

    (a) Pilomotor muscle contraction

    (b) Increases sweating

9. Spleen

    (a) Contraction of capsule

    (b) Increases number of circulating erythrocytes and platelets

10. Liver

    (a) Increases glycogenolysis

    (b) Increases gluconeogenesis

III. PARASYMPATHETIC NERVOUS SYSTEM (PNS)

a. The PNS is devoted primarily to repleting the energy stores of the body (decreasing unnecessary energy expenditures and maximizing energy intake)

b. Energy-conserving/building responses

1. Bradycardia

2. Decreased cardiac output

3. Bronchoconstriction

4. Miosis (pupillary constriction)

5. Increased salivation

6. Increased peristalsis

c. General anatomy of the PNS

1. Parasympathetic nerves exit the CNS via cranial nerves (CN) III, VII, IX, and X and S2–S4

2. Parasympathetic nerves have long preganglionic neurons and short postganglionic neurons that innervate the effector organs

3. Some discrete ganglia are present

III. Parasympathetic nervous system; c. General anatomy of the PNS (continued)

(a) CN III: ciliary

(b) CN VII: sphenopalatine

(c) CN VII/IX: otic

4. Preganglionic parasympathetics do not activate large numbers of postganglionic fibers and there is no mass reflex as with the SNS

d. Organs affected by the PNS

1. Heart
   (a) Innervated by the vagus (CN X) nerve
   (b) Parasympathetic (cholinergic) tone predominates over sympathetic (adrenergic) tone in the heart
   (c) Decreased heart rate and contractility

2. Vascular
   (a) No clinically significant parasympathetic innervation; however, the vasculature does contain muscarinic cholinergic receptors
   (b) Stimulated by Ach
   (c) Produces vasodilation

3. Pulmonary
   (a) Bronchoconstriction
   (b) Increases secretions

4. Ocular
   (a) Miosis (pupillary constriction)
   (b) Improved near vision

5. Stomach and intestinal tract
   (a) Increased motility
   (b) Increased secretions
   (c) Relaxation of sphincter tone

IV. INFORMATION TRANSMISSION IN THE ANS

a. Neurotransmitters

1. Acetylcholine (Ach)
   (a) Degraded by circulating acetylcholinesterase

2. Epinephrine (EPI)
   (a) Reuptake into nerve terminals

3. Norepinephrine (NE)
   (a) Recycled for reuse by SNS reuptake

4. Dopamine (D)

b. Nerves using Ach as a neurotransmitter

1. Skeletal (motor)

2. Preganglionic sympathetic and parasympathetic

3. Postganglionic parasympathetic

4. Few postganglionic sympathetic

c. Nerves using NE/EPI as a neurotransmitter

1. Most postganglionic sympathetic
2. Adrenal medulla

d. ANS receptors

1. Muscarinic
2. Nicotinic
3. Alpha
4. Beta
5. Dopamine

e. Ach receptors

1. Muscarinic: postganglionic parasympathetic
   (a) Five molecular subtypes but only three, M_1–M_3, delineated pharmacologically
   (b) M_1
       (1) Located in autonomic ganglia and CNS
       (2) Produces neuronal depolarization
   (c) M_2
       (1) Located in the heart
       (2) SA node: slows spontaneous depolarization
       (3) Atrium: decreases contractility
       (4) AV node: decreases conduction
       (5) Ventricle: decreases contractility
   (d) M_3
       (1) Smooth muscle: contraction
       (2) Secretory glands: increases secretion
2. Nicotinic
   (a) N_M (muscle)
       (1) Neuromuscular junction
       (2) End-plate depolarization
       (3) Skeletal muscle contraction
   (b) N_N (neuronal)
       (1) Autonomic ganglia
       (2) Adrenal medulla

f. Adrenergic receptors

1. Alpha
   (a) Vasoconstriction
   (b) Pupillary dilation
   (c) Intestinal relaxation
   (d) Piloerector muscle contraction in the skin
   (e) Stimulated by NE
   (f) Types of alpha receptors
       (1) $Alpha_1$
           [a] Postsynaptic
           [b] Epi greater than NE stimulation
           [c] Contracts vascular smooth muscle
           [d] Contracts genitourinary smooth muscle

IV. Information transmission in the ANS; f. Adrenergic receptors (continued)

        [e] Liver
            i) Glycogenolysis
            ii) Gluconeogenesis
        [f] Intestinal smooth muscle relaxation
        [g] Heart
            i) Increased contractility (significant in congestive heart failure (CHF) with down-regulation of beta receptors)
            ii) Arrhythmias
    (2) Alpha$_2$
        [a] EPI greater than NE stimulation
        [b] Presynaptic
            i) Feedback inhibition (decreased NE release)
            ii) CNS sympathetic suppression
        [c] Postsynaptic
            i) Platelet aggregation
            ii) Decreased insulin secretion
            iii) Vasoconstriction

2. Beta
  (a) Beta$_1$
    (1) Increases heart rate
    (2) Increases contractility
  (b) Beta$_2$
    (1) Bronchodilatation
    (2) Increases mucociliary clearance
    (3) Decreases bronchopulmonary secretions
    (4) Increases hepatic glycogenolysis/gluconeogenesis (produces hyperglycemia)
    (5) Uterine relaxation
    (6) Increases insulin secretion
    (7) Increases renin secretion
    (8) Increases skeletal muscle tremor
    (9) Peripheral vasodilation
    (10) Intracellular potassium shift (receptor stimulation can be used to treat hyperkalemia)
  (c) Beta$_3$
    (1) Adipose tissue
        [a] Lipolysis

3. Dopamine
  (a) Renal vasodilation
  (b) Mesenteric vasodilation

V. ANS PHARMACOLOGY

a. Alpha agonists

1. Nonselective stimulation of both alpha$_1$ and alpha$_2$
  (a) Epinephrine (see "Beta agonists")
  (b) Norepinephrine
    (1) Natural catecholamine
    (2) Clinically increases systemic vascular resistance (SVR) and mean arterial pressure (MAP) with compensatory bradycardia in the presence of an intact baroreceptor reflex

      (3) Also stimulates beta$_1$

      (4) Dose: 4 mg/250 ml; 0.01–1.0 μg/kg/min

      (5) Onset: immediate

      (6) Duration of action: minutes due to in vivo metabolism

      (7) Perioperative indications: as an inotrope in postcardiopulmonary bypass if increased SVR also desired; septic shock

      (8) Caution: increased afterload may exacerbate myocardial dysfunction in CHF or coronary artery disease, splanchnic (including renal) vasoconstriction

2. Alpha$_1$ stimulation (phenylephrine greater than NE greater than EPI [high dose])

  (a) Phenylephrine

      (1) Noncatecholamine vasoconstriction

      (2) Clinically produces abrupt increases in SVR and MAP with compensatory bradycardia in patients with intact baroreceptor reflexes

      (3) 50–100 μg and infuse at 0.15–0.5 μg/kg/min (10 mg/250 [40 μg/ml])

      (4) Immediate onset

      (5) Half-life is 2 minutes, with duration of action about 20 minutes

      (6) Perioperative indications: maintenance of coronary or cerebral perfusion pressure (during carotid artery cross-clamp, spinal-induced hypotension, initial hypotension on cardiopulmonary bypass, treatment of symptoms in tetralogy of Fallot to reverse right to left shunt)

      (7) Caution: avoid in obstetrics because of uterine arterial vasoconstriction and compromise of placental perfusion; acute increases in SVR may cause myocardial failure in patients with compensated therapeutic dilation for CHF; concern about vasoconstriction of internal mammary graft in bypass surgery, and renal arteriolar vasoconstriction may occur in patients with decreased renal blood flow

  (b) Methoxamine

  (c) Metaraminol

3. Alpha$_2$ stimulation (dexmedetomidine greater than clonidine greater than NE greater than Epi)

  (a) Dexmedetomidine

      (1) Produces decreased sympathetic outflow leading to decreases in blood pressure, heart rate, and catecholamines; sedation, anxiolysis, and anesthesia (decrease MAC); analgesia (parenteral, neuraxial, and probably nerve trunk)

      (2) A 5-minute onset of action with a half-life of 90 minutes

      (3) 0.5–1.0 μg/kg

      (4) Perioperative indications: premedication (decreases MAC and anesthetic requirements); attenuates opioid-induced rigidity; decreases postoperative shivering; analgesia (decreases opioid requirements and prolongs LA block); attenuates stress response (intubation, CAD [favorably affects myocardial oxygen balance]); treatment of drug withdrawal states

      (5) Caution: produces perioperative bradycardia and hypotension, overdose may unmask peripheral alpha$_1$-mediated vasoconstriction, dry mouth

  (b) Clonidine

      (1) Central (alpha$_2$) stimulation decreases sympathetic outflow, thus lowering blood pressure

      (2) Well absorbed orally with onset in 30–60 minutes and maximum effect at 2–4 hours

      (3) Dosing

         [a] Oral: 0.1–0.3 mg (5 μg/kg), 60–90 minutes prior to surgery

         [b] IV: 2–7 μg/kg

         [c] Transdermal: 1–3 mg

         [d] Neuraxial: 0.15 mg (2 μg/kg)

V. ANS pharmacology; a. Alpha agonists (continued)

    (4) Perioperative indications and caution similar to dexmedetomidine
- (c) Guanabenz
- (d) Guanfacine

b. Alpha antagonists

1. Nonselective blockade of both alpha$_1$ and alpha$_2$
   - (a) Phenoxybenzamine
     - (1) Noncompetitive (alpha$_1$ greater than alpha$_2$) blocker with irreversible binding to the receptor for 24 hours
     - (2) Only clinical use is preparation of pheochromocytoma patients for adrenalectomy
     - (3) Initial dose of 10 mg increased over 7–14 days until clinical effect documented with mild postural hypotension, nasal stuffiness, and absence of ischemia or premature ventricular complexes (PVC) on ECG
     - (4) Caution: first dose effect, especially in patients with contracted peripheral vasculature; with prolonged duration of effect, it has been recommended to take only half the usual dose on the morning of surgery
   - (b) Phentolamine
     - (1) Competitive alpha$_1$ and alpha$_2$ antagonist
     - (2) Advantages of alpha$_1$ blockade often decreased by presynaptic alpha$_2$ blockade, causing increased NE release. Hypotensive effects, therefore, are often accompanied by tachycardia
     - (3) Parenteral dosing in 1–2-mg increments
     - (4) Clinically indicated to treat hypertension in pheochromocytoma, control of MAP during cardiopulmonary bypass (after ensuring anesthesia), clonidine withdrawal, MAO inhibitors
     - (5) A 19-minute half-life (IV)
     - (6) Hepatic metabolism
   - (c) Ergot alkaloids
2. Alpha$_1$ blockade
   - (a) Prazosin
     - (1) Selective competitive blocker
     - (2) Well absorbed orally
     - (3) Half-life of 2.5 hours
     - (4) Decreased SVR and MAP
     - (5) Increased stroke volume and cardiac output
     - (6) Efficacy as an antihypertensive enhanced with the addition of a diuretic
     - (7) Initial dose of 0.5 mg, can be increased to 20 mg
     - (8) Perioperative indication: usually related to continuation of preoperative antihypertensives; if for pheochromocytoma preparation, then be aware of competitive nature of the alpha blockade (compare phenoxybenzamine)
     - (9) Caution: first-dose effect with postural hypotension
   - (b) Terazosin
   - (c) Labetalol
     - (1) Selective alpha$_1$ and nonselective beta blockade
     - (2) 0.25 mg/kg IV bolus, repeat every 5–10 minutes to a maximum dose of 300 mg
     - (3) Infuse at 2 mg/min
     - (4) Half-life of 5.5 hours
     - (5) Hepatic metabolism
     - (6) Decreases SVR and MAP, little change in HR or cardiac output

3. Alpha$_2$ blockade
   (a) Yohimbine

---

c. Beta agonists (no pure beta$_1$ agonist) (Isoproterenol greater than EPI = dobutamine greater than NE greater than dopamine [dose dependent])

1. Nonselective stimulation of both beta$_1$ and beta$_2$
   (a) Isoproterenol
      (1) Pure beta agonist
      (2) Produces increased heart rate and cardiac output by stimulation of beta$_1$
      (3) Vasodilatation (decreased SVR and pulmonary vascular resistance) and bronchodilatation via beta$_2$ stimulation
      (4) Cardiac output increases but MAP may decrease due to dramatic decreases in SVR
      (5) 0.4 mg IV bolus; infuse at 1 mg/250 ml (4 μg/ml) at 0.01–0.1 μg/kg/min
      (6) Onset within 1–5 minutes with duration of 0.5–2.0 hours
      (7) Perioperative indications: complete heart block while awaiting pacing, bronchospasm, weaning from cardiopulmonary bypass if chronotropy required or pulmonary hypertension present
      (8) Caution: deleterious effects on myocardial oxygen supply/demand, arrhythmogenic, hypotension
   (b) Epinephrine
      (1) Natural sympathomimetic with dose-dependent effects
         [a] 0.01–0.03 μg/kg/min (pure beta$_{1\&2}$)
         [b] 0.03–0.15 μg/kg/min (mixed alpha$_{1\&2}$ and beta$_{1\&2}$)
         [c] Over 0.15 μg/kg/min (pure alpha$_{1\&2}$)
      (2) In emergency situations, use 0.5–1.0 mg IV or via ETT
      (3) Clinical effect depends on dose, but at beta doses, heart rate and contractility increase with an increase in venous return. In the alpha dose range, SVR is increased with splanchnic (including renal) vasoconstriction and potential myocardial impairment in patient with poor ventricular function
      (4) Perioperative indications: anaphylaxis, cardiac arrest, life-threatening bronchospasm (all IV bolus); most effective, proved, and least expensive inotrope for cardiopulmonary bypass weaning; prolongation of LA effect (neuroaxial and peripheral blocks)(most effective for agents of shorter duration, e.g., lidocaine, mepivicaine)
   (c) Dobutamine
      (1) Synthetic modification of isoproterenol molecule with beta$_1$ greater than beta$_2$
      (2) Increased inotropy and chronotropy (at higher doses) with less vasodilatation than isoproterenol
      (3) Hepatic metabolism/renal excretion
      (4) Short half-life of 2 minutes
      (5) Infuse at 2–20 (up to 40) μg/kg/min
      (6) Perioperative indications: expensive, poorer alternative to epinephrine for cardiopulmonary bypass weaning, slight theoretical advantage in myocardial failure due to ischemia (if tachycardia avoided)
      (7) Caution: decreased MAP if vasodilation occurs, increased myocardial oxygen consumption if tachycardia occurs, tachyphylaxis if infused for longer than 72 hours (as for most sympathomimetics)
   (d) Norepinephrine (see "alpha")
   (e) Dopamine
      (1) Natural precursor of NE with dose-dependent effects

V. ANS pharmacology; c. Beta agonists (continued)

   (2) 2–5 μg/kg/min: dopaminergic-mediated increase in renal blood flow with some beta$_{1\&2}$ effect

   (3) 5–10 μg/kg/min: beta$_{1\&2}$ effects with some alpha-mediated vasoconstriction

   (4) Over 10 μg/kg/min: overriding alpha effect (action similar to NE at this dose)

   (5) Perioperative indications: renal and mesenteric vasodilatation for patients at risk for renal dysfunction; theoretically useful when aortic cross-clamp anticipated and hepatorenal dysfunction possible. Inotropy (as for epinephrine)

   (6) Caution: may have unwanted alpha effects at high doses and deleterious effects on myocardial oxygen consumption (same as for epinephrine)

  (f) Dopexamine

   (1) Synthetic dopamine analogue with selective DA$_{1\&2}$ effect (less than dopamine) and beta$_2$ stimulation. Beta$_1$ activity is weak, with the mild inotropic effects ascribed to inhibition of catecholamine reuptake

   (2) Marked vasodilation, increased renal perfusion, weak inotropy, and absence of alpha activity

   (3) Infused at 1–5 μg/kg/min

   (4) Perioperative indication: unloading in CHF (may benefit left and right ventricles); support of renal perfusion (as for dopamine); increased renal and splanchnic flow

   (5) Caution: tachycardia with dose over 4 μg/kg/min

 2. Beta$_2$ agonists

  (a) Ritodrine

   (1) Structurally related to EPI with beta$_2$ greater than beta$_1$

   (2) Uterine smooth muscle relaxation accompanied by decreased SVR, decreased systolic and diastolic blood pressure, increased heart rate/stroke volume/cardiac output

   (3) Infused at 0.05–0.1 mg/min

   (4) Caution: hypokalemia, hyperglycemia, hypotension, tachycardia, dysrrhythmias, pulmonary edema (especially in conjunction with steroids given to enhance fetal lung maturation)

  (b) Terbutaline

   (1) Inhaled, nebulized, PO, SC

   (2) Onset within 5–60 minutes (depends on route of administration)

   (3) Duration of action: 2–8 hours

   (4) Clinically indicated for treatment of bronchospasm, promotion of uterine relaxation

  (c) Albuterol

   (1) Inhaled, PO, nebulized

   (2) Onset: 5–45 minutes

   (3) Duration of action: 3–8 hours

---

d. Beta antagonists

 1. Nonselective blockade of both beta$_1$ and beta$_2$

  (a) Propranolol

   (1) Hepatic metabolism

   (2) Renal excretion

   (3) Onset: immediate (IV)

   (4) Duration of action: 2.5 hours

  (b) Timolol

  (c) Pindolol

   (1) Has intrinsic sympathomimetic activity

(d) Nadolol

2. Beta$_1$ blockade

    (a) Acebutolol

    (b) Atenolol

    (c) Metoprolol

        (1) Relatively beta$_1$-specific antagonist but with beta$_2$ effects at high doses. No intrinsic sympathomimetic activity or membrane stabilizing effect

        (2) Hepatic metabolism with renal excretion

        (3) Onset immediate (IV) with duration of 3–7 hours

        (4) Perioperative indications: premedication in patient at risk for CAD or hypertension (one dose has this effect); intraoperative heart-rate control and supraventricular tachycardia (SVT) treatment/prophylaxis

        (5) Caution: *all* beta antagonists can potentially exacerbate obstructive airway disease or peripheral vascular disease, or mask the symptoms of hypoglycemia in diabetics; negative inotropy may be significant in the presence of CHF and a volatile anesthetic

    (d) Esmolol

        (1) Very short acting

        (2) Metabolized by red blood cell esterase

        (3) Half-life of 9 minutes

        (4) Bolus of 0.5–1.0 mg/kg; infused at 50–300 µg/kg/min

        (5) Perioperative indications: blunting of sympathetic responses to intubation, incision, and extubation; control of heart rate, MAP, and tachydysrhythmias; used in combination with nitroprusside in dissecting aortic aneurysms

        (6) Caution: short action may be a disadvantage in that rebound postoperative hypertension may be a problem after adequate intraoperative control

3. Nonselective beta blockade plus alpha blockade

    (a) Labetalol (see "Alpha antagonists")

---

e. Cholinergic agonists (parasympathomimetics)

1. Nonselective stimulation of muscarinic and nicotinic receptors

    (a) Acetylcholine

        (1) Intraocular solution

    (b) Carbachol

        (1) Ophthalmic solution used to produce miosis during ocular surgery

2. Direct-acting muscarinics

    (a) Methacholine

        (1) 100–200 mg PO or 10–25 mg SC

        (2) Undergoes less rapid destruction than endogenous Ach with a longer duration of action

        (3) Decreases HR, SVR, and useful in treatment of SVT

        (4) Adverse effects: increased secretions and bronchial hyperreactivity

    (b) Pilocarpine

        (1) Ophthalmic solution used to treat glaucoma

        (2) Minimal systemic effects, although can produce hypersecretion

3. Indirect-acting muscarinics (anticholinesterases)

    (a) Increase Ach by attaching to the anionic and exteratic binding sites and inactivating the enzyme acetylcholinesterase. The binding is reversible (clinical agents for anesthesiologist) or irreversible (toxins and ophthalmologic agents)

    (b) Increase parasympathetic output

    (c) Primary therapeutic uses
- (1) Treatment of atony of the smooth muscle of the intestinal tract and urinary bladder
- (2) Glaucoma
- (3) Myasthenia gravis
- (4) Termination of the effects of competitive neuromuscular blocking drugs

    (d) Neostigmine
- (1) Parenterally administered reversible anticholinesterase with onset at 7–11 minutes and half-life of 1–2 hours at 0.05 mg/kg
- (2) Actively secreted into renal tubule, so prolonged elimination in renal failure can occur (often matching the prolonged duration of action of many nondepolarizing muscle relaxants)
- (3) Nicotinic effects desired for reversal of muscle relaxant, so muscarinic effects blocked with coadministered antimuscarinic
- (4) Important muscarinic effects include bradycardia, salivation, increased bowel motility, relation to postoperative nausea, and increased airway resistance
- (5) Useful for treatment of abdominal distention (postoperative ileus), bladder atony, and myasthenia

    (e) Edrophonium
- (1) Onset of action (1–2 minutes) and elimination (2 hours) faster than neostigmine
- (2) Useful in diagnosis of myasthenia and suggested for reversal of muscle blockade with short- to intermediate-acting agents and when some spontaneous reversal is already present (train-of-four greater than 3)

    (f) Pyridostigmine
- (1) Patients with myasthenia are often maintained on anticholinesterases (60 mg PO three to four times daily) and preoperative assessment should exclude underdosage (myasthenic crisis) and overdosage (cholinergic crisis) as causes of weakness. The morning-of-surgery dose can either be omitted or only a half dose given

    (g) Physostigmine
- (1) Relevant because its tertiary amine structure allows for passage through the blood–brain barrier
- (2) Useful for treatment of atropine intoxication, phenothiazine and tricyclic antidepressant overdoses, and glaucoma

    (h) Ecothiopate
- (1) Topical irreversible anticholinesterase inhibitor used in the treatment of glaucoma
- (2) Effects last for 2–3 weeks after discontinuation, although topical absorption is variable

    (i) Organophosphates
- (1) Irreversibly bind and inhibit cholinesterases
- (2) Exposure produces the following clinical syndrome
  - *S*—salivation
  - *L*—lacrimation
  - *U*—urination
  - *D*—defecation
- (3) Treatment
  - [a] Atropine
    - i) 2–4 mg IV push
    - ii) 2 mg IV every 5–10 minutes until muscarinic symptoms resolve
    - iii) More than 200 mg may be required in first 24 hours

[b] Pralidoxime
    i) Cholinesterase reactivator
    ii) 1–2-gram IV push
    iii) Repeat in 20–60 minutes

f. Cholinergic antagonists

1. Muscarinic receptor blockade

  (a) Atropine
    (1) Rapid onset of action (1 minute) with a duration of action of 0.5–1.0 minute
    (2) Produces tachycardia by blocking M_2 receptor on SA node. Can produce paradoxic bradycardia if inadequate dose is given. Also decreases secretions in the salivary, respiratory, and GI systems while producing bronchial and lower esophageal sphincter smooth muscle relaxation
    (3) Usual dose is 0.5–1.0 mg IV or via ETT
    (4) Perioperative indications: infant premedication, antisialogogue, hemodynamically significant bradycardia, used with edrophonium for reversal of nondepolarizing relaxant, and pupillary dilation for ophthalmic surgery and examination
    (5) Caution: central anticholinergic syndrome, especially in the elderly (delirium and hyperthermia); avoid tachycardia in those patients at risk (i.e., CAD)

  (b) Glycopyrrolate
    (1) Slower onset (2–3 minutes) and longer duration of action (2–4 hours) than atropine, which is more appropriate for use with neostigmine. This compound does not cross the blood–brain barrier
    (2) Perioperative indications: antisialagogue (e.g., awake fiberoptic airway instrumentation), with neostigmine for reversal of nondepolarizing muscle relaxants (0.01–0.015 mg/kg), to decrease parasympathetically mediated changes in heart rate, such as occurs with peritoneal traction

  (c) Scopolamine
    (1) Tertiary amine that does cross the blood–brain barrier. Prolonged duration of action after IM administration (4–6 hours)
    (2) Main difference is CNS depression with sedation and anxiolysis, especially in combination with opioid as premedication. Limiting dose to 0.2 mg often avoids tachycardia; however, and as with low-dose atropine, may slow heart rate
    (3) Effective in preventing motion sickness/emesis
    (4) Caution: in elderly, may produce a central anticholinergic syndrome

2. Nicotinic receptor blockade

  (a) Hexamethonium
  (b) Trimethaphan
  (c) Curare
  (d) Pancuronium
    (1) Dose: 0.08–0.1 mg/kg
    (2) Onset: 3.0–5.0 minutes
    (3) Time to 25% recovery: 90–100 minutes
    (4) Renal metabolism
    (5) Tachycardia and hypertension
    (6) No histamine release

  (e) Vecuronium
    (1) Dose: 0.08–0.1 mg/kg
    (2) Onset: 2.0–4.0 minutes
    (3) Time to 25% recovery: 25–40 minutes
    (4) No histamine release

V. ANS pharmacology; f. Cholinergic antagonists (continued)

        (5) Hepatic metabolism
        (6) Possible myopathy with long-term use, especially if receiving steroids concurrently

    (f) Atracurium
        (1) Dose: 0.4–0.5 mg/kg
        (2) Onset: 2.0–2.5 minutes
        (3) Time to 25% recovery: 40–60 minutes
        (4) Not affected by renal/hepatic dysfunction
        (5) Histamine release leads to hypotension

    (g) Metocurine
        (1) Dose: 0.4 mg/kg
        (2) Onset: 3.0–5.0 minutes
        (3) Time to 25% recovery: 70–90 minutes
        (4) Histamine release with occasional hypotension

    (h) Mivacurium
        (1) Dose: 0.15–0.25 mg/kg
        (2) Onset: 1.5–2.0 minutes
        (3) Time to 25% recovery: 16–23 minutes
        (4) Some histamine release
        (5) Renal/hepatic dysfunction may increase duration of blockade

    (i) Rocuronium
        (1) Dose: 0.6–1.2 mg/kg
        (2) Onset: 0.7–1.0 minute
        (3) Time to 25% recovery: 31–67 minutes
        (4) No histamine release
        (5) Hepatic metabolism

    (j) Succinylcholine
        (1) Depolarizing
        (2) Dose: 0.6–1.0 mg/kg
        (3) Onset: 0.5–1.0 minute
        (4) Time to 25% recovery: 4–10 minutes
        (5) Increased intragastric and intraocular pressure, potential for hyperkalemia, tachyphylaxis, and rarely malignant hyperthermia

VI. CLINICAL

a. Induced hypotension

    1. Definition: lowering of MAP to decrease blood loss during surgery and to provide a dry surgical field for the surgeon

    2. Indications

        (a) To control bleeding
            (1) To improve surgical conditions
                [a] Cerebral aneurysm clipping
                [b] Middle ear microsurgery
            (2) To reduce blood loss and thereby reduce the need for blood transfusions
                [a] Orthopedic surgery
                [b] In patients with rare blood groups or antibodies
                [c] In Jehovah's Witnesses or patients subject to other religious constraints on receiving blood products
        (b) To decrease the risk of vessel rupture
            (1) Resection of cerebral aneurysm

(2) arterio-venous malformation surgery

(3) Aortic dissection

3. Contraindications

(a) Vascular occlusive disease of the brain, heart, or kidneys

(b) Myocardial dysfunction (unless the decrease in afterload improves cardiac output)

(c) Anemia

(d) Fever

(e) Hypovolemia

(f) Prolonged retractor pressure

(g) Intracerebral hematoma

(h) Chronic uncontrolled hypertension

    (1) Relative contraindication

    (2) May consider gentle reduction of 50 mm Hg or less below the patient's MAP

4. General guidelines

(a) Reduction of MAP in association with parallel decreases in organ vascular resistance

(b) MAP = 50–60 mm Hg in young healthy patients

(c) MAP = 60–70 mm Hg in suitable older patients

(d) Myocardial ischemia necessitates termination of technique

(e) Careful volume assessment and replacement (hypotensive technique abolishes normal compensatory reactions)

(f) Position patient with operative site least dependent

(g) Control ventilation

    (1) Positive airway pressure decreases venous return and potentiates hypotension

    (2) Maintain normocarbia (vasoconstriction associated with hypocarbia in addition to hypotension increases the risk of ischemia)

5. Monitoring considerations

(a) Standard monitors

(b) Indwelling bladder catheter

(c) Arterial line

(d) Central venous catheter if large blood loss is expected

(e) EEG—monitor for cerebral ischemia

(f) SSEPs—monitor for spinal cord ischemia

6. Methods and drugs used to achieve deliberate hypotension

(a) Preoperative: adequate premedication to decrease excessive circulating catecholamines

(b) Intraoperative

    (1) Controlled hemorrhage

    (2) Preganglionic blockade

        [a] Spinal anesthesia

        [b] Epidural anesthesia

    (3) Inhaled anesthetics

    (4) IV anesthetics

        [a] Sodium nitroprusside (0.5–10 μg/kg/min) (NTP)

        [b] Nitroglycerin (1–2 μg/kg/min)

        [c] Trimethapan (0.5–6.0 mg/min)

        [d] Hydralazine

        [e] Labetalol/esmolol

        [f] Calcium channel blockade

        [g] Prostaglandin E_1

        [h] Adenosine

7. Reversal

   (a) MAP should normalize before surgical completion to facilitate hemostasis
   (b) Resuscitation drugs: calcium chloride, inotropes, and vasopressors should be available

8. Complications

   (a) General
       (1) Cerebral
           [a] Increased intracranial pressure
           [b] Cerebral ischemia, thrombosis, or edema
       (2) Myocardial
           [a] Infarction, CHF
           [b] Tachycardia, bradycardia, cardiac arrest
       (3) Reactive hemorrhage with hematoma
       (4) Acute tubular necrosis
       (5) Shock liver
       (6) Spinal cord ischemia
   (b) Specific
       (1) Accumulation of toxic metabolites (NTP, adenosine)
       (2) Rebound systemic and pulmonary hypertension (NTP)
       (3) Pulmonary shunting (NTP, NTG)
       (4) Bronchospasm (TMP)
       (5) Severe acidosis (NTP)
       (6) Hypothyroidism (NTP)
       (7) Blood coagulation abnormalities (NTP)

9. Alternatives in neurosurgical procedures

   (a) Ipsilateral carotid artery tamponade
   (b) Temporary clips

b. Temperature and temperature regulation

1. Mechanisms

   (a) Body temperature homeostasis is mediated by the preoptic anterior hypothalamus and is normally maintained within a narrow range (36.5–37.5°C) by a number of physiologic mechanisms
       (1) Heat production
           [a] Shivering (most potent and effective), which is centrally, but not sympathetically, mediated muscle activity
           [b] Nonshivering thermogenesis mediated by thyroid and catecholamine-mediated brown fat metabolism
       (2) Heat loss
           [a] Active regulation of cutaneous blood flow to shunt heat to the skin
           [b] Sweating to increase cutaneous heat loss through evaporation
       (3) The most important factor in thermal balance is behavioral—seeking a thermoneutral environment through clothing, shelter, and activity level
           [a] This mechanism is not available to the anesthetized patient
       (4) Anesthetic effects
           [a] Active thermoregulation is attenuated during general anesthesia
           [b] Heat-conserving mechanisms are not activated until 35°C

2. Hypothermia

   (a) Heat is lost via four distinct mechanisms

        (1) Radiation losses (40–50% of total) are proportional to body/environment temperature difference (normal operating room is 19–24°C)

        (2) Convection losses (25–35% of total) result from direct heat transfer to air currents (wind chill)

        (3) Evaporative losses can occur from skin preparation, body cavity moisture, and respiratory loss

        (4) Conduction loss (less than 10%) occurs from direct skin contact with objects

    (b) Hypothermia is categorized as

        (1) Mild (32–36°C)

        (2) Moderate (30–32°C)

        (3) Severe (27–30°C)

3. Clinical effects

    (a) Metabolic

        (1) Decreased metabolic rate (5–7%/°C) and O_2 consumption

        (2) Slower hepatic drug metabolism

    (b) Cardiovascular

        (1) Decreased cardiac output (30–40% at 30°C)

        (2) Peripheral vasoconstriction

        (3) Cardiac conduction abnormalities (less than 31°C)

    (c) Hematologic

        (1) Left shift of HbO_2 dissociation curve

        (2) Platelet sequestration at less than 32°C

        (3) Increased blood viscosity

        (4) Immune suppression?

        (5) Increased incidence of venous thrombosis and thromboembolism

    (d) Endocrine

        (1) Decreased insulin release (hyperglycemia)

        (2) Plasma catecholamines initially elevated, then depressed

    (e) Musculoskeletal

        (1) Increased sensitivity to neuromuscular blockade

        (2) Shivering (400–500% increase in metabolic rate)

    (f) GI/renal

        (1) Decreased GFR (50% at 30°C) and tubular depression

        (2) Decreased GI motility or ileus

    (g) Cerebral

        (1) Cerebral blood flow decrease of 7%/°C

4. Temperature measurement

    (a) Core body temperature reflects essential organ (heart, brain) temperature

        (1) Sites—in order of desirability

            [a] Central intravascular (pulmonary artery catheter)

            [b] Esophageal

            [c] Tympanic (risk of tympanic membrane trauma)

            [d] Nasopharyngeal

            [e] Bladder

            [f] Rectal

            [g] Axillary

        (2) Multiple probes desirable for critical situations

    (b) Peripheral temperature monitoring is a useful addition for estimating core/skin gradients

        (1) The presence of a gradient implies peripheral vasoconstriction and active intrinsic thermoregulation

5. Heat conservation and rewarming
   (a) Conservation
       (1) Minimize radiant/convective loss by
           [a] Warming the environment (heating the operating room)
           [b] Covering the patient
           [c] Using reflective material for procedures lasting more than 2 hours
           [d] Minimize pharmacologic vasodilation
       (2) Minimize conductive/evaporative loss by
           [a] Heating and humidifying gases
           [b] Heating IV fluids (especially in resuscitation)
           [c] Warming skin preparation solutions
   (b) Rewarming
       (1) Techniques
           [a] Lavaging body cavities
           [b] Forced-air blankets
           [c] Heating and humidifying gases
       (2) Caveats
           [a] Aggressive rewarming of deep hypothermia may aggravate cerebral edema
           [b] Open lavage of pleura or pericardium may precipitate arrhythmias in severe hypothermia
           [c] Ventilatory support may be necessary at temperatures under 35°C

c. Malignant hyperthermia

1. Introduction
   (a) A rare and serious clinical syndrome, classically observed during general anesthesia, that results from uncontrolled increases in skeletal muscle metabolism that may proceed to severe rhabdomyolysis
   (b) Incidence
       (1) Children, 1 in 15,000
       (2) Adults, 1 in 50,000
   (c) Mortality less than 10–70% (dependent on early recognition and aggressive treatment)
   (d) Etiology: inherited disorder of variable penetrance and expression
2. Clinical characteristics
   (a) Onset
       (1) Acute/rapid on anesthesia induction
       (2) Delayed for hours—overt in recovery room
   (b) Triggering agents
       (1) Succinylcholine
       (2) Volatile anesthetics
       (3) Decamethonium
   (c) Metabolic features
       (1) Increased aerobic/anaerobic metabolism
           [a] Intense production of heat, CO_2, and lactate
           [b] Associated respiratory and metabolic acidosis
       (2) Initial increase in serum K^+, Ca^{2+}, CPK, myoglobin, and Na^+ from rhabdomyolysis—late decrease in serum K^+ and Ca^{2+}
       (3) Increased cellular permeability with generalized and acute cerebral edema

3. Theory
   (a) The precipitating cellular event is a marked increase in intracellular ionized calcium and blockage of calcium reuptake secondary to a defect in the sarcoplasmic reticulum, mitochondria, sarcolemma, or transverse tubule
   (b) Increased intracellular calcium combines with troponin to form actin-myosin cross-bridges that contract; rigidity may result
   (c) Continuous muscle contraction requires constant energy supply of ATP
      (1) Activation of glycogenolysis and phosphorylase kinase
      (2) Muscular hypermetabolic state that exhausts aerobic metabolism
      (3) Anaerobic metabolism results in lactate accumulation and heat production
4. Clinical syndrome: signs and symptoms
   (a) Cardiovascular (sympathetic hyperactivity)
      (1) Tachycardia—early sign
      (2) Arrhythmias—PVCs/VT
      (3) Hemodynamic instability—initial hypertension followed by hypotension secondary to cardiac depression from acidosis, conduction abnormalities, and hyperkalemia
   (b) Respiratory
      (1) Hypercarbia
      (2) Pulmonary edema—late event
      (3) Cyanosis—secondary to increased O_2 consumption or cardiopulmonary failure (dark blood in surgical field)
   (c) Cutaneous
      (1) Reddish to mottled purple rash
      (2) Diaphoresis
   (d) CNS abnormalities are usually the result of cerebral hypoxia and ischemia
      (1) Cerebral edema
      (2) Permanent coma
      (3) Paralysis
   (e) Renal
      (1) Dysfunction secondary to myoglobin within tubules and inadequate renal perfusion
   (f) Hematopoietic
      (1) DIC secondary to release of tissue thromboplastin during fever, acidosis, hypoxia, hypoperfusion, and gross alterations in membrane permeability of various body tissues
   (g) Neuromuscular
      (1) Diffuse muscular rigidity
         [a] 75% incidence
         [b] Not relieved by neuromuscular blocking agents
      (2) Trismus
         [a] Etiologies
            i) Malignant hyperthermia
            ii) Myotonia
            iii) Normal response to halothane and succinylcholine—1% incidence
            iv) Unknown etiology
         [b] Incidence of malignant hyperthermia and trismus is 50%
         [c] Recommended treatment
            i) Stop anesthetic/cancel elective surgery
            ii) Continue emergency surgery with nontriggering agents
            iii) Careful monitoring: ET-CO_2, A-line
            iv) Consideration of prophylactic dantrolene. Dantrolene may not be given if rigidity resolves quickly without other clinical evidence of the disorder

      v) Mask ventilate with 100% FiO_2

     vi) Do not repeat succinylcholine

    vii) Monitor temperature, CPK, every 4–6 hours; myoglobin and potassium every 12–24 hours

   viii) Hydrate to maintain adequate urine output

    ix) Patient/family counseling

5. Treatment of acute malignant hyperthermia

    (a) Call for help

    (b) Discontinue all halogenated agents

    (c) Hyperventilate with 100% O_2 at high gas flows to maintain normocarbia (produces a clean anesthesia machine)

    (d) Inform surgeon

    (e) Administer dantrolene sodium 2.5 mg/kg IV (20-mg bottle with 50–60 ml sterile water)

    (f) Additional IV access (possibly central venous access)

    (g) Place intra-arterial line

    (h) STAT labs (arterial and venous blood gases, electrolytes, CPK)

    (i) Initiate cooling as needed

    (j) Maintain urine output—2 ml/kg/hr (helps remove urine myoglobin)

    (k) Treat dysrhythmias resistant to dantrolene with procainamide

    (l) Admit to intensive care

   (m) Counsel patient and family

6. Associated disorders

    (a) King-Denborough syndrome
       (1) Always involves malignant hyperthermia
       (2) Short stature with growth retardation
       (3) Muscular-skeletal abnormalities

    (b) Duchenne's muscular dystrophy
       (1) Inconsistent association

    (c) Others: inconsistent association
       (1) Muscular dystrophy
       (2) Central core disease
       (3) Sudden infant death syndrome
       (4) Neuroleptic malignant syndrome
       (5) Heat stroke

d. Autonomic hyperreflexia

1. A syndrome of reflex generalized sympathetic activity, seen in spinal cord injury patients, in response to stimulation below the level of the cord injury that is uninhibited by higher centers

2. Triggering events

    (a) Distention of hollow viscus
       (1) Bladder
       (2) Gut

    (b) Noxious skin stimuli

    (c) Labor

    (d) Hypotension during induction of anesthesia

3. Population/incidence

    (a) Quadriplegics (85%)

    (b) High paraplegics (66%)

        (1) Above T5–6 (full blown)
        (2) T6–10 (mild)

  4. Natural history

    (a) Syndrome may develop in a patient 1–3 weeks after a spinal cord injury as chronic reflex activity is developing

    (b) Occurs acutely in response to stimulation below the level of the cord injury

    (c) Regression can occur suddenly

  5. Manifestations

    (a) Acute generalized sympathetic activity (below the level of the spinal cord injury)
        (1) Paroxysmal hypertension
        (2) Cardiac dysrhythmias

    (b) Parasympathetic countereffects (glossopharyngeal plus vagus)
        (1) Bradycardia
        (2) Flushing
        (3) Sweating

  6. Acute treatment

    (a) Remove the stimulus

    (b) If this occurs during anesthesia, deepen the sedation

    (c) Short-acting pharmacologic intervention
        (1) Nitroprusside infusion (0.01% solution)

  7. Prevention

    (a) Deep general anesthesia

    (b) Dense epidural blockade

    (c) Spinal blockade

    (d) Long-term pharmacologic control (limited by orthostatic hypotension)
        (1) Ganglionic blockers
        (2) Alpha adrenergics (oral clonidine)
        (3) Catecholamine depleters
        (4) Direct vasodilators

e. Neuroleptic malignant syndrome

  1. A rare complication of antipsychotic therapy whose clinical presentation is similar to that of malignant hyperthermia

  2. Incidence: 0.5–1% of all patients who receive neuroleptics

  3. Population: most common in young adult males

  4. Onset

    (a) Days to weeks

    (b) Not related to duration of exposure to triggering agent

  5. Triggering agents

    (a) Phenothiazines

    (b) Butyrophenones

    (c) Thioxanthenes

    (d) Miscellaneous antipsychotics

    (e) Abrupt withdrawal of levodopa

  6. Etiology

    (a) Central defect, possibly in dopamine receptor blockage

  7. Clinical features

    (a) Hyperthermia

    (b) Muscular rigidity and akinesia

    (c) Altered conciousness

VI. Clinical; e. Neuroleptic malignant syndrome (continued)

    (d) Autonomic instability
    (e) Multiorgan failure
  8. Laboratory abnormalities
    (a) Increased CPK
    (b) Leukocytosis
    (c) Increased liver function tests
    (d) Myoglobinuria
  9. Treatment
    (a) Cessation of triggering drug
    (b) Dantrolene
    (c) Dopamine agonists
      (1) Bromocriptine
      (2) Amantadine
      (3) Levodopa with carbidopa
    (d) Supportive therapy
 10. Mortality of 20–30%

II Pharmacologic Principles

A. INTRODUCTION

I. PHARMACOKINETICS

II. DISTRIBUTION AND ELIMINATION

III. PHARMACODYNAMICS

IV. CHARACTERISTICS

V. PROTEIN BINDINGS

VI. UPTAKE AND DISTRIBUTION

B. INHALED ANESTHETICS

I. HALOTHANE

II. ENFLURANE

III. ISOFLURANE

IV. DESFLURANE

V. SEVOFLURANE (APPROVED BY FOOD AND DRUG ADMINISTRATION)

C. INTRAVENOUS INDUCTION AGENTS

I. THIOPENTONE (INTRODUCED 1934)—A THIOBARBITURATE

II. METHOHEXITONE (INTRODUCED 1957)—OXYBARBITURATE

III. DIPRIVAN (INTRODUCED 1977)

IV. ETOMIDATE (INTRODUCED 1973)

V. KETAMINE (INTRODUCED 1957)—PHENCYCLIDINE DERIVATIVE

VI. DIAZEPAM (INTRODUCED 1964)

VII. MIDAZOLAM (INTRODUCED 1978)

VIII. FLUMAZENIL (INTRODUCED 1979)

IX. FENTANYL

X. SUFENTANIL

XI. NALOXONE—OPIOID ANTAGONIST

D. INTRAVENOUS ANESTHETICS

    I. OPIOIDS
   II. OPIOID AGONISTS
  III. OPIOID ANTAGONISTS
  IV. NONSTEROIDAL ANTI-INFLAMMATORY DRUGS
   V. BENZODIAZEPINES
  VI. BENZODIAZEPINE ANTAGONISTS
 VII. ANTIEMETICS

E. LOCAL ANESTHETICS (LAS)

    I. STRUCTURE
   II. MECHANISM OF ACTION
  III. PHARMACOKINETICS
  IV. SIDE EFFECTS
   V. REPRESENTATIVE LOCAL ANESTHETIC AGENTS

F. MUSCLE RELAXANTS

    I. NEUROMUSCULAR JUNCTION
   II. CLASSIFICATION OF NEUROMUSCULAR BLOCK
  III. NONDEPOLARIZING MUSCLE RELAXANTS
  IV. DEPOLARIZING MUSCLE RELAXANTS
   V. REVERSAL OF NEUROMUSCULAR BLOCKADE
  VI. NEUROMUSCULAR BLOCKADE MONITORING

G. IMMUNOSUPPRESSIVES AND ANTIREJECTION DRUGS

    I. INTRODUCTION
   II. CYCLOSPORIN
  III. STEROIDS
  IV. CYTOTOXICS
   V. DOXORUBICIN (ADRIAMYCIN)
  VI. BLEOMYCIN

H. DRUG REACTIONS: HYPERSENSITIVITY/ALLERGY

   I. DRUG REACTIONS
  II. ANAPHYLAXIS
 III. ANAPHYLACTOID REACTION
 IV. CLINICALLY IMPORTANT REACTIONS

A. INTRODUCTION

I. PHARMACOKINETICS

a. Definition: the time course of drugs and their metabolites in the body

b. Parameters

1. Mathematically derived
2. Theoretical (volume of distribution, clearance, relationship between blood flow and drug distribution)
3. Experimentally determined (protein binding, drug metabolic pathways)

c. Source

1. Serial blood sampling
   - (a) 10–20 serial samples from a small number of patients
   - (b) Limited samples obtained from a large population (100–300)
2. Urine and body fluid
3. Organ tissues
4. Affected by numerous factors: gender, race, age, pathologic conditions (liver, renal, and cardiac failure), food, smoking
5. Should be taken as relative rather than absolute indicators for adequately dosing anesthetics and other drugs

d. Elimination

1. Linear (first order)—constant clearance
2. Zero order—clearance becomes dependent on drug concentration

I. DISTRIBUTION AND ELIMINATION

a. Noncompartmental

1. Time delay of drug concentration is described as a whole

b. Compartmental approach

1. Drug concentration time course relationship is described as a series of linear relationships
2. Allows the best fit of the curve
3. Theoretical approach
4. None of the compartments has any anatomic meaning
5. None of the parameters translates in any physiologic concept

6. Definitions: volume of distribution (V)—volume in which a drug is homogeneously distributed; clearance (Cl)—the volume of plasma from which drug is completely removed per unit of time; half-life ($T_{1/2}$)—time required for plasma concentration to decrease by 50%; constant fraction of drug eliminated by unit of time (Kel)

7. Elimination

   (a) After four half-lives, 94% of a drug is being eliminated
   (b) After five half-lives, 95% of a drug is being eliminated

8. One-compartment model

   (a) Simplest
   (b) Assumptions
      (1) At the time of drug administration, there is an instantaneous dilution and distribution of a drug (X) given in a dose (D) into the volume of distribution (Vd), allowing it to reach an instantaneous measurable concentration C
      (2) At any time, since the distribution is homogeneous, the concentration of drug in the plasma (Cp) is an exact reflection of drug in the volume in which the drug is distributed (Vd)

9. Two-compartment model

   (a) Central compartment—drug is initially introduced
   (b) Peripheral compartment—tissue distribution
   (c) Distribution phase
      (1) Alpha (distribution phase)—from central to peripheral compartment
         [a] From central to peripheral compartment
         [b] Plasma concentration drops rapidly until equilibrium is reached between the two compartments
      (2) Beta (elimination phase)
         [a] Drug's total clearance and half-life are defined by these parameters

III. PHARMACODYNAMICS

a. Definition: relationship between drug effect and dose administered

1. Sigmoid curve

   (a) Threshold (no effects produced)
   (b) Maximum (maximum response regardless of dose administered)
   (c) Linear (between threshold and maximum response)

2. Receptors

   (a) Agonist
   (b) Antagonist
   (c) Partial agonist

3. Receptor binding

   (a) Michaelis kinetics
   (b) Allosteric kinetics

4. Drug combinations

   (a) Additive
   (b) Synergistic
   (c) Antagonistic

IV. CHARACTERISTICS

a. Drug absorption

1. Drug transport
   - (a) Passive diffusion
     - (1) Along a concentration gradient
     - (2) Across a membrane
     - (3) Drug absorption depends on lipid solubility, molecular size, surface area of absorption
   - (b) Facilitated diffusion
     - (1) Along a concentration gradient
     - (2) Selective and saturable carrier
     - (3) No energy requirement (glucose)
   - (c) Active transport
     - (1) Against a concentration gradient
     - (2) Specific and saturable carrier
     - (3) Energy required (ions, amino acids, vitamins, sugars)
2. Ionization
   - (a) pKa
   - (b) pH
   - (c) pH gradient

V. PROTEIN BINDINGS

a. Plasma drugs

1. Free
   - (a) Available for passive diffusion and binding to receptor sites
   - (b) Responsible for pharmacologic response
2. Bound
   - (a) Characteristics
     - (1) Reversible and dependent on drug and concentration of proteins
     - (2) Binding affinity and capacity of plasma proteins is variable
   - (b) Proteins
     - (1) Albumin
       - [a] Preferentially binds a large number of drugs (warfarin, diazepam, lidocaine, valproate, phenytoin)
       - [b] Decreased in patients with burns, liver disease, and nephrotic and malnutrition syndromes, as well as in neonates, the elderly, and in pregnancy
       - [c] A decrease may be associated with an increase in unbound drug
     - (2) Alpha glycoproteins
       - [a] Concentration is usually low
       - [b] Elevated in burns, Crohn's disease, colitis, trauma, surgery, myocardial ischemia and necrosis, rheumatoid arthritis, lupus, trauma, and chronic pain
       - [c] Binds such drugs as antibiotics, beta-blockers, hormones, calcium channel blockers, antiarrhythmics, antidepressants, and narcotic analgesics
       - [d] An increase in AAG will decrease the amount of free drug

b. Elderly

1. Physiologic changes

    (a) CV: decreased cardiac index
    (b) Blood flow: decreased regional blood flow (splanchnic, renal, hepatic)
    (c) Respiratory: decreased function
    (d) Renal: decreased RBF, GFR
    (e) Decreased plasma albumin concentration

2. Increased drug half-life secondary to decreased metabolism and excretion

c. Pregnancy

1. Physiologic changes

    (a) Increased plasma volume (maximum at 30 weeks)
    (b) Increased red blood cell mass
    (c) Increased liver blood flow, renal blood flow
    (d) Increased cardiac output
    (e) Increased GFR (maximum in first 20 weeks) with a parallel decrease in filtration fraction

2. Drug distribution

    (a) Mother (absorption, distribution, elimination)
    (b) Placenta
    (c) Fetus (umbilical cord, amniotic fluid)
    (d) Five-compartment model required to account for drug distribution

d. Liver failure

1. Reduced liver cell mass and function—may reduce the maximal rate of drug metabolism (drug with low extraction ratio)

2. Decrease in intrahepatic perfusion and the formation of extrahepatic portosystemic shunts—reduced drug uptake for highly extracted drugs

3. Liver diseases alter protein synthesis (synthesis of albumin, alpha globulins, glycoproteins, and gamma globulins)

e. Renal failure

1. Renal diseases can decrease urinary excretion of active drugs and their metabolites

2. Renal disease may also alter plasma protein concentrations

3. Nephrotic syndrome may result in a decrease in the fraction bound to plasma proteins

4. Alters drug biotransformation (acetylation of several drugs is decreased and plasma hydrolysis of procaine is slowed)

VI. UPTAKE AND DISTRIBUTION

a. Uptake and distribution during induction and recovery from anesthesia

1. Introduction of gas anesthetics into the ventilatory circuit (inspired concentration, Fi)

2. Lung uptake of anesthetics by the lung (alveolar concentration, Fa)

VI. Uptake and distribution; a. Uptake and distribution during induction and recovery from anesthesia (continued)

   3. Introduction of the gas into the intravascular compartment, e.g., transfer from the lung to the circulation (blood concentration, Cb)

   4. Tissue distribution, e.g., transfer from the blood to the brain and other organs (tissue concentration, Ct)

b. Rate of induction

   1. Rate of anesthetic uptake by the lung

      (a) Equilibrium between inspired and alveolar concentration
      (b) Rate at which gas concentration increases in the circuit
      (c) Relationsip between gas vapor pressure and rate of increase in inspired gas concentration
      (d) Kinetic of lung uptake is dependent on minute ventilation (tidal volume and rate)

   2. Development of an adequate anesthetic concentration in the brain

c. Rate of recovery

   1. Determined by the rate of removal of anesthetic from the brain and lung

   2. Indirect relationship between time of recovery and

      (a) Concentration gradient between the anesthetic gas in the circuit and the alveoli
      (b) Concentration of nitrous oxide (second gas effect)
      (c) Vapor pressure coefficient
      (d) Blood:tissue partition coefficients
      (e) Proportion of anesthetic being metabolized

   3. Direct relationship between time of recovery and the blood:gas partition coefficient (the lower the anesthetic solubility in blood to gas [higher vapor pressure], the shorter is the time of recovery from anesthesia)

d. Distribution

   1. Fa/Fi ratio

      (a) Anesthetic alveolar concentration (Fa) is initially dependent on Fi
      (b) With time, the amount of anesthetic gas dissolved in blood limits the increase in Fa/Fi
      (c) At equilibrium, the Fa/Fi ratio remains constant

   2. Regional blood flow

      (a) Direct relationship between tissue uptake and degree of regional perfusion
          (1) Highly perfused tissues (liver, heart, kidney, brain) have greater anesthetic uptake
          (2) Intermediate uptake: muscle
          (3) Low perfusion: fat
      (b) Equilibrium is more rapid in highly perfused organs
      (c) Recovery: anesthetic decreases more rapidly in the highly perfused tissues

B. INHALED ANESTHETICS

Table 1. Characteristics of Inhaled Anesthetics

	Halothane	Enflurane	Isoflurane	Desflurane	Sevoflurane
MAC with 100% O_2 (volumes, %) (33–50 years)	0.75	1.68	1.15	6.00	1.71
Vapor pressure (mm Hg at 20°C)	241	175	238	669	160
Boiling point (760 mm Hg) °C	50.2	56.5	48.5	22.8	58.5
Oil and gas partition coefficient (37°C)	224	98	98	18.7	47.2
Blood and gas partition coefficient (37°C)	2.4	1.9	1.4	0.42	0.69

Clinical correlates: lower oil:gas partition coefficient—higher MAC; lower blood:gas partition coefficient—more rapid wash-in and wash-out.

Table 2. Effects on Systems

	Halothane	Enflurane	Isoflurane	Desflurane	Sevoflurane
Cardiovascular					
CO	↓	↓	O	O or ↓	↓
SVR	O	↓	↓ ↓	↓ ↓	↓ ↓
HR	O	↑	↑	O or ↑	O
MAP	↓ ↓	↓ ↓	↓ ↓	↓ ↓	↓
Respiratory					
VT	↓	↓	↓	↓	↓
RR	↑ ↑	↑ ↑	↑	↑	↑
$PaCO_2$	↑	↑ ↑	↑	↑	↑
Cerebral					
CBF	↑ ↑	↑	↑	↑	↑
ICP	↑ ↑	↑ ↑	↑	↑	↑
Neuromuscular					
Nondepolarizing blockade	↑ ↑	↑ ↑ ↑	↑ ↑ ↑	↑ ↑ ↑	↑ ↑
Renal					
RBF	↓ ↓	↓ ↓	↓ ↓	? ↓	? ↓
GFR	↓ ↓	↓ ↓	↓ ↓	? ↓	? ↓
Urine output	↓ ↓	↓ ↓	↓ ↓	? ↓	? ↓
Hepatic					
Blood flow	↓ ↓	↓	↓	↓	? ↓

I. HALOTHANE

a. Physical properties

1. Halogenated alkane

```
      F   Cl
      |   |
  F—C—C—H
      |   |
      F   Br
```

I. Halothane; a. Physical properties (continued)

2. Pungent odor
3. Thymol preservative and amber-colored bottles to retard spontaneous oxidative decomposition

b. Effects on organ systems

1. Cardiovascular

    (a) Decreases arterial blood pressure
    (b) Decreases cardiac output, decreases myocardial contractility
    (c) Inhibits baroreceptor-mediated reflex tachycardia so no change in heart rate
    (d) Slows sinoatrial node conduction—may result in junctional rhythm
    (e) Sensitizes the heart to the dysrhythmogenic effects of epinephrine; avoid doses over 1.5 μg/kg
    (f) Systemic vascular resistance—unchanged

2. Respiratory

    (a) Rapid shallow breathing
    (b) VT decreased
    (c) RR increased
    (d) Resting Pa_{CO_2} is elevated
    (e) Central (medullary) and peripheral (intercostal muscle dysfunction) mechanism of action for respiratory effects
    (f) Depresses hypoxic drive even with 0.1 MAC
    (g) Bronchodilator
    (h) Depresses mucociliary function

3. Cerebral

    (a) Decreases cerebral vascular resistance
    (b) Increases cerebral blood flow the most
    (c) Autoregulation impaired
    (d) Decreases cerebral metabolic rate the least
    (e) Decreases rate of CSF production but increases resistance to reabsorption
    (f) Dose-related decrease amplitude and increased latency of cortical components of somatosensory-evoked potentials

4. Renal

    (a) Renal blood flow generally decreases secondary to increased renal vascular resistance or decreased MAP or decreased CO or both
    (b) Autoregulation of blood flow in the kidney is maintained during halothane anesthesia

5. Neuromuscular: potentiates depolarizing and nondepolarizing relaxants
6. Uterus: myometrial relaxation
7. Hepatic

    (a) Decreases hepatic blood flow in proportion to depression of cardiac output
    (b) Reported hepatic artery vasospasm

c. Biotransformation and toxicity

1. Some 20–40% of the absorbed drug undergoes metabolism
2. Preferentially undergoes oxidative metabolism via cytochrome p450 enzymes

    (a) Major metabolite—trifluoroacetic acid; excreted in the urine; other metabolites— chloride and bromide

   (b) Trifluoroacetic acid—no adverse effects
   (c) Bromide toxicity (rare)
      (1) Somnolence and mental confusion occur with bromide levels greater than 6 mEq/L
      (2) Serum bromide concentrations will increase approximately 0.5 mEq/L/MAC hour of halothane
3. Reductive metabolism (hypoxic conditions) yields fluoride and reactive intermediary metabolites. Increase fluoride concentrations after administration of halothane to obese but not to nonobese patients
4. Toxicity
   (a) "Halothane hepatitis"
   (b) Unknown etiology
   (c) Allergic reaction versus familial factor that predisposes patient
   (d) Two entities
      (1) One mild form—transient
      (2) Other is full-blown fulminant hepatitis
   (e) Diagnosis of exclusion
   (f) One in 35,000 anesthetics
   (g) Middle-aged, obese women with repeated exposure to halothane

II. ENFLURANE

a. Physical properties

1. Halogenated ether
2. Mild, sweet ethereal odor

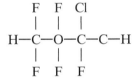

3. Colorless

b. Effects on organ systems

1. Cardiovascular
   (a) Decreases arterial blood pressure
   (b) Decreases cardiac output, decreases myocardial contractility
   (c) Decreases SVR (systemic vascular resistance)
   (d) Increases heart rate
   (e) Sensitizes the heart to the dysrhythmic effects of epinephrine (doses over 4.5 μg/kg)
2. Respiratory
   (a) Like halothane, VT is decreased and RR is increased
   (b) Increases resting $PaCO_2$ the most
   (c) Depresses hypoxic drive
   (d) Bronchodilator
   (e) Depressed mucociliary function
3. Cerebral
   (a) Increases cerebral blood flow
   (b) Increases intracranial pressure

II. Enflurane; b. Effects on organ systems (continued)

    (c) Increases secretion of CSF fluid and increases resistance to CSF reabsorption

    (d) In the presence of hypocapnia, deep enflurane anesthesia has been associated with high-voltage, fast-frequency EEG changes—seizures

    (e) Hyperventilation is not recommended

    (f) Decreases cerebral metabolic rate (CMR) unless there is seizure activity

    (g) Decreases amplitude and increases latency of SSEP

4. Renal

    (a) Decreases renal blood flow

    (b) Decreases GFR

    (c) Decreases urine output

5. Neuromuscular: potentiates muscle relaxation

6. Uterus: myometrial relaxation

7. Hepatic: decreases hepatic blood flow

c. Biotransformation and toxicity

1. Minimal oxidative metabolism in humans (2.4–8.5%)

2. Elimination primarily by ventilation of the lungs

3. Most important metabolite is fluoride

4. Defluorination of enflurane increased in patients being treated with isoniazid

5. Also increased with ethanol in rats but not with enzyme induction by Pb

6. Serum fluoride concentrations are higher in obese patients

7. Fluoride-induced nephrotoxicity

    (a) Inability to concentrate urine

    (b) Fluoride levels over 50 mm/L

    (c) After prolonged administration (9.6 MAC hours), may have transient decrease in urine-concentrating ability

III. ISOFLURANE

a. Physical properties

1. Isomer of enflurane

2. Halogenated ether

```
        F   H   F
        |   |   |
   H—C—O—C—C—F
        |   |   |
        F   Cl  F
```

3. Pungent ethereal odor

4. Colorless

b. Effect on organ systems

1. Cardiovascular

    (a) Lowers arterial blood pressure

    (b) Mild beta-adrenergic stimulation

    (c) Lowers systemic vascular resistance

    (d) Increases heart rate 20% above awake levels (more likely to occur in young than in elderly patients)

    (e) Least depression in cardiac output

    (f) Twofold to threefold increase in skeletal muscle blood flow that contributes to decreased SVR

    (g) Coronary steal syndrome

    (h) Normal coronary arteries are dilated, thus diverting blood away from fixed stenotic lesions

    (i) Conflicting evidence about whether coronary steal syndrome causes regional myocardial ischemia during episodes of tachycardia

2. Respiratory

    (a) Irritant to upper airway

    (b) Good bronchodilator

    (c) Less increase in RR compared with other volatile anesthetic agents

    (d) Depressed hypoxic drive

3. Cerebral

    (a) Decreases cerebral metabolic rate (CMR) the most

    (b) Autoregulation is better preserved with isoflurane

    (c) Smallest increase in CBF and CBV

    (d) No significant change in CSF production or reabsorption

    (e) Can produce isoelectric EEG at 2 MAC

    (f) Dose-related decrease in amplitude and increase in latency of cortical components of somatosensory-evoked potentials

4. Renal

    (a) Decreased RBF

    (b) Decreased GFR

    (c) Decreased urine output

5. Neuromuscular

    (a) Relaxes skeletal muscle

    (b) Potentiates nondepolarizing muscle relaxants

6. Hepatic

    (a) Total hepatic blood flow is reduced

    (b) Hepatic artery perfusion is better maintained with isoflurane

7. Uterus: relaxes uterine musculature

c. Biotransformation and toxicity

1. Insignificant oxidative metabolism 0.17% of the absorbed drug

2. Ventilation of lungs is primary route of elimination

3. Metabolites are trifluoroacetic acid and difluromethanol. Difluromethanol (unstable) → formic acid + fluoride

4. No enzyme induction even with isoniazid

5. Minimal increase in serum fluoride levels

IV. DESFLURANE

a. Physical properties

1. Very similar structure to isoflurane
2. Substitution of fluorine for chlorine atom on the alpha carbon of isoflurane

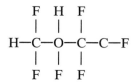

3. Colorless
4. Fluorinated methyl-ethyl ether
5. Pungent odor—not recommended for mask inductions
6. Low solubility—more rapid wash-in and wash-out
7. Vapor pressure of desflurane increases with increasing temperature. Desflurane boils at 23°C at sea level

b. Effect on organ systems

1. Cardiovascular
   (a) Similar to isoflurane
   (b) Decreased SVR, decreased arterial blood pressure
   (c) Increased HR, increased CVP, increased PA pressures that become apparent with high doses
   (d) No coronary steal
   (e) No sensitization of myocardium to epinephrine-induced dysrhythmias
2. Respiratory
   (a) Irritating to airway
   (b) VT decreased
   (c) RR increased
   (d) $PaCO_2$ increased
3. Cerebral
   (a) Significant dose-related suppression of EEG activity—similar to equipotent levels of isoflurane
   (b) Increased cerebral blood flow
   (c) Increased intracranial pressure
   (d) Recommended dose 0.8 MAC desflurane after a barbiturate induction for neurosurgery on space-occupying lesions
   (e) Hyperventilation desflurane can lower ICP
4. Renal
   (a) No reports of nephrotoxicity
   (b) No change in serum creatinine or blood urea nitrogen
5. Neuromuscular
   (a) Similar to isoflurane
   (b) Resists degradation by soda lime and the liver
   (c) 0.02% metabolized

V. SEVOFLURANE (approved by Food and Drug Administration)

a. Physical properties

1. Fluorinated methyl isopropyl ether
2. Pleasant odor
3. Not pungent
4. Colorless

$$H \diagdown \quad \diagup CF3$$
$$F—C—O—C—H$$
$$H \diagup \quad \diagdown CF3$$

5. Smooth mask induction
6. Blood/gas solubility coefficient 0.63–0.69

b. Effect on organ systems

1. Circulatory
   (a) Decreased heart rate at doses less than 2 MAC
   (b) Decreased myocardial contractility less than halothane
   (c) Decreased systolic blood pressure (slight)
   (d) In dogs, appears to be coronary artery dilator
   (e) Does not appear to be arrythmogenic
2. Respiratory
   (a) Increased RR similar to other inhaled agents
   (b) Increased $PaCO_2$ similar to other inhaled agents
   (c) Not irritating to airway
   (d) Bronchodilator
3. Cerebral
   (a) In rats, dose-related increase in CBF
   (b) In rabbits, isoflurane and sevoflurane decrease ICP and decrease $CMRO_2$ the same
4. Neuromuscular: potentiates muscle relaxants
5. Renal
   (a) Not recommended for use in patients with preexisting renal insufficiency (creatinine over 1.5 g/dl)—see below

c. Biotransformation

1. Sevoflurane not stable in vivo or in vitro
2. Decomposes in soda lime and baralyme
   (a) Compound A (pentafluoroisopropenyl fluoromethyl ether)
       (1) Baralyme causes more production of compound A than soda lime
   (b) Trace amounts of compound B (pentafluoromethoxy isopropyl fluoromethyl ether PMFE $C_5J_6F_6O$)
   (c) Concentration of degradants is inversely correlated with the fresh gas flow rate
       (1) At FGF of 1 L/min, mean maximum concentrations of compound A are approximately 20 ppm with soda lime and 30 ppm with baralyme
   (d) Compound A has been shown to be nephrotoxic in rats at various concentrations and lengths of exposure

  (e) Compound A concentration increases with increasing absorber temperature and low FGF
    (1) FGF rates greater than 2 L/min in a circle absorber system are recommended

d. Metabolism

1. By cytochrome p450 2E1
 (a) Metabolites
   (1) Hexafluoroisopropanol (HFLP) with release of inorganic fluoride and CO_2
   (2) HFLP is conjugated with glucuronic acid and eliminated
 (b) Inducible by chronic exposure to isoniazid and ethanol but not by exposure to barbiturates

2. Fluoride concentration ranges between 12 μM and 90 μM in anesthetics maintained with sevoflurane
 (a) Peak concentrations occur within 2 hours of the end of the anesthetic
 (b) In clinical trials, no reports of toxicity associated with elevated fluoride ion levels

C. INTRAVENOUS INDUCTION AGENTS

I. THIOPENTONE (introduced 1934)—a thiobarbiturate

a. Preparation

1. Water-soluble sodium salt dissolved in water or 0.9% saline
2. 2.5% solution, pale yellow, pH > 10
3. Stable for 2 weeks if refrigerated
4. Precipitation in lactated Ringer's solution or acid solution with water-soluble drugs

b. Mechanism of action

1. Interacts with gamma aminobutyric acid (GABA) receptor complex
2. Leads to membrane hyperpolarization
3. Main effect may be on reticular activating system

c. Termination of action

1. Redistribution to larger, less well-perfused compartments, e.g., muscle, skin
2. $T_{1/2}\alpha$: redistribution half-life (time to redistribute half of central distribution to total distribution volume) = 3 minutes
3. Eventually metabolized

d. Metabolism—liver

1. Hydroxythiopental + carboxylic acid derivative (not active)
2. Very high dose may be metabolized to pentobarbital
3. $T_{1/2}\beta$: clearance half-life (time to clear one half of distribution volume of circulating drugs) = 12 hours

e. Excretion—renal excretion of water-soluble metabolites

f. Dose

1. 3–6 mg/kg IV depending on age, ASA status, other medication: onset = 60 seconds; recovery = 5–10 minutes
2. 30–60 mg/kg PR in children; onset 5–10 minutes

g. Pharmacologic actions

1. CNS
   (a) EEG
      (1) Increased slow-wave high-amplitude activity
      (2) Burst suppression at very high concentrations
   (b) Anticonvulsant activity
   (c) Cerebral metabolic rate ($CMRO_2$), cerebral blood flow (CBF), intracranial pressure (ICP) are decreased

I. Thiopentone; g. Pharmacologic actions (continued)

(d) Cerebral perfusion pressure (CPP) will depend on arterial pressure

$$CPP = MAP - ICP$$

2. Cerebrovascular system (CVS)
   (a) Venous dilation with cardiac depression decreases cardiac output and arterial pressure
   (b) Heart rate—slight increase

3. Respiratory
   (a) Depression of medullary centers decreases rate and tidal volume
   (b) May be transient apnea

4. Hepatic—none; chronic exposure may affect enzyme systems

5. Renal
   (a) Change in cardiac output may affect renal blood flow
   (b) Increased antidiuretic hormone may decrease urine output

h. Adverse effects

1. Allergy—very uncommon but histamine levels may rise 300% with induction dose

2. Fixed cardiac output syndromes (e.g., aortic, mitral stenosis) may lead to profound hypotension

3. Intra-arterial injection
   (a) Clinical symptoms: spasm, thrombosis of vessel
   (b) Treatment
       (1) Lidocaine, papaverine 40 mg in 20 mg/ml saline intra-arterially
       (2) Consider sympathetic block
       (3) Consider heparinization

4. Subcutaneous injection—necrosis, consider lidocaine, hyaluronidase

5. Acute intermittent porphyria/variegate porphyria precipitation of episode (increased porphyrin)

II. METHOHEXITONE (introduced 1957)— oxybarbiturate

a. Preparation—water-soluble sodium salt 1% solution clear color pH > 10

b. Mechanism of action

1. Interacts with GABA receptor complex—inhibition of transmission
2. Probably mainly at reticular activating system

c. Termination of action

1. Redistribution
2. $T_{1/2}\alpha$: 5 minutes

d. Metabolism—liver

1. Water-soluble hydroxy derivatives excreted by kidney

2. Cleared three time as fast as thiopentone

3. $T_{1/2}\beta$ 4 hours

e. Excretion—renal

f. Dose

1. 1–3 mg/kg IV; lower dose with old age
2. Hypovolemia, poor ASA status
3. 25 mg/kg rectally in children
4. 10% solution available
5. Onset = 1 arm–brain circulation time = 60 seconds
6. Recovery in less than 10 minutes

g. Pharmacologic actions

1. CNS
   (a) Increased low-frequency, large-amplitude waves. Burst suppression at high dose
   (b) May be epileptogenic in psychomotor epilepsy
   (c) Myotonus at induction—pretreat with benzodiazepine
2. CVS
   (a) Venous dilation with cardiac depression decreases cardiac output and arterial pressure
3. Respiratory—decreased rate and tidal volume, may be transient apnea
4. Hepatic—none at usual dosage
5. Renal—RBF may decrease with decreased cardiac output

h. Adverse effects

1. Venous irritation
2. Myoclonus
3. Precipitation of porphyria
4. Intra-arterial injection, spasm, thrombosis
5. Caution in fixed cardiac output stages

III. DIPRIVAN (introduced 1977)

a. Preparation—2,6 di-isopropylphenol; 1% solution in egg white lecithin emulsion

b. Mechanism of action—may be at GABA receptor

c. Termination of action

1. Redistribution
2. $T_{1/2}\alpha$ 3 minutes

III. Diprivan (continued)

d. Metabolism—liver

1. Possibly lung
2. Very high clearance
3. $T_{1/2}\beta$ 2 hours

e. Excretion—renal

f. Dose

1. 2–3 mg/kg IV induction
2. 100–200 μg/kg/min maintenance
3. Loading dose = plasma concentration μg/ml × volume distribution ml/kg = 5 × 300 μg/kg
4. Maintenance infusion
   (a) Plasma concentration μg/ml × clearance ml/kg/min = 5 × 30 μg/kg/min
   (b) Sedation: 25–100 μg/kg/min

g. Pharmacologic actions

1. CNS
   (a) EEG—similar to barbiturates
   (b) $CMRO_2$ decrease; CBF decrease; CPP decrease; ICP decrease
   (c) CPP decrease may exceed decrease in ICP
   (d) May have anticonvulsant effect
   (e) Occasional excitatory activity, e.g., myoclonic movements, hiccupping
   (f) Less residual CNS impairment than barbiturates
2. CVS
   (a) Venous dilation, decreased peripheral vascular resistance and cardiac depression lead to hypotension
   (b) May be greater CVS depression than with thiopentone
   (c) Heart rate may decrease
3. Respiratory
   (a) May be transient apnea
   (b) Decreased rate and tidal volume
   (c) Depression of laryngeal reflexes more than barbiturates
4. Hepatic—none
5. Renal
   (a) Decreased cardiac output may decrease renal blood flow
6. Miscellaneous
   (a) Less postoperative nausea than barbiturates
   (b) Possible antipruritic effect at low dose

h. Adverse effects

1. Very low incidence of anaphylaxis; caution with history of egg allergy (usually due to yolk component)

2. Caution if lipid disorder present
3. Preservative-free—possibility of contamination of solution if exposed for prolonged time
4. Occasional myoclonic movements
5. Caution where cardiac output compromised
6. Pain on injection—pretreat with lidocaine 20 mg IV or in propofol itself, use large vein

IV. ETOMIDATE (introduced 1973)

a. Preparation

1. Introduced in 1972
2. Imidazole compound
3. Water soluble in acidic solutions, lipid soluble in physiologic solutions
4. Clear, 0.2% solution in propylene glycol

b. Mechanism of action—may act at GABA receptor at level of reticular activating system

c. Termination of action

1. Redistribution
2. $T_{1/2}\alpha$ 3 minutes

d. Metabolism

1. Hepatic
2. Plasma hydrolysis ($T_{1/2}\beta$ 4 hours)

e. Excretion—renal

f. Dose

1. 0–3 mg/kg IV induction
2. Onset 30–60 seconds
3. Recovery = 5 minutes

g. Pharmacologic actions

1. CNS
   (a) EEG—similar to barbiturates, may increase EEG activity in those with epilepsy
   (b) Myoclonic movements on induction, reduced with opioid pretreatment
2. CVS—minimal
   (a) Slight decrease in PVR
   (b) May decrease BP

IV. Etomidate; g. Pharmacologic actions (continued)

3. Respiratory
   (a) Transient apnea
   (b) Decreased rate and tidal volume
   (c) Depression may be less than barbiturates
4. Hepatic—none
5. Renal—none
6. No histamine release

h. Adverse effects

1. Pain on injection due to propylene glycol; pretreat with lidocaine, use large vein
2. Myoclonic movement at induction
3. Relatively high incidence of associated nausea/vomiting
4. Adrenal suppression of cortisol, aldosterone production, even with single dose; increased mortality where infusion used in ITU

V. KETAMINE (introduced 1957)—phencyclidine derivative

a. Preparation—water soluble, 1% or 10% solution, racemic mixture

b. Mechanism of action

1. May act on *N*-methyl–*D*-aspartate (NMDA) receptor
2. May also act on opioid and cholinergic receptors
3. Causes dissociation between limbic and thalamocortical systems

c. Termination of action

1. Redistribution
2. $T_{1/2}\alpha$ 15 minutes

d. Metabolism—hepatic

1. High liver uptake
2. By-product norketamine—one-fifth potency of ketamine
3. $T_{1/2}\beta$ 3 hours

e. Excretion—renal

f. Dose

1. 1–2 mg/kg IV induction
2. 4–6 mg/kg IM induction
3. 10 mg/kg PR in children
4. 15–45 µg/kg/min with O_2/N_2O maintenance

5. 0.2–0.8 mg/kg IV sedation followed by 5–20 mg/kg/min

6. Onset 30–60 seconds IV and 5–10 minutes IM

7. Recovery 15 minutes

g. Pharmacologic actions

1. CNS

   (a) $CMRO_2$ increase, CBP increase, ICP increase
   (b) CPP increase/decrease depending on effect on ICP
   (c) EEG—may activate foci in patients with seizure disorders
   (d) Analgesia
   (e) Myoclonic activity

2. CVS

   (a) MAP increase, CO increase, heart rate increase, primarily by central sympathetic stimulation
   (b) If catecholamine depleted or autonomic blockade, may depress myocardium

3. Respiratory

   (a) Minimal depression
   (b) Bronchodilation—sympathetically mediated
   (c) Relative preservation of laryngeal reflexes

4. Hepatic—none

5. Renal—may increase RBF

h. Adverse effects

1. Emergence delirium

2. Unpleasant dreams for up to 24 hours in 10–30% of patients, reduced by benodiazepine premedication

3. Increased oropharyngeal secretions; preoperative glycopyrrolate

4. Myoclonic movements

5. Nystagmus; IOP increase—caution in ocular surgery

6. Myocardial work plus increased blood pressure may adversely affect those with hypertension or ischemic heart disease

VI. DIAZEPAM (introduced 1964)

a. Preparation

1. Not soluble in water

2. Formulated in propylene glycol or lipid emulsion; 0.5% solution

b. Mechanism of action—modifies GABA receptor activity

c. Termination of action

1. Redistribution

VI. Diazepam (continued)

d. Metabolism—hepatic

1. Desmethyldiazepam—active
2. Hydroxydiazepam—active: $T_{1/2}\beta$ 3 hours

e. Excretion—renal

f. Dose

1. 0.3–0.5 mg/kg IV induction
2. 0.05–0.1 mg/kg p.r.n. IV maintenance
3. 1–2 mg p.r.n. IV sedation
4. Onset = 60 seconds
5. Duration = 15–30 minutes

g. Pharmacologic actions

1. CNS

   (a) Slight increase in $CMRO_2$, CBF, CPP, ICP
   (b) Muscle relaxant effect at spinal level
   (c) Anterograde amnesia
   (d) Potent anticonvulsant

2. CVS

   (a) Venous/arterial dilation—slight decrease
   (b) Slight increase in heart rate

3. Respiratory

   (a) Depression of CO_2 response
   (b) Mild but caution when used with other depressants

4. Hepatic—none
5. Renal—none

h. Adverse effects

1. Variation in response
2. Prolonged residual sedation
3. Pain on injection with propylene glycol preparation, use large vein
4. Caution with use in pregnant patients—possibility of teratogenesis, neonatal depression

VII. MIDAZOLAM (introduced 1978)

a. Preparation

1. Undergoes structural rearrangement with pH change

   (a) Physiologic pH—closed structure; lipid soluble
   (b) pH < 4, water soluble—open structure; clear 0.2/0.5% solution

b. Mechanism of action—modifies GABA receptor activity

c. Termination of action

1. Redistribution
2. Rapid hepatic clearance
3. $T_{1/2}\alpha$ 10 minutes

d. Metabolism

1. Highly metabolized—hydroxymidazolam
2. Clearance rate = ten times that of diazepam
3. $T_{1/2}\beta$ 3 hours

e. Excretion—renal

f. Dose

1. Induction = 0.15–0.3 mg/kg
2. Onset = 60 seconds variable
3. Duration = 20 minutes
4. Maintenance = 1 µg/kg/min
5. Sedation = 0.5–1 mg repeated to effect

g. Pharmacologic actions

1. CNS
   (a) Anxiolysis
   (b) Amnesia—dose related
   (c) Central muscle relaxant effects
   (d) Anticonvulsant properties
2. CVS
   (a) SVR and blood pressure—slight decrease; greater if concurrent use of opioids
   (b) Heart rate—slight increase
3. Respiratory
   (a) Dose-related respiratory depression; may be greater with chronic obstructive airway disease
   (b) High potency needs careful titration

h. Adverse effects—high safety profile but steep dose-response effect

VIII. FLUMAZENIL (introduced 1979)

a. Preparation

1. Water soluble
2. Clear 0.1% solution

VIII. Flumazenil (continued)

b. Mechanism of action

1. Competitive antagonist of benzodiazepine site on GABA complex
2. Similar in structure to benzodiazepines

c. Termination of action

1. Redistribution
2. Rapid clearance
3. Possibility of resedation
4. $T_{1/2}\alpha$ 15 minutes

d. Metabolism

1. Liver to glucuronide
2. $T_{1/2}\beta$ 1 hour

e. Excretion—renal

f. Dose

1. Incremental 100 μg up to 1 mg
2. Up to 3 mg in diagnosis of coma
3. Infusion 0.5–1 μg/kg/min

g. Pharmacologic actions

1. Antagonizes all benzodiazepines' effects
2. Some evidence for differential dose effect; e.g., reversal of respiratory depression with preservation of anxiolysis

h. Adverse effects

1. Possibility of withdrawal reaction with chronic benzodiazepine use
2. Short action—possibility of resedation

IX. FENTANYL

a. Preparation

1. Synthetic opioid agonist related to phenylpiperidine derivative of morphine
2. Highly lipid soluble
3. Clear 0.05% solution

b. Mechanism of action

1. μ_1/μ_2 agonist at pre- and postsynaptic sites (brain stem/spinal cord)
2. May block afferent input to CNS by direct stimulation of opioid receptors

c. Termination of action

1. Low-dose redistribution less than 1 hour
2. $T_{1/2}\alpha$ 13 minutes
3. > 20 µg/kg—metabolism much slower
4. Large doses may be sequestered in lung/gastric fluid
5. $T_{1/2}\beta$ 5 hours

d. Metabolism

1. Liver
2. Inactive metabolites, including norfentanyl excreted in bile and urine

e. Excretion

1. Biliary
2. Renal

f. Dose

1. Analgesia 1/2 mg/kg IV as needed
2. Blunting of hemodynamic response to intubation 2–10 mg/kg IV
3. Anesthesia 50–100 mg/kg IV

g. Pharmacologic actions

1. CNS
   (a) EEG
       (1) High dose—slow high-voltage delta waves
       (2) Ceiling effect—does not give flat EEG
   (b) CBF—may decrease
   (c) $CMRO_2$ may decrease
   (d) Intracranial pressure—little effect but some reports raise possibility of increase
   (e) Even in high dose may not reliably prevent awareness
   (f) Stimulation of chemoreceptor trigger zone—nausea/vomiting
2. CVS
   (a) Minimal myocardial depression
   (b) Little effect on preload/afterload
   (c) Heart rate may decrease due to central vagal effect
   (d) When used with benzodiazepines/nitrous oxide may depress cardiovascular system
3. Respiratory—depression of CO_2 response
4. Ocular—stimulation of Edinger-Westphal nucleus of oculomotor nerve, miosis
5. Gastrointestinal—increased smooth-muscle tone

6. Hepatobiliary—may cause spasm of sphincter of Oddi, antagonized by naloxone

7. Genitourinary increase—muscle tone may cause urinary retention

h. Adverse effects

1. Respiratory depression, particularly when used with other central depressants

2. Cardiovascular depression with nitrous oxide/benzodiazepine

3. Pruritus—not histamine mediated, reversed by naloxone

4. When used as primary anesthetic agent

    (a) Slow induction
    (b) Possibility of awareness
    (c) Does not reliably block hemodynamic response to surgery
    (d) Muscle rigidity
    (e) Prolonged ventilation postoperatively

X. SUFENTANIL

a. Preparation

1. Thienyl analogue of fentanyl

2. More lipid soluble than fentanyl

3. μ_1/μ_2 agonist

4. Five to 10 times the potency of fentanyl

b. Mechanism of action—may block afferent input to CNS by direct stimulation of opioid receptors

c. Termination of action

1. Low dose—redistribution

2. High dose—elimination

3. $T_{1/2}\alpha$ 17 minutes

d. Metabolism

1. Liver

2. Small amounts of weakly active desmethylsufentanil produced

3. $T_{1/2}\beta$ 2.5 hours—smaller volume of distribution; greater hepatic clearance than fentanyl

e. Excretion

1. Renal

2. Biliary

f. Dose

1. Analgesia 0.5–3 μg/kg IV
2. Anesthesia 8–30 μg/kg IV

g. Pharmacologic actions—similar to fentanyl

1. May allow faster induction of anesthesia than fentanyl
2. May have greater hemodynamic stability than fentanyl
3. May allow earlier extubation compared with fentanyl-based anesthesia

h. Adverse effects—similar to fentanyl

XI. NALOXONE (opioid antagonist)

a. Preparation—*N*-alkyl derivative of oxymorphone

b. Mechanism of action

1. Competitive antagonist at all opioid receptors
2. Possibly greater affinity for μ receptors

c. Termination of action

1. Redistribution
2. $T_{1/2}\alpha$ 1 hour

d. Metabolism

1. Liver
2. $T_{1/2}\beta$ 1–4 hours

e. Excretion—renal

f. Dose

1. 1 μg/kg increments IV
2. More than 400 μg rarely needed
3. 5 μg/kg per hour infusion
4. Onset 1–2 minutes
5. Duration less than 1 hour
6. May be possible to reverse respiratory depression while preserving some analgesia

g. Pharmacologic actions—reversal of all opioid-mediated effects

XI. Naloxone—opioid antagonist (continued)

h. Adverse effects

1. Short half-life—possibility of renarcotization
2. Reversal of analgesia
3. Rarely, hypertension, arrhythmias, pulmonary edema, probably due to reversal of narcotic effect
4. Antagonism of clonidine effects

D. INTRAVENOUS ANESTHETICS

I. OPIOIDS

a. Structure

1. Endorphins: naturally occurring opioids
2. Formed following hydrolysis of β-lipotropin and dynorphin in the anterior pituitary

b. Mechanism of action

1. Opioids in their ionized, *levo* form bind to anionic opioid receptors
   (a) Inhibit adenylate cyclase in the neuron
   (b) Neuronal hyperpolarization and suppression of evoked responses
2. Analgesic potency correlates with opioid receptor affinity
   (a) Opioid receptors are found at many sites in the CNS
       (1) From the dorsal horn to higher centers
       (2) Postulated to exist in peripheral tissues, such as synovium
   (b) Supraspinal receptor activation activates descending pathways
       (1) Modulate unmyelinated, slowly conducting C-fiber activation in the substantia gelatinosa
   (c) Spinal cord level receptors
       (1) Inhibit presynaptic substance P release
       (2) Reduction in afferent nociceptive transmission
       (3) Spinal administration of opioids
           [a] Analgesia
           [b] No autonomic, sensory, or motor blockade
   (d) May also alter the cognitive processing of unpleasant afferent nociceptive stimuli
       (1) Limbic level
       (2) Cortical level

c. Opioid receptors

	Effect	Agonists	Antagonists
μ_1	Supraspinal analgesia	β-endorphin, morphine	Naloxone, nalbuphine, pentazocine
μ_2	Hypoventilation, bradycardia, ileus, euphoria, physical dependence	Meperidine, fentanyl, sufentanil, alfentanil	
κ	Analgesia, sedation, miosis	Pentazocine, butorphanol, nalorphine, nalbuphine, buprenorphine	Naloxone
ρ	Dysphoria, hypertonia, mydriasis, tachycardia, tachypnea	? Pentazocine	Naloxone
δ	Modulates μ activity	*Leu*-enkephalin	Naloxone

1. Opioid side effects
   (a) Nausea and vomiting
       (1) Direct stimulation of chemoreceptor trigger zone
       (2) Sensitization of vestibular system to movement
   (b) Pruritus
       (1) Mast cell μ_1 receptor activation with peripheral histamine release
       (2) Urticaria
       (3) Late-onset (2–4 hours) pruritus
           [a] Seen after spinal administration
           [b] Blockade of receptors in the medulla
   (c) Visceral smooth muscle
       (1) Constipation
       (2) Biliary spasm
       (3) Ureteral spasm
   (d) CVS
       (1) Hypotension (arteriolar and venous dilatation)
       (2) Bradycardia
   (e) Reduction of respiratory rate
       (1) Reduced sensitivity of respiratory center to Pa_{CO_2}
       (2) Suppression of the cough reflex
   (f) Chest wall rigidity
   (g) Urinary retention, some antidiuretic effects
   (h) Blunting of the adrenocortical response to surgical stress (at high doses)
2. Absorption
   (a) Parenteral
       (1) Rapid IV
       (2) IM injection: proportional to blood flow
   (b) Oral
       (1) Good
       (2) Significant first-pass effect with some agents
   (c) Rectal
       (1) Good, but variable
       (2) Avoids first-pass effect
   (d) Transmucosal
       (1) Rapid
       (2) Early peak levels
   (e) Transdermal
       (1) Slow
       (2) Best for low-molecular-weight, lipid-soluble agents, such as fentanyl
   (f) Transplacental
       (1) Dependent on lipophilicity
       (2) Expressed in breast milk
3. Metabolism
   (a) Conjugation by the liver
       (1) Function of hepatic blood flow
       (2) Wide therapeutic margin
   (b) Renal elimination of the resultant water-soluble molecule
       (1) Accumulation of active metabolites in renal failure
       (2) May need to alter dose in renal failure to avoid toxic side effects

II. OPIOID AGONISTS

a. Morphine

1. Structure

    (a) Poorly lipid soluble
    (b) Naturally occurring alkaloid of opium
    (c) Standard by which all opioids are judged
    (d) Potent analgesic agent without a ceiling effect for analgesia
    (e) Colorless, odorless solution

2. Onset

    (a) IV: immediate
    (b) IM: 2–5 minutes
    (c) Spinal: 15–60 minutes

3. Metabolism

    (a) Hepatic: conjugation to morphine-6-glucuronide
    (b) Excretion: 10% in feces

4. Volume of distribution: 3.2–3.4 L/kg

5. Half-life: 120–240 minutes

6. Clearance: 15–23 ml/kg/min

7. Protein binding: 30%

8. Dosages

    (a) Induction: 1 mg/kg IV
    (b) Analgesia: 0.05–0.2 mg/kg IV
    (c) Intrathecal: 200–10,000 µg (preservative-free)
    (d) Epidural
        (1) Bolus: 40–100 µg/kg
        (2) Infusion: 2–20 µg/kg/hr
    (e) Intra-articular: 500–1,000 µg preservative-free

b. Fentanyl

1. Structure

    (a) $C_{22}H_{28}N_2O.C_6H_8O_7$
    (b) Highly lipid-soluble phenylpiperidine derivative of the phenanthrene morphine nucleus
    (c) Potency is 75–125 times that of morphine
    (d) Minimal histamine release and maintains cardiovascular stability
    (e) Blunts the reflex hypertension and tachycardia associated with laryngoscopy and intubation
    (f) Decreased sensitivity to $Paco_2$ may persist longer than depression of respiratory rate
    (g) Colorless, odorless solution
    (h) May be prepared in a laminate for transdermal delivery or as lozenge for oral delivery

2. Onset

    (a) IV: immediate (duration 30–60 minutes)
    (b) IM: 6–8 minutes
    (c) Epidural: 4–10 minutes
    (d) Transdermal: 12–18 hours
    (e) PO: 5–15 minutes

3. Metabolism: Liver transformation (high first-pass clearance)
4. Volume of distribution: 4 L/kg
5. Half-life: 185–219 minutes
6. Clearance: 10–20 ml/kg/min
7. Protein binding: over 80%
8. Dosages
    (a) Induction
         (1) Bolus: 5–50 μg/kg IV
         (2) Infusion: 3–12 μg/kg/hr
    (b) Analgesia
         (1) IV: 0.5–2 μg/kg
         (2) Transmucosal: 5–20 μg
    (c) Epidural
         (1) Bolus: 1–2 μg/kg
         (2) Infusion: 0.4–0.6 μg/kg/hr
    (d) Transmucosal: 5–15 μg/kg every 4–6 hours

---

c. Sufentanil

1. Structure

    (a) Thienyl analogue of fentanyl
    (b) Parenteral analgesic potency 5–10 times greater than fentanyl
    (c) Spinal analgesic potency 2–5 times greater than fentanyl
    (d) Highly lipophilic
    (e) Rapidly penetrates the blood–brain barrier
    (f) Redistribution rapidly reduces the effects of small doses
    (g) Cumulation can be seen with higher doses
    (h) Recovery from 8–30 μg/kg of sufentanil is quicker than from an equipotent dose of fentanyl

2. Onset

    (a) IV: immediate
    (b) Spinal: 4–10 minutes
    (c) Intranasal: less than 5 minutes

3. Metabolism: hepatic, small bowel
4. Half-life: 148–164 minutes, independent of liver function
5. Volume of distribution: 2.86 L/kg
6. Clearance: 13 ml/kg/min
7. Protein binding: 92.5%
8. Dosages:

    (a) Analgesia
         (1) 0.2–0.6 μg/kg IV/IM
         (2) 1.5–3 μg/kg intranasal
    (b) Intranasal: 1.5–3 μg/kg
    (c) Epidural
         (1) Bolus: 0.2–1 μg/kg
         (2) Infusion: 0.1–0.6 μg/kg/hr
    (d) Intrathecal: 0.02–0.08 μg/kg
    (e) IV PCA
         (1) Bolus: 0.05–2 μg/kg IV
         (2) Infusion: 0.04–0.4 μg/kg/hr

d. Alfentanil

1. Characteristics

   (a) Fentanyl analogue
   (b) Potency: 20% of fentanyl
   (c) Duration: 35% of fentanyl
   (d) Higher incidence of bradycardia and hypotension than with fentanyl/sufentanil
   (e) 90% of drug un-ionized at physiologic pH
   (f) Brief duration is due to redistribution

2. Onset of action

   (a) IV: immediate
   (b) IM: less than 5 minutes
   (c) Epidural: 5–15 minutes

3. Metabolism: hepatic

4. Volume of distribution: 0.4–1 L/kg

5. Half-life: 90–111 minutes

6. Clearance: 5 ml/kg/min

7. Protein binding: 92%

8. Dosages

   (a) Induction: 50–150 μg/kg IV
   (b) Analgesia: 10–25 μg/kg
   (c) Infusion: 0.1–3 μg/kg/min
   (d) Epidural
       (1) Bolus: 10–20 μg/kg
       (2) Infusion: 100–250 μg/hr

e. Meperidine

1. Characteristics

   (a) Synthetic opioid agonist
   (b) Phenylpiperidine derivative
   (c) Structure similar to atropine
   (d) Some vagolytic and antispasmodic effects
   (e) Potency: 10% that of morphine
   (f) Duration of action: 120–240 minutes
   (g) Less sedation, nausea, vomiting, euphoria, and respiratory depression than morphine
   (h) Only opioid with direct myocardial depressant effects at high doses
   (i) Active metabolite
       (1) Normeperidine
       (2) Cerebral stimulant
       (3) May accumulate with repetitive/prolonged administration/renal impairment
   (j) Confusion/hallucinations if given longer than 3 days
   (k) Local anesthetic effects
   (l) Neuraxial administration: autonomic, sensory, and motor blockade
   (m) Well absorbed from the GI tract, but less effective orally
   (n) Withdrawal has fewer autonomic side effects

2. Presentation

   (a) Colorless, aqueous solution
   (b) IV/IM injections: 10, 25, 50, 75, 100 mg/ml
   (c) Tablets: 50 and 100 mg

II. Opioid agonists; e. Meperidine (continued)

        (d) Oral syrup: 50 mg/ml

   3. Onset of action

        (a) PO: 15–45 minutes
        (b) IV: less than 1 minute
        (c) IM: 1–5 minutes
        (d) Spinal: 2–12 minutes

   4. Metabolism

        (a) Hepatic
        (b) 90% demethylated to normeperidine

   5. Volume of distribution: 3–4.5 L/kg

   6. Half-life

        (a) 180–264 minutes
        (b) Normeperidine: 15–40 hours

   7. Clearance: 5–6.5 ml/kg/min

   8. Protein binding: 70%

   9. Dosages

        (a) Analgesia: 0.5–2 mg/kg IV/IM/PO
        (b) Spinal: 0.2–1 mg/kg
        (c) Epidural
            (1) Bolus: 1–2 mg/kg
            (2) Infusion: 10–20 mg per hour

III. OPIOID ANTAGONISTS

a. Structure

   1. Pure antagonist

        (a) No agonist activity
        (b) Naloxone, naltrexone
            (1) Act by displacing agonists from receptor binding sites
            (2) Bind to these sites to prevent activation

   2. Agonist-antagonist

        (a) Partial agonism
        (b) Levorphanol, nalorphine, pentazocine, buprenorphine, butorphanol
            (1) Bind to mu receptors
            (2) Produce either a limited response (partial agonism) or no effect (competitive antagonism)
            (3) May also have effects at kappa and delta receptors
            (4) Can reduce the clinical efficacy of pure agonists
            (5) Advantages
                [a] Provides analgesia
                [b] Less respiratory depression
                [c] Lower potential to produce dependence

b. Naloxone

   1. Characteristics

        (a) Prevents or reverses the effects of opioid agonists

   (1) Such effects include respiratory depression, hypotension, sedation, analgesia, pruritus, biliary spasm

   (b) Can also reverse the psychomimetic and dysphoric effects of agonist-antagonists

   (c) Can precipitate withdrawal symptoms in the physically dependent

   (d) No pharmacologic effect in the absence of opioids

2. Presentation

   (a) Colorless solution

   (b) IV, IM, and SC injection in 0.02-, 0.04-, and 1.0-mg concentrations

   (c) With or without preservatives

3. Elimination: hepatic

4. Onset of action

   (a) IV: 1–2 minutes

   (b) SC: 2–5 minutes

5. Duration of action: 1–4 hours

6. Half-life

   (a) Adults: 30–81 minutes

   (b) Neonates: 2.6–3.6 hours

7. Clearance: 30 ml/kg/min

8. Volume of distribution: 1.8 L/kg

9. Dosages

   (a) Adult opioid overdose
       (1) 0.1–0.2 mg IV/IM/SC
       (2) Repeat every 2–3 minutes to a maximum of 10 mg

   (b) Adult infusion: 5–15 μg/kg/hr

   (c) Pediatric overdosage: 10–100 μg/kg

   (d) Pediatric infusion: 10–150 μg/kg/hr

   (e) Treatment of opioid side effects (adult)
       (1) 0.01–0.8 mg IV/IM/SC
       (2) Infusion: 1–5 μg/kg/hr

c. Naltrexone

1. Characteristics

   (a) Thebaine derivative

   (b) Congener of oxymorphone

   (c) Properties similar to naloxone

   (d) Administered orally

   (e) Active metabolite
       (1) 6-β-naltrexol
       (2) Long elimination half-life
       (3) Prolongs the duration and effect of naltrexone

2. Bioavailability

   (a) 5%

   (b) Extensive first-pass metabolism

3. Elimination: hepatic

4. Presentation: 50-mg tablets

5. Half-life

   (a) Naltrexone: 3.9 hours

   (b) 6-β-naltrexol: 12.9 hours

III. Opioid antagonists; c. Naltrexone (continued)

6. Dosages

    (a) Treatment of side effects: 12.5–50 mg/day as necessary

    (b) Opioid cessation: 12.5 mg/day, increasing to effect

    (c) Maintenance: 50 mg/day

IV. NONSTEROIDAL ANTI-INFLAMMATORY DRUGS

a. Characteristics

1. Analgesic, antipyretic, and anti-inflammatory properties

2. Acetylate cyclooxygenase

3. Inhibit the first step in the conversion of arachidonic acid to prostaglandins

4. Reduction in prostaglandins may also inhibit norepinephrine release

5. Narrow therapeutic range

6. Higher doses result in side effects without improvement in analgesia

7. Antipyretic effects may arise from

    (a) Inhibition of pyrogen-induced release of prostaglandins in the CNS

    (b) Centrally mediated peripheral vasodilatation

8. Most are available in oral or rectal forms

9. Indications

    (a) Mild to moderate pain (arthritis)

    (b) Adjunct to opioids in moderate to severe pain

b. Pharmacokinetics

1. Oral route

    (a) High bioavailability (85–100%)

    (b) Peak levels within 2 hours of ingestion

2. Highly protein-bound

    (a) Albumin

    (b) 80–95%

    (c) Low volume of distribution

3. Metabolism: oxidation and glucuronide conjugation in the liver

4. Excretion: kidney

5. Conjugated moiety

    (a) Can be converted to parent compound

    (b) May act as a drug reservoir when excretion is reduced

c. Side effects

1. Gastrointestinal

    (a) Direct gastric mucosal irritation

    (b) Gastritis and GI bleeding due to a reduction in cytoprotective PGE_2 and PGI_2

2. Renal

    (a) Renal vasoconstriction due to prostaglandin inhibition

    (b) Renal papillary necrosis and chronic interstitial nephritis (in excessive doses or elderly)

3. Hemostasis

    (a) Reversible inhibition of platelet aggregation

    (b) Prolongation of bleeding time (normal PT, PTT)

d. Ketorolac

1. Characteristics

    (a) Weak anti-inflammatory

    (b) Good analgesic properties (30 mg IM equipotent to MSO_4 9 mg)

    (c) Use with caution in hepatic/renal insufficiency

    (d) Administer for no longer than 5 days

2. Presentation

    (a) Clear, yellowish solution

    (b) Racemic mixture of ketorolac trimethamine

    (c) 15 or 30 mg/ml for IV or IM injection

    (d) 10-mg tablets

3. Absorption

    (a) Complete after IM injection

    (b) Peak levels after 50 minutes

4. Bioavailability: 100%

5. Half-life: 3.5–9 hours

6. Metabolism

    (a) Hepatic conjugation

    (b) Parahydroxy metabolite

7. Volume of distribution: 0.15–0.33 L/kg

8. Dosage

    (a) Loading: 0.5–1 mg/kg IM/slow IV

    (b) Maintenance: 0.25–0.5 mg/kg IM/slow IV every 6 hours

    (c) PO: 10 mg every 4–6 hours

    (d) Maximum dosages

        (1) 2–3 mg/kg per day for day 1

        (2) 1.5–2.5 mg/kg per day thereafter

        (3) Parenteral use 5 days only

        (4) PO use 7 days only

V. BENZODIAZEPINES

a. Characteristics

1. Benzene ring linked to a diazepine ring

2. Metabolites

    (a) Members share metabolites

    (b) Many are active

3. Receptors

    (a) Modulatory structures found on/near the alpha subunit of the GABA receptor

    (b) Found mostly on postsynaptic nerve endings in the CNS

    (c) Presence suggests the existence of an endogenous, benzodiazepinelike molecule

    (d) Highest concentrations found in the cortex, with decreasing numbers through the limbic system, thalamus, hypothalamus, cerebellum, midbrain, and medulla to the spinal cord

4. Facilitate binding of GABA to its receptors
   (a) Results in hyperpolarization of cell membranes
   (b) Reduced neuronal excitability
5. Abuse potential
   (a) Much less than opioids
   (b) Physiologic dependence can occur after prolonged use
   (c) Rare psychological dependence
   (d) Withdrawal symptoms may not occur for up to 7 days
6. No analgesic properties
7. Minimal effects on cardiorespiratory function when used alone
8. Effective anticonvulsants
9. Produce anxiolysis, skeletal muscle relaxation, anterograde amnesia

b. Side effects

1. CNS: drowsiness, fatigue, ataxia, confusion, dysarthria, headache
2. Respiratory: vent depression (especially with opioids and in those with COPD)
3. CVS: bradycardia, hypotension (in hypovolemic patients)
4. GU: incontinence, urinary retention, changes in libido
5. Ocular: blurred vision, diplopia, nystagmus, aggravation of glaucoma
6. General: urticaria, neutropenia, jaundice, changes in salivation, hiccups

c. Metabolism

1. Hepatic
2. Microsomal enzyme system (oxidation/*N*-demethylation)
3. Active metabolites
4. Enterohepatic recirculation may prolong clinical effects
5. Do not stimulate enzyme induction

d. Elimination

1. Renal
2. Oxidized and glucuronide-conjugated metabolites

e. Diazepam

1. Characteristics
   (a) Highly lipid soluble
       (1) Insoluble in water
       (2) Crosses blood–brain/placental barriers
       (3) Solubilized in propylene glycol, ethyl alcohol, sodium benzoate and benzoic acid
   (b) Can cause pain on injection (IM or IV)
   (c) Does not alter mechanics of respiration
   (d) No sympatholytic effects
   (e) Minimal cardiovascular actions

    (f) Causes skeletal muscle relaxation (effect on spinal internuncial neurons)

2. Presentation
   (a) Oral: 1 mg/ml
   (b) Tablets: 2, 5, 10 mg; sustained release: 15 mg
   (c) IV injection: 5 mg/ml

3. Metabolism
   (a) Desmethyldiazepam
   (b) Oxazepam

4. Elimination: renal

5. Half-life: 21–37 hours

6. Clearance: 0.2–0.5 ml/kg

7. Protein binding: 96–98%

8. Volume of distribution: 1–1.5 L/kg

9. Dosages
   (a) Premedication
       (1) 0.1–0.2 mg/kg IV/PO
       (2) 0.4 mg/kg IM
   (b) Induction: 0.3–0.5 mg/kg IV
   (c) Seizure management: 0.1–0.2 mg/kg every 10 minutes IV
   (d) Withdrawal effects
       (1) 0.1–0.2 mg/kg every 3–4 hours IV
       (2) 5–10 mg every 6–8 hours PO

---

f. Midazolam

1. Characteristics
   (a) Imidazole ring structure
       (1) Highly water soluble at low pH
       (2) Lipophilic at physiologic pH (minimizes venous irritation)
   (b) Compared with diazepam
       (1) Affinity for receptors is twice as great
       (2) Clinical potency is three times greater
       (3) More rapid onset
       (4) Greater amnestic and sedative potencies
       (5) Shorter duration of action
           [a] Mainly due to its lipid solubility
           [b] Rapid redistribution to inactive tissue sites
   (c) Uses
       (1) Premedication
       (2) Conscious sedation
       (3) Induction of anesthesia

2. Presentation
   (a) Colorless injectable solution
   (b) Concentrations: 1 and 5 mg/ml IV/IM injection; PO, PR, and intranasal

3. Metabolism
   (a) Hepatic
   (b) Hydroxylation to 1-hydroxy midazolam (some pharmacologic activity)
   (c) High first-pass effect

4. Elimination: renal

5. Half-life: 1–4 hours

6. Clearance: 6–8 ml/kg/min
7. Protein binding: 96–98%
8. Volume of distribution: 1–1.5 L/kg
9. Dosages
   (a) Premed
       (1) Oral: 0.5–0.75 mg/kg
       (2) IV: 0.025–0.1 mg/kg
       (3) IM: 0.07–0.08 mg/kg
       (4) Intranasal: 0.25–0.3 mg/kg
       (5) PR: 0.3–0.35 mg/kg
   (b) Induction: 0.3–0.6 mg/kg IV

g. Lorazepam

1. Characteristics
   (a) Highly insoluble analogue of oxazepam
   (b) Potent amnestic properties
   (c) Other clinical effects resemble diazepam
   (d) Uses
       (1) Sedation
       (2) Ability to respond to simple commands
       (3) Anterograde amnesia lasting for up to 6 hours
       (4) Effective in the treatment of chemotherapy-related nausea
   (e) Binds avidly to its receptor, prolonging its clinical effects
   (f) Effective premedication
   (g) Prolonged duration of effect limits usefulness as an induction/sedating agent in the operating room
   (h) Less painful on injection than diazepam
2. Presentation
   (a) Solution for injection
   (b) Concentrations
       (1) 2 or 4 mg for injection
       (2) 1- and 2-mg tablets
   (c) Solubilized in polyethylene glycol, propylene glycol, and benzyl alcohol
3. Metabolism
   (a) Hepatic conjugation
   (b) Inactive metabolites
4. Elimination: renal (80%)
5. Half-life: 10–20 hours
6. Clearance: 0.7–1.0 ml/kg/min
7. Volume of distribution: 0.8–1.3 L/kg
8. Dosages
   (a) Sedation
       (1) 0.02–0.08 mg/kg IV/IM
       (2) 2–3 mg PO every 6–12 hours
   (b) Antiemesis
       (1) 0.01–0.02 mg/kg IV
       (2) 1–2 mg PO every 6–12 hours

VI. BENZODIAZEPINE ANTAGONISTS

a. Flumazenil

1. Characteristics

    (a) Competitive antagonist
    (b) High affinity for the benzodiazepine receptor
    (c) Weak agonist effects
        (1) Attenuate anxiety, hypertension, and tachycardia following reversal of benzodiazepine effects
        (2) May prevent seizures after administration to patients with seizure disorder
    (d) Uses
        (1) To reverse the effects of short-acting benzodiazepines after surgery
        (2) For the treatment of benzodiazepine overdose
    (e) Short half-life requires redosage or infusion to minimize patient risk

2. Presentation

    (a) Colorless solution
    (b) 0.1 mg/ml solubilized in methylparaben, editate disodium, sodium chloride, or acetic acid

3. Metabolism

    (a) Hepatic
    (b) Deethylation and glucuronidation

4. Elimination

    (a) Renal (90%)
    (b) Hepatic

5. Half-life: 41–79 minutes

6. Clearance: 0.7–1.4 ml/kg/min

7. Protein binding: 50%

8. Dosage

    (a) Bolus
        (1) 0.2 mg over 30 seconds IV
        (2) May repeat dose of 0.3 mg after 30 seconds if no response
        (3) Repeat doses of 0.5 mg over 30 seconds at 1-minute intervals
        (4) Cumulative dose maximum: 3 mg
        (5) Repeat doses can be given every 20 minutes to a maximum of 1 mg
        (6) Hourly maximum: 3 mg
    (b) Infusion
        (1) 0.5–1 μg/kg/min
        (2) Maximum of 3 mg per hour
        (3) Lack of response after 5 mg implies that benzodiazepines are unlikely as the cause of sedation

VII. ANTIEMETICS

a. Promethazine

1. Structure

    (a) $C_{17} H_{20} N_2 S.HCl$
    (b) Phenothiazine derivative

2. Mechanism of action

    (a) Minimal antipsychotic or neuroleptic properties at standard doses

    (b) Competitive H1 histamine receptor antagonist (does not prevent histamine release)

    (c) Has anticholinergic, sedative, and antimotion-sickness properties

    (d) Difficult to separate the contribution of antihistamine effects to antiemetic potency from its central anticholinergic effect

    (e) Has 10% the antidopaminergic potency of chlorpromazine

3. Uses

    (a) Prevention and control of perioperative nausea

    (b) Active treatment of nausea and vomiting

    (c) Perioperative and intrapartum sedation

    (d) An adjunct to epinephrine in the treatment of anaphylaxis

    (e) An adjunct to opioids in the treatment of postoperative pain

    (f) Relief of allergic reactions to blood products

4. Presentation

    (a) Clear solution

    (b) Concentrations

        (1) 25 or 50 mg/ml for deep IM/IV injection

        (2) 12.5-, 25-, or 50-mg tablets and suppositories

        (3) 6.25 mg/5 ml in a flavored syrup base

5. Metabolism: hepatic

6. Elimination: renal

7. Dosage

    (a) Adults: 25–50 mg PO/PR/IV/deep IM

    (b) Children: 12.5–25 mg PO/PR/IV/deep IM

8. Side effects

    (a) Sodium metabisulfite

        (1) Anaphylactic reactions

        (2) Asthma attacks

    (b) Use with caution in glaucoma, prostatic hypertrophy, and bladder neck obstruction

    (c) Intra-arterial injection: vasospasm, ischemia, and distal gangrene

---

b. Droperidol

1. Characteristics

    (a) Inhibits transmission at postsynaptic dopaminergic, serotonergic, alpha-adrenergic, and GABAergic sites in the CNS

    (b) Butyrophenone

    (c) May increase sedation or prolong recovery if more than 2.5 mg is given

    (d) Short elimination half-life, but antiemetic effects may last up to 24 hours

    (e) No effect on motion (vestibular-induced) vomiting

    (f) Potentiates the effects of opioids

        (1) Neuroleptanalgesia/neuroleptanesthesia

        (2) Characterized by immobility in an outwardly tranquil patient/indifferent to surroundings

        (3) Intense analgesia at the expense of CNS depression and incomplete suppression of the autonomic response to the procedure

2. Effects

    (a) Respiratory

        (1) Does not alter the ventilatory response to CO_2

        (2) May augment the response to arterial hypoxemia

(b) CNS
  (1) Cerebral vasoconstrictor
  (2) Does not reduce $CMRO_2$
  (3) Does not produce amnesia
  (4) Produces extrapyramidal reactions in 1% of patients
  (5) Can reduce shivering associated with deliberate hypothermia
  (6) May exhibit dysphoria and akathisia (usually restless legs)
(c) CVS
  (1) Adrenergic blockade
    [a] Slight hypotension
    [b] Transient falls in systemic and pulmonary vascular resistances
  (2) Protects against catecholamine-induced dysrhythmias
  (3) Sudden death reported after injection of high (over 25-mg) doses

3. Presentation
  (a) Colorless solution (2.5 mg/ml)
  (b) In combination (2.5 mg/ml) with fentanyl (50 μg/ml) for IV injection

4. Metabolism
  (a) Hepatic
  (b) Renal

5. Half-life: 1.7–2.1 hours

6. Volume of distribution: 2.04 L/kg

7. Clearance: 14.1 ml/kg/min

8. Dosage
  (a) Premedication: 2.5–10 mg IV/IM
  (b) Antiemesis: 15 μg/kg IV
  (c) Neuroleptanalgesia/anesthesia
    (1) Droperidol 0.2 mg/kg
    (2) Fentanyl 4 μg/kg IV

E. LOCAL ANESTHETICS (LAs)

I. STRUCTURE

a. Subunit I

1. Aromatic portion of molecule
2. Substituted benzene nucleus
3. Confers lipid solubility
   (a) Introduction of lipid-soluble groups attached to the nucleus enhances lipid solubility of the parent compound
4. Rate of hydrolysis and pKa also influenced by substitutions here
5. Planarity of aromatic portion important in conferring compatibility with neural sites of action ("receptors")

b. Subunit II

1. Ester (—CO—) or amide (—HNC—) linkage
2. Contributes to stability of the molecule with respect to in vitro or enzymatic hydrolysis
3. Amino esters
   (a) Extensively and rapidly metabolized in plasma by pseudocholinesterase
   (b) Cocaine—only amino ester that undergoes significant hepatic degradation
4. Amino amides
   (a) Not significantly hydrolyzed by plasma pseudocholinesterase
   (b) Extensively metabolized by hepatic mixed-function oxidase system
   (c) Oxidative dealkylation—primary metabolic pathway for bupivacaine, etidocaine, lidocaine, mepivacaine, and ropivacaine

c. Subunit III

1. Hydrocarbon chain connecting ester or amide group with terminal amine group
2. Enhancement of lipid solubility occurs by increasing the length of this hydrocarbon chain
3. Substitution of a side-chain alkyl group also enhances lipid solubility

d. Subunit IV

1. Terminal, tertiary amine group
2. Governs hydrophilicity of the compound
3. Important in determining membrane solubility and affinity for plasma and tissue proteins

II. MECHANISM OF ACTION

a. Conduction blockade of neural impulses

1. LAs prevent increases in permeability of neural membrane to sodium ions
2. Failure to increase membrane's permeability to sodium ions slows rate of depolarization so that threshold potential is never reached and no action potential is propagated

3. LAs do not alter resting transmembrane potential or threshold potential
4. LAs stabilize and maintain sodium channels in their inactive (closed) state by binding to specific receptors located in inner portion of the sodium channels
5. LAs may also obstruct sodium channels near their external openings

b. Frequency-dependent blockade

1. LAs gain access to sodium channels only when they are in their activated (open) state
2. Rapidly firing nerves are more sensitive to LA block and therefore are blocked first
3. Cardiac effects
    (a) Small molecules with modest lipid solubility (e.g., lidocaine)
        (1) Bind and dissociate rapidly from sodium channels
        (2) Frequency dependence appears only at high frequencies
        (3) Drugs may act as antiarrhythmics
    (b) Large molecules with high lipid solubility (e.g., bupivacaine)
        (1) Dissociate slowly from sodium channel receptors
        (2) Frequency dependence appears at slow rates of channel activation
        (3) Drugs potently depress cardiac conduction

c. Nerve fiber classification

1. Fiber diameter
    (a) Cm—minimum concentration of LA required to block nerve conduction, analogous to MAC
        (1) Greater in large-diameter nerve fibers
        (2) Cm for motor fibers is approximately twice that of sensory fibers (therefore, sensory blockade may not be accompanied by motor blockade)
    (b) Selective blockade of preganglionic SNS type B fibers with low- concentration LA does not interrupt conduction in motor fibers

2. Myelination
    (a) Peripheral nerves are made up of a combination of myelinated type A and B and unmyelinated type C fibers
    (b) Myelinated fibers
        (1) Conduction blockade produced if three successive nodes of Ranvier are exposed to adequate concentrations of LA
        (2) Both types of pain-conducting fibers (myelinated type B and unmyelinated type C) are blocked by similar concentrations of LA, despite differences in diameters/myelination of these fibers
        (3) Preganglionic type B fibers are more readily blocked by LAs than any other fiber type, even though these fibers are larger in diameter than type C fibers
            [a] Presence of myelin
            [b] Small diameter

3. Position of nerve in a bundle
    (a) LAs diffuse from the outer surface (mantle) toward the center (core of the nerve) along a concentration gradient
    (b) Nerve fibers located in the mantle of a mixed nerve are blocked first
    (c) Mantle fibers are often distributed to proximal anatomic structures in contrast to distal anatomic structures (innervated by nerve fibers located near the core of the nerve)
    (d) This explains the development of proximal analgesia initially with subsequent distal spread

II. Mechanism of action; c. Nerve fiber classification (continued)

    (e) Skeletal muscle paralysis may precede sensory blockade if motor fibers are distributed peripherally to sensory fibers in the mixed peripheral nerve

  4. Fiber types

    (a) Type A alpha
      (1) Diameter: 12–20 μm
      (2) Myelinated
      (3) Function: proprioception/motor

    (b) Type A beta
      (1) Diameter: 5–12 μm
      (2) Myelinated
      (3) Function: proprioception/motor

    (c) Type A gamma
      (1) Diameter: 3–6 μm
      (2) Myelinated
      (3) Function: muscular tone

    (d) Type A delta
      (1) Diameter: 2–5 μm
      (2) Myelinated
      (3) Function: pain/temperature/touch

    (e) Type B
      (1) Diameter: less than 3 μm
      (2) Myelinated
      (3) Function: preganglionic autonomic

    (f) Type C
      (1) Diameter: 0.3–1.2 μm
      (2) Unmyelinated
      (3) Function: pain/postganglionic autonomic

  5. Summary

    (a) Smaller-diameter nerves are more susceptible to LA blockade than are larger-diameter ones
    (b) Myelinated nerve fibers are more susceptible to LA blockade than are unmyelinated ones
    (c) Active (rapidly firing) nerves are more susceptible to LA blockade than are inactive ones
    (d) Peripherally located nerve fibers (within a nerve bundle) are blocked first
    (e) A combination of these factors will ultimately determine whether a given nerve can be effectively blocked with a given concentration of LA agent

III. PHARMACOKINETICS

a. pKa—speed of onset

  1. pKa = pH at which 50% of drug is ionized

  2. LAs possess pKa's, such that less than one half the total LA exists in a lipid-soluble, nonionized form at physiologic pH

  3. Only the nonionized form of the LA is capable of crossing the lipophilic nerve sheath to access the sodium channels on the neural membrane

  4. Speed of onset

    (a) The lower the pKa, the faster the onset
    (b) Actual values
      (1) Bupivacaine, 8.1

      (2) Tetracaine, 8.6

      (3) Lidocaine, 7.7

      (4) Procaine, 8.9

      (5) Mepivacaine, 7.6

      (6) Etidocaine, 7.7

  5. Consistent with the observation that local tissue acidosis, produced by infection, is associated with poor-quality local anesthesia

    (a) Low pH results in increased LA drug ionization

    (b) Poor penetration of lipophilic nerve sheath

    (c) Limited amount of drug reaches sodium channels on the neural membrane

b. Lipid solubility—potency

  1. Primary determinant of potency

  2. Higher solubility, lower concentration needed to produce effect

c. Protein binding

  1. Primarily influences duration of effect

  2. Actual amount of protein binding

    (a) Bupivacaine, 95%

    (b) Etidocaine, 95%

    (c) Lidocaine, 65%

    (d) Prilocaine, 55%

    (e) Procaine, 6%

d. Clearance

  1. Hydrolysis (plasma pseudocholinesterase)—esters

  2. Hepatic metabolism (hepatic microsomal enzymes)—amides

  3. Rate of metabolism influences systemic toxicity

    (a) Rapid metabolism prevents accumulation of LA in plasma with decreased risk of systemic toxicity

    (b) Normal patients: esters may be less likely to produce sustained plasma concentrations with resultant toxicity than the more slowly metabolized amides

    (c) Hepatic metabolism of lidocaine is extensive

      (1) Plasma clearance of lidocaine closely parallels hepatic blood flow

      (2) Hepatic disease or decreased hepatic blood flow can reduce the metabolic rate of lidocaine

  4. Poor water solubility of LAs limits the renal excretion of unchanged drug to less than 5% of the injected dose

e. Vasoconstrictors

  1. Epinephrine: 1:200,000 or 5 μg/ml

  2. Phenylephrine: 1:20,000

  3. Produce localized vasoconstriction

    (a) Limit systemic absorption

    (b) Prolong duration of effect by keeping LA in contact with nerve fibers

  4. Less effective with high-lipid-solubility agents (bupivacaine/etidocaine)

  5. High lipid solubility causes these agents to avidly bind to tissues

III. Pharmacokinetics; e. Vasoconstrictors (continued)

6. Systemic absorption of epinephrine may contribute to cardiac dysrhythmias or accentuate hypertension in vulnerable patients

IV. SIDE EFFECTS

a. Systemic toxicity

1. Due to excess plasma concentrations (usually secondary to inadvertent intravascular injection)
2. Less often may result from excess absorption from tissue sites
3. Magnitude of systemic absorption from tissue injection sites depends on
   (a) Dose injected
   (b) Vascularity of injection site
   (c) Inclusion of vasoconstrictor in LA solution
   (d) Estimation of maximal acceptable doses for uses during performance of regional blocks attempts to limit plasma concentrations resulting from systemic absorption of injected LAs
   (e) Relative amount of absorbed LA by injection site: intercostal > interpleural > caudal > epidural > brachial plexus

b. CNS signs/symptoms of LA toxicity

1. Restlessness
2. Vertigo
3. Tinnitus
4. Slurred speech
5. Generalized tonic-clonic seizures
6. Apnea
7. Death: onset of seizures may reflect depression inhibitory cortical neurons leaving excitatory pathways unopposed
8. Treatment of LA-induced seizures
   (a) Airway management
      (1) Supplemental O_2 (decreased arterial oxygen content occurs rapidly)
      (2) ET intubation
         [a] Facilitates oxygenation of lungs and hyperventilation
         [b] Decreases likelihood of pulmonary aspiration of GI contents
      (3) Hyperventilation
         [a] Reduces delivery of additional LA to the brain (decreases cerebral blood flow)
         [b] Associated respiratory alkalosis and decreased potassium ion concentration result in hyperpolarization of neural membranes with decreased LA effects
   (b) Administration of drugs to control seizures
      (1) Diazepam
         [a] IV dosage: 0.1 mg/kg
         [b] Effectively stops LA-induced seizures
         [c] Specific effects on the limbic system
      (2) Thiopental
         [a] IV dosage: 0.5–2 mg/kg
         [b] Effectively stops central seizure activity

[c] Shorter duration of effect than diazepam

[d] Nonspecific site of action

(3) Muscle relaxants

[a] Do nothing to stop central seizure activity

[b] Stop peripheral manifestation of seizure activity

[c] May be necessary to facilitate endotracheal intubation

---

c. CV system toxicity

1. CV system is more resistant to toxic effects of LAs than the CNS

2. High LA concentration can produce

   (a) Profound hypotension

   (1) Relaxation of arteriolar smooth muscle

   (2) Direct myocardial depression

   (b) Impaired cardiac conduction

   (1) ECG changes

   (2) Prolonged P-R interval

   (3) Widened QRS complex

3. Bupivacaine has a greater potential to cause complications than lidocaine

4. Pregnancy may increase sensitivity to cardiotoxic effects of bupivacaine

---

d. Methemoglobinemia

1. Large doses of prilocaine (over 8 mg/kg) may result in accumulation of the metabolite ortho-*o*-toludine, an oxidizing compound capable of changing Hgb to *met*Hgb

2. Produces cyanosis and chocolate-colored blood

3. Treatment: IV administration of methylene blue

---

e. Neurotoxicity

1. LAs are not neurotoxic when administered at recommended concentrations, except chloroprocaine

2. Chloroprocaine

   (a) Not recommended for subarachnoid block or IV regional secondary to potential for irritant effects

   (b) Neurotoxic effects possibly related to low pH (3.0) and sodium bisulfite (antioxidant)

---

f. Allergic reactions

1. Rare—less than 1% of all adverse reactions associated with LA administration

2. Ester LA

   (a) Produce metabolites related to para-amino benzoic acid (PABA)

   (b) More likely to produce allergic reactions than amides

3. Allergic reactions following LA administration may be related to methylparaben (or other preservative), which resembles PABA, resulting in antibody production and subsequent allergic reaction unrelated to the LA

4. Cross-sensitivity does not exist between the classes of LAs (therefore, patients known to be allergic to ester LA may safely receive amide LAs)

5. Documentation of LA allergy

   (a) Clinical history (rash, laryngeal edema, hypotension, bronchospasm)

IV. Side effects; f. Allergic reactions (continued)

(b) Intradermal test with preservative-free LA solution (Syncope, tachycardia, or brady-cardia when epinephrine-containing solutions are used is more suggestive of accidental IV injection or psychogenic vagally mediated reaction than allergic reaction)

V. REPRESENTATIVE LOCAL ANESTHETIC AGENTS

a. Chloroprocaine

1. Ester
2. pH (plain solution): 2.7–4.0
3. pKa: 8.7
4. Maximum single dose/kg: 15

b. Tetracaine

1. Ester
2. pH (plain solution): 4.5–6.5
3. pKa: 8.6
4. Maximum single dose/kg: 2.5

c. Lidocaine

1. Amide
2. pH (plain solution): 6.5
3. pKa: 7.9
4. Maximum single dose/kg: 7

d. Mepivacaine

1. Amide
2. pH (plain solution): 4.5
3. pKa: 7.6
4. Maximum single dose/kg: 7

e. Bupivacaine

1. Amide
2. pH (plain solution): 4.5–6
3. pKa: 8.1
4. Maximum single dose/kg: 3

f. Etidocaine

1. Amide
2. pH (plain solution): 4.5
3. pKa: 7.7
4. Maximum single dose/kg: 4

F. MUSCLE RELAXANTS

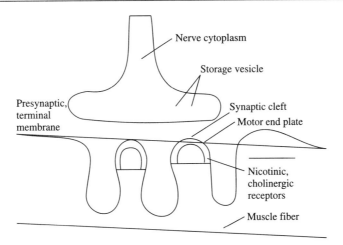

Nerve cytoplasm

Storage vesicle

Presynaptic, terminal membrane

Synaptic cleft

Motor end plate

Nicotinic, cholinergic receptors

Muscle fiber

I. NEUROMUSCULAR JUNCTION

a. Components

1. Motor nerve terminal
   - (a) Nonmyelinated
   - (b) Mitochondria
   - (c) Endoplasmic reticulum
   - (d) Synaptic vesicles

2. Motor end plate
   - (a) Highly folded membrane
   - (b) Situated opposite the motor nerve terminal

3. Synaptic cleft
   - (a) Gap of 200–300 A
   - (b) Filled with extracellular fluid
   - (c) Contains plasma cholinesterase

4. Cholinergic receptors
   - (a) Located on presynaptic/postsynaptic membranes

5. Acetylcholine receptor
   - (a) Glycoprotein
   - (b) Molecular weight 250,000 daltons
   - (c) Five subunits arranged around a central cationic channel
   - (d) Subunits consist of four proteins: alpha (two), beta (one), gamma (one), delta (one)

6. Binding sites for acetylcholine
   - (a) Located in the alpha subunit
   - (b) Unidentical
   - (c) May explain differential binding

7. Central channel
   - (a) Undergoes a conformational change when agonist binds to the alpha subunits
   - (b) Allows the flow of ions down a concentration gradient
   - (c) Membrane becomes depolarized
   - (d) Neuromuscular transmission occurs
   - (e) Succinylcholine

(1) Binds to both alpha subunits
(2) Channel remains open
(f) Competitive antagonists
(1) Bind to the alpha subunits
(2) Channel remains closed
(3) Access of acetylcholine to receptor is prevented

8. Acetylcholine synthesis and hydrolysis

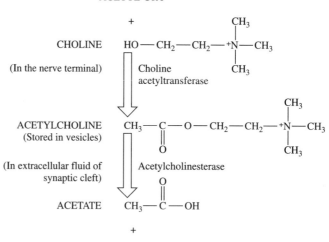

II. CLASSIFICATION OF NEUROMUSCULAR BLOCK

a. Three kinds of neuromuscular block

1. Nondepolarizing

   (a) Competitive, antagonist
   (b) Characteristics
       (1) Absence of fasciculation
       (2) Fade after twitch or tetanic stimulation
       (3) Fade with train-of-four stimulation at 2 Hz
       (4) Posttetanic facilitation
       (5) Antagonism by anticholinesterases
       (6) Potentiation by nondepolarizing relaxants
       (7) Antagonism by depolarizing relaxants

2. Depolarizing block

   (a) Agonist
   (b) Phase I block
   (c) Characteristics
       (1) Muscle fasciculations preceding the onset of relaxation
       (2) Absence of fade after twitch and tetanic stimulation
       (3) No posttetanic facilitation
       (4) Potentiation by anticholinesterases
       (5) Antagonism by nondepolarizing relaxants
       (6) Potentiation by depolarizing relaxants

3. Phase II

   (a) Dual block
   (b) Desensitization block

    (c) Large or repeated dose of a depolarizing relaxant can cause the block to change from depolarizing to nondepolarizing

    (d) Characteristics

        (1) Poorly sustained tetanus

        (2) Posttetanic facilitation

        (3) Train-of-four ratio of less than 0.3

        (4) Reversal of block by anticholinesterases

        (5) Develops more commonly in neonates, myasthenia gravis, atypical plasma cholinesterase

b. Factors affecting neuromuscular blockade

1. Drug interactions

    (a) Antibiotics

        (1) Increase the action of nondepolarizing relaxants

            [a] Aminoglycosides

            [b] Polymixins A and B

            [c] Coliston

            [d] Lincomycin

            [e] Tetracycline

        (2) Increase the action of succinylcholine

            [a] Aminoglycosides

            [b] Polymixin B

            [c] Coliston

        (3) Devoid of neuromuscular effects

            [a] Penicillin

            [b] Chloramphenicol

            [c] Cephalosporins

    (b) Anticholinesterases (inhibit plasma cholinesterase)

        (1) Echothiophate

        (2) Tetrahydroaminoacrine

        (3) Procaine

        (4) Trimethaphan

        (5) Phenelzine

        (6) Chlorpromazine

        (7) Some insecticides

    (c) Cardiovascular drugs

        (1) Diuretics (furosemide)

        (2) Increase the actions of nondepolarizing relaxants

        (3) Possibly due to hypokalemia

    (d) Local anesthetics

        (1) Procaine and lidocaine

        (2) Increase the action of nondepolarizing relaxants

    (e) Other drugs

        (1) Lithium

            [a] Increases the actions of both depolarizing and nondepolarizing relaxants

            [b] Postulated mechanisms

                i) Substitution of lithium for sodium

                ii) Interference with acetylcholine synthesis or release

                iii) Postsynaptic effects

        (2) *D*-Penicillamine (myasthenia gravis–like syndrome)

        (3) Azathioprine

            [a] Antagonizes nondepolarizing block

            [b] Possibly inhibits phosphodiesterase

II. Classification of neuromuscular block; b. Factors affecting neuromuscular blockade (continued)

        (4) Ketamine
            [a] Prolongs nondepolarizing neuromuscular blockade
            [b] Decreased acetylcholine release
            [c] Decreased receptor sensitivity to acetylcholine

2. Inhalational anesthetic agents (all increase the action of nondepolarizing relaxants)

3. Electrolytes

    (a) Increased actions of nondepolarizing relaxants
        (1) Decreases in plasma potassium
        (2) Decreases in plasma calcium
        (3) Increases in plasma magnesium
    (b) Increased action of succinylcholine
        (1) Increases in plasma magnesium

4. Acid-base balance

    (a) Increased action of nondepolarizing relaxants
    (b) Oppose reversal by neostigmine
    (c) Respiratory acidosis and metabolic alkalosis

5. Hypothermia

    (a) Increases the magnitude and duration of depolarizing block
    (b) Diminishes the response to nondepolarizing relaxants

6. Disease states

    (a) Renal disease
        (1) Atracurium: no effect
        (2) Vecuronium: modest accumulation
        (3) Long-acting nondepolarizing relaxants: accumulation
    (b) Hepatic disease
        (1) Pancuronium
            [a] 15–40% hepatically metabolized
            [b] Increased volume of distribution
            [c] Decreased elimination
            [d] Larger initial dose required
            [e] Prolonged duration of action
        (2) Atracurium: unaffected
        (3) Vecuronium
            [a] 30–50% elimination in bile
            [b] Prolonged duration of action
        (4) Succinylcholine and mivacron
            [a] Reduced levels of plasma cholinesterase in advanced liver disease
            [b] Prolonged action
    (c) Neuromuscular disease (neuromuscular function monitoring essential)
        (1) Myasthenia gravis
            [a] Sensitive to nondepolarizing relaxants
            [b] Resistant to depolarizing relaxants
            [c] Responsive to anticholinesterases
            [d] Readily develops phase II block
        (2) Myasthenic syndrome
            [a] Sensitive to nondepolarizing relaxants
            [b] Sensitive to depolarizing relaxants
            [c] Not responsive to anticholinesterases
        (3) Upper motor neuron lesions (affected muscles resistant to nondepolarizers)
        (4) Lower motor neuron lesions (exaggerated response to nondepolarizers)

  (5) Malignant hyperthermia myopathy (depolarizers: hyperpyrexia, myoglobin-uria, hyperkalemia, acidosis, and renal failure)
  (6) Muscular dystrophy
    [a] Sensitive to nondepolarizing agents
    [b] Depolarizers: rhabdomyolysis, myoglobinuria, and renal failure
  (7) Familial periodic paralysis: unpredictable response
  (d) Burns
    (1) Succinylcholine
      [a] May cause massive hyperkalemia
      [b] May lead to arrhythmias or cardiac arrest
    (2) Nondepolarizing relaxants
      [a] Increased requirements
      [b] Possible mechanism: increased number of extrajunctional cholinergic receptors

7. Age
  (a) Neonates
    (1) Sensitive to nondepolarizing relaxants
    (2) Resistant to succinylcholine
  (b) Elderly
    (1) Reduced requirement for nondepolarizing relaxants
    (2) Decreased plasma clearance
    (3) Prolonged elimination half-life

c. Properties of the ideal muscle relaxant

1. Nondepolarizing

2. Fast in action

3. Free of cardiovascular side effects

4. Easily antagonized

5. Stable pharmacokinetics and pharmacodynamics in the presence of renal or hepatic disease

III. NONDEPOLARIZING MUSCLE RELAXANTS

a. Atracurium (Tracrium)

ATRACURIUM

1. Characteristics
  (a) Ultrashort-acting nondepolarizing muscle relaxant
  (b) Independent of liver and kidney for termination of effect
  (c) Minimal side effects

II. Classification of neuromuscular block; a. Atracurium (continued)

2. Chemistry

    (a) *Bis*-quaternary ammonium compound
    (b) Mixture of 16 steric isomers but behaves as a single substance
    (c) Water soluble; stable at pH 3.5
    (d) Stable for 2 years at 5°C (solutions stored at room temperature (20°C) for more than 2 weeks should be discarded)

3. Metabolism

    (a) Ester hydrolysis (two thirds)
    (b) Hofmann elimination (one third)
        (1) Spontaneous decomposition of a quaternary ammonium compound
        (2) Elimination of a molecule of water
        (3) Originally described in 1851 by A.W. Hofmann
        (4) Chemical reaction took place at high temperature (over 100°C) and alkaline pH of 14
        (5) Occurs at body pH and temperature

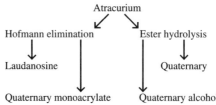

        (6) Metabolites are devoid of neuromuscular or cardiovascular effects
        (7) Laudanosine
            [a] CNS stimulant
            [b] Shown to cause strychninelike convulsions
            [c] Unlikely to reach convulsive levels after clinical doses of atracurium

4. Pharmacokinetics

Dose (mg/kg)	Distribution Volume (L/kg)	Plasma Clearance (ml/kg/min)	Elimination Half-life $T_{1/2}\beta$ (minutes)
Normal			
0.3	0.153	5.5	20
0.6	0.16	5.5	20
0.7	0.16	5.3	21
Renal/hepatic failure			
0.7	0.2	6.5	22

5. Neuromuscular block

    (a) Potency—ED_{95} = 0.25 mg/kg
        (1) Vecuronium is five times as potent as atracurium
        (2) Pancuronium is four times as potent as atracurium
    (b) Onset and intubation
        (1) At a dose of 0.2 mg/kg (ED_{95}), onset time to maximum twitch depression is 4 minutes
        (2) At a dose of 0.6 mg/kg (three times ED_{95}), patients can be intubated at between 30 and 120 seconds
    (c) Duration of action
        (1) Related to dose

        (2) When equipotent doses are administered, duration of block is similar to that of vecuronium but only approximately one third that of pancuronium and *d*-tubocurarine

        (3) Duration is prolonged by inhalational anesthetic agents

        (4) Repeated doses demonstrates little or no accumulation

    (d) Recovery and reversal

        (1) Recovery rate from 75–25% neuromuscular block is rapid: 11–23 minutes

        (2) Recovery may be accelerated by anticholinesterases

6. Cardiovascular effects

    (a) Cardiovascular stability when bolus dose is less than twice ED_{95}

7. Histamine release

    (a) At doses over 0.4 mg/kg, hypotension and tachycardia may occur

    (b) Cardiovascular changes—dose dependent, related to histamine release

    (c) Cutaneous reactions, e.g., rash, frequently reported, seldom associated with severe reactions

    (d) Histamine release may be reduced by slow IV injection

    (e) Anaphylactoid reactions have been described

8. Intracranial and intraocular pressures—no effect

9. Lower esophageal sphincter tone—no effect

10. Effect of age

    (a) Pediatric age group

        (1) Onset time is reduced

        (2) Infusion requirements: 5–7 µg/kg/min

    (b) Elderly: no change in drug requirements

11. Drug interactions

    (a) Potentiation of block seen with inhalational agents and antibiotics

    (b) Antagonized by epinephrine

    (c) Can be used to decrease succinylcholine myalgia and fasciculations

    (d) Decreases the potency of succinylcholine

    (e) Potentiated by other nondepolarizing neuromuscular blocking drugs

12. Use in obstetrics

    (a) Used to provide maintenance relaxation following intubation facilitated by succinylcholine

    (b) Small quantities cross the placenta but no problems have been reported in the fetus

13. Use in disease states

    (a) Renal and hepatic disease—unaffected

    (b) Myasthenia gravis

        (1) Requirements vary but usually are approximately 50% of normal

        (2) Metabolism ensures a normal rapid rate of recovery

    (c) Malignant hyperthermia—does not trigger malignant hyperthermia

    (d) Myotonic dystrophies—patients respond normally

14. Use in the burned patient

    (a) Patients show resistance to atracurium

    (b) Maximal at 15–40 days postburn injury

    (c) May last up to a year

15. Modes of administration

    (a) Bolus of 0.4–0.5 mg/kg gives good intubating conditions in 2–3 minutes

    (b) Surgical relaxation lasts 30–40 minutes with repeated doses of 0.05–0.1 mg/kg/hr

    (c) Diluted in normal saline (versus more alkaline Ringer's lactate degradation more likely)

    (d) Recovery is rapid on stopping the infusion

III. Nondepolarizing muscle relaxants (continued)

b. Cisatracurium (Nimbex)

CISATRACURIUM

1. Characteristics

   (a) Intermediate acting
   (b) Independent of liver and kidney for termination of action
   (c) Minimal side effects

2. Chemistry

   (a) Atracurium isomer
   (b) Water soluble, pH 3.25–3.65
   (c) Relatively stable potency when stored cool

3. Metabolism

   (a) Hofmann elimination
   (b) Laudanosine production one third of atracurium

4. Pharmacokinetics

	Distribution Volume L/kg	Plasma Clearance ml/kg/min	Elimination Half-life $t_{1/2}\beta$ (minutes)
Adult	133 + 15	5.3 + .9	22.1 + 2.5
ESRD*	160 + 32	4.2 + .6	32.3 + 6.3
ESLD†	195 + 38	6.6 + 1.1	24.4 + 2.9

   *ESRD = End stage renal disease.
   †ESLD = End stage liver disease.

5. Neuromuscular block

   (a) Potency (ED_{95}) = 0.05 mg/kg
   (b) Onset and intubation
       (1) $2 \times ED_{95}$ (0.1 mg/kg) onset time to maximal twitch depression is 5 minutes.
       (2) $3 \times ED_{95}$ (0.15 mg/kg) time to maximal twitch depression is 3.5 minutes.
   (c) Duration of action
       (1) Related to dose
       (2) Once recovery begins rate is independent of dose
       (3) Continuous infusion of up to 3 hours is not associated with tachyphylaxis
   (d) Recovery and reversal
       (1) Recovery rate from 25–75% 41–81 minutes
       (2) Readily antagonized by anticholinesterase agents once recovery has begun

6. Side effects

   (a) Bradycardia (0.4%)
   (b) Hypotension (0.2%)
   (c) Flushing (0.2%)
   (d) Bronchospasm (0.2%)
   (e) Rash (0.1%)

7. Effect of age

   (a) Faster onset and recovery in ages 2–12

   (b) Nonsignificant variations in elderly

8. Drug interactions

   (a) Potentiation with inhalation agents, antibiotics, magnesium, lithium, local anesthetics, procainamide, and quinidine

   (b) Unknown effect on succinylcholine-induced myalgias and fasciculations

   (c) May be used as long-term agent in ICU

9. Disease states

   (a) Does not trigger hyperthermia

   (b) Safe to use in renal and hepatic failure patients in normal doses

---

c. Doxacurium

1. Chemistry

   (a) *Bis*-quaternary benzyl-isoquinolinium diester

   (b) Mixture of three stereoisomers

2. Metabolism

   (a) Excreted unchanged in the urine (35%) and bile—overall extent of biliary excretion is unknown

   (b) Minimal hydrolysis by human plasma cholinesterase (6% of the rate of hydrolysis of succinylcholine)

   (c) Plasma protein binding: 30%

DOXACURIUM

3. Pharmacokinetics

Distribution Volume (L/kg)	Plasma Clearance (ml/kg/min)	Elimination Half-life $T_{1/2}\beta$ (minutes)
Normal		
0.22	2.66	99
Renal transplant patients		
0.27	1.23	221
Liver transplant patients		
0.29	2.3	115

4. Neuromuscular blockade

   (a) $ED_{95} = 25$ mg/kg

   (b) Potency

      (1) Two and a half to three times more potent than pancuronium

      (2) Ten to 12 times more potent than metocurine

III. Nondepolarizing muscle relaxants; c. Doxacurium (continued)

    (c) Onset and intubation
        (1) With a single dose (40 mg/kg), time to maximum block is 9 minutes
        (2) After a larger dose of 80 mg/kg, tracheal intubation can be accomplished after 5 minutes
    (d) Duration of action

Dose (mg/kg)	Duration of Clinical Relaxation (minutes)
40	77
50	120
60	122
80	164

5. Cardiovascular effects

    (a) Doxacurium has no dose-related effects on heart rate or blood pressure

6. Histamine release: no

7. Effect of age: prolonged

    (a) Onset time to the occurrence of maximal block
    (b) Time to 25% recovery

8. Interactions

    (a) Potentiated by volatile anesthetics, enflurane more than isoflurane more than halothane
    (b) Antagonized by anticonvulsants phenytoin and carbamazepine

9. Use in malignant hyperthermia

    (a) In a study of malignant hyperthermia–susceptible pigs, doxacurium did not trigger malignant hyperthermia
    (b) Doxacurium has not been studied in malignant hyperthermia–susceptible humans

10. Use in obstetrics

    (a) Duration of action of doxacurium exceeds the usual duration of surgical obstetrics
    (b) Not routinely recommended for use in patients undergoing cesarean section

11. Modes of administration

    (a) 80 mg/kg: intubation may be accomplished after 5 minutes
    (b) Subsequent block has a clinical duration of 150 minutes
    (c) Maintenance: (5–10 mg/kg) give further relaxation of 30–60 minutes' duration
    (d) Use in infusion is not recommended

d. Gallamine (Flaxedil)

$$OCH_2CH_2N^+ (C_2H_5)_3$$
$$OCH_2CH_2N^+ (C_2H_5)_3$$

GALLAMINE

$$OCH_2CH_2N^+ (C_2H_5)_3$$

1. Characteristics

    (a) First widely used synthetic muscle relaxant
    (b) Contains three positively charged nitrogen atoms
    (c) Not metabolized but excreted unchanged almost entirely by the kidneys
    (d) After a bolus dose of 2.5 mg/kg, 15–100% was found in the urine after 24 hours

2. Pharmacokinetics

	Distribution Volume (L/kg)	Plasma Clearance (ml/kg/min)	Elimination Half-life $T_{1/2}\beta$ (minutes)
Normal	0.2	1.2	134
Biliary obstruction	0.26	1.2	160
Renal failure	0.28	0.24	752

3. Neuromuscular blockade
   (a) $ED_{95} = 3$ mg/kg
   (b) Onset, duration, and recovery
       (1) With equipotent doses, onset of action is similar to that of pancuronium and *d*-tubocurarine
       (2) Maximum block with ED_{95} dose occurs in 5–7 minutes
       (3) Time to recovery from 95% to 25% is 27 minutes
       (4) Rapidly reversed by anticholinesterases
4. Cardiovascular effects
   (a) Causes vagal blockade—tachycardia (dose related)
   (b) Increased cardiac output
   (c) Increased systemic arterial blood pressure
5. Histamine release
   (a) None known
   (b) Anaphylactoid reactions have been reported
6. Use in disease states
   (a) Renal failure
       (1) Clearance of gallamine is markedly reduced
       (2) Large or repeated doses produce prolonged neuromuscular blockade
7. Mode of administration
   (a) Too slow to use for intubation
   (b) Intubation may be facilitated with succinylcholine
       (1) Relaxation can be maintained with a dose of 1–2 mg/kg
       (2) Repeated doses of 0.25–0.5 mg/kg

e. Metocurine (Metubine)

1. Chemistry
   (a) Formed by the methylation of two hydroxy groups of *d*-tubocurarine
2. Metabolism and excretion
   (a) No measurable metabolism

III. Nondepolarizing muscle relaxants; e. Metocurine (continued)

(b) Excretion
  (1) 46–58% in urine
  (2) 2% in bile
  (3) The remainder is distributed to body storage depots, e.g., cartilage and mucopolysaccharide
(c) Protein binding is approximately 35%

3. Pharmacokinetics

Distribution Volume (L/kg)	Plasma Clearance (ml/kg/min)	Elimination Half-life $T_{1/2}\beta$ (minutes)
Adults		
0.4	1.34	216
> 70 years		
0.28	0.36	530
Renal failure		
0.35	0.38	684

4. Neuromuscular blockade

(a) Potency
  (1) ED_{95} 0.28 mg/kg
  (2) Twice as potent as *d*-tubocurarine
(b) Onset and intubation are similar to that of pancuronium
(c) Maximum block after 0.3 mg/kg is approximately 5 minutes
(d) Duration of block
  (1) Recovery from 95% to 25% twitch height after 0.3 mg/kg occurs in 80 minutes
  (2) Recovery can be accelerated with anticholinesterases

5. Cardiovascular effects

(a) No change in heart rate or blood pressure until doses exceed ED_{95}
(b) Produces less histamine release than *d*-tubocurarine

6. Intracranial and intraocular pressures—no effect

7. Mode of administration

(a) Slow in onset and, therefore, is not used for tracheal intubation
(b) Maintenance: 0.2–0.3 mg/kg, with the resultant block lasting 40–60 minutes

---

f. Mivacurium (Mivacron)

MIVACURIUM

1. Chemistry

(a) Bisbenzylisoquinolinium diester compound

2. Metabolism
   (a) Rapidly hydrolyzed by plasma cholinesterase
   (b) Approximately 88% of the rate of hydrolysis of succinylcholine
   (c) Abnormal responses have been reported in some patients with atypical enzymes
3. Pharmacokinetics

Distribution Volume (L/kg)	Plasma Clearance (ml/kg/min)	Elimination Half-life $T_{1/2}\beta$ (minutes)
0.15	55	16.9

4. Neuromuscular blockade
   (a) Potency: $ED_{95} = 0.07$ mg/kg
   (b) With a dose of twice the ED_{95}, time to maximum block is approximately 2 minutes
   (c) Spontaneous recovery of the twitch response from 25% to 75% of control amplitude
       (1) 6 minutes following an initial dose of 0.15 mg/kg
       (2) 7–8 minutes following initial doses of 0.2 or 0.25 mg/kg of mivacurium
   (d) Accumulation does not occur
   (e) No development of phase II blockade
5. Cardiovascular effects
   (a) (Twice ED_{95}): no hemodynamic side effects or release of histamine
   (b) At doses of 0.2 mg/kg or greater
       (1) Histamine release is seen occasionally
       (2) Can be prevented by slowing the rate of injection to 30 seconds or more
6. Use in children
   (a) Require higher bolus doses and infusion rates than adults on a milligram-per-kilogram basis
   (b) Onset times for dose two to two and a half times ED_{95} (0.2–0.25 mg/kg)
       (1) Shorter in children
       (2) May allow intubation within 1 to 2 minutes
7. Use in renal or hepatic disease
   (a) Reduction in plasma cholinesterase activity may prolong neuromuscular block
8. Use in obstetrics
   (a) Use of mivacurium during labor or cesarean section has not been studied in humans
   (b) Not known whether mivacurium administered to the mother has any effects on the fetus
9. Malignant hyperthermia
   (a) In a study of malignant hyperthermia–susceptible pigs, mivacurium did not trigger malignant hyperthermia
   (b) Mivacurium has not been studied in malignant hyperthermia–susceptible humans
10. Dosage and administration
    (a) Initial dose
        (1) 0.15 mg/kg administered over 5 to 15 seconds
        (2) Produces good to excellent intubating conditions in 2.5 minutes
    (b) Maintenance dose
        (1) 0.10 mg/kg each
        (2) Provides approximately 15 minutes of additional clinical block
    (c) Infusion
        (1) Wait for early evidence of spontaneous recovery from an initial dose
        (2) Start an initial infusion rate of 9–10 mg/kg/hr

III. Nondepolarizing muscle relaxants (continued)

---

g. Pancuronium (Pavulon)

PANCURONIUM

1. Chemistry
    (a) *Bis*-quaternary ammonium salt
2. Metabolism
    (a) Theoretically metabolized to 3-OH, 17-OH, 3,17-$(OH)_2$ derivatives
    (b) Only the 3-OH compound has been identified in humans
3. Elimination
    (a) Mainly by the kidneys, with some biliary excretion
    (b) Protein binding is approximately 25%
4. Pharmacokinetics

	Distribution Volume (L/kg)	Plasma Clearance (ml/kg/min)	Elimination Half-life $T_{1/2}\beta$ (minutes)
Normal	0.26	123	133
Renal failure	0.29	53	257
Biliary obstruction	0.42	102	208

5. Neuromuscular blockade
    (a) ED_{95}: 0.06–0.07 mg/kg
    (b) Potency: five times as potent as *d*-tubocurarine
    (c) Onset and intubation
        (1) With nitrous/oxygen/halothane anesthesia
        (2) After 0.1 mg/kg pancuronium
        (3) Endotracheal intubation can be achieved within 2 minutes
    (d) Duration of action
        (1) With doses of 0.04–0.05 mg/kg: 1 hour
        (2) Increased dose prolongs the block
        (3) Duration of second similar dose is longer; repeat doses: 20–25% of the initial dose
        (4) Accumulation can occur
    (e) Recovery and reversal
        (1) Once recovery has commenced, it proceeds rapidly
        (2) Can be accelerated with anticholinesterases
6. Cardiovascular effects
    (a) Vagolytic at postganglionic nerve terminal—tachycardia
        (1) Increased cardiac output

(2) Increased blood pressure

(b) Sympathomimetic activity due to blockade of muscarinic receptors

7. Histamine release

(a) Pancuronium does not normally cause an increase in plasma histamine levels

8. Intracranial and intraocular pressures—no effect

9. Lower esophageal sphincter tone

(a) Causes an increase in barrier pressure that persists for approximately 5 minutes

10. Effect of age

(a) Infants (under 1 year) and children are slightly more resistant to pancuronium than adults

(b) Plasma clearance of the drug is reduced with age, causing duration of action to be prolonged

11. Use in cardiopulmonary bypass

(a) Can be used to counteract bradycardia seen with use of high-dose narcotics in cardiac surgery

12. Use in obstetrics

(a) Used to provide surgical relaxation following intubation facilitated with succinylcholine

(b) Pancuronium passes to the fetus but fetal amounts are not clinically relevant

13. Use in renal failure

(a) Duration of action and rate of recovery prolonged

(b) Due to decreased plasma clearance

14. Use in hepatic failure

(a) Patients with chronic liver disease are resistant to pancuronium

15. Use in neuromuscular disease

(a) Myasthenia gravis—not recommended

16. Use in malignant hyperthermia

(a) Pancuronium has not been implicated as a triggering agent

17. Modes of administration

(a) Onset of action is slow

(b) Increasing doses (over 0.15 mg/kg)
    (1) Give intubating conditions similar to that seen with succinylcholine
    (2) Prolonged blockade occurs
    (3) Usually given after endotracheal intubation with succinylcholine

(c) Maintenance
    (1) Initial dose of 0.03 mg/kg
    (2) Subsequent doses of 0.01–0.03 mg/kg
    (3) Continuous infusion—0.4–0.6 mg/kg/hr

h. Pipecuronium (Arduan)

PIPECURONIUM

III. Nondepolarizing muscle relaxants; h. Pipecuronium (continued)

1. Chemistry
   (a) *Bis*-quaternary ammonium compound
   (b) Analogue of pancuronium
   (c) Plasma protein binding: 32%

2. Metabolism and excretion
   (a) Hepatic metabolism
   (b) Renal excretion

3. Pharmacokinetics

Distribution Volume (L/kg)	Plasma Clearance (ml/kg/min)	Elimination Half-life $T_{1/2}\beta$ (minutes)
0.3	2.4	137

4. Neuromuscular blockade
   (a) ED_{95}: 45 mg/kg
   (b) Approximately 20–25% more potent than pancuronium
   (c) Time to onset of block is dose dependent
   (d) At 45–50 μg/kg, onset of block is 3.5–5 minutes
   (e) Duration of clinical relaxation: 29–40 minutes
   (f) At 70–85 mg/kg, complete block occurs in 2–2.5 minutes
   (g) Duration of clinical relaxation: 1.5–2 hours

5. Cardiovascular effects
   (a) Doses as high as 0.2 mg/kg: no effects on heart rate, mean arterial pressure, or cardiac index

6. Histamine release—no

7. Effect of age
   (a) Infants and children: relaxation is shorter by about 25%
   (b) Older children and adults: there is no significant difference
   (c) Elderly (over 60 years old): the ED_{95} is approximately 35 mg/kg

i. Rocuronium (Zemuron)

1. Chemistry: acetoxy analogue of vecuronium

2. Metabolism and excretion
   (a) Not metabolized
   (b) Excretion
      (1) Bile (80%)
      (2) Urine (under 10%)

3. Pharmacokinetics

	Distribution Volume (L/kg)	Plasma Clearance (ml/kg/min)	Elimination Half-life $T_{1/2}\beta$ (minutes)
Normal	0.17	2.8	73
Hepatic dysfunction	0.32	2.0	173

4. Neuromuscular blockade
   (a) ED_{95} = 0.3–0.4 mg/kg
   (b) Time to 90% block after a dose of 0.25 mg/kg is 4.6 minutes
   (c) Doses of 0.6–0.8 mg/kg
       (1) Good to excellent intubating conditions in about 90–110 seconds
       (2) Duration of clinical relaxation of between 27 and 45 minutes
   (d) No significant accumulation has been observed

5. Cardiovascular effects: none with dose ranges of 0.5–0.6 mg/kg

6. Histamine release: none with doses of up to 1.2 mg/kg

7. Effect of age

	ED_{95}	Duration of Action	Time to 90% Recovery
Children	0.4 mg/kg	32 minutes	46.9 minutes
Adults	0.3 mg/kg	40 minutes	54 minutes
Elderly	0.3 mg/kg	45 minutes	137 minutes

8. Malignant hyperthermia: does not trigger malignant hyperthermia

9. Dose and mode of administration
   (a) Initial dose
       (1) 0.5 mg/kg: good to excellent intubating conditions exist after 60 seconds
       (2) 1.5 mg/kg: intubating conditions are similar to succinylcholine at 60 seconds
   (b) Maintenance
       (1) 2 mg/kg: further blockade of approximately 30 minutes' duration
       (2) Infusion: 5–10 mg/kg/min

j. *d*-Tubocurarine (Tubarine)

d-TUBOCURARINE

1. Chemistry
   (a) Originally thought to be a *bis*-quaternary ammonium compound
   (b) Now realized that one of the nitrogen atoms is tertiary
   (c) At body pH, it becomes protonated to give two positively charged centers

2. Metabolism and excretion
   (a) Undergoes minimal metabolism in the body
   (b) 24 hours after administration

III. Nondepolarizing muscle relaxants; j. d-*Tubocurarine (continued)*

                (1) 12% can be recovered in the bile

                (2) 44% in the urine

                (3) Remainder is bound at inaccessible sites and released slowly into the circulation

            (c) Protein binding: 35–44%, is not affected by renal, hepatic, or cardiac disease

      3. Pharmacokinetics

Distribution Volume (L/kg)	Plasma Clearance (ml/kg/min)	Elimination Half-life $T_{1/2}\beta$ (minutes)
0.3–0.6	100–300	1–3

           The wide spread of values is due to individual variation

      4. Neuromuscular blockade

            (a) ED$_{95}$: 0.5 mg/kg

            (b) Potency: approximately one sixth as potent as pancuronium

            (c) Onset and intubation

                (1) After 0.6 mg/kg, maximum block develops in approximately 6 minutes

                (2) Seldom used for intubation

            (d) Duration of action

                (1) Similar to an equipotent dose of pancuronium

                (2) After a dose of 0.6 mg/kg, twitch height returns to 25% of normal in about 80 minutes

            (e) Recovery and reversal

                (1) Recovery from 75% to 25% block occurs in 25–35 minutes

                (2) May be accelerated with anticholinesterases

      5. Cardiovascular effects

            (a) Autonomic blockade at parasympathetic and sympathetic ganglia occurs

            (b) Hypotension and tachycardia/bradycardia

      6. Histamine release

            (a) Does occur at clinical doses

            (b) Dose related

            (c) May be more important than ganglionic blockade

                (1) Hypotension

                (2) Reduced perfusion of stomach, kidneys, liver, and spleen

      7. Intracranial and intraocular pressures: no effect

      8. Effect of age

            (a) Neonates

                (1) Increased elimination half-life, volume of distribution

                (2) Increased sensitivity of the neuromuscular junction

                (3) Therefore, dose requirements stay the same

            (b) Infants

                (1) Reduction of glomerular filtration rate

                (2) Longer duration of action of *d*-tubocurarine

            (c) Elderly

                (1) Decreased renal clearance

                (2) Prolongation of neuromuscular block

      9. Modes of administration

            (a) Not used for intubation

            (b) Initial dose of 0.25–0.5 mg/kg

(c) Maintenance: subsequent bolus doses are one fourth to one half of the initial dose

(d) Can also be used for precurarization in a dose of 3 mg/70 kg adult

---

k. Vecuronium (Norcuron)

VECURONIUM

1. Chemistry
   (a) Diester monoquaternary compound
   (b) Unstable in aqueous solution
2. Metabolism and excretion
   (a) Undergoes spontaneous deacetylation similar to pancuronium
   (b) May produce 3-OH, 17-OH, and 3,17-$(OH)_2$ derivative amounts
   (c) 20% excreted by the kidneys
   (d) 12% excreted in the bile in the first 24 hours
3. Pharmacokinetics

Distribution Volume (L/kg)	Plasma Clearance (ml/kg/min)	Elimination Half-life $T_{1/2}\beta$ (minutes)
Normal		
0.26	4.6	62
Renal failure		
0.24	2.5	97
Cirrhosis		
0.23	2.7	73
Elderly		
0.18	3.7	58

4. Neuromuscular blockade
   (a) ED_{95} = 0.05 mg/kg
   (b) Potency
      (1) Similar to pancuronium
      (2) Some 4.4 times as potent as atracurium
   (c) Onset: with a single dose 0.05 mg/kg (one times ED_{95}), maximum blockade develops in 5–6 minutes
   (d) Intubating conditions: after 0.1 mg/kg, good intubating conditions exist in 90 seconds
   (e) Duration of action
      (1) At a dose of one times ED_{95}, vecuronium lasts 20 minutes
      (2) At three times ED_{95}, vecuronium lasts 53 minutes
   (f) Accumulation does not occur
   (g) Recovery can be accelerated with the use of anticholinesterases
5. Cardiovascular effects: no action at autonomic ganglia or the sympathetic nervous system

III. Nondepolarizing muscle relaxants; k. Vecuronium (continued)

    6. Histamine release

        (a) No increase in plasma histamine levels at doses up to 0.2 mg/kg

        (b) Anaphylactoid reactions can occur

    7. Intracranial and intraocular pressure: no effect

    8. Effect of age

        (a) Onset of action is more rapid in infants than in children

        (b) Onset of action is more rapid in children than in adults

    9. Use in obstetrics

        (a) Maintain surgical relaxation following intubation facilitated with succinylcholine

        (b) Crosses the placenta but fetal levels of the drug have no clinical significance

    10. Modes of administration

        (a) Intubation: two to three times ED_{95}, 0.1–0.15 mg/kg

        (b) Maintenance: 0.01–0.02 mg/kg to maintain relaxation

        (c) Infusion

            (1) 1 µg/kg/min will result in 50% blockade of receptors

            (2) 1–1.7 µg/kg/min causes 90% blockade

---

l. ANQ 9040

    1. Experimental nondepolarizing muscle relaxant, steroidal class

    2. Preclinical investigations in animals

        (a) Onset of action at least as fast as that of succinylcholine

        (b) Short duration of action

        (c) Cardiovascular effects primarily vagolytic

    3. In human studies

        (a) Twice the ED_{95} dose is associated with significant histamine release and tachycardia

        (b) Indicates an inadequate safety margin for clinical practice

---

m. ORG 9487

    1. New steroidal nondepolarizing muscle relaxant

    2. 16-*N*-allyl-17-*b*-propionate analogue of vecuronium

    3. Rapid onset

        (a) 1.5 mg/kg

            (1) Time to maximum block is 67 seconds

(2) Intubating conditions at 1 minute similar to those seen following the administration of succinylcholine, 1 mg/kg

4. Recovery

(a) Complete spontaneous recovery occurs in 24 minutes
(b) May be accelerated with the use of anticholinesterases

5. Low potency: ED_{95} is 1.15 mg/kg

6. Metabolism: thought to be via the liver; renal excretion appears to be of minor importance

7. Cardiovascular effects: no information available

n. 51W89

1. Chemistry: 51W89 is one of the stereoisomers of atracurium

2. Potency

(a) Approximately three to four times more potent than atracurium in humans
(b) Has weaker side effects
(c) ED_{95}: 0.05 mg/kg

3. Dosage

(a) Intubating: 0.15–0.2 mg/kg has a duration of action of 40–75 minutes
(b) Maintenance: 0.01–0.02 mg/kg gives a further 15–20 minutes of relaxation
(c) Infusion rate: 1–2 mg/kg/min

4. Metabolism and elimination: undergoes Hofmann degradation

5. Histamine release: does not affect plasma histamine concentrations in doses as high as eight times the ED_{95}

6. Not yet available for clinical use

IV. DEPOLARIZING MUSCLE RELAXANTS

a. Characteristics

1. Imitate the action of acetylcholineDepolarizing muscle relaxants

2. Bind to and stimulate the postsynaptic receptor

3. Cause depolarization of the postsynaptic membrane

4. Depolarization

(a) Lasts longer than that produced by acetylcholine
(b) Maintained and repolarization prevented

IV. Depolarizing muscle relaxants (continued)

b. Succinylcholine (Anectine)

$$
\begin{array}{l}
O \\
\| \\
COCH_2CH_2N^+(CH_3)_3 \\
| \\
(CH_2)_2 \qquad\qquad \text{SUCCINYLCHOLINE} \\
| \\
COCH_2CH_2N^+(CH_3)_3 \\
\| \\
O
\end{array}
$$

1. Chemistry
    (a) Dicholine ester of succinic acid
    (b) Active part of the molecule is the cation
    (c) Unstable when mixed with alkalis
2. Metabolism
    (a) Undergoes rapid hydrolysis by pseudocholinesterase, an enzyme of the liver and plasma
        (1) Step 1 (rate-limiting step)

        Pseudocholinesterase
        Succinylcholine → Succinylmonocholine + Choline

        (2) Step 2

        Pseudocholinesterase

        Succinylmonocholine → Succinic acid + Choline
        Specific liver esterase

    (b) Pseudocholinesterase
        (1) Enormous capacity to hydrolyze succinylcholine
        (2) Very small fraction of initial IV dose actually reaches the neuromuscular junction
        (3) Prolonged by a reduced quantity of normal enzyme or by an atypical form of pseudocholinesterase
        (4) Factors that lower cholinesterase levels
            [a] Inherited: cholinesterase variants
            [b] Acquired: hepatic disease, uremia, malnutrition, carcinoma, acute infection, burns
            [c] Iatrogenic: plasmapheresis, extracorporeal circulation
            [d] Medications: anticholinergic drugs, alkylating antineoplastic drugs, oral contraceptive pill, echothiphate, esmolol, propranolol, monoamine oxidase inhibitors, and pancuronium
        (5) Atypical cholinesterase
            [a] Low affinity for succinylcholine
            [b] Does not bind to succinylcholine in the pharmacologic range
            [c] Nerve end plate receives a 50–100-fold overdose of succinylcholine
    (c) Cholinesterase
        (1) Has no effect on succinylcholine once the drug is at the nerve end plate
        (2) Commercially purified, concentrated cholinesterase
            [a] Used to treat succinylcholine apnea
            [b] Has been extensively tested in Denmark
            [c] Although this treatment is effective, it is not recommended for routine use
            [d] Injected cholinesterase only works if it is given at the right time
            [e] Given late, it has little or no effect
            [f] Expensive

> [g] Risk of infection from a human blood product

(d) Genetic variants of pseudocholinesterase

	Abbreviation	Dibucaine No.	Incidence
Normal activity			
Usual	UU	70–85	96.2%
Reduced activity			
Atypical	AA	16–25	1/3,000
Silent-1	SS		
Fluoride	FF		
Quantitative variant J	JJ		1/150,000
Quantitative variant K	KK		1%
Quantitative variant H	HH	Found in two families	
Newfoundland		Found in one family in Newfoundland	
		High % inhibition by dibucaine	
Increased activity			
C5 +: associated with up to 30% increased activity			
Incidence: approximately 40,000 people have been tested			
Present in 9% of Europeans			
3% of Asians			
5% of Africans			
7% of Americans			
Cynthiana variant: increased activity; increased amount of cholinesterase protein			
Johannesburg: twice the normal activity; normal number of enzymes			

Only one gene for human cholinesterase (long arm, chromosome 3)
Homozygotes—UU, AA, SS, FF, KK, JJ, HH
Heterozygotes—e.g., UA for usual-atypical, etc.
Silent (called Silent-1)—anticipated that additional silent variants will be identified

(e) Dibucaine number: percentage inhibition of plasma cholinesterase activity by dibucaine (Cinchocaine) under standardized conditions

3. Cardiovascular effects

(a) Stimulates all cholinergic autonomic receptors
(b) Bradycardia, junctional arrhythmias, and even cardiac arrest have been reported
(c) Sinus bradycardia occurs particularly in nonatropinized, sympathatonic patients, especially children
(d) In adults, appears more commonly after a second dose
(e) May be prevented by thiopental, atropine, ganglion blockers
(f) Nodal (junctional) rhythms commonly occur, probably due to emergence of the A-V node as the pacemaker
(g) Ventricular arrhythmias
  (1) Threshold of the ventricle lowered to catecholamine-induced arrhythmias
  (2) May be enhanced by endotracheal intubation, hypoxia, hypercarbia, surgical stimulation

4. Histamine release

(a) Antigenic group lies in the quaternary ammonium group
(b) True anaphylaxis can occur

5. Hyperkalemia

(a) Plasma potassium level rises by approximately 0.7 mmol/L in the normal patient
(b) May be greatly increased in the following conditions
  (1) Burns
    [a] May increase to levels as high as 13 mEq/L
    [b] Susceptibility to hyperkalemia exists only between days 10 and 60 postburn
    [c] Is dose related
    [d] Varies with the extent of the burn

IV. Depolarizing muscle relaxants; b. Succinylcholine (continued)

    (2) When infection is present, the time period for development of hyperkalemia may be extended

    (3) Trauma

        [a] Potassium levels may be increased from about 1 week to 60 days postinjury

        [b] Until adequate healing of damaged muscle has occurred

    (4) Nerve damage/neuromuscular disease

        [a] Susceptible patients—patients with hemiplegia, paraplegia, or progressive disease, such as muscular dystrophy

        [b] Vulnerable period: within the first 6 months following the onset of hemiplegia/paraplegia and in a longer period in patients with progressive disease

        [c] Degree of hyperkalemia is associated with the degree and extent of muscle affected

    (5) Intra-abdominal sepsis

        [a] Kohlschutter et al. found that four of nine patients with intra-abdominal sepsis had an increase in plasma potassium following succinylcholine

        [b] May be due to generalized muscle wasting from prolonged bed rest and immobility as opposed to a direct effect of sepsis

6. Muscle pains

    (a) Incidence: 0.2–89%

    (b) Occur in young, healthy patients (mainly females) who mobilize early on the day of surgery

    (c) Site: shoulder girdle, rib cage, and neck

    (d) Postulated mechanism: due to fasciculations

    (e) Attenuated by pretreatment with a small dose of nondepolarizing muscle relaxant

7. Intraocular pressure

    (a) Increased; manifested 1 minute after injection

    (b) Peaks between the second and fourth minute

    (c) Subsides by the sixth minute

    (d) Mechanism unclear, involves contraction of tonic myofibrils

    (e) Recommended that succinylcholine be avoided in penetrating eye injuries

    (f) Attenuated by calcium channel blockers, nondepolarizing muscle relaxants

8. Intragastric pressure

    (a) Increased, related to the intensity of fasciculations

    (b) May also be a reactive increase in esophageal pressure above the sphincter

    (c) Thus, no net decrease in pressure across the sphincter

9. Intracranial pressure

    (a) Increased

    (b) Mechanism and clinical significance of transient increase unknown

10. Malignant hyperthermia

    (a) One of the drugs most commonly implicated in triggering malignant hyperthermia

    (b) Incidence: 1:100,000 anesthetics

11. Mode of administration

    (a) IV: 1 mg/kg

    (b) IM

        (1) 2 mg/kg in adults

        (2) 1.5 mg/kg IV in children

12. Characteristics

    (a) Good intubating conditions after 60 seconds

    (b) Depolarizing block lasts approximately 5–10 minutes

    (c) Full recovery is complete after 12–15 minutes

c. Decamethonium

1. Chemistry

    (a) *Bis*-methylammonium decane dihalide

    (b) Little used today because tachyphylaxis and a phase II block readily occur

    (c) Soluble in water

    (d) Neutral in solution

    (e) Stable

    (f) Resistant to heat

    (g) Nonirritant to tissues

2. Pharmacology

    (a) Causes depolarization of postjunctional membrane of the motor end plate in skeletal muscles

    (b) May cause fasciculations

    (c) Not antagonized by anticholinesterases

    (d) Repeated use may lead to nondepolarizing block, which can be reversed by anticholinesterases

    (e) Side effects are minimal

    (f) Excreted by the kidneys

3. Dosage

    (a) 3–10 mg/kg in adults

    (b) Duration of effect is approximately 15–30 minutes

d. Dantrolene

DANTROLENE

1. Characteristics

    (a) Lipid-soluble hydantoin

    (b) Introduced as a skeletal muscle relaxant for use in chronic disorders of muscle spasticity, e.g., spinal cord injury, stroke, cerebral palsy

    (c) Also used in the management of malignant hyperthermia

    (d) Poorly soluble in water

    (e) Supplied in ampules

        (1) 20 mg of lyophilized dantrolene sodium (powder)

        (2) Mannitol 3 g (to improve solubility)

        (3) Sodium hydroxide to give a solution of pH 9.5 when the contents are dissolved in 6 ml of water

        (4) Final concentration of the parenteral preparation is 0.33 mg/ml

    (f) Azumolene

        (1) New investigational dantrolene analogue

        (2) Antagonizes halothane and caffeine contracture

        (3) Has greater water solubility than dantrolene

2. Mechanism of action

    (a) Inhibits SR calcium release without affecting reuptake

IV. Depolarizing muscle relaxants; d. Dantrolene (continued)

- (b) May interact at the level of the DHP receptor and block electrical transmission to the ryanodine receptor
- (c) Dantrolene also has effects on heart muscle, as well as on skeletal muscle

3. Pharmacokinetics
   - (a) Oral administration
     - (1) 20% of the dose is absorbed
     - (2) Peak plasma levels occur in about 6 hours
   - (b) Metabolism
     - (1) Liver microsomal oxidase system
     - (2) Oxidative and reductive pathways

4. Suggested dosage and administration
   - (a) During a crisis
     - (1) Initial dose of 2.4 mg/kg
     - (2) May be repeated at 15-minute intervals until clinical improvement is seen or to a total dose of 10 mg/kg
     - (3) Second dose of 2.4 mg/kg 12 hours after the first dose as malignant hyperthermia may recur in the postoperative period
   - (b) Preanesthetic medication to malignant hyperthermia–susceptible individuals
     - (1) Controversial
     - (2) Preoperative oral administration is no longer advocated
     - (3) If dantrolene is to be given to prevent the occurrence of malignant hyperthermia, it should be given in a dose of 2.4 mg/kg IV during induction of anesthesia

5. Toxicity and precautions
   - (a) May cause dizziness, dysarthria, lightheadedness, and drowsiness
   - (b) Hepatic dysfunction has been reported after chronic oral therapy
   - (c) May induce pronounced prolonged weakness in myopathic patients
   - (d) Dantrolene causes serum potassium elevation

V. REVERSAL OF NEUROMUSCULAR BLOCKADE

a. Anticholinesterase pharmacology

NEOSTIGMINE

EDROPHONIUM

PYRIDOSTIGMINE

1. Mechanism of action
   - (a) Neostigmine, pyridostigmine, and edrophonium inhibit acetylcholinesterase
   - (b) Neostigmine and pyridostigmine are hydrolyzed by acetylcholinesterase

(1) Hydrolytic process

(2) Carbamylated enzyme is produced, which is not capable of further action

(c) Acetylcholinesterase does not break down edrophonium

(1) Interaction is competitive and reversible

(2) Different mechanisms of action have little significance in clinical practice

(d) Neostigmine block

(1) Massive doses of anticholinesterases produce a form of neuromuscular blockade

(2) Mechanism of foregoing is uncertain

(3) Theory: an excess of acetylcholine, produced by acetylcholinesterase inhibition at the neuromuscular junction, causes desensitization

2. Pharmacokinetics

Distribution Volume (L/kg)	Plasma Clearance (ml/kg/min)	Elimination Half-life $T_{1/2}\beta$ (minutes)
1) 0.7	9.2	77
2) 1.6	7.8	181
3) 1.1	9.6	110
4) 0.7	2.7	206
5) 1.1	8.6	112
6) 1.0	2.1	379

1) Neostigmine in normal patients
2) Neostigmine in renal failure patients
3) Edrophonium in normal patients
4) Edrophonium in renal failure patients
5) Pyridostigmine in normal patients
6) Pyridostigmine in renal failure patients

3. Onset of action

(a) Edrophonium—1–2 minutes

(b) Neostigmine—7–11 minutes

(c) Pyridostigmine—16 minutes

4. Duration of action

(a) Constant infusion

(1) 90% block

(2) Equipotent doses of neostigmine, edrophonium, and pyridostigmine

(3) Effect of 1–2 hours, with no clinically important differences among them

5. Dose

(a) Neostigmine: 0.03–0.07 mg/kg

(b) Edrophonium: 0.5–1 mg/kg

(c) Pyridostigmine: 0.21 mg/kg

6. Suggested choice of reversal agent

TOF count < 2	Neostigmine	0.07 mg/kg
TOF count 3	Edrophonium	1 mg/kg
TOF count 4 + fade	Edrophonium	0.5 mg/kg
TOF count 4 − fade	Edrophonium	0.25 mg/kg

7. Complications of reversal agents

(a) Neuromuscular block

(1) Neuromuscular weakness in patients with myasthenia gravis when the administered dose is too high

(2) Relatively high doses of neostigmine are administered in the presence of little residual nondepolarizing block; tetanic fade is sometimes seen

V. Depolarizing muscle relaxants; a. Anticholinesterase pharmacology (continued)

    (b) Cardiovascular effects
        (1) Vagal effects
            [a] Bradyarrhythmias
            [b] Attenuated by anticholinergic drugs
    (c) Alimentary effects
        (1) Increased salivation
        (2) May be blocked by atropine
        (3) Increased bowel motility (? blocked by atropine)
        (4) Combination of atropine and neostigmine
            [a] Decreases cardiac sphincter pressure
            [b] Greater incidence of postoperative vomiting
    (d) Respiratory effects
        (1) Increased airway resistance due to bronchoconstriction
        (2) Anticholinergics tend to reduce this effect
    (e) Use of anticholinesterases in special situations
        (1) Renal failure
            [a] Clearance of anticholinesterases is reduced to a greater extent than with most muscle relaxants
            [b] Rate and extent of recovery from nondepolarizing blockade after administration of anticholinesterases are not impaired in renal failure
            [c] Accumulation does not occur
        (2) Myasthenia gravis
            [a] All of the anticholinesterase have been used to successfully reverse neuromuscular block in myasthenia gravis
            [b] Goal is to achieve adequate reversal of blockade while avoiding a cholinergic crisis
            [c] Atracurium may be the preferred muscle relaxant

---

b. Anticholinergic drugs

    1. Structure

ATROPINE

GLYCOPYRROLATE

    2. Characteristics
        (a) Block muscarinic receptors
        (b) Have no activity at nicotinic receptors
        (c) Given to prevent the cardiovascular changes brought about by the administration of anticholinesterases

    3. Atropine

        (a) Rapid onset of action, approximately 1 minute

    (b) Duration of action: 30–60 minutes
    (c) Crosses the blood–brain barrier
    (d) Associated with an increased incidence of memory deficit following anesthesia as
         compared with glycopyrrolate
    (e) Dose
         (1) 20 μg/kg with neostigmine or pyridostigmine
         (2) 10–15 μg/kg with edrophonium
  4. Glycopyrrolate
    (a) Slower onset of action, approximately 2–3 minutes
    (b) Duration of action: 30–60 minutes
    (c) Does not cross the blood–brain barrier
    (d) Dose: 8 μg/kg

VI. NEUROMUSCULAR BLOCKADE MONITORING

a. Types of monitoring

  1. Clinical
    (a) During anesthesia
         (1) Spontaneous movement
         (2) Triggering of the ventilator
         (3) Change in inflation pressures
         (4) Paradoxical respirations
         (5) "Tight" abdomen—reported by the surgeon
    (b) Patients recovering from anesthesia
         (1) Head lift for 5 seconds (most sensitive)
         (2) Tongue protrusion
         (3) Eye opening
         (4) Hand grip
         (5) Ability to lift the leg off the bed
  2. Evoked responses: a peripheral nerve is stimulated and a muscle response is quantified
  3. Applications
    (a) Characteristics
         (1) Simple, clinical perioperatively
         (2) Long-term paralysis in the ICU, extended perioperatively
         (3) Closed-loop systems for relaxant administration
         (4) Research into neuromuscular physiology and pharmacology
    (b) Stimulus
         (1) Square waveform of shorter duration than the refractory period of the
              neuromuscular junction
         (2) 0.1–0.3 ms
    (c) Current
         (1) Supramaximal current should be used
         (2) That is, that current above which no further increase in response is seen
              = 2.75 times the current that first produced an identifiable twitch in that
              particular patient
         (3) Usually in the range of 15 to 40 mA
    (d) Stimulus/patient interface
         (1) Rounded tip or ball electrodes—protrude from most hand-held stimulators
         (2) Applied to the skin
         (3) Position of the electrodes over the nerve is critical
         (4) Needle electrodes

VI. Depolarizing muscle relaxants; a. Types of monitoring (continued)

             [a] May be placed subcutaneously
             [b] Current required for supramaximal stimulation is reduced
             [c] Use may be associated with infection, broken needles, or intraneural placement
             [d] May be useful in obese patient
        (5) Surface pregelled, self-adhesive electrodes commonly used
    (e) Site of stimulus
        (1) Any accessible nerve
        (2) Ulnar nerve
             [a] Most commonly used
             [b] At the wrist
             [c] Superficial, accessible
             [d] Easy to stimulate
             [e] Always supplies adductor pollicis muscle
             [f] Muscle response is easily visible
        (3) Facial nerve
             [a] Electrodes may be placed over the main trunk of the facial nerve or one of its major branches
             [b] Usually the temporal branch supplying orbicularis oculi and frontalis muscle
             [c] Response—movement of the eyebrow and around the mouth
        (4) Posterior tibial nerve
             [a] Electrodes are placed over the course of the nerve posteriorly to the medial malleolus
             [b] Muscle response is from flexor hallucis brevis and abductor hallucis
    (f) Electrode polarity
        (1) Electrode placed over the nerve is termed the active electrode
        (2) Electrode distant to the nerve is termed inactive or indifferent
        (3) Greater twitch results if the negative electrode (cathode) is used over the ulnar nerve at the wrist, provided that the inactive electrode is placed at some distance from the nerve
        (4) Alterations in polarity produce no change in twitch response if both electrodes are placed within a few centimeters of each other along the nerve

---

b. Nerve stimulators

    1. Ideal characteristics of nerve stimulators

        (a) Constant-current design
        (b) Adjustable currents up to 70–80 mA
        (c) Square-wave stimulus, duration 0.1–0.3 ms
        (d) Stimulator/patient interface by fixed rounded-tip electrodes and availability of sockets for leads to surface electrodes
        (e) Polarity of electrodes marked
        (f) Display of current passing
        (g) Stimulation at 1 Hz, 50 Hz, train-of-four
        (h) Repeated stimulation possible at preset intervals
        (i) Visual (and audible, if desired) alert at time of stimulation
        (j) Robust, inexpensive
        (k) Battery operated with low battery alert
        (l) Conform to recommended safety standards

    2. Pattern of stimulation

        (a) Single twitch

        (1) Frequency of 1 Hz or 0.1 Hz
        (2) Duration of less than 0.2 ms
        (3) Current over 50 mA
        (4) Transmission failure commences when 70% of receptors are occupied with relaxant and will be completed when 90% are occupied

   (b) Train-of-four stimulation (TOF)
        (1) 2 Hz for 2 seconds every 10–12 seconds
        (2) Train-of-four count
           [a] Counting the number of responses to TOF stimulation
           [b] Correlates well with first twitch height
        (3) TOF ratio
           [a] The ratio of the magnitude of the fourth to the first response
           [b] Does not require preparalysis train
           [c] Impossible to determine by visual or tactile evaluation of thumb movement
           [d] Ratio of 0.6–0.7 is consistent with recovery of respiratory and airway musculature to safe levels

   (c) Tetanus
        (1) High-frequency stimulation, at 50 Hz, 100 Hz, and 200 Hz
        (2) Usually applied for 5 seconds
        (3) Sustained tetanus for 5 seconds correlates with a TOF ratio greater than 0.7

   (d) Posttetanic facilitation
        (1) With dense neuromuscular block, there is no response to single stimuli, TOF, tetanic stimulation
        (2) Posttetanic facilitated count (PTC)
           [a] Stimulation at 1 Hz for 1 minute
           [b] 50-Hz tetanus is applied for 5 seconds
           [c] An interval of 3 seconds
           [d] Stimulation at 1 Hz
           [e] A count is made of the number of single twitches elicited
           [f] For each relaxant, a correlation exists between the posttetanic count and the time before the first response of the TOF reappears

   (e) Double-burst stimulation
        (1) Two short trains (three stimuli each train at 50 Hz)
        (2) An interval of 750 ms
        (3) Enables fade to be detected more easily
        (4) The two responses of the double-burst stimulation do not appear to be equal until the measured TOF ratio is 0.5–0.7

3. Recording of the response
   (a) Response to nerve stimulation is a muscle response
   (b) The magnitude of the response is an indication of the degree of blockade
   (c) There are six ways in which the muscle response may be determined
        (1) Visual observation
           [a] Inaccurate
           [b] In clinical practice, the presence or absence of a response can be seen easily, the number of PTC or TOF responses determined, and appropriate changes made
        (2) Tactile assessment
           [a] Of the force of contraction
           [b] Gives more reliable information
           [c] Should always be used in preference to visual observation when knowledge of the force of contraction is required
        (3) Visual observation of the preloaded thumb

VI. Depolarizing muscle relaxants; b. Nerve stimulators (continued)

[a] Reliability of visual observation can be enhanced by attaching a spring with a compliance of 400 g/cm to the thumb, producing an abducting load

(4) Mechanomyography

[a] This is undertaken when the force of contraction is measured with a force displacement transducer

[b] Transducer should

i) Measure isometric force in the correct vector

ii) Give a linear output over the range of forces encountered (2 kgf and 7 kgf for single twitch and tetanus)

iii) Hold the thumb in a constant position relative to the hand with a constant and known degree of preload (200–400 g)

[c] Advantages

i) Measures the required parameter, i.e., force of contraction

ii) Calibration, determination of recording system, and linearity are easily accomplished

[d] Disadvantages

i) Hand and thumb immobilization may be difficult

ii) The system is susceptible to physical knocking

iii) Constancy of preload is vital

iv) Systems are generally only suitable for the thumb

v) Adaptations are possible

4. Electromyography

(a) Characteristics

(1) Measures the compound muscle action potential in response to nerve stimulation

(2) Uses needle or surface electrodes

(3) Stimulation—peak voltage 0.5–0.7 mV

(4) Duration of action potential: 20 ms

(5) Recording system must possess a fast response time

(6) By direct measurement of the height of the action potential, changes in the electromyograph can be quantified

(7) Developments using computer technology led to the production of the Relaxograph and other systems

[a] Incorporates stimulator unit, patient leads, analysis of the waveform by integration, digital display of T1: control and the TOF ratio, and a printer

(b) Advantages of electromyography

(1) Possible to record from otherwise inaccessible muscles

(2) Less dependent on accurate fixation of preload

(3) Less susceptible to knocking

(c) Disadvantages of electromyography

(1) Difficulties in production and analysis of waveform

(2) Difficulties in interpretation of the relationship between the electromyograph and the mechanomyograph

(3) Some studies suggest that a drug-specific electromyograph/mechanomyograph correlation may exist

5. Accelerography

(a) Quantifies the degree of neuromuscular blockade by measurement of the acceleration of a digit in response to nerve stimulation

(b) Force = mass × acceleration; thus, the force of contraction will be directly

proportional to the magnitude of acceleration, provided that the effective mass of the thumb remains constant
- (c) Consists of an acceleration transducer with stimulating and computing units
    - (1) Acceleration transducer is small (0.5 by 1 cm)
    - (2) Consists of a piezoelectric ceramic wafer with an electrode on each side
    - (3) Voltage difference develops between these electrodes when the transducer experiences acceleration
    - (4) Voltage of the initial positive deflection, approximately 20 mV, is a measure of the maximal acceleration
- (d) Output currents of 60 mA will be maintained with skin resistances up to 5 kΩ
- (e) In addition to 1 Hz and TOF patterns of stimulation, posttetanic counts are possible
- (f) A printer may be attached for a permanent record

G. IMMUNOSUPPRESSIVES AND ANTIREJECTION DRUGS

I. INTRODUCTION

a. **Used to control the rejection reaction resulting from antigenic differences remaining after**

   1. Tissue typing
   2. Donor–recipient matching

b. **Primarily responsible for clinical transplantation success**

c. **Nonspecific (making overwhelming infection the leading cause of death in transplant recipients)**

d. **Intensive immunosuppression is required for first few weeks posttransplant or with rejection crisis**

e. **Maintenance**

   1. Relatively small doses
   2. Decreased side effects (graft may become accommodated)
   3. Rarely can be stopped completely

II. CYCLOSPORIN

a. **Fungal metabolite**

b. **More selectively inhibits T-cell proliferation/activation**

c. **Molecular mechanism is unknown (helper-cell activity is inhibited, suppressor is not)**

d. **Usually used in combination with other drugs (steroids)**

e. **Dose**

   1. Transplant: 6–12 mg/kg/day orally
   2. Maintenance: 3–5 mg/kg/day orally
   3. Effective therapeutic dose undetermined

f. Toxicity

1. Nephrotoxicity with irreversible failure
2. Hepatotoxicity
3. Refractory hypertension
4. Increased neoplasms
   (a) B-cell lymphomas
   (b) EBV activation at higher doses

III. STEROIDS

a. Prednisone (oral)/methylprednisolone (IV)

b. Dose

1. Transplant: 2–20 mg/kg
2. Maintenance: 0.2 mg/kg/day indefinitely
3. Late after transplant: dose on alternate days to reduce side effects

c. Allograft rejection: dose is sharply increased

d. Adrenal suppression during stress

IV. CYTOTOXICS

a. Used in treatment of neoplastic disease not amenable to surgery/local radiation

b. 75% of cases receive chemotherapy at some point

c. Cure achieved in small fraction

d. Palliation/regression occurs in most cases

e. Indications

1. Disseminated disease
2. Surgical supplement

f. Response determined by number of cells in replicative cycle

g. Classification

1. Antimetabolites
2. Antibiotics

3. Alkylating agents

4. Mitotic spindle poisons

5. Hormones

6. Other

V. DOXORUBICIN (ADRIAMYCIN)

a. Anthracycline antibiotic (blocks RNA, DNA synthesis)

b. Mechanism

1. Reduction by cytochrome p450 reductase

2. Produces superoxide activity and hydrogen peroxide accumulation (DNA strand breaks)

3. Cardiotoxicity from low superoxide dismutase activity and lack of catalase in cardiac tissue

4. Tumors are low in superoxide dismutase activity

c. Therapeutic applications

1. Carcinomas (breast and lung cancer)

2. Sarcomas

3. Acute lymphocytic leukemia

4. Hodgkin's disease

d. Absorption and distribution

1. Must be given IV

2. Extravasation causes tissue necrosis

3. Does not penetrate the CNS

e. Metabolism

1. Products are also cytotoxic

2. Liver (bile) major route of excretion

3. Modify dose for patients with impaired liver function

4. Some kidney excretion

5. No modification for renal failure

6. Gives urine a red color

f. Adverse effects

1. Irreversible

2. Dose-dependent cardiotoxicity

3. Increased with irradiation of thorax

4. Alopecia

5. Transient bone marrow suppression
6. Stomatitis
7. GI disturbances

VI. BLEOMYCIN

a. Mixture of different copper chelating glycopeptides

b. Mechanism

1. Causes strand breaks of DNA by oxidation involving superoxide/hydroxide radicals
2. Cell-cycle specific (cells accumulate in phase G2)

c. Therapeutic applications

1. Testicular tumors (with vinblastine)
2. Response rate 90% (higher if cisplatin is added)
3. Effective, not curative, for squamous cell carcinomas and lymphomas

d. Absorption and distribution

1. Effective SC, IM, IV, and intracavitary
2. Localized in epithelial organs (skin, lung, peritoneum, and lymphatics)

e. Metabolism

1. Most is excreted unchanged by glomerular filtration
2. Modify dose in renal failure

f. Adverse effects

1. Pulmonary toxicity (progresses from cough, coarse crackles, and infiltrate to potentially fatal fibrosis)
2. Anaphylactoid reactions
3. Fever
4. Hypertrophic skin changes
5. Hyperpigmentation of the hands

H. DRUG REACTIONS: HYPERSENSITIVITY/ALLERGY

I. DRUG REACTIONS

a. Exaggerated immune response

b. Antibody production

1. First contact with antigen
2. Antigen sensitizes
3. Antibody production
4. Subsequent contact elicits the allergy response

c. Types of reactions

1. Type I
   (a) Anaphylaxis
   (b) IgE mediated
2. Type II
   (a) Cytotoxic
   (b) Cell lysis
       (1) Antibody attached to AG
       (2) Complement-activated cell lysis
   (c) Example: ABO, Rh reactions
3. Type III
   (a) Immune complex
   (b) Antigen—antibody deposits in tissues
   (c) Example: autoimmune diseases, serum sickness, Arthus reactions
4. Type IV
   (a) Delayed—cell mediated
   (b) Antigen sensitizes T lymphocytes
   (c) Example: tuberculin or contact hypersensitivity

II. ANAPHYLAXIS

a. Definition

1. Life-threatening reaction
2. Occurs in 1:3,500–7,000 anesthetics
3. 90% of these reactions occur within 5–10 minutes after administration

b. Mechanism

1. Antigen-induced formation of IgE antibodies
2. IgE antibodies bind to basophils and mast cells
3. Reexposure induces degranulation and release of pharmacologically active mediators

c. Types of mediators

1. Histamine

   (a) Mucus secretions, increase of vasopermeability
   (b) CVS
       (1) HR increase/chronotropic effect
       (2) Antidromic effect
       (3) Increase of fibrillation threshold
       (4) Decrease of SVR as much as 80% mediated directly through H receptors
   (c) Bronchoconstriction

2. Prostaglandins

   (a) Bronchoconstriction
   (b) Vasodilation
   (c) Increased capillary permeability

3. Leukotrienes

   (a) Bronchoconstriction
   (b) Increased capillary permeability
   (c) Negative inotropy
   (d) Coronary artery constriction

4. Eosinophil and neutrophil chemotactic factor

5. Platelet activating factor

6. Serotonin—minor impact

d. Clinical manifestations of anaphylaxis

1. CVS

   (a) Cardiovascular collapse (68%)—hypotension, arrhythmias, cardiac arrest (11%)
   (b) Often sudden
   (c) Follow drug administration and cannot be explained otherwise

2. Respiration

   (a) Bronchoconstriction (only 25%)
   (b) Increased peak airway pressure
   (c) Cyanosis
   (d) Laryngeal edema
   (e) Dyspnea

3. Skin

   (a) Widespread flush (50%)
   (b) Edema
   (c) Urticaria

4. Other emergencies in anesthetized patient

   (a) Myocardial infarction
   (b) Pulmonary embolism
   (c) Edema
   (d) Aspiration

e. Diagnosis

1. Detailed history and drug administration sequence

2. In vitro tests = skin tests

3. In vitro

II. Anaphylaxis; e. Diagnosis (continued)

     (a) RAST (radioallergosorbent test) and ELISA
         (1) Commercially available antigens
         (2) Combine with antibodies in patient plasma
         (3) Specific antibody testing
     (b) Total serum IgE
     (c) Plasma histamine level
         (1) Normal under 1 ng/ml
         (2) Significant when greater than 2 ng/ml EDTA tube
         (3) Short plasmatic half-life

f. Treatment

1. Stop drug administration

2. Airway maintenance, 100% oxygen

3. Epinephrine if hypotension

     (a) Start with 0.1-mg bolus
     (b) Set up for infusion
     (c) Double dose can be given intratracheally in l cc of hypotonic solution

4. Volume expansion—2–4 liters initially

5. Other

     (a) Steroids will only act several hours after administration
         (1) Hydrocortisone, 5 mg/kg
         (2) Prednisone, 1 mg/kg
     (b) Aminophylline
         (1) Bolus: 5–6 mg/kg
         (2) Infusion up to 0.9 mg/kg/hr
     (c) H_1 and H_2 blockers IV
     (d) $NaHCO_3$ according to ABG
     (e) Hemodynamic monitoring
     (f) Patient observation for 24 hours

g. Prophylaxis

1. Careful history, observation of the patient after each drug administration

2. Alter speed of administration of drugs with allergic potential

3. Prefer drugs causing minimal or no histamine liberation

4. Caution in atopic patients and multidrug allergy individuals

5. Obtain immunologic consultation if necessary

6. Pharmacologic prevention unreliable

     (a) $H_{1,2}$ antagonists taken the night before and the morning of exposure
     (b) Prednisone, 1 mg/kg every 6 hours for four doses

III. ANAPHYLACTOID REACTION

a. Non-IgE mediated, clear mechanism uncertain

b. Clinically similar to anaphylactic reaction

1. Drug directly induced release of mediators by mast cells and basophils
2. Iodinated contract media, morphine, atracurium, tubocurarine

IV. CLINICALLY IMPORTANT REACTIONS

a. Thiopental

1. Can cause anaphylactic (1:30,000) or anaphylactoid reaction
2. Skin tests available

b. Propofol—life-threatening reactions after first exposure or reexposure

c. Muscle relaxants

1. Most frequent cause of allergic reaction in preoperative period
2. Anaphylactic reaction by IgE mechanism

   (a) Directed against the quartenary or tertiary ammonium ion of muscle relaxants
   (b) The ammonium groups are present in cosmetics, disinfectants, soaps
   (c) Can cause cross-sensitivity

3. Some relaxants can cause direct histamine release

   (a) Usually mild and brief hemodynamic and skin manifestations
   (b) Amount of histamine depends on the speed of injection of a total dose
   (c) DTC, metocurine, atracurium, succinylcholine

d. Narcotics

1. Most reactions are self-limiting
2. Cutaneous or mild hypotension
3. Caused by nonimmunologically mediated histamine release

e. Local anesthetics

1. True allergic reactions

   (a) Very rare
   (b) Lower incidence in amides (bupivacaine and lidocaine)

2. Ester-allergic patients

   (a) Preparations should be preservative-free
   (b) Ester-based parabens used as preservatives

3. Skin test available if history is positive

f. Protamine

1. True allergy

   (a) Patients with fish allergies

IV. Drug reactions: hypersensitivity/allergy; f. Protamine (continued)

      (b) Diabetic on insulin-containing protamine

      (c) Vasectomy patients and those with previous exposure

  2. Other reactions

      (a) Hypotension from rapid injection—predictable

      (b) Catastrophic pulmonary vasoconstriction—rare

g. Latex/natural rubber

1. Up to 70% of operating room staff

2. 40% of spina bifida patients (frequent bladder catheter exposure)

3. Especially if in contact with mucosa membranes

4. Cause IgE antibodies synthesis

5. RAST test available

6. Clinical manifestation often severe (delayed, unexplained hypotension during general anesthesia)

7. Polyvinyl or polyethylene gloves are available for health-care personnel

8. Avoid contact with IV tubing, catheters, etc. containing latex

h. Antibiotics

1. Penicillin—most common (90%) medication causing allergic reaction

      (a) Up to 8% of patients treated will experience allergic reaction

      (b) Mortality 1:100,000 cases treated with PNC

      (c) Threefold to fourfold risk of experiencing an allergic reaction to other drugs

      (d) Should not receive penicillin or cephalosporin

2. Vancomycin

      (a) Direct myocardial depression

      (b) Nonimmunologically mediated histamine release causing hypotension if infused rapidly

      (c) "Red man's syndrome"—erythematous discoloration of upper body

3. Radiocontrast media

      (a) Severe anaphylactoid reactions occur in 2% of patients

      (b) Fatal reactions in 1:50,000 administrations

      (c) 500 deaths a year

      (d) Previous reaction: increased risk on reexposure

      (e) Reaction might be decreased by pretreatment

          (1) $H_{1,2}$ antagonists

          (2) Steroids

III Principles of Technology and Measurement

A. DEVICES FOR MEASUREMENT OF FLOW RATES OF FLUID (LIQUID OR GAS)

I. ROTAMETER

II. ELECTROMAGNETIC

III. ULTRASONIC

IV. PNEUMOTACHOMETER

V. SPIROMETER

B. BLOOD (DISSOLVED) GASES

I. GENERAL

II. BENCH-TOP ANALYZER

III. POINT-OF-CARE ANALYZERS

IV. "EX VIVO" MONITORS

V. CONTINUOUS IN VIVO ARTERIAL BLOOD GAS MONITORS

C. INSPIRED, EXPIRED GASES

I. MASS SPECTROSCOPY

II. GAS CHROMATOGRAPHY

D. OXYGEN/HYPOXIA MONITORING

I. PULSE OXIMETRY

II. TRANSCUTANEOUS P_{O_2} MONITORING

E. PRESSURES

   I. GENERAL
  II. LUNG
 III. VASCULAR
 IV. INTRACRANIAL PRESSURE

F. CARDIAC FUNCTION

   I. OSCILLOMETRY
  II. DIAGNOSTIC (ECHO) ULTRASOUND
 III. DOPPLER ULTRASOUND

G. PATIENT SAFETY

   I. SEE "GAS SUPPLY"
  II. U.S. FOOD AND DRUG ADMINISTRATION
 III. PATIENT ELECTRICAL SAFETY
 IV. OTHER PATIENT SAFETY STANDARDS AND AGENCIES
  V. EXPLOSION AND FIRE HAZARDS

H. ELECTRICITY, ELECTRONICS, INSTRUMENTATION

    I. VOLTAGE
   II. CURRENT
  III. RESISTANCE
  IV. CAPACITANCE
   V. ALTERNATING CURRENT
  VI. BASIC CONCEPTS
 VII. ELECTRONIC (MEDICAL) INSTRUMENTS
VIII. COMPUTER NETWORKS
  IX. WIRELESS TELECOMMUNICATION
   X. BATTERIES
  XI. MEDICAL IMAGING SYSTEMS

I. STATISTICS

I. STATISTICAL ANALYSIS PROGRAMS

II. DESCRIPTIVE

III. PROBABILITY

IV. INFERENCE ON POPULATION MEANS FROM QUANTITATIVE DATA

V. INFERENCE ON POPULATION MEANS FROM ENUMERATION (OR ATTRIBUTE) DATA

VI. REGRESSION AND CORRELATION

VII. CLINICAL TRIALS

J. OTHER APPLIED MATHEMATICS

I. FUNCTION

II. ASYMPTOTE

III. INCREMENT

IV. DERIVATIVE OF f

V. DEFINITE INTEGRAL

VI. INDEFINITE INTEGRAL

VII. DIFFERENTIAL EQUATION

VIII. TRANSCENDENTAL FUNCTIONS

IX. INFINITE SERIES

X. COMPLEX VARIABLE

XI. TRANSFORM ANALYSIS

XII. BIOLOGIC CURVES

A. DEVICES FOR MEASUREMENT OF FLOW RATES OF FLUID (LIQUID OR GAS)

I. ROTAMETER™: device for manual control and monitor of gas flow rates

a. Description

1. Gas flows through needle valve (at bottom of Rotameter) and through vertical, transparent tube with tapered cross-sectional area and calibrated flow rate markings; position of "float" free to move inside the tapered glass tube varies up or down with gas flow rate
2. Gas flow rate controllable with needle valve
3. Accuracy approximately (plus or minus) 5% of indicated flow

b. Principle

1. Pressure drop in tube is constant
2. Cross-sectional flow area between float and tube wall varies to accommodate different flow rates: $F_D = F_G - F_B = V_f(\rho_f - \rho)g/g_c$, where F_D is drag force on float, F_G is gravity force on float, F_B is buoyant force acting to raise float, V_f is volume of float, ρ_f is density of float, ρ is density of gas, g/g_c is gravitational constant

c. Applications

1. Operating room: typically three Rotameters attached to a block: O_2, CO_2, N_2O (left to right)
2. PACU, ICU: O_2 Rotameter at wall outlet to set and monitor O_2 flow rate to patient

d. Use: read flow rate (typically ml/min [milliliters per minute] or L/min [liters per minute]) by viewing position of float relative to calibration markings (ball float—read across diameter; other shape—read across top flat surface)

e. Problems

1. Static charge accumulation—float "sticks"
2. Use each Rotameter for only the gas indicated (e.g., O_2, not N_2O)
3. Use only with medical-grade gases (condensation or contamination can cause inaccurate measurement)
4. Needle valve delicate; leak if forced
5. In operating room manifold, breakage of one glass flow tube or leak in one needle valve will cause inaccurate flow rates of other gases

II. ELECTROMAGNETIC: electronic probe most commonly used to monitor blood flow invasively

a. Description

1. Probe with pair of measuring electrodes to directly contact fluid of interest or conduit through which fluid flows (e.g., outside artery wall), and coil(s) to produce magnetic field (induces a potential [voltage] difference normal to the magnetic field vector)
2. Electrical potential proportional to flow rate; alternating magnetic fields provide stability

b. Principle: magnetic field across flow field of a fluid with magnetic susceptibility induces electrical potential across flow field proportional to flow rate

c. Application: measurement of flow rate of H_2O solutions (e.g., blood plasma)

d. Use: continuous monitoring of blood flow rate through artery around which placed

e. Problems

1. Electrodes must contact fluid or artery to obtain flow rate measurement; probe diameter must match artery diameter (if arterial pressure decreases, contact can be lost)
2. Invasive monitor requires sterile probe and surgical placement
3. Requires gas with a molecular magnetic moment: O_2, CO_2, N_2O, or liquid with molecular magnetic moment: H_2O, O_2

III. ULTRASONIC

a. Description: probe with piezoelectric crystals acoustically coupled with the fluid (liquid or gas) of interest to detect or monitor flow

b. Principle: voltage pulses converted to displacement (vibration) pulses and vice versa by piezoelectric crystals (piezoelectric effect of certain materials [e.g., lead zirconate, barium titanate]: voltage pulse causes mechanical strain or vice versa)

1. Blood flow
    (a) Two basic types
        (1) Transit time (pulsed)—does not require reflective particles, due to up- and downstream placement of crystals
            [a] Short bursts of ultrasonic energy (e.g., eight cycles of 3 MHz repeated 12,000 times per second) carried by the bloodstream

[b] Upstream and downstream crystals, positioned outside the blood vessel (artery or vein), produce and detect pulses; switch between upstream and downstream crystals as transmitter and receiver of pulse at, e.g., 800 Hz

[c] Difference between up- and downstream transit times linearly proportional to flow velocity

[d] Recently developed: absolute flow rate (milliliters per minute) from precalibrated perivascular probe (Transonic Systems Inc., Ithaca, N.Y.)

(2) Doppler (frequency) shift—requires reflective particles (e.g., blood cells) to obtain shift in return frequency

[a] Continuous ultrasound beam produced by one crystal, e.g., 5 MHz, reflected from particles or regions of density difference to a second crystal mounted in the same probe

[b] Audible signal generated by comparing incident and reflected signals (0–3,500 Hz for 0–100 cm/s change in flow velocity)

[c] Rugged, cheap probe—instrument design from early 1960s is in common use to detect blood flow in extremities noninvasively

2. Gas flow—vortices caused by vane in flow stream are sensed by a Doppler ultrasound transducer as changes in density of the gas; frequency of oscillation of vortices across flow stream proportional to flow rate (Ohmeda ventilation monitor)

IV. PNEUMOTACHOMETER
(or pneumotachograph)

a. Description: fast-response intermittent-flow-rate measurement; conduit of circular cross section with metal screen (or gauze) or bundle of small flow channels

1. Screen or bundle serves as a resistance across which pressure drop is measured by external pressure transducer

2. Screen or tube bundle large enough in area (typically larger than the breathing circuit) to introduce a very small airway resistance

3. Heater maintains gas temperature and viscosity and prevents condensation on screen or bundle

4. Fleisch, Lilly: well-known, early manufacturers

b. Principle

1. Flow rate proportional to pressure drop across orifice

2. Screen presents many tiny orifices "in parallel"

3. Approximately linear pressure–flow relation across screen or bundle element: $Q = \Delta P / R(T, [F(x)])$, where Q is flow rate measured by pneumotachometer (L/min), ΔP is differential pressure across screen or bundle, R is gas constant, T is absolute temperature, and $[F(x)]$ is gas mixture with species molar fractions $[N_1/N, N_2/N, \ldots, N_x/N]$

c. Application

1. Research or special studies for which breath flow-rate waveform is of interest

2. Typically used in applications requiring several consecutive breaths; used to determine flow rate and volume (integration of flow rate with time)

d. Use

1. Use with gas indicated (different gas or mixture has a different viscosity and heat capacity)

2. Use with size of breathing circuit indicated or provided (pediatric, adult)

3. Maintain clean (with methods indicated)

V. SPIROMETER: gas volume measurement

a. Displacement from calibrated vessels—lightweight bell suspended over water with pulley counterweight

b. Calibrated disposable expired volume collector

c. Special-purpose devices for measurement of vital capacity, force expired volume in 1 second (great variation among instruments)

d. Wright Respirometer™—early convenient mechanical anemometer (velocity meter with rotating vane) used to measure tidal volumes (milliliters) or minute volumes (16–60 L/min) with clinical accuracy (plus or minus 10%); delicate

B. BLOOD (DISSOLVED) GASES

I. GENERAL

a. A 40-year-old technology developed for routine clinical use during the polio epidemics of early 1950s (automated positive pressure ventilator technology developed soon thereafter)

b. Currently, about 170 million ABGs/year; about 30 million patients/year have two or more ABGs per hospital stay (U.S.)

c. Change from clinical laboratory to bedside (or point of care) may occur with new technology introduced during early 1990s, cost and regulatory experience pending

II. BENCH-TOP ANALYZER

a. Complex, automated instrument developed and refined over past 40 years

b. Usually operated and maintained in clinical laboratories (central and satellite) and at points of care (ICUs, emergency rooms, and operating rooms)

c. Separate, stand-alone instrument, not incorporated with (other) clinical chemical analyzers; whole blood oximeters may be connected (requires sample introduction to each instrument), or included as part of the analyzer (requires one sample)

d. Typically, two analyzers maintained in any clinical laboratory facility to accommodate occasional electrode maintenance or fluid flow path plugging

e. Description

1. Measures partial pressure of dissolved oxygen, P_{O_2}, partial pressure of dissolved carbon dioxide, P_{CO_2}, and pH of whole blood at 37°C (can also be used to determine P_{O_2}, P_{CO_2}, pH of other fluids [e.g., CSF, urine] or P_{O_2} of gas samples)

2. Highly dependent engineered systems, dependent on careful maintenance

   (a) Electrode sensors (maintained at constant temperature, 37°C)
   (b) Solid-state electrometers (microvolt and microamp meter)
   (c) Small-volume gas and liquid conveyance devices to and from electrode sensors (tubing, pumps, valves, reservoirs), and electric power supply and data display

3. Measurements of P_{O_2}, P_{CO_2}, pH of plasma fraction of whole blood

4. Sample volume

   (a) 0.2 ml or less "used" by instrument
   (b) Approximately 0.5–1.0 ml is adequate from the patient
   (c) Sample must be anticoagulated to prevent clogging of instrument fluid path

5. Small sample of whole blood (or any fluid, gas, or liquid) introduced to the instrument and, via pumps and tubing, to the sensors for measurement

6. Sensors are electrode systems carefully maintained by the instrument fluid system and by technicians

   (a) pH—glass membrane ion-selective electrode cell
       (1) Made practical for blood pH by McInnes and Belcher (1930s); Astrup, Schrøder, and Siggaard-Anderson (1950s)
       (2) Special glass is selective for H^+; bulb of this thin glass separates solution of interest (blood plasma) from internal solution of known pH (KCl)
       (3) "Nernstian" response H^+ activity is measured across this membrane
           [a] 60 mV/pH unit
           [b] Measured relative to a separate reference electrode (i.e., electrode with stable half-cell potential; other half of potentiometric cell)
       (4) Reference electrode
           [a] Isolated from solution of interest
           [b] Contacts the solution through a reference solution (saturated KCl) and a porous plug or fiber (minimizes diffusion of either sample or reference solution)
       (5) $pH = pK + \log[HCO_3^-]/[CO_2]$, where pK is dissociation constant of carbonic acid (= 6.1), $[HCO_3^-]$ is activity of bicarbonate ion (= 24 mEq/L, typical), $[CO_2]$ is concentration of dissolved CO_2 (= 40 mm Hg × 0.03 = 1.2 mmol/L, typical) (therefore, $pH = 6.1 + \log 24/1.2 = 7.4$)
   (b) P_{CO_2}—ion-selective electrode cell based on pH electrode, with voltage measured relative to reference electrode
       (1) pH electrode in bicarbonate buffer contained by CO_2-permeable, ion-impermeable membrane (Stow and Severinghaus invention, 1950s)
       (2) Log P_{CO_2} and pH linear over range of P_{CO_2} 10–90 mm Hg
       (3) $H_2O + CO_2 \rightleftarrows H_2CO_3 \rightleftarrows H^+ + HCO_3^-$
           $[CO_2] = a(P_{CO_2})$, a = 0.0301 mmol/L/mm Hg CO_2
           $k = [H^+][HCO_3^-]/[CO_2] = [H^+][HCO_3^-]/a(P_{CO_2})$
           $\log k = \log[H^+] + \log[HCO_3^-] - \log a - \log P_{CO_2}$
           $\log P_{CO_2} = \log[HCO_3^-] - \log k - \log a - pH$, $pH = -\log[H^+]$
   (c) P_{O_2}—redox reaction consumes O_2, producing current in proportion to the amount (concentration) of O_2 present at the cathode
       (1) When 600–800 mV applied between cathode and anode
           [a] At cathode (platinum; reduction rxn)
               $O_2 + 2H_2O + 4e^- \rightarrow 2H_2O_2 + 4e^- \rightarrow 4OH^-$
               $4OH^- + 4KCl \rightarrow 4KOH + 4Cl^-$
       (2) At anode (Ag-AgCl; oxidation)
               $4Ag + 4Cl^- \rightarrow 4AgCl + 4e^-$
       (3) Electrodes are covered with polymeric membrane permeable to O_2, impermeable to proteins (contaminate electrode system; Clark invention (1950s)

f. Calibration

1. P_{O_2}, P_{CO_2}: typically two point, based on 2-cal gas mixtures contained in compressed gas cylinders. (Note: Point-of-care systems use solutions packaged with dissolved gases and known pH.)

2. pH: typically two point; two buffer solutions contained in separate bottles

g. Sample, syringe, and time to analysis

1. Sample must represent blood volume of interest, not fluid in catheter, cannula, connectors, etc., i.e., "dead space"
    - (a) Pull back four times dead space into separate syringe to obtain representative blood sample for analysis; reinfuse plus flush catheter, cannula, connector, etc., after sample obtained
    - (b) Sample syringe must contain adequate heparin (10–100 U, i.e., 1 drop of 1,000 U/ml heparin solution) and no dead space: be sure that some heparin solution is visible in syringe tip prior to sampling
2. Preheparinized blood gas syringes, with cap to prevent uptake/loss of dissolved gas from/to ambient environment
    - (a) Preferred device for sample acquisition; individually packaged syringe
    - (b) Heparin solution or dry heparin
        - (1) Specification of heparin amount is difficult
        - (2) Chelates Ca^{++}, contributes to Ca^{++} analysis errors
3. Analyze within 15 minutes to avoid significant changes

h. Manufacturers: Radiometer, Ciba-Corning, Instrumentation Laboratories, AVL

III. POINT-OF-CARE ANALYZERS:
available from various manufacturers with clinically useful menus that include Po_2, Pco_2, pH, Hb, K^+, Ca^{++}, glucose

a. Disposable cartridge electrode systems: single analysis—throw away; 50–75 analyses—throw away

b. Technology: disposable electrodes based on printed circuit and thin-film chemical indicator-membrane deposition. Integral calibration fluid packages. Portable instruments (some hand held, battery powered)

c. Calibration: automatic, prior to each analysis; uses carefully packaged solutions of known Po_2, Pco_2, and pH

d. Manufacturers: Mallinckrodt, I-STAT, PPG (or successor), Diametrix

IV. "EX VIVO" MONITORS (not analyzers)

a. Technology

1. Optical (see below) or electrode sensors

2. Semidisposable sensor module in series with arterial line, connected to physiologic monitor module

3. Closed system: blood is withdrawn through arterial cannula and proximal tubing to contact sensors; reinfused following analysis

4. ABG analysis on demand by bedside clinician

5. No discrete sample volume or disposal

b. Application: cardiac surgery bypass pump system (3M/Cardiovascular Devices Inc., Irvine, Calif.); critical care systems (1996; Optical Sensors Inc., Minneapolis, Minn.; 1987: VIA Medical Corp., San Diego, Calif. (to include electrolytes, hematocrit (hct), glucose)

V. CONTINUOUS IN VIVO ARTERIAL BLOOD GAS MONITORS: new sensor technology; optical sensors for Po_2, Pco_2, pH

a. Technology

1. Optical fiber conducts light to chemical indicator at or near distal (patient) end of fiber in fluid of interest

2. Multisensor probes (Po_2, Pco_2, pH, plus thermocouple temperature sensor)

3. In development since early 1980s; limited availability during 1994–1995; commercial success pending

b. Application: intra-arterial (radial artery; femoral artery placement likely to be approved)

c. Manufacturers: Pfizer/Biomedical Sensors Ltd., Optex Biomedical Inc., Puritan Bennett/FOxS Division (or successors)

C. INSPIRED, EXPIRED GASES

I. MASS SPECTROSCOPY: separates charged particles (ions) in a gas stream into a spectrum according to their mass-to-charge ratio; determines relative concentration of each ionic species present

a. Description: sample inlet assembly, ionization chamber, dispersion chamber, ion detector (collector)

1. Sample inlet—heated or unheated capillary (approximately 0.25 mm inner diameter) and inlet chamber; rotary vacuum pump draws gas into and through capillary and produces inlet chamber pressure of about 20–25 mm Hg (1.3–1.7 kPa) absolute; porous plug permits diffusion ("leak") of some of the gas in the inlet chamber into the ionization chamber

2. Ionization chamber

   (a) Evacuated to very low pressure of about 10^{-7} mm Hg (10^{-5} Pa) by high-vacuum, high-capacity pump

   (b) At entrance, electron beam bombards gas molecules and atoms entering the ionization chamber; causes them to lose electrons; creates positive ions

   (c) Positive ions are focused into beam, accelerated by an electric field into a dispersion chamber

3. Dispersion chamber—ions in the beam are dispersed using a magnetic field or a quadrupole electric field, or dispersion occurs following acceleration and during "time of flight" across dispersion chamber to ion detector(s); lighter ions are deflected or accelerated most

4. Ion detector(s)—ions collected and detected using two methods; both measure current proportional to partial pressure of corresponding component in the gas mixture

   (a) Single collector—impinged by component beams and scanned at high frequency for ions of different mass

   (b) Multiple collectors—adjusted for continuous impingement by ions of only one component

b. Characteristics

1. Range of molecular weight for most respiratory measurements: four (He) to 44 (CO_2) atomic mass units

   (a) Expanded range for monitoring halothane

   (b) Gases with same atomic mass units

       (1) CO_2 and N_2O have same AMU = 44; distinguish by detecting NO fragments produced from N_2O on electron-beam exposure

       (2) O_2, CO_2 cannot be distinguished in presence of N_2O

       (3) CO interferes with N_2

       (4) Use IR-based instruments to distinguish CO and N_2O

2. Response time: less than 100 ms; transport delay (through capillary): approximately 200 ms

3. Eight or more components; sequential sampling from different inlet capillaries (catheters) available in early to mid-1980s

c. Applications: operating room, pulmonary diagnostics lab, clinical chemistry lab

II. GAS CHROMATOGRAPHY: detects presence and determines quantities and concentrations of (trace) analytes

a. Based on differential solubility of gases in mixture as mixture flows through stationary column containing a liquid phase to separate mixture into components

b. Description: mobile phase (carrier gas), stationary phase (liquid with solid support medium), injection port, detector

1. Mobile phase

   (a) Carrier gas, typically Ar, He, or N_2
   (b) Compressed source with accurate flow control
   (c) Carrier gas flows through stationary phase

2. Stationary phase

   (a) Chromatographic column packed with inert support material (e.g., silica-alumina particles) coated with inert liquid (e.g., polyethylene glycol, silicone oil)
   (b) Typically coiled glass tube to provide length for improved separation

3. Injection port

   (a) Located at column inlet
   (b) Gas mixture to be analyzed is introduced from a gas-tight syringe through a rubber septum
   (c) Heated port may be incorporated for vaporization of liquids and analysis of volatile components (e.g., blood plasma or serum, urine samples)
   (d) Gas sampling valve alternative to syringe

4. Detector—outlet of separation column connected to a detector

   (a) Flame ionization for detection of organics—polarizing voltage across H_2/O_2 flame detects ions; increases with ionizable component
   (b) Thermal conductivity (katharometer) for detection of inorganics (e.g., N_2O, O_2)—heated wire changes resistance in presence of thermally conductive component in column eluent (sample)
   (c) Electron capture for halogenated compounds—polarizing voltage across ionization chamber causes current, which decreases in presence of halogenated compounds due to electron capture

5. Analysis

   (a) Retention time (time after injection for sample component to appear at detector)
   (b) Peak heights, areas for quantitative analysis (intensity versus time record)
   (c) Quantitative analysis requires comparison with known amounts of the analyte of interest (i.e., calibration samples)

c. Characteristics: identification, measurement of small concentrations of drugs and mixtures; requires sampling; requires calibration using known amounts of substance of interest for quantitative analysis

II. Gas chromatography (continued)

d. Applications

1. Operating room—volatile anesthetic agents (anesthetic concentration and trace amounts in operating room)

2. Clinical chemistry lab—barbiturates, phenothiazines, benzodiazepines, steroids, catecholamines

D. OXYGEN/HYPOXIA MONITORING

I. PULSE OXIMETRY

a. Clinical standard hypoxia monitor in operating room and ICU

b. Continuous noninvasive monitor of arterial O_2 saturation, Sp_{O_2} (estimate of bench-top instrument measurement of Sa_{O_2} in whole blood sample)

c. About 20 manufacturers

d. Principle

1. Distinguish Hb_{O_2} (oxyhemoglobin) and Hb (deoxyhemoglobin) by measuring absorption of light at two wavelengths that can be reliably obtained from a small, cheap light source and at which absorption by Hb_{O_2} and Hb differs

   (a) 660 nm (red)—Hb_{O_2} absorbs less red than Hb (red color)
   (b) 940 nm (infrared [IR])—Hb absorbs less IR than Hb_{O_2}
   (c) Light sources are LEDs (light-emitting diodes)
   (d) Detector (photodiode) cannot distinguish wavelengths—light sensed is from LED that is on, plus artifact
   (e) LEDs on/off at frequency, typically less than 1 kHz

2. Distinguish arterial–venous blood

   (a) Diastole—venous blood, other tissue/pigments
   (b) Systole—increased light absorption due to influx of arterialized blood
   (c) Ratio: red/IR absorption determined during diastole and systole, compared
   (d) Calibration using empirical Sa_{O_2} versus $A_{660\,nm}/A_{940\,nm}$ (lab) data

3. Limitations

   (a) Sp_{O_2} over 70%: best accuracy
   (b) Detectable plethysmographic pulsation: absent or minimal in hypothermia, hypovolemia, cardiogenic shock
   (c) Approximately 30 seconds' transition at fingertip to rapid change in arterial saturation
   (d) Pa_{O_2} is more sensitive indication of deterioration of pulmonary function than Sa_{O_2}
       (1) Sp_{O_2} is continuous monitor, however
       (2) Tissue O_2 delivery is proportional to Sa_{O_2}, so that Sp_{O_2} will detect changes in pulmonary gas exchange before tissue oxygenation is impaired
   (e) Interference
       (1) Intrinsic
           [a] MetHb, COHb in abnormally high concentrations (i.e., approximately 5–10%); COHb similar to Hb_{O_2} $\Rightarrow$ Sp_{O_2} overestimated; MetHb 1:1 absorption at 660 and 940 nm $\Rightarrow$ decreased sensitivity (same absorption at 660 and 940 nm)
           [b] Diagnostic dyes: methylene blue, indocyanine green; strong absorption at 660 nm $\Rightarrow$ artifactually low Sp_{O_2} until dye redistributed to nonpulsatile compartments
           [c] Nail polish—blue may cause artifactually low Sp_{O_2}

(2) Extrinsic
   [a] Patient motion can cause orientation of probe relative to tissue (finger) to change
   [b] Electrosurgery—interference varies with manufacturer; weak pulse gives poor signal
   [c] Intense ambient light—broad spectrum; sensed by detector; can introduce noise, cause error signal
(f) Accuracy
   (1) Standard deviation 2–3% over SpO_2 range of 70–100%
   (2) 95% confidence limit $\pm 6\%$ (i.e., 95% chance that $SpO_2 = 90\%$ corresponds to $84 < SaO_2 < 96\%$)
(g) Recent: estimation of PaO_2 based on SpO_2
   (1) Estimate Hb—O_2 dissociation curve shift using SaO_2 and PaO_2 from most recent arterial blood gas analysis (PO_2, PCO_2, pH, T, SaO_2)
   (2) Correct for offset between SaO_2 and SpO_2 at time of sampling

---

e. Some manufacturers: Catalyst Research Division, Mine Safety Appliances Corp. (Owings Mills, Md.); Nellcor Inc. (Hayward, Calif.); Ohmeda-Biox Division, British Oxygen Corp. (Boulder, Col.); SensorMedics Corp. (Anaheim, Calif.)

II. TRANSCUTANEOUS PO_2 MONITORING

a. Noninvasive continuous monitor of partial pressure of O_2 dissolved in arterial blood plasma, PaO_2

---

b. O_2 dissolved in arterialized blood of skin capillaries is made available to skin surface PO_2 electrode by moderate local heating to 43–44°C sufficient to

1. Cause flow needed for heat removal to exceed that needed for metabolism
2. Melt fat/wax crystallites to increase gas permeability

---

c. Transcutaneous PO_2 electrode is Clark polarographic electrode design (see "Blood gas analysis" above) that incorporates a heater and temperature sensors to warm the skin in contact with electrode to maximum temperature without thermal injury

---

d. Limitations and inaccuracies

1. Hb—O_2 curve shift with temperature
2. Skin thermal injury with prolonged exposure to temperature approximately 43–45°C $\Rightarrow$ change location every 3–6 hours
3. Edema with thermal injury decreases permeability
4. Response to step change in PaO_2 approximately 2 minutes
5. Adhesive attachment ring must be in place and not permeable to O_2

e. Most common uses

1. Neonate P_aO_2 monitoring
2. Hyperbaric/hyperoxic therapy monitoring of wound tissue periphery

f. Manufacturer: Radiometer (Copenhagen, Denmark)

E. PRESSURES

I. GENERAL

a. **Force applied over surface area; force/unit area; $P = f/a$**

b. **Absolute pressure = gauge pressure + atmospheric pressure**

c. **$1\ Pa = 1\ N/1\ m^2$; $100\ kPa = 1\ bar = 750\ mm\ Hg = 14.7\ psi \simeq$ 1 atm at sea level ($101.3\ kPa = 1\ atm = 760\ mm\ Hg$)**

d. **$10.2\ cm\ H_2O = 7.5\ mm\ Hg$ (density Hg = $13.6 \times$ density H_2O)**

e. **Vacuum: 1 torr = 1 mm Hg; 7.5 torr = 1 kPa**

II. LUNG

a. **Note:** pressures of compressed gases used with anesthesia machines and with other mechanical ventilator support devices range from about 745 to 2,200 psig, depending on size and gas; in-house gas supplies of O_2 and air range from 50 to 60 psig. Pressure regulators with mechanical (Bourdon tube) pressure gauges are used to provide a reliable step-down to physiologic range. See "Gas supply" for pressure regulator and gauge description

b. **Inspiratory**

1. Peak (or end) inspiratory pressure (PIP)
   (a) Monitored by positive-pressure ventilator
   (b) Used to calculate dynamic compliance: $C_{dyn} = V_t/[PIP\text{-}PEEP]$, $V_t =$ delivered tidal volume
   (c) PIP increased due to
      (1) Lung edema
      (2) Artificial airway obstruction
      (3) Lung (over)expansion to elastic limit
         [a] Excessive PEEP
         [b] Intrinsic (auto) PEEP
         [c] Excessive peak flow
         [d] Excessive tidal volume (V_t over 15 ml/kg)
   (d) Maximum "pop off" valve setting 50–70 cm H_2O, depending on V_t

2. Plateau pressure (P_p)
   (a) Monitored by positive-pressure ventilator
   (b) Temporary occlusion of airway at end expiration
   (c) Inflation pressure needed to overcome elastic recoil of respiratory system
   (d) Estimation of maximum alveolar pressure
   (e) Used to calculate static compliance: $C_{st} = V_t/[P_p - PEEP]$,
       $V_t =$ delivered tidal volume

3. Maximum inspiratory pressure (MIP; P_I max); negative inspiratory pressure (NIP); negative inspiratory force (NIF)

    (a) Negative pressure (i.e., $P_{atm} > P_{insp}$)

    (b) As weaning parameter, MIP ≤ -30 cm H_2O indicates adequate inspiratory force

    (c) Maximum pressure exerted by patient with temporary occlusion of airway (less than 30 seconds) with in-line manometer gauge

    (d) Normal: -60 to -80 cm H_2O

c. Expiratory

1. Positive end expiratory (PEEP)

    (a) Physiologic PEEP due to resistance of airway: approximately 5 cm H_2O

    (b) Set as needed: 5–25 cm H_2O

    (c) Created by resistance in expiratory limb of breathing circuit, with manually adjusted valve or automatic expiratory control

    (d) Promotes recruitment of under- or unexpanded alveoli

    (e) Used to improve oxygenation

    (f) Potential benefits

        (1) Increased function residual capacity

        (2) Increased compliance

        (3) Decreased FiO_2

        (4) Decreased shunt fraction

        (5) Decreased physiologic dead space

    (g) Potential problems

        (1) Decreased oxygenation

        (2) Decreased ventilation

        (3) Decreased venous return (increased intrathoracic pressure)

            [a] Decreased right ventricular preload

            [b] Increased right ventricular afterload

            [c] Increased cerebral edema

        (4) Barotrauma

2. Continuous positive airway pressure (CPAP)

    (a) Provided by continuous gas flow, not expiratory limb resistance

    (b) Patient provides inspiratory force, regulates tidal volume, minute volume

    (c) Used to

        (1) Treat atelectasis

        (2) Maintain nondependent lung for one-lung ventilation

        (3) Wean from mechanical ventilatory support

III. VASCULAR

a. Arterial

1. Dependent on

    (a) Method, accuracy, site of measurement

    (b) Patient (temperature, hemodynamic status, movement, cardiovascular disease)

    (c) Location of sensor (transducer) or cuff relative to heart (hydrostatic effects)

        (1) Should be located at level of heart

        (2) Standing man: 50 mm Hg in head, 90 mm Hg at heart, 200 mm Hg in feet

2. Noninvasive

    (a) Sphygmomanometer: Korotkoff's sounds (stethoscope), Riva-Rocci (palpation)

III. Vascular; a. Arterial (continued)

       (1) Cuff width: important to obtain rounded pressure front (gradient) in tissue surrounding artery ($\sim 0.4 \times$ circumference of arm, or $1.2 \times$ diameter of arm)

       (2) Deflation (2–3 mm Hg per second); discrimination of diastolic pressure problematic

       (3) Manual, intermittent

       (4) Most common and inexpensive

       (5) Inaccurate with infants, hypotensive or hemodynamically unstable patients

       (6) ± 20 mm Hg error compared with invasive radial artery site

    (b) Automated

       (1) Oscillometry (oscillotonometry)

          [a] Von Recklinghausen discovery (1931)

          [b] Onset of pulsations distal to occluding cuff sensed with a distal cuff-pressure transducer; pressure in occluding cuff slowly discharged (~ 2 mm Hg per second); distal sensing cuff pulsates once the proximal occluding cuff pressure is low enough to allow the pressure wave to pass under it

          [c] Single cuff system: cuff inflated (20–30 mm Hg per second, to 160 mm Hg or 25 mm Hg over previous SBP measured) and deflated stepwise; cuff pressure monitored at same frequency (cycles per second); pressure waves are transmitted via tubing to a pressure transducer in instrument; at SBP, transient (oscillometric) pressure wave sensed and recorded; good correlation between MAP and maximum amplitude of transient wave; DBP taken when transient waves abruptly decrease in amplitude

          [d] SBP is highest cuff pressure at which oscillations detected; MAP is cuff pressure at which oscillations have greatest magnitude; DBP is cuff pressure at which oscillations no longer decrease in magnitude

          [e] Compared with direct intra-arterial measurement: 95% confidence interval for SBP: ± 13.7 mm Hg (regarded as fairly accurate); MAP 95% confidence interval ± 17.3 mm Hg; DBP 95% confidence interval ± 38.1 mm Hg (diastolic end-point controversial)

          [f] DINAMAP™ (device for indirect noninvasive mean arterial pressure, J&J/Critikon, Tampa, Fla.): oscillometric pulsations detected as spike of cuff pressure at particular step; confirmed by searching for repeat pulsation within certain time interval (e.g., 1.5 seconds); pulses accepted if similar amplitudes, hence problems if the patient is moving or has irregular pulse (e.g., atrial fibrillation); DBP calculated from systolic and mean, but more accurate than auscultation; reported accuracy: ± 3 mm Hg or 2% of full scale

          [g] Frequency of noninvasive BP measurement: set interval should be over 1 minute (approximately 5 minutes OK) for incompetent patient to avoid nerve damage

          [h] Reliable and convenient monitor for stable patient; incorporated as module in bedside physiologic monitor systems

          [i] Sources of error: cuff leak, dysrhythmias, patient movement, wrong size cuff

          [j] Manufacturers: J&J/Critikon, Tampa, Fla. (DINAMAP™); Ohmeda, Madison, Wis.

          [k] Inaccurate if patient hemodynamically unstable

       (2) Peñaz (Finapres, Ohmeda, Madison, Wis.)

          [a] Continuous, noninvasive

          [b] Small cuff exerts pressure $\simeq$ arterial pressure; inflates, deflates around mid-phalanx of thumb or other finger to reflect arterial pressure

           [c] Light source (LED; IR) and photodetector across finger just distal to cuff; based on photodetector signal (propor- tional to blood volume in finger), cuff pressure adjusted continuously to be equal to internal artery pressure

           [d] Electronic-pneumatic system with high-frequency response (over 50-Hz bandwidth) and sophisticated control algorithm (proportional–integral–derivative)

           [e] Inaccuracy due to vasoconstrictor drugs, hemodynamic instability

3. Invasive

  (a) Arterial

    (1) Arterial waveform

        [a] Varies with patient, cardiovascular performance, site of measurement

        [b] 0–50-Hz signal frequency range; represented well by six harmonic (sinusoidal) components (sixth harmonic is $\sim 12\%$ of fundamental amplitude)

    (2) Extravascular transducer: arterial cannula–pressure tubing– external pressure transducer–display instrument (waveform and numeric readout of SBP, MAP, DBP) is gold standard with which other (e.g., noninvasive) systems compared

    (3) Sterile, precalibrated, disposable pressure transducer is standard: deflection, resistance of metallized film (strain gauge)

    (4) Other components

        [a] Patient vasculature

        [b] Arterial cannula

        [c] Pressure tubing to connect cannula to transducer

        [d] Transducer–tubing–cannula flush fluid and pressure source

        [e] Instrument connections, amplifiers

    (5) Transducer mounted on IV pole or attached to patient: requires positioning at elevation of heart for accurate measurement

    (6) Dynamics

        [a] Transducer (with fluid chamber)—instrumentation (low mass, low compliance); bandwidth ≥ 0–50 Hz

        [b] Entire mechanical system (fluid column mass, fluid-tubing friction, tubing compliance, air bubbles)—bandwidth can be less than 10 Hz; use stiff tubing, length under 4 feet

        [c] Damping ratio—overdamped (loss of trace detail): blood clot, bubbles, crimping of cannula, tubing, number of connectors—low SBP indicated (about 10%), delay (150 ms; noticeable); underdamped (too responsive): tubing too stiff—high SBP (about 10–20%), low DBP; check by crimping tubing to make overdamped

        [d] Check response with rapid flush pressure spike: if ringing (many cycles of oscillation), then system is underdamped and/or frequency response too low—remove air bubbles, use shorter, stiffer tubing

    (7) Arterial site

        [a] Affects dynamics: more peripheral site has higher frequency components of pressure waveform—overestimation of SBP; additional inaccuracy if frequency response degraded by tubing, bubbles, etc.

        [b] Radial—20 gauge, 1.5 inches (Note: 1 mm outer diameter, 100-cm cannulas for central arterial monitoring placed via radial artery are still in limited use; these devices minimize fluid column mass, peripheral artifact, potential to dislodge art line with patient movement or bleed-out)

        [c] Femoral—20 or 18 gauge, 6 inches

        [d] Dorsalis pedis—20 gauge, 1.5 inches

        [e] Axillary—20 gauge, 6 inches

III. Vascular; a. Arterial (continued)

               [f] Aorta—lower frequency content than radial or brachial
    (b) Central venous (CVP line)
        (1) Monitor right-side filling pressure: 1–8 mm Hg (normal range)
        (2) Seldinger placement technique
        (3) One-, two-, three-lumen catheters
            [a] One lumen—rapid fluid resuscitation; 8.5 Fr
            [b] Three lumen (two 18 gauge, one 16 gauge), 20 or 30 cm: for administration of incompatible drugs
        (4) Sites
            [a] Internal jugular
            [b] External jugular
            [c] Femoral vein (no risk of pneumothorax)
            [d] Subclavian
    (c) Pulmonary artery catheter (PAC; Swan-Ganz; S-G)
        (1) Provides
            [a] Estimate of left ventricular end diastolic pressure (LVEDP; also, pulmonary artery wedge pressure [PAWP], pulmonary capillary wedge pressure [PCWP], pulmonary capillary occlusion pressure [PCOP])
            [b] Cardiac output (CO)
            [c] Mixed venous O_2 saturation (Svo_2)
            [d] Hemodynamic waveforms, R intracardiac pressures (RA, RV, PA)
            [e] Sample port for mixed venous blood gas analysis
        (2) Placement: flow-directed balloon-tipped catheter; site same as (in place of) CVP catheter; confirm with chest x-ray
        (3) Normal pressures

Site	Range (mm Hg)
RA	1–8
RV systolic	15–30
RV diastolic	1–8
PA systolic	15–30
PA diastolic	5–15
PA mean	10–20
LA	2–12
LVEDP	4–12

        (4) Insertion site versus PAC tip location

PAC Tip Location	Insertion Site	Insertion Length (cm)
SVC/RA	Internal jugular vein	15–20
	Subclavian vein	10–15
	Femoral vein	30–40
RV	Internal jugular vein	30–40
	Subclavian vein	25–30
	Femoral vein	45–55
PA	Internal jugular vein	40–55
	Subclavian vein	35–45
	Femoral vein	55–70

IV. INTRACRANIAL PRESSURE (ICP)

a. Normal—5–15 mm Hg in supine patient (uniform throughout cranial vault, although different monitors may indicate different ICPs)

b. ICP over 20 mm Hg reflects intracranial pathology (e.g., traumatic brain injury and edema); does not reflect neurologic status

c. Methods (all ICP monitors are placed by neurosurgeon in operating room or at ICU bedside; used by intensivist to monitor ICP and cerebral perfusion pressure)

1. Ventriculostomy (intraventricular)
   (a) Catheter inserted through brain parenchyma into lateral ventricle
   (b) Placed via scalp incision, skull burr hole (typically about 1 cm anterior to coronal suture, about 3 cm from midline, about 1 cm in diameter), dura incision, through brain parenchyma, and into lateral ventricle (penetration 6–7 cm from scalp surface; indicated by free CSF flow from catheter)
   (c) Connected via sterile fluid-filled tubing with external pressure transducer at definite elevation relative to the head (i.e., 20 mm Hg $\times$ 13.6 cm H_2O/ mm Hg = 27 cm above auditory canal to maintain maximum normal ICP; no leakage, air bubbles)
   (d) Advantages
       (1) Accurate measurement of cranial vault pressure
       (2) Reliable ICP waveforms for analysis
       (3) Removal of CSF (a screening tool for infection, prescribed for ICP over 20 mm Hg)
       (4) Route for intraventricular antibiotics
   (e) Potential problems, complications (during placement, setup of tubing and transducer, or catheter maintenance)
       (1) Collapse of ventricle around catheter tip obstructing further CSF drainage, distorting ICP measurement—adjust height of pressure transducer
       (2) Height adjustment (recalibration)
           [a] Transducer drift
           [b] After patient repositioning
           [c] After patient transport
           [d] After tubing change
       (3) Catheter tip obstruction with intraventricular blood, brain debris, cell debris produced during CNS infection or inflammation
       (4) Infection
           [a] Ventriculitis (typical rate 22%)
           [b] Requires sterile placement of the catheter
           [c] Incidence increases with catheter duration, use of antibiotic flush solutions, older patients, steroid use, open trauma or hemorrhage
           [d] Rate of infection very low on days 1–4; infection rate approximately 50% by day 9
           [e] To prevent infection, change tubing every 24 hours; CSF sample for Gram stain, culture, cell count with differential, glucose, and protein every 48 hours

    (f) Contraindications
        (1) Massive midline shift and/or collapsed ventricles evident from head CT scan
        (2) Coagulopathy (risk of extra- and intraparenchymal hemorrhage associated with skin, skull preparation, and passage of the catheter through brain parenchyma)

2. Subarachnoid (Richmond) bolt (obsolete)
    (a) Bolt with external threads and lumen through its shaft
    (b) Placed via small craniotomy (drill hole); skin incision (about 1 cm anterior to the coronal suture in mid-pupillary line); bolt extends about 1 mm below skull inner table; small incision to open dural and subarachnoid membranes at the tip of the bolt; continuous fluid path (bolt lumen should fill spontaneously with CSF; if not, fill with sterile saline)
    (c) Bolt connected to a closed pressure tubing–transducer system similar to ventriculostomy catheter system (transducer elevation adjusted to be equal to middle ear)
    (d) No air bubbles, fluid leakage
    (e) Advantages over ventriculostomy
        (1) Simpler, less risky placement
        (2) Useful in patients with distorted or collapsed ventricles
    (f) Potential problems, complications (fewer than with ventricular catheters)
        (1) Surface bleeding if the bolt is advanced too far
        (2) Infection at insertion site, osteomyelitis, and meningitis (incidence of 0–10%)
        (3) Inadequate CSF drain or sample port
        (4) Pressure differential between ventriculostomy and subarachnoid bolt ($ICP_{subarachnoid\ bolt}$ less than $ICP_{ventriculostomy}$, especially if ICP is greater than 20 mm Hg due to brain swelling and herniation of brain tissue to occlude bolt tip)

3. Fiberoptic pressure probe—bolt (subdural–intraparenchymal)
    (a) Currently most convenient, least hazardous ICP monitor
    (b) Probe tip pressure transducer; disposable probe approximately 1 mm in diameter
    (c) Advantages
        (1) Accurately monitors ICP at any sensor location: lateral ventricle, brain parenchyma, subarachnoid space (no need to place probe tip pressure transducer in ventricle system)
        (2) Less artifact than fluid-filled tubing systems (e.g., ventriculostomy)
        (3) No adjustment of external pressure transducer elevation, no concern about air bubbles or occlusion of catheter
        (4) Lower incidence of infection (closed, nonflushed system; manufacturer [Camino Laboratories Inc., San Diego, Calif.] reports an infection rate of under 5% if probe is in place for 5 days)
    (d) Placement
        (1) Site similar to ventriculostomy; craniotomy (2.7 mm burr hole), dura incision, bolt placed
        (2) Make probe optical–electrical connector–bedside display connections (ICP waveform and mean ICP displayed)
        (3) Adjust to 0 mm Hg offset prior to placement in bolt
        (4) Place to 5-cm mark (probe tip protrudes 0.5 cm beyond bolt tip)—probably extends into brain parenchyma (can advance 2–3 cm further)
    (e) Potential problems, complications
        (1) No recalibration after placement
        (2) Drift ± 0.6 mm Hg per day, 5-day drift of ± 2.1 mm Hg (maximum of ± 6 mm Hg), compared with ventriculostomy $\Rightarrow$ use for less than 5 days

        (3) No CSF drain

        (4) Probe can be dislodged during nursing procedures, patient transport, rotation

4. Epidural ICP monitoring (ICP monitoring from the epidural space [obsolete])

    (a) May present less risk to the patient (dura intact)

    (b) Placed during surgery or at ICU bedside via a small craniotomy (burr hole): dura detached from the skull along 0.5 by 2–3-cm tract to provide a space for sensor-tipped probe or catheter; probe inserted into the space between the dura and skull

    (c) Disadvantages

        (1) Thick, nonelastic dura dampens and/or distorts ICP signal

        (2) Stripped dura becomes rigid—decreased sensitivity

        (3) Increased ICP $\Rightarrow$ increased artifact

        (4) Accuracy problems; trend, not ICP

        (5) No CSF drain

F. CARDIAC FUNCTION

I. OSCILLOMETRY (see section: E, "Vascular pressures")

II. DIAGNOSTIC (ECHO) ULTRASOUND

a. Human ear can hear frequencies of 20–20,000 Hz; ultrasound is the term used for frequencies above 20 kHz (1 kHz = 1,000 Hz)

b. Diagnostic ultrasound

1. Most common frequencies are 1–10 MHz (1 MHz = 1 million Hz)
2. Waves move about 1,500 m/s in tissue $\Rightarrow$ wavelength = 1.5 mm for 1-MHz frequency; 0.15 mm for 10-MHz frequency
3. Better resolution at higher frequencies
4. Depth of penetration reduced with higher frequency

c. Transducers

1. Piezoelectric crystals for generation and sensing of ultrasound
   (a) Ceramic materials, disk shape, thickness determines the operating frequency
   (b) Metalized front and back surfaces, wire leads to connect to amplifier or voltage pulse circuitry (to sense voltage generated by reflected pressure waves of characteristic frequency, or to apply voltage pulse to generate pressure wave)

d. Ultrasound absorbed by tissues, reflected and refracted at tissue interfaces (absorption of ultrasound by tissues generates heat; may explain physiotherapy use)

e. Reflection: echo generated if the characteristic impedances of two adjacent tissues differ

1. Characteristic impedance: (density of the tissue) × (speed of sound in that tissue)
2. Differences between tissues are small: bone impedance is very high, air very low
3. Angle of reflection from the tissue interface = angle of the incidence
   (a) Ultrasound beam needs to be perpendicular to tissue planes examined for greatest reflection
   (b) Dispersion at imperfect interface causes reflection in path wider than incident beam
4. Scanning techniques
   (a) A scan (amplitude scan, or A mode)
      (1) Crystal is transmitter and receiver
      (2) Echoes reflected back to the crystal are delayed by time intervals determined by the distance away from the transducer and the speed of sound in the tissues
      (3) Most useful where anatomic structures are not complex and accurate dimensions are not required (e.g., fetal dimensions)

    (b) B scan (brightness modulation of the display)
        (1) Brightness of spot on the display is proportional to intensity of echo at spot from which it is reflected
        (2) Helps identify the site of reflection of all the echoes received
    (c) M mode (time-position)
        (1) Vertical axis displays the depth of the reflecting surfaces from the transducer with varying degrees of brightness
        (2) Any movement is shown as spots moving up and down on the vertical axis
        (3) If time is added on the horizontal axis, a display across a screen can be read
    (d) Real-time scan
        (1) Pulsed ultrasound
            [a] A pulse of ultrasound is emitted from a transducer at the characteristic frequency of the transducer
            [b] Maximum pulse repetition rate is limited by the time taken for the echoes and their reverberations to return to the transducer
            [c] For penetration of 15 cm, one sweep takes 0.2 second, and this is followed by a dead period of about 0.1 second for the reverberations to die down
            [d] Maximum pulse repetition rate is about 3,000 per second
        (2) Phased arrays of transducers
            [a] Emission of pulses from a matrix of transducers is timed so that signals from each transducer are able to be recognized
            [b] From a single transducer, each pulse can contribute only a single line to a B scan
        (3) Real-time image
            [a] When images scanned at greater than 20 frames per second, they appear to the human eye to be moving and thus are seen to be "real time"
            [b] For satisfactory resolution, approximately 100 scan lines are needed (U.S. television has 625)
            [c] For pulse repetition rate of 3,000 per second, an image from 100 scan lines can be scanned completely 30 times a second; i.e., real time
        (4) Real-time scanners
            [a] Differ only in the array of their transducers, which may vary from 50 to several hundred
            [b] TEE (transesophageal echocardiography) probes use phased array transducers with some 50 transducers (crystals) arranged in parallel; time delay circuits steer ultrasound beam through scan sector

III. DOPPLER ULTRASOUND

a. Doppler effect

  1. When an ultrasound beam is reflected from a stationary object, the frequency of the reflected wave equals that of the transmitted wave
  2. If the reflector is moved toward the transmitter, it encounters more waves in a given time than does a stationary reflector so that the frequency of the waves impinging on the reflector appears to be increased

b. Simple continuous-wave Doppler ultrasound instrument

  1. Transmitting and receiving crystals are mounted side by side in a hand-held probe
  2. Although the receiver senses echoes from both static and moving objects, output is related to frequency shift; static reflections not detected
  3. These probes cannot detect depth accurately

c. Duplex scanners

1. Combine Doppler detection with real-time pulse echo imaging
2. Color flow Doppler (CFD) developed to interrogate a much larger volume of tissue
   - (a) Pulsed-wave technology
     - (1) Samples at multiple points along each ultrasound beam
     - (2) Much slower sampling rate
   - (b) Typically, blood flowing toward the probe is displayed in shades of red and that moving away is shown as blue
   - (c) Intensity of color reflects the velocity of the fluid movement

G. PATIENT SAFETY

I. NOTE: See "Gas supply" for patient safety issues regarding compressed gases

II. U.S. FOOD AND DRUG ADMINISTRATION (FDA) (medical device amendments [1976] to Federal Food Drug and Cosmetic Act [1938])

a. Mission

1. Premarket clearance
2. Monitoring (inspection, investigation, surveillance)
3. Compliance
4. Promulgation of regulations
5. Bioresearch monitoring
6. Health protection activities

b. Department of Health and Human Services

1. Public Health Service
   (a) FDA Policy Board
       (1) Commissioner
           [a] Center for Devices and Radiological Health (medical device classification, investigational device exemption, premarket notification, premarket approval, medical device reporting, radiologic health)
           [b] Center for Drugs and Biologics
           [c] Center for Food Safety and Applied Nutrition
           [d] Center for Veterinary Medicine
           [e] Center for Toxicological Research
           [f] Ten regional offices

c. Class I, general controls: registration of manufacturers, good manufacturing practice; record keeping and reporting; restriction of sale to certain professionals; notification of risks, repair, replacement, redesign; possible banning

d. Class II, performance standard: development of standards to provide assurance of safety and efficacy

e. Class III, premarket approval: for devices used to support or sustain human life and prevent impairment of human health

f. New devices

1. Premarket notification (510k)
   (a) Substantially equivalent to device existing prior to 1976

      (b) Contents of submission: device name, establishment registration number, classification, compliance with performance standard, proposed labeling, information to show substantial equivalency, additional information

      (c) Review process

         (1) 90 days (stated; actual is more than 120 days)

         (2) Cost is $100–300k

         (3) Preparation time about 4 months

2. Premarket approval

      (a) New device, class III

      (b) Contents of submission (24 topics, including intended use; device description; adverse effects; experimental design; data collection and reduction procedures; laboratory, animal, clinical data; software flowcharts and algorithms; standard compliance; labeling; company organization; samples)

      (c) Review process

         (1) 180 days (stated; actual over 250 days)

         (2) Cost

            [a] PMA with clinical trials: $0.6–1.5M

            [b] PMA without clinical trials: $300–600k

         (3) Preparation time about 1 year

3. Investigational device exemption (IDE)

      (a) Encourages discovery and development of useful devices intended for human use while protecting the public health

      (b) Applies to all clinical investigations of devices to determine safety and effectiveness

      (c) Significant risk device study

         (1) Institutional review board (IRB) approval of investigational plan and report of prior investigations

         (2) IDE application to FDA for review, obtain FDA approval of IDE, IDE number

            [a] Labeling

            [b] Distribution to qualified investigators

            [c] Informed consent

            [d] Monitoring

            [e] Prohibition of commercialization, promotion, misrepresentation

            [f] Records and reports to IRBs, investigators, FDA

         (3) Select qualified investigators, obtain signed agreements from them

         (4) Begin study

         (5) Significant-risk device

            [a] Presents significant risk to health safety, welfare of a subject, and

            [b] An implant (30 days or more), used in supporting or sustaining human life, or

            [c] Substantially important in diagnosing or treating disease

      (d) Nonsignificant-risk-device study

         (1) IRB review of investigational plan and reports of prior investigations; statement of why device does not present significant risk

         (2) Approval by IRB as nonsignificant-risk-device at its institution

         (3) Begin study

4. Near future/now

      (a) Software regulations

      (b) User fees

      (c) Preproduction quality assurance

III. PATIENT ELECTRICAL SAFETY

a. Distribution of electric power in hospitals

1. 4,800 V (volts), 60 Hz from substation via underground cables
2. Two stepdown transformers: 240 vac (volts alternating current) with grounded center tap to provide two 120-volt circuits
3. Essential electrical system for health care facilities
   (a) Normal source—one- or two-substation feed
   (b) Alternate source (e.g., generator on premises)—startup in 10 seconds or less of failure of normal source
4. Patient environments
   (a) 120-vac receptacles, wired with correct polarity, each with separate insulated ground conductor
       (1) Six or more receptacles for each patient bed location in critical care areas
       (2) Four or more in general care areas
       (3) 20 A (amperes) or more in each patient bed area
       (4) Receptacle retention force of grounding blade is 115 g or more (4 ounces)
       (5) Checked regularly
           [a] General care areas: 12 months
           [b] Critical care areas: 6 months
   (b) Ground system
       (1) Integrity throughout normal and essential power distribution
       (2) Criteria: voltage and impedance between reference points in or near room under test and ground contacts
           [a] 500 mv general care areas, 40 mv critical care areas (20 mv new construction)
           [b] 0.2 ohm impedance (0.1 ohm new construction)
       (3) Ground fault: short circuit between hot (high-voltage) and ground conductors (injects large current into ground conductor, causes voltage differences)
   (c) Electrical devices (instruments) used in patient care areas
       (1) Metal chassis and case (common design)
           [a] Macroshock hazard (uncommon occurrence): insulation failure (short circuit) between "hot" power supply lead and chassis or case
           [b] If chassis and case connected to ground wire, fault current conducted safely to ground
       (2) Leakage current—small ($\sim$ 1 mA [milliampere; 0.001 ampere]) resulting from
           [a] More than one instrument on same patient
           [b] Poor isolation of patient–instrument connections
           [c] Ground wire with high resistance
       (3) Safety checked regularly (NFPA requirement)
           [a] General care areas: 12 months
           [b] Critical care areas: 12 months
           [c] Wet locations: 6 months
   (d) Isolated power system (IPS)
       (1) Present in most operating rooms, theaters
       (2) NFPA requirement (1990) in "wet location patient care areas, Class W" (interpreted to include operating rooms)
       (3) Isolation transformer isolates both hot and neutral current conductors from ground
       (4) Line isolation monitor (LIM) detects occurrence of leakage of current from either hot or neutral conductor to ground conductor

           [a] Set point for alarm: 1.7–2 mA
           [b] Alarm does not shut off power; other current limiters (fuses, circuit breakers) must trip
           [c] Corrective action: check for offending instrument; call biomed technician or electrician; do not overreact

(e) Ground fault circuit interrupter (GFCI) system
    (1) Monitors current in hot and neutral conductors; if different, then ground fault is assumed and power to the circuit is shut off
    (2) Interrupts power if ground fault current exceeds set point (NFPA: 6 mA)
    (3) Acceptable system in wet-location patient care areas where power can be interrupted

b. Physiologic effects of electricity

1. Major effects

    (a) Resistive heating of tissue
    (b) Electrical stimulation of excitable tissue (nerve and muscle)
    (c) Electrochemical burns

2. Skin and body impedance

    (a) Skin
        (1) Major resistance to current flow through body if contact voltage source
        (2) Range: 15 to 1,000,000 ohms/cm^2, depending on moisture (e.g., sweat) content, anatomy
    (b) Body (skin broken, penetrated or wet; e.g., IV catheter, ECG electrode paste)
        (1) Each limb, about 200 ohms; trunk, about 100 ohms
        (2) Two limbs plus trunk, about 500 ohms

3. Perception of current: 70-kg man; 60 Hz applied for 1–3 seconds to wet hands, each grasping copper wire (i.e., macroshock)

    (a) 0.5 mA minimum, 1.1 mA mean; 2–10 mA direct current
    (b) Let-go current
        (1) Maximum current at which subject can withdraw voluntarily
        (2) 10 mA minimum (6 mA women); 16 mA mean

4. Respiratory paralysis, pain, fatigue: 20 mA or greater

5. Ventricular fibrillation

    (a) Point of entry
        (1) Macroshock—applied at two surface points; 75–400 mA minimum; if both points on same extremity, low risk of fibrillation
        (2) Microshock—internally applied at heart via intracardiac catheter; high current density; about 100 μA (microampere, 10^{-6} ampere), less than 1 second

6. Sustained myocardial contraction: 1–6 A (normal rhythm returns when current stopped; no irreversible damage)

7. Burns, physical injury: burns due to resistive heating, especially at current entry points over 10 A; may cause muscle–bone detachment due to excessive contraction; skin puncture over 240 volts ac

8. Frequency effects

    (a) 5 Hz: approximately 25 mA
    (b) 50–60 Hz (utility power supplies): approximately 15 mA
    (c) 400 Hz (aircraft power supplies): approximately 20 mA
    (d) 1 kHz: approximately 25 mA

c. Safe current limits for electromedical apparatus (American National Standards Institute [ANSI]/Association for the Advancement of Medical Instrumentation [AAMI] ES1-1993 [third edition; previous editions 1978, 1985])

1. Primarily United States, but with consideration of International Electrotechnical Commission Standard; Medical Electrical Equipment—Part 1: General Requirements for Safety (IEC 601-1, 1988)

2. Risk current—background

   (a) If grounding is lost or other safety methods fail, risk current from the enclosure (box) should not be a hazard to the patient
   (b) Survey of published data
      (1) Humans: mechanically induced ventricular fibrillation (VF) during cardiac catheterization (no current) has been observed; 15 μA smallest current reported to cause VF
      (2) Not all patients are equally susceptible to current-induced VF; normal distribution for currents to 300 μA (0.003 A); about 1% probability of fibrillation at 30 μA
      (3) Perception of current affected by contact location, pressure and area, skin condition, moisture content; range 300–500 μA
      (4) Worldwide, since advent of risk current standards, concern about grounding, better practice in handling catheters and invasive cardiac connections, no report of incidents involving risk current through the patient

3. Does not address composite risk current (from several devices used simultaneously)

4. Specifications for testing of electromedical apparatus intended for use in the patient care vicinity

5. Risk categories of electromedical apparatus

   (a) With isolated patient connection—intended to be connected to the patient with patient circuit isolated from power ground, utility power, other circuitry
   (b) With nonisolated patient connection—intended to be connected to the patient
   (c) Likely to contact patient—no patient-applied part, but intended for use in patient care vicinity
   (d) No patient contact—intended for use outside the patient care vicinity and without patient connections

6. Battery-powered equipment tested with charger connected to line power

7. Definitions

   (a) Enclosure—exterior surface of the electromedical apparatus, including all accessible parts, knobs, grips, shafts
   (b) Isolated patient connection—connection between the patient and the electromedical apparatus that is isolated from power (earth) ground, the utility power system, and other supporting circuitry such that current through the connection does not exceed established limits (below)
   (c) Patient-applied risk current—flows between any patient-applied part and power ground, exposed chassis conductive surfaces, a 200-cm^2 foil in contact with a nonconducting enclosure, or any other patient-applied part
   (d) Patient care vicinity—6 feet (1.8 meters) beyond normal location of bed, chair, table, treadmill, or other device that supports the patient during examination and treatment; 7.5 feet (2.3 meters) vertical extension above the floor
   (e) Patient connection—deliberate connection that can carry current between electromedical apparatus and a patient (e.g., skin surface electrode, implanted catheter); not casual contact (e.g., push-button, bed surface)
   (f) Risk current—nontherapeutic current that can flow through the patient, medical staff, or bystander

III. Patient electrical safety; c. Safe current limits for electromedical apparatus (continued)

    8. Risk current limits

       (a) 100 μA: from contact with enclosure (cord connected, battery powered, or permanently installed)

       (b) 10 μA: through patient connection

    9. Risk current limits versus frequency

       (a) Direct current to 1 kHz as above

       (b) Over range 1–100 kHz: limit is increased proportionally to a maximum of 100 times limit at 1 kHz (perception and lethality decrease as frequency increases; beyond 100 kHz, no reliable data for sinusoidal currents)

IV. OTHER PATIENT SAFETY STANDARDS AND AGENCIES

(standards useful for general information about devices, safety issues; voluntary compliance standards for U.S. manufacturers; applied by individual hospitals)

a. Other AAMI safety, labeling, and performance standards

    1. Blood pressure transducers

    2. Nonautomated sphygmomanometers

    3. Ambulatory electrocardiographs

    4. Automatic external defibrillators and remote control defibrillators

    5. Electrosurgical devices

    6. Pacemaker emergency intervention system

    7. Cardiovascular implants—vascular prostheses

    8. Intracranial pressure monitoring devices

b. Underwriters Laboratories Inc. (Melville, N.Y.; Standard for Medical and Dental Equipment, UL544)

c. National Fire Protection Association Inc. (Quincy, Mass.; Health Care Facilities, NFPA 99)

d. Compressed Gas Association (Arlington, Va.)

e. International Organization for Standardization (ISO; Geneva, Switzerland)

f. Deutscher Normenausschuss (DIN; Berlin, Germany)

V. EXPLOSION AND FIRE HAZARDS

a. Fuel + O_2 + spark $\rightarrow$ reaction products + energy (heat); combustible agent + oxidizing agent + activation energy $\rightarrow$ reaction products + energy

b. Inhalational anesthetic agents isoflurane and halothane are nonflammable (actually retard fire), but pure, compressed O_2 and/or N_2O in the presence of a fuel material is an extreme fire hazard

c. Potential fuels

1. Alcohol (skin preparations)
2. Degreasing agents
3. Paper drapes
4. Polymeric (disposable) devices
5. Bowel gas

d. Excessive temperature can cause oxidation reaction to be self-sustaining (i.e., combustion or explosion)

e. Activation energy and ignition temperature

1. Energy to cause molecules of flammable mixture to increase proximity
2. Temperature for combustion to start (400°C for many explosive mixtures)
3. Spark from voltage source (e.g., electrosurgery) can provide sufficient energy and temperature, because energy is concentrated
4. Spark from static charge (static electricity)
   (a) Important spark source, especially in low-humidity environments (i.e., relative humidity less than 50%)
   (b) Caused by charge separation due to dissimilar materials rubbing together
   (c) Causes static charge to dissipate with
       (1) Conductive contacts (wheels) for mobile equipment
       (2) Antistatic shoes/covers
       (3) Cotton clothes
       (4) Drapes treated with conductive polymer
       (5) Humidity
   (d) Conductive floors no longer required in operating rooms that use nonflammable anesthetic agents

f. Flammability limits

1. Mixture concentrations of combustible material or oxidizer in great excess of stoichiometric concentrations so that combustion cannot occur (e.g., cyclopropane 2.5–63% in O_2)
2. Modified with presence of other molecules (e.g., N_2, in air; cyclopropane 2.5–10% in air)

g. N_2O is oxidizing agent: explosion or fire can be more violent with mix of N_2O and O_2 than with only O_2

V. Explosion and fire hazards (continued)

h. Risk zones with flammable anesthetic agent

1. Anesthesia machine
2. Patient airway
3. 5-cm and 25-cm ranges around breathing systems, patient head (extended under drapes if used)
4. 5–25-cm range: anesthetic proof (AP) equipment; 0–5 cm: anesthetic proof category G (APG)
5. No electrical spark

i. Oxygen, compressed O_2

1. Especially high risk of fire and explosion
2. O_2 oxidizes all/most materials; concentrated, high-pressure O_2 oxidizes all/most materials rapidly; fires start more easily, burn hotter in presence of O_2-enriched atmosphere
3. With ignition source, very high-temperature fire can result
4. No oil, grease, polymeric fittings, organic material in O_2 supply systems, pressure regulators
5. Defective or contaminated equipment replaced, repaired

H. ELECTRICITY, ELECTRONICS, INSTRUMENTATION

I. VOLTAGE: movement of electrons in materials in other than random directions caused by a "voltage" across the material (e.g., flashlight battery voltage is approximately 1.5 volt; wall outlet voltage is approximately 110 volts in the United States, approximately 220 volts in Europe)

II. CURRENT: rate of flow of electrons through a conductor, measured in amperes (approximately 1 A through 100-watt light bulb)

III. RESISTANCE: measure of difficulty of electron movement (resistance of human body with intact skin approximately 5,000 times that of power cord wire; skin provides about 10–100 times the resistance of blood and internal tissues)

IV. CAPACITANCE: if two conductive surfaces are close, but not touching each other, charge can accumulate at the surfaces, building up voltage and energy between them

V. ALTERNATING CURRENT: voltage and resulting current continually reverse direction, at 60 hertz (Hz; cycles per second) in the United States, at 50 Hz in Europe

VI. BASIC CONCEPTS

a. Materials and physics

1. Electric charge—two kinds (named by Benjamin Franklin)
   (a) Positive (+): accumulates on glass rubbed with silk
   (b) Negative (−): accumulates on rubber rubbed with fur
2. Materials are electrically neutral; charge separation occurs to some extent on dissimilar materials when brought into contact
3. Classifications of materials
   (a) Conductors—electric charges free to move
      (1) Metals—(−) charge (only) is free to move; (+) charge immobile; free electrons (electrons in outer orbitals of metal atoms) are (−) charge carriers
      (2) Electrolytes—(+) and (−) charges free to move
   (b) Insulators (also called dielectrics)—electric charge immobile
      (1) No perfect insulators—charge conductance of materials in an electric field varies greatly with temperature (temperature coefficient)
      (2) Ceramic, polymeric materials
      (3) Dielectric constant (permittivity): $F = q_1q_2/4$
4. Properties of materials
   (a) Resistivity, ρ—basic electrical property; uniform material, voltage applied across it: $R = v/i$ (Ohm's law), $\rho = RA/L \,[=]\, \Omega\text{-cm}$, where L = length and A = cross-sectional area of material sample

VI. Basic concepts; a. Materials and physics (continued)

(b) $\rho \lesssim 10^{-2}$ Ω-cm—conductor (e.g., $\rho_{aluminum} \sim 10^{-6}$ Ω-cm); $\rho \gtrsim 10^5$ Ω-cm-insulator (e.g., $\rho_{epoxy} \sim 10^{-18}$ Ω-cm); $10^{-2} \lesssim \rho \lesssim 10^5$ Ω-cm-semiconductor: ρ can be varied greatly by design under precise control

5. Circuit elements
   (a) Resistance (passive—dissipates energy)
       (1) $v = iR$ (Ohm's law), where v = voltage across resistance (volts), i = current in resistance (amperes, A), R = resistance (ohms, Ω)
       (2) Macroscopic description of conducting materials in terms of voltage and current
   (b) Inductance (active—accumulates or dissipates energy)
       (1) $v = L\, di/dt$, where v = voltage across inductance, L = inductance (henrys), i = current in inductance, t = time
       (2) Relates current and voltage without need for magnetic field description
   (c) Capacitance (active)
       (1) $I = C\, dv/dt$, where I = current in capacitance, C = capacitance ([micro] farads, μF), v = voltage across capacitance, t = time (seconds)
       (2) Current in C is directly proportional to the time rate of change of voltage across C
       (3) dv/dt not infinite: no instantaneous change in voltage across a capacitance
       (4) Relates current induced in a conductor by a time-varying electric field and the voltage producing the field (without need for electric field description)
   (d) Voltage source (active)
   (e) Current source (active)

6. Impedance
   (a) Resistance to current flow due to circuit combination of active and passive elements
   (b) Series: $Z_{eq} = Z_1 + Z_2 + \ldots + Z_n$, Z_{eq}—equivalent impedance of circuit, Z_i—impedance of circuit element I
   (c) Parallel: $1/Z_{eq} = 1/Z_1 + 1/Z_2 + \ldots + 1/Z_n$
   (d) Input impedance (general)
       (1) Want to maximize input impedance to minimize disturbance (i.e., energy withdrawn) of quantity being measured
       (2) Ratio of input "effort variable" to input "flow variable"

b. Power and energy

1. Description
   (a) Joule is unit of energy (200–400 J is energy stored in capacitors of defibrillator transferred to patient)
   (b) Watt is unit of power (rate of energy transfer, joules per second; horsepower)
   (c) Work is power delivered (consumed) for a time (watt-second; kilowatt-hours)
2. Instantaneous power in circuit: $p = vi$, where p = power (watts), v = voltage across circuit element (volts); i = current in circuit element (amperes)
   (a) Resistor (or resistive circuit): $p = iR \cdot i = i^2R$
   (b) Capacitor: $p = v \cdot C\, dv/dt$
   (c) Inductor: $p = L\, di/dt \cdot i$

c. Semiconductor materials, devices

1. Energy band model of crystalline solids
   (a) Band gap for insulators 5 eV or over (e.g., silicon dioxide [SiO_2] about 9 eV;

silicon nitride [Si_3N_4] about 4.7 eV); for semiconductors; $0.5 \lesssim E_g \lesssim 2.5$ eV
(1 eV $= 1.6 \times 10^{-19}$ joule)

  (b) Apply electric field: electron jumps to next higher energy (conduction) band, leaves hole in lower (valence) band; electrons $+$ n $=$ total charge carriers

  (c) Vary number of charge carriers in semiconductor material by incorporating impurities (dopant atoms)

    (1) n-type—dopant adds extra electrons in conduction band (e.g., phosphorus)

    (2) p-type—dopant causes electron vacancies in valence band (e.g., boron)

    (3) 10^{15}–10^{20} dopant atoms/cm^3 (Si contains approximately 5×10^{22} atoms/cm^3)

2. Some devices able to be formed on (within) planar surface of semiconductor materials (primarily Si)

  (a) Resistor

  (b) Diode

  (c) Junction field effect transistor (JFET)

  (d) Metal oxide semiconductor field effect transistor (MOSFET)

  (e) Bipolar junction transistor

  (f) MOS capacitors, charge-coupled device (CCD)

  (g) Insulated gate field effect transistor (IGFET)

  (h) Light-emitting diode (LED)

  (i) Lasers

  (j) Typical dimensions: a few micrometers by a few micrometers

3. Commercial semiconductor materials

  (a) Si

    (1) Cheap, large band gap (compared with Ge), good processing and dopant properties

    (2) Formation of high-quality insulator layers, SiO_2, Si_3N_4

    (3) Selective etch process: hydrofluoric acid etches SiO_2, but not Si

    (4) Dope as p- or n-type in very localized regions of Si surface

  (b) Ge

    (1) Less reactive than Si (more easily processed)

    (2) Higher-frequency devices (high electron mobility)

    (3) Large devices only (poor dopant properties)

  (c) GaAs

    (1) Expensive

    (2) Important for high-frequency device operation (high electron mobility)

    (3) Solar cell performance, light emission

d. Integrated circuits (chips)

1. Typically hundreds to millions of semiconductor electronic devices in one integrated circuit (IC)

2. Need pure Si (i.e., dopant impurity 10^{13} cm^{-3} or less, or approximately one impurity atom per billion Si atoms—extreme purity required)

3. Molten Si with dopant (e.g., P or B, 0.1 mg/kg Si) grown into single crystal ingot (boule; 5–7 inches in diameter)

4. Slice (diamond saw) into wafers (10–20 mil thick)

5. Planar process technology, starting with IC design

  (a) Multiple mask—chemical etch—oven or ion implant, diffuse steps

  (b) Form hundreds of separate ICs on surface of 5- or 7-inch wafer; form millions of resistor, transistor, capacitor devices per integrated circuit

  (c) Cut (dice) wafer into separate ICs

  (d) Attach chip to package, form microscopic wire connections to macroscopic metal connectors, seal with encapsulant, ceramic or metal cover

VI. Basic concepts; d. Integrated circuits (continued)

  6. Some types of ICs
    (a) Linear (analog)
      (1) Operational amplifiers
        [a] 20–50 transistors
        [b] Voltage gain
        [c] Signals: dc, ac
      (2) Analog–digital (A-D) converters
        [a] Convert analog signals from pressure, temperature, other sensors to digital form for transmission, computer processing, numeric display
        [b] D-A converter needed to operate analog controller
      (3) Audio amplifier (FM receivers, sound equipment)
      (4) Television receiver (220- by 175-micrometer dimensions)
      (5) Voltage regulator
      (6) Regulated power supplies
    (b) Digital
      (1) Memories (millions of transistors)
        [a] Static random access memory (RAM)
        [b] Serial memory
        [c] Dynamic RAM (DRAM)
        [d] Read-only memory (ROM)
      (2) Central processor unit (CPU)
      (3) Floppy disk controller
      (4) Modem
      (5) Clock (MHz)

VII. ELECTRONIC (MEDICAL) INSTRUMENTS

a. Interface between transducer (sensor, actuator) and user

b. Transducers

  1. Pressure

    (a) Strain gauge—calibrated change of dimension (length of wire, area of membrane)
    (b) Membrane deflection—optical transducer

  2. Piezoelectric crystal

    (a) Ultrasound instruments: Doppler flow probe, transesophageal echography (TEE), imaging ultrasound
    (b) Vibration detection: noninvasive blood pressure instruments

  3. Temperature

    (a) Thermocouple
      (1) EMF across junction of two dissimilar metals (Peltier and Thomson effects); voltmeter circuit
      (2) Need reference junction temperature; moderate sensitivity (6.5–80 μV/°C)
      (3) Very small (to 12 micrometers in diameter); fast response; stable long term; accuracy 0.25–1%
    (b) Thermistor
      (1) Semiconductor material; resistor with large ($-$) temperature coefficient
      (2) Constant-voltage source; measure current through thermistor; bridge circuit

(3) Small (to 0.5 mm in diameter); large temperature sensitivity (-3 to $-5\%/°C$)

(4) Nonlinear—need linearizing circuit—slow response

(5) For example, oral temperature (IVAC)

4. Optical filters—control distribution of radiant power or wavelength

(a) Neutral density

(b) Color—transmit certain wavelengths

(c) Diffraction grating—provide wavelength spectrum in spectrophotometer

(d) Interference—reflective stack of layers on both sides of spacer; multiple reflection and interference effects; sharp-edge bandpass filters (below 0.5–200 nm)

5. Light sources

(a) Tungsten wire filament lamps

(1) Radiant output varies with temperature (low temperature—IR lamp; high temperature—blue flood lamp)

(2) Tungsten-halogen (iodine or bromine added to gases to fill bulb; tungsten combines with halogen in gas and redeposits on filament—bulb retains 90% of initial radiant output over life of bulb (nonhalogen about 50%)

(b) Arc discharge (fluorescent)

(1) Low-pressure Ar-Hg mix

[a] Electrons accelerate, collide with gas atoms, excite atoms, which emit light on transition to lower energy state; Hg maximum emission at 250 nm (UV)

[b] Phosphor on inside of bulb absorbs UV, emits visible

[c] Low radiant power/cm^2—not used in optical instruments

(2) High pressure

[a] Used in optical instruments

[b] Hg lamp (bluish); Na lamp (yellow); Xe lamp (white)

6. Optical fiber

(a) Transparent glass or polymer coated with second material with lower refractive index; total internal reflection

(b) Glass approximately 60% transmission, 50 cm, 400–1,200 nm; polymer approximately 70% transmission, 50 cm, 500–850 nm

(c) Noncoherent bundle—no precise fiber alignment; used to transmit light (e.g., intravascular oximetry [Svo_2]); diameter—10–100 μm (1 micrometer = 1,000 nm)

(d) Coherent bundle—transmit image from one end to the other

(e) Endoscope—coherent bundle with lens for image; noncoherent bundle for illumination

7. Radiation detectors

(a) IR (heat)—thermistor, thermocouple with appropriate package (slow response; no spectral selectivity)

(b) Quantum (photon)

(1) Phototube—photo cathodes coated with alkali metals; electrons emitted (if photon energy sufficient; λ less than 1,200 nm), attracted to anode

(2) Photomultiplier—multiple phototube elements; most sensitive detectors (individual photons)

(3) Photo resistor—photosensitive crystal material (CdS, PbS) on ceramic substrate with electrode contacts; photon causes electron to "jump" energy (band) gap with resultant electron-hole current

(4) Photo junction (silicon p-n junction) devices—optical isolator devices (electrical safety)

8. (Wheatstone) bridge circuits (see figure)

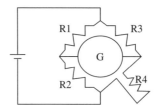

(a) Measure small changes in resistance of resistive-type transducer
(b) Null balance: calibrated variable resistor changed to balance change in transducer resistance
(c) Deflection balance: bridge imbalance is measure of change of transducer resistance
(d) G-voltmeter readout; R_4-transducer, R_3-variable resistor
(e) Elements may be reactive elements; ac voltage may energize bridge; dc battery indicated; $R_1/R_2 = R_3/R_4$ is balance condition

---

c. Amplifiers, signal processing

1. Operational amplifier (op amp) (see figure)

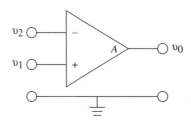

(a) High-gain dc differential amplifier
(b) Voltage at v_1 (inverting input) is greatly amplified and inverted with output at v_0; voltage at v_2 (noninverting input) is greatly amplified to give in-phase output at v_0; no current into either terminal
(c) Combined with other elements (resistors, capacitors, diodes, transistors) to provide many basic analog functions (e.g., inverter, adder, differentiator, integrator)

---

d. Microprocessor (microcomputer)

1. Reduces complexity of instrument by reducing number of op amps, ICs, printed circuits
2. Provides
    (a) Self-calibration, error detection (storage of empirical data)
    (b) Automated, specified sequencing of events (controller function)
    (c) Computing
3. Data acquisition, handling
    (a) A-D converter (separate IC)—converts conditioned (amplified, filtered) analog signal to digital format
    (b) Central processor unit (CPU)
        (1) Accepts data, transfers data, performs some arithmetic operations, all under direction of a program
        (2) Registers store instructions (program steps), keep place in program

(c) Memory
  (1) Random access memory (RAM; read-write)—volatile (temporary data storage; lost when power off); current instructions, data, file
  (2) Read-only memory (ROM)—permanent storage of data, instructions, program
  (3) System memory
    [a] Configured for DOS applications (see figure)

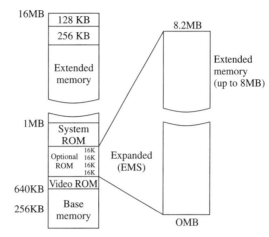

    [b] Windows 95 integrates DOS and application software
(d) Bus
  (1) Transfers data, instructions to different elements of microcomputer
  (2) Set of 4 (original), 8, 16, 32 (current standard), or 64 lines, each of which carries a bit, and together carry a digital word (byte)
(e) Clocks—create uniform operating cycle for all microcomputer elements; bytes transfer at clock rate (e.g., 166 MHz, or a million times per second)
(f) Program (software)
  (1) Reprogram instead of rewire
  (2) Sequential set of instructions executed in order without (human) operator
  (3) Coded in machine language (compiled from a higher-order programming language, e.g., C or C++)
  (4) Instructions transfer data to and from CPU, operate on data in CPU (increment, decrement, compare, add, subtract), move to another place in program (jump, "go to" instruction)
  (5) "Interrupt" allows external device to stop program execution and process new input data

e. Modular components

1. Power supply
2. Amplifier, signal conditioner
3. Microcomputer(s)
4. Controls, switches
5. Display
6. Each component may include integral electronics, microcomputer

f. Evolution

1. Monitor instruments
   (a) Stand-alone instrument ⇒ physiologic monitor module

VII. Electronic (medical) instruments; f. Evolution (continued)

    (b) Product of startup corporation (miniaturized) $\Rightarrow$ larger corporation (license to, for example, HP, Marquette, Spacelabs)

2. Time

    (a) 1950s: mechanical switches; discrete electrical components mounted on plates, frames; soldered wire connections; CRT, indicator light displays

    (b) 1960s: semiconductor solid-state electronic devices mounted on printed circuit boards; solderless connectors; modular components; color CRT, gas plasma discharge (Nixie) tubes

    (c) 1970s: integrated circuit chips, semiconductor devices, hybrid printed circuit boards; edge connectors; modular components; portable equipment, rechargeable batteries; color CRT, LED segment display, liquid crystal display (LCD)

    (d) 1980s: microcomputers (all/most electronic equipment), ICs, printed circuits; CRT, flat-panel LCD

    (e) 1990s: high-capacity memory, optical memory, high-speed microcomputers, networks, wireless data communication

VIII. COMPUTER NETWORKS

a. Local area network (LAN)

1. Data communication network over limited area (a few square miles at most)

2. Original idea: share expensive devices (printers, mass memory)

3. Now: essential information transfer system; all forms of stored information (image, text, voice)

4. Types of LANs

    (a) Baseband: typical in office environment

        (1) Ethernet

        (2) Arcnet

        (3) Token Ring

    (b) Broadband (similar to cable TV)

5. LAN topology

    (a) How LAN cabling is organized, arranged to connect scattered computers, other devices

    (b) Bus, ring, star: determines media access control method (e.g., Ethernet or Token Ring)

    (c) Buses easily expanded; require a lot of cable

    (d) Ring; popularized by IBM as Token Ring (introduced 1984): token (electronic signal; series of data bits) is passed from station to station on the ring; enables network access and data packet transmission (16 Mbs); reliable, expandable

    (e) Star: typical mainframe or minicomputer environment; system of terminals wired directly to central processor (AT&T: Starlan and PBX [private branch exchange]–based network); each workstation connected via dedicated cable to central concentrator

6. LAN protocols

    (a) Protocol stack: set of rules for communicating between computers

    (b) Format, timing, sequence, error control; packetizing of file

    (c) Software (program) that resides in network interface card or in PC; protocol software executed when instruction for data transmission is issued; standard or proprietary

    (d) Standard

(1) Widely agreed upon set of rules to allow PCs from different vendors to communicate

(2) Open System Interconnection (OSI)

[a] Set of protocols

[b] Divides communication process into seven "layers": 1. physical (cable, interconnect specs) →→→→ 7. application (interface between software running in PC and network, e.g., e mail, file transfer)

[c] Modular; each layer works with others; more than one protocol can exist at any layer

[d] Middle layers developing: TCP/IP (Transmission Control Protocol/ Internet Protocol; TCP is transport, IP is session protocol; Department of Defense developed); NetBIOS (Network Basic Input/Output System; IBM developed); APPC (Advanced Program to Program Communication; IBM developed)

[e] Applications written for TCP/IP: FTP (File Transfer Protocol); SMTP (Simple Mail Transfer Protocol); SNMP (Simple Network Management Protocol)

[f] Supported by most computer and network vendors, most governments, including the United States

[g] Promulgated by International Standards Organization (ISO)

(e) Proprietary (e.g., AppleTalk [Apple Computers, Inc.]; Network Filing System [Sun Microsystems, Inc.])

7. Network interface card: provides physical and functional connection to network

(a) Functions

(1) Data to and from PC via network card

(2) Buffering

(3) Packetization (packet formation)

[a] Packet is basic unit of data for transmission

[b] Header, data, trailer

[c] Ethernet 4KB packet size

(4) Parallel-serial conversion

[a] From PC in parallel format: 8, 16, or 32 bits, depending on bus width

[b] Cable transit in serial form (1 bit at a time)

(5) Encode–decode (encode into 1s and 0s after parallel-to-serial conversion)

[a] Manchester encoding (Ethernet)

[b] Differential Manchester encoding (Token Ring)

(6) Cable access: protocol (e.g., token) generation circuitry, firmware reside on network card

(7) Handshaking

[a] To send data, a second network card must be waiting to receive

[b] Transmitting card sends signal to receiving card, sets parameters (e.g., maximum packet size, number of packets, buffer sizes, etc.)

(8) Transmission (network card's transceiver provides power to send data along cable; transceiver in receive mode accepts data for decoding, serial-parallel conversion, depacketizing)

(b) Fits into expansion slot of computer

(c) Laptops may need external interface box or desktop expansion (docking) station

8. Physical network: connects network devices

(a) Cable

(1) Coaxial

[a] Standard Ethernet

[b] Thin Ethernet (black; about ¼ inch in diameter; uses biconic [BNC] connector)

             [c] Thick Ethernet (yellow jacket; about ½ inch in diameter; uses vampire tap; 2,000-foot range between PCs

        (2) Twisted pair
           [a] Commonly used for telephone voice transmission
           [b] Lighter, thinner, cheaper, easier to install than coaxial
           [c] Shielded, unshielded (mainstay of office environment)

    (b) Optical fiber
        (1) Broad bandwidth, very long-distance transmission without loss, no electromagnetic interference
        (2) Secure: difficult to tap directly
        (3) Expensive
        (4) Backbone for subnetwork connection
        (5) Image communication
        (6) Standards in process: IEEE standard for fiberoptic Ethernet; ANSI Fiber Distributed Data Interface (100-Mbs network)

  9. Network operating systems (NOS)

    (a) Analogous to DOS; operates more than one computer
    (b) Allows LAN users to share files, peripherals; provides security, data integrity; internetworking support
    (c) Redirector software
        (1) Operations across network (e.g., copy c:fileA f:fileA—"f" resides on another computer attached to the network)
        (2) Applies to peripherals (e.g., modems)
    (d) Server software
        (1) Computer running server software
        (2) Dedicated (not used as workstation)
        (3) Nondedicated (users do administrative functions, e.g., backup of data, security)
    (e) File service
        (1) Extension of local PC
        (2) Map to logical (virtual) drive
           [a] Drive f: typically designated as file server's hard drive
           [b] Process of accessing virtual drive: mounting, mapping
        (3) Applications, files that reside on server disk transfer to local (user's) PC (e.g., f:WINWORD loads from server to user's PC; if multiple license, another user can load and run WINWORD at the same time)
        (4) File server computer, internal hardware, software
        (5) Gigabyte (Gb) hard drives
    (f) File backup (tape cartridges; optical disks)

 10. Mainframe gateways

    (a) Physical link between PCs and host mainframe
    (b) VTAM (virtual telecommunications access method) resides in mainframe; has information about every device that is connected
    (c) SDLC (synchronous data link control) gateway: card in a designated network PC for connection of network PCs to mainframe

b. Internet

  1. Global, nonproprietary information infrastructure

  2. 1964: Rand Corp proposal addressing how to maintain communication of U.S. authorities after a nuclear war

(a) Decentralized (no central authority; designed from the beginning to operate while in "tatters"; assumed unreliable at all times)

(b) Separate nodes with equal authority

(c) Messages divided into packets, each separately addressed, tossed like hot potatoes from node to node, reassembled at destination address

(d) Secure system, difficult to eavesdrop

(e) Different from telephone circuit switch technology (connection made from phone to phone for duration of call; no other user of that circuit)

3. 1973: Defense Advanced Research Project Agency (DARPA) research program to develop communication protocols to let networked computers communicate transparently across multiple linked packet switching networks of various kinds

(a) Called internetting project; networks that were linked were called the Internet

(b) System of interconnection protocols developed
    (1) TCP (transmission control protocol)
    (2) IP (internet protocol)
    (3) TCP/IP "suite": about 100 protocols

4. 1986: National Science Foundation initiated NSFnet

(a) Current communication backbone of Internet

(b) 45-Mbs fiberoptic telephone line facilities leased from AT&T, MCI, and Sprint

(c) Total about $20M NSF funding: funding of network backbone stopped April 30, 1995; funding of 17 regional networks goes to $0 by 1998; move to private backbone service providers

(d) Individual user has had no cost, no capacity limit

(e) Some 25,000 networks linked worldwide; about 30 million users; approximately 10% per month increase in users

5. 1983: Internet Activities Board

(a) Internet Engineering, Research Task Forces (standards development; new concepts)

(b) Internet Registry: Domain Name System (DNS) root database
    (1) Distributed database associates host and network names with Internet addresses (critical to higher-level TCP/IP protocol operation, including e mail)
    (2) Connectivity is now bundled as standard function of new PCs

6. European Internet: CERN largest Internet site in Europe

7. Internet access, software industry: three lanes on the information highway

(a) Electronic mail (e mail)
    (1) Send, receive messages, documents
    (2) e mail address
        [a] User id@host computer name .subdomain.subdomain. subdomain.domain
        [b] Internet maintains registry (see "Internet registry" above)

(b) Bulletin boards
    (1) Post messages, notes, documents for interested subscriber to read, respond
    (2) Usenet newsgroups: many, many subjects, including anesthesiology: listserv@mcon00.med.nyu.edu
    (3) Subscriber address and user address

(c) WWW (World Wide Web), Web browsers, servers
    (1) Graphic user interface (GUI) to Internet: no need to type instructions
    (2) Responsible for much recent interest in Internet
    (3) Body of software, set of protocols and conventions; hypertext and multimedia techniques
    (4) CERN (Conseil Européen pour la Recherche Nucleaire; Swiss–French border near Geneva) initiative; started about 1990

            (5) WWW consortium
              [a] Development of common standards for WWW evolution
              [b] Industry funded consortium directed by MIT Laboratory for Computer Science, collaboration with CERN, INRIA (French Institut National de Recherche en Informatique et en Automatique)
            (6) HTTL (Hypertext Transfer Protocol): object-oriented application-level protocol for hypermedia information systems
            (7) HTML (Hypertext Markup Language)
              [a] Format for documents and data
              [b] Make easily using Microsoft Word or WordPerfect editor (save as HTML)
       (d) Bandwidth limits of Internet
            (1) Since about 1993, powerful PCs and SWs enable transmission of high-resolution color images, sound files, full-motion video
              [a] Transmission delay not tolerable
              [b] Anyone with camcorder—multimedia PC video conference causes overload of parts of Net
            (2) Expect technology improvements from 2.4 Gbs (billion bits per second, present state of art) to 40 Gbs transmission rate by 1998
       (e) Commerce on Internet embryonic
            (1) SW delivery
            (2) Advertising
            (3) Publication

IX. WIRELESS TELECOMMUNICATION

a. Microwave, satellite, infrared, radio frequency (RF), laser; wider and deeper than regional digital networks or LANs

b. Channel: width of a RF spectrum band, typically 30 kHz for cellular phones

c. RF spectrum is "land rush of '90s"

1. Low frequency (30–300 Hz [about 3-km wavelength]; marine and aeronautical navigational equipment)

2. Medium frequency (300–3 MHz [about 300-meter wavelength]; AM radio, long-distance marine, aeronautical navigation)

3. High frequency (3–300 MHz [about 30-meter wavelength]; short wave, citizens' band, amateur radio)

4. Very high frequency (30–300 MHz [about 3-meter wavelength]; TV (channels 2–13), FM radio, private mobile land radio [police, fire dispatch])

5. Ultrahigh frequency (300 MHz–3 GHz [about 30-cm wavelength]; cellular phone, personal communication services, wireless data networks, UHF TV, microwave long-distance phone transmission)

6. Superhigh frequency (3–30 GHz [about 3-cm wavelength]; radar, microwave and satellite transmission)

d. Cells

1. Geographic area divided into sections called "cells," 1–20 miles wide
2. Callers in different cells use same frequencies
3. Microcells about 1–300 feet wide; developing for digital wireless pocket-size communicators

e. Pagers: about 18 million (United States; 1993); about 3 million (China; 1993)

f. Cellular phones

1. Hand-held cellular radio phone (radio transceiver on 2-inch by 3-inch circuit board), $2,500: Motorola, 1986
2. About 30 million (1994); about 100 million (2000)
3. Basic function
   (a) Cellular phone→cell site→mobile telephone switching office (MTSO)→local phone exchange
   (b) Wire (noncellular) phone→MTSO→broadcast to all cells→ destination cellular phone
   (c) For moving cellular phone "hand off" to adjacent cell and open frequency as MTSO detects signal weakening
4. Analog mobile phone service (AMPS; AT&T/Bell Labs)
   (a) Current standard for cellular phones
   (b) RF analog of sound waves is transmitted

g. Digital cellular phone services (developing; wireless regional networks; personal communication service [PCS])

1. Digital wireless services; make calls from pocket phones, send data from personal data assistant (PDA)
2. Expected to be widely available by late 1990s
3. Microcells, low-power transceivers, higher frequency channels than current cell phones
4. Digital data compression (about eight times): different proposed standards
   (a) TDMA (time division multiple access)
   (b) CDMA (code division multiple access; spread spectrum)

h. Developing technology

1. Frequency hopping (portable communicators search for empty channel every 0.5 second; regional wireless network)
2. Higher frequencies (RF signals of 3 GHz or higher behave like light beams; move in straight lines, bounce off objects, do not penetrate walls)
   (a) 28-GHz video transmission for interactive video, cable TV alternative (Cellular Vision, Bell Atlantic Corp.)
   (b) 1.8-GHz LAN based on GaAs semiconductor devices, sophisticated antenna (Altair, Motorola Inc.)

i. Earth orbit communication systems (developmental; FCC licenses approved)

1. Satellite network in low or high earth orbit to extend cell system over most of earth's surface
2. High-power portable phones with direct satellite connect
3. Voice, data, fax, physical location, monitoring from hand-held portable device
4. Several companies (e.g., Iridium Inc. [66 satellites]; Teledesic. Corp. (McCaw–Microsoft [840 satellites])

X. BATTERIES

a. Primary (no recharge): electrochemical energy converter with internal storage of reactants

1. Carbon-zinc (1.5 volts)
2. Alkaline-manganese-zinc (1.5 volts)
3. Mercuric oxide (1.35 or 1.4 volts)
4. Silver oxide (1.5 volts)
5. Lithium (about 10 times NiCd energy density)

b. Secondary (rechargeable): input electric energy converted to chemical energy and stored; accumulator

1. Rechargeable alkaline-manganese dioxide (50–60 charge–discharge cycles)
2. Nickel cadmium (NiCd; sealed; 1.2 volts)
    (a) 10–14-hour charge
    (b) Hundreds of charge–discharge cycles
    (c) Memory effect
        (1) After several shallow discharges, cell will not discharge fully
        (2) Battery will charge, discharge rapidly; will not deliver designed Wh capacity
        (3) Prevent by allowing to discharge completely until recharge (e.g., recharge cellular telephone when "lo bat" message displayed)
    (d) Sealed lead acid (e.g., Gel Cell)—rapid charge

c. Capacity—ampere-hours

d. Energy density

1. Energy (watt-second; ampere-volt-seconds per weight [kg] [or per volume])
2. NiCd approximately 40 Wh/kg; Ag_2OZn approximately 100 Wh/kg
3. Depends on weight of active materials, electrode current density
4. Varies with power (rate of energy delivery)

e. Power density

1. Rate of energy delivery (watts; ampere-volts) per weight (kg) or per volume

2. Limited by current density at electrodes (diffusional and resistive effects)
3. High energy density $\Rightarrow$ low power density

XI. MEDICAL IMAGING SYSTEMS

a. Information content—number of pixels (picture elements) × number of amplitude levels of each pixel

b. Number of amplitude levels—signal-to-noise ratio (S/N)

c. Resolution

1. Surface of some dimension with number of line pairs per millimeter (lp/mm)
2. Objects and spaces between object count equally
3. One object requires ≥ 1 lp, 2 pixels on each axis
4. If n objects, need $2n\sqrt{2}$ scan lines to detect them and the spaces between them
5. Blanking time

   (a) Time for camera and monitor tube scanning electron beams to magnetically reposition to start point for each horizontal scan line and each vertical field; about 18% of total horizontal time for each line

   (b) 525-line U.S. standard TV

   (1) About 480 lines visible, vertical resolution about 180 objects

   (2) Each 1/30-second image frame is 2-1/60 seconds, 262.5-line frames interlaced; retrace and blanking about 8% of frame time

   (3) Horizontal resolution about 240 objects

   (4) Bandwidth $= n_h n_v 2\sqrt{2}/F_h F_v T = (240)(180)2\sqrt{2}/(.82)(.92)(1/30)$
   $= 4.85$ MHz, T-frame scan time, $F_{h,\,v}$-fraction scan time spent on picture (1.0-blank fraction), $n_{h,\,v}$-number objects in horizontal, vertical scan

   (c) Matrix of independent detectors or visual field elements (e.g., charge-coupled device, CCD)

   (1) Solid-state detectors (e.g., 512×512 photo diodes)

   (2) Light partially discharges each diode; scan process transfers remaining charge to storage part of detector

   (3) Charge transferred from detector to detector (shift register) to output bus, amplified

   (4) Resolution, 512×512 matrix: $512(2\sqrt{2}) \times 512(2\sqrt{2}) = 181 \times 181$ (similar to TV)

6. Modulation transfer function (MTF)

   (a) Needed in addition to spatial resolution to account for contrast

   (b) Amplitude response of imaging system as function of spatial frequency

d. Radiography

1. High-voltage generator, x-ray tube, collimator, object (patient), grid, intensifier screen, photographic film
2. Typical: 80 kVp (kilovolts peak), 300 mA, 0.1 second; power $\simeq 100$ kW
3. Patient absorbs 95–99% of radiation; some scattered as secondary radiation, 1–4% transmitted to detector (lead grid with ribs aligned with source to block secondary radiation from film)

XI. Medical imaging systems; d. Radiography (continued)

    4. Intensifying screen (polymeric substrate coated with scintillation powder, e.g., $CaWO_4$) placed against double emulsion film—reduce exposure requirement (choose film–screen combination to minimize exposure)

e. Computed tomography (CT; computer assisted tomography, CAT)

1. Originally developed for brain imaging
2. Plane-film transmission radiography is projection of information in one direction; large range of electron density along beam path
3. Anatomic information reconstructed from x-ray transmission data projected from many directions
4. Scan x-ray beam source and detector about 160 evenly spaced points; rotate source-detector 1 degree, repeat through 180 degrees $\Rightarrow$ about 29,000 measurements of x-ray absorption
5. Two-dimensional function is determined by its projections in all directions $\Rightarrow$ reconstruct two-dimensional image of x-ray absorption as function of position as 160×160 matrix of square picture elements
6. Image reconstruction during data acquisition
   (a) Iterative model array
   (b) Analytic back projection
7. Rapid CT (cine CT)
   (a) No mechanical scan of x-ray source-detector
   (b) Magnetically deflected x-ray beam $\Rightarrow$ obtain multiple slices simultaneously $\Rightarrow$ decrease scan time (cardiac imaging—right, left ventricular volumes, wall thickness; chest, abdomen) $\Rightarrow$ image available within minutes

f. Emission computed tomography

1. Same principles as x-ray CT
2. Image distribution of radioactivity
3. Measure sums of activity along straight lines
   (a) Single photon emission computed tomography (SPECT)
      (1) Count rate of nuclear particles
      (2) Cardiac studies—thallium-201 (^{201}Tl); technetium 99m pyrophosphate (^{99m}TcPYP)
      (3) Cerebral blood flow—^{133}Xe
   (b) Positron emission tomography (PET)
      (1) Positron (antielectron) from decaying nucleus travels few millimeters in tissue
      (2) Annihilation with atomic electron
      (3) Produces two gamma rays in opposite directions $\Rightarrow$ two opposed detectors
      (4) Coincidence count rate (gamma ray emitted at same time) proportional to total activity along line of two detectors
      (5) Image information—absorption of radiation between decay event and detector (based on modeled and measured absorption)
      (6) No radiation scatter
      (7) Expensive, cumbersome equipment
      (8) Isotopes of O_2, carbon, nitrogen, and fluorine
      (9) Cerebral physiology, lung tomography, estimation of lung water

g. Magnetic resonance imaging (MRI; developed late 1960s)

1. Atomic nuclei with unpaired nuclear protons (odd number of protons or neutrons, e.g., H nuclei) have spin axes

2. In externally applied magnetic field, spin axes align with "wobble" (i.e., precess around the axis parallel to magnetic field)

3. Apply second excitation field at radio frequency (RF) $\Rightarrow$ shift alignment or precession

4. Realign $\Rightarrow$ emit electromagnetic signal with specific frequency

   (a) Time constants

       (1) T1 (spin lattice time constant)

           [a] Rate at which nuclei align

           [b] Function of element, temperature, viscosity, interaction of nuclei with surrounding tissue

           [c] Tissue resolution: T1 short—protein bound water; T1 long—free water; T1 intermediate—water in fat; absence of bone artifact

       (2) T2 (spin—spin time constant; interaction of nuclei; characteristic of tissue)

   (b) T1,2 determine excitation field and measurement frequency for optimum image

   (c) ^{31}P, ^{13}C—other nuclei abundant in tissue with resonant frequencies that can be detected

5. Computer analysis to create image

6. Intense magnetic fields limit equipment and personnel access

   (a) Equipment near scanner ferrometal-free

   (b) Batteries in nonmetallic laryngoscopes cause problems

   (c) Signal degradation in patients with metal-based prosthetic devices (dental bridgework, pacemakers, aneurysm clips, ventricular shunts, prosthetic heart valves)

   (d) These devices can also cause injury to the patient if any movement or heating

7. Full-body imager—long image acquisition times (30–60 minutes), claustrophobia may require patient sedation or full general anesthesia

8. Partial-body imager—designed for anatomic parts (e.g., knee)

9. Rapid image acquisition—cardiac imaging (LV volume, ejection fraction) using cardiac cycle synchronized pulse; construct image over several cycles

I. STATISTICS

I. STATISTICAL ANALYSIS PROGRAMS are commonly available

a. With spread sheet programs (e.g., Microsoft Excel, Borland Quattro Pro)

b. Specialty statistics packages (e.g., StatSoft Statistica; Abacus Concepts Statview; SAS Institute Inc. Statistical Analysis System)

c. Choice of "right" analysis requires basic knowledge

II. DESCRIPTIVE: organization, presentation, summarization of data

a. Vital: describe health status of populations; derived from official recording of vital events (births, deaths, occurrences of communicable diseases)

1. Mortality rates
2. Morbidity rates
3. Adjusted rates
4. Population life table

   (a) Hypothetical population
   (b) Summary of mortality experience at particular time or period, e.g., particular year

b. Statistical inference: logical basis for conclusions regarding populations drawn from results obtained in a sample of the population; based on mathematical theory of probability

1. Target population: that population about which an investigator wants to draw a conclusion
2. Population sampled: that population from which the sample was drawn and about which a conclusion can be drawn
3. Bias: way(s) in which target and sampled populations differ
4. Selective factors: distinguish the target and sampled populations

c. Scales of measurement

1. Nominal

   (a) Unordered, dichotomous; either–or (lived, died); 0–1 scale
   (b) Unordered, multichotomous (no ordering, e.g., blood groups)

2. Ordered classification (predetermined order, e.g., improved, no change, deteriorated)

3. Ranks: full ranking scale—arrays members of group from high to low according to magnitude of observations
4. Numeric discrete data: observations are integers (count, e.g., number of heartbeats within a time interval, RBCs in a grid)
5. Numeric continuous data: most clinical measurements (e.g., BP, serum glucose, height, age)

d. Frequency distribution: series of predetermined classes presented together with counts of number of observations that fall within interval for each class

1. Tabular presentation (table often clearer than prose)
2. Graphs: aid reader in comprehending data (e.g., histogram—area of bar depicts frequency)

e. Summarization of data

1. Averages (location; central tendency)
   (a) Mean (arithmetic): $\bar{x} = \Sigma x/n$; seriously affected by extreme values; easiest for mathematical treatment
   (b) Median: "middlemost" observation; one half of observations exceed median and one half are less than median; unaffected by extreme observations; better descriptive measure if data are skewed; if even number of observations, median is halfway between observation $n/2$ and $n/(2+1)$
   (c) Mode: most frequently occurring observation; used rarely
2. Spread (variation)
   (a) Range: largest minus smallest number
   (b) Mean deviation
   $$\Sigma|x - \bar{x}|/n$$
   (c) Variance, $V(x)$
   $$\Sigma(x - \bar{x})^2/(n - 1)$$
   (d) Degrees of freedom (df)
      (1) For a series of numbers, df is number of independent quantities among entire series; or df is total number of quantities in series minus number of restrictions imposed on quantities
      (2) For deviations about the mean (series $x - \bar{x}$): n deviations, one restriction
      $$(\Sigma(x - \bar{x}) = 0) \Rightarrow n - 1 \text{ df}$$
   (e) Standard deviation (SD)
      (1) $SD(x) = \sqrt{V(x)} = \sqrt{\Sigma(x - \bar{x})/(n - 1)}$
      (2) $V(x)$ readily calculated; disadvantage is squares of units of measure
      (3) Mean ± 1 SD includes approximately 67% of observations
          Mean ± 2 SD includes approximately 95% of observations
          Mean ± 3 SD includes approximately 99% of observations
   (f) Coefficient of variation (CV)
      (1) $CV = 100\% \, SD/mean$
      (2) Used to compare relative spread of distributions
   (g) Standard error of mean (SE)
      (1) Applies to sample data (repeated samples, means of each sample of size n)
      (2) SD of sampling distribution of means
      (3) $SE(\bar{x}) = \sigma/\sqrt{n}$

II. Descriptive (continued)

f. Variability of clinical measurements

1. Unbiasedness—tendency to obtain "true" value

2. Precision—spread of series of observations (medical data may be unbiased but imprecise, or vice versa)

3. Accuracy—unbiased and precise (inaccurate measurements may be biased, imprecise, or both)

4. Skewness (symmetry)

5. Sources of variation

   (a) True biologic—make individuals different
   (b) Temporal—produce variation in observations in an individual over time
   (c) Measurement error—produce differences among measurements (observers, instruments, stability of reagents, technician error, ambient conditions)
   (d) To separate true biologic and measurement sources—replicate measurements (duplicate, triplicate, etc.)
       (1) Intersubject variability (true biologic source)—calculate means of repeated measurements in each subject; calculate variance of these means
       (2) Intrasubject variability (measurement error source)—calculate variance of replicate measurements on each subject; calculate mean variance
       (3) Use source of variation that is most relevant to the goals of the analysis
       (4) Basis of analysis of variance (ANOVA)—isolate and assess contribution of different factors to variation of data

6. Variation and interpretation of clinical data

   (a) Reproducibility by different researchers, physicians, institutions, laboratories (effect of measurement error)
   (b) Measurement distribution in normal and abnormal (sick) individual (what is true biologic variation, or physiologic norm?)
   (c) Unusual occurrences (temporal variation and other effects, e.g., patient agitation, temperature; time of day)

III. PROBABILITY: long-run relative frequency of an event in repeated trials under similar conditions, Pr(A); complementary event—probability that the event does not occur, $1 - Pr(A)$

a. Additive law: for mutually exclusive events

$$Pr(A \text{ or } B \text{ or } C \text{ or } \ldots) = Pr(A) + Pr(B) + Pr(C) + \ldots$$

b. Conditional probability: depends on outcome of other event(s); probability of event B if A has already occurred, $Pr(B|A)$ (e.g., survival next year, $Pr[B]$, depends on survival this year, $Pr[A]$)

c. Multiplicative law: chance that two independent events A and B both happen

$$Pr(A \text{ and } B) = Pr(B|A)Pr(A)$$

d. Independent events

$$Pr(B|A) = Pr(B), Pr(A \text{ and } B) = Pr(A)Pr(B)$$

e. Bayes' theorem

1. Logic system for medical diagnosis
2. For mutually exclusive diagnoses, A1, A2, . . . Ak, and a particular complex of symptoms, signs, and lab results, B: Pr(Ai|B) is chance of occurrence of ith diagnosis, given patient presents symptoms B (must be known for each of k mutually exclusive diagnoses); Pr(Ai) is fraction of patients with ith diagnosis (must be known for each of k diagnoses; $\Sigma Pr(Ai) = 1$)

f. Random variables and distributions

1. Probability distribution—mathematical function, $f(x)$, that indicates the probability of exactly x events occurring in n trials with chance π; $\Sigma f(x) = 1$ for all x
2. Random variable—number of successes, x, among n independent trials with constant probability π for each
3. Chance of x successes among n independent trials with chance π of success with each trial—probability of success, π; probability of failure, $(1 - \pi)$ (e.g., x heads in n coin tosses; x boys in n children; x deaths among n patients; x cures from treatment of n patients)
   (a) Two trials (n = 2)
       (1) Success followed by success
$$(\pi)(\pi) = \pi^2$$
       (2) Success followed by failure or failure followed by success
$$(\pi)(1 - \pi) = (1 - \pi)(\pi)$$
       (3) Failure followed by failure
$$(1 - \pi)(1 - \pi) = (1 - \pi)^2$$
       (4) Σ(all probabilities) $= 1 = \pi^2 + 2(1 - \pi)(\pi) + (1 - \pi)^2 = [(1 - \pi) + \pi]^2$
       (5) Probability of one success in two trials is $2(\pi)(1 - \pi)$
   (b) Three trials (n = 3)
       (1) $1 = [(1 - \pi) + \pi]^3$
       (2) Probability of one success in 3 trials is $3(\pi)(1 - \pi)^2$
   (c) n trials
       (1) $1 = [(1 - \pi) + \pi]^n$ (binomial expansion)
       (2) Probability of x successes in n trials is $^nC_x\pi^x(1 - \pi)^{n-x}$,
           $^nC_x \equiv$ combination of n objects taken x at a time $\equiv$
           $n!/x!(n - x)!$
   (d) Binomial distribution
$$f(x) = {}^nC_x\pi^x(1 - \pi)^{n-x}, 0 < x < n; \Sigma^nC_x\pi^x(1 - \pi)^{n-x}$$
$$= [(1 - \pi) + \pi]^n = 1, \text{where } 0 = x = n$$
   (e) Poisson probability distribution
       $f(x) = e^{-\lambda}\lambda^x/x!, 0 < x < \infty$
       (e.g., probability of x cells randomly distributed in suspension in small sample of a large volume)
   (f) Uniform probability distribution
$$f(x) = \text{constant}, x = 0, 1, 2, \ldots n; \Sigma f(x) = 1$$

III. Probability; f. Random variables and distributions (continued)

4. Continuous probability distributions
    (a) Exponential: $f(x) = \theta e^{-\theta x}, 0 < x < \infty$ (time intervals between successive random events, e.g., disintegration of radionuclide, time to failure of a part, time between epidemics, disasters)

    $$1 = \int f(x)dx, \infty < x < \infty, = \int \theta e^{-\theta x}, 0 < x < \infty$$

    (b) Normal (Gaussian) distribution
        (1) $f(x) = (\sigma \sqrt{(2\pi)})^{-1} e^{-1/2(x-\mu)^2/\sigma^2}, -\infty < x < \infty$
        (2) Determined by μ (mean) and σ (SD)
        (3) Bell shaped, symmetric about $x = \mu$
        (4) Distribution of many medical measurements in populations is approximately "normal"
        (5) Standardized normal curve $\mu = 0, \sigma = 1$; widely used for statistical inference by finding area under curve corresponding to ranges along the x axis
            $\mu \pm 1\sigma$: approximately two thirds of observations
            $\mu \pm 2\sigma$: approximately 95% of observations
            $\mu \pm 3\sigma$: approximately 99% of observations
        (6) Nonstandardized normal curve: critical ratio (or standardized value), $z = (x - \mu)/\sigma$, permits use of tables of standardized normal distribution
        (7) Can adjust raw data to yield derived data that are closer to normal, e.g., log transform (log of each observation, analysis done is log units: pharmacology—log dose; epidemiology—log incubation period)

IV. INFERENCE ON POPULATION MEANS FROM QUANTITATIVE DATA

a. Strength of inference

1. Sample size, n: larger $\Rightarrow$ stronger inference
2. Variability, σ: less $\Rightarrow$ stronger inference

b. Population distribution: distribution of characteristics in defined populations

c. Sampling distribution of means of sample of size n

1. Obtained from repeated samples of n observations from a large population
2. Mean determined from each sample

d. Properties

1. μ, σ are population mean and SD; $\bar{x}$ and s are mean and SD of single sample of size n
2. Mean of sampling distribution of means is same as population mean, μ
3. Standard error of mean—SD of sampling distribution of means is $\sigma/\sqrt{n}$, called standard error of the mean, $SE(\bar{x})$
4. Shape of sampling distribution of means is approximately normal, although population distribution may not be normal (if n is large enough)

5. n "large enough"
   (a) Normal population—n = 1 is large enough
   (b) Nonnormal population
       (1) n at which sampling distribution of means is approximately normal in shape
       (2) Depends on how "nonnormal" the underlying population is
       (3) If underlying population is known (e.g., Poisson, exponential, etc.), guidelines exist for sample size n to assure normal distribution of means
       (4) Use critical ratio, redefined as $z = (\bar{x} - \mu)/\sigma/\sqrt{n}$, to relate sampling distribution of means to standardized normal distribution
           [a] What sample size is required so that 5% of means of samples differ from population mean by specified amount? (Use table of standard normal curves to find z = 1.65 corresponding to 5%; $\bar{x} - \mu$ = [specified amount]; calculate n)
           [b] One- or two-tailed normal curve depending on whether difference more and/or less than population mean is needed

---

e. Statistical test of significance on a mean (statistical inference to accept or reject claimed survival, performance, etc., based on a single sample mean)

1. A population mean, μ_o, is claimed or hypothesized; the actual population mean, μ, is unknown (e.g., survival of ARDS patients treated with surfactant is 80%)
   (a) Reject the claim (there is enough evidence to doubt its validity)
   (b) Do not reject the claim (there is not enough evidence to doubt its validity)

2. A probability, α, is specified that μ_o is not the true population mean; α is "sufficiently small"
   (a) Compare $\bar{x}$ and μ_o, where $\bar{x}$ is sample mean from random sample of n observations from the population
       (1) Is chance sampling variation likely to cause a discrepancy between a $\bar{x}$ and μ_o?
           [a] If no, then a discrepancy is not likely due to chance, and $\bar{x}$ differs from μ_o because $\bar{x}$ is probably not from a population for which μ_o is the population mean, i.e., the difference is *statistically significant*
           [b] If yes, then a discrepancy between $\bar{x}$ and μ_o is likely due to chance, and $\bar{x}$ is representative of μ_o, i.e., the difference is *not statistically significant*
   (b) Significance level: is the chance (relative frequency) sufficiently small?
       (1) Willing to accept a (small) chance of rejecting the claimed or hypothesized μ_o when it is true
       (2) α = 5% (1 in 20) or 1% (1 in 100) for most medical situations (convention)
       (3) Statistically significant?
           [a] Statistically significant (P < .05 or P < .01)
           [b] Not statistically significant (P > .05), where P indicates probability
           [c] Statistically significant versus medically important
   (c) Inference is made based on comparison of a single sample mean with a population mean

3. Deviation from μ_o in one or two directions: determines use of one- or two-tailed normal curve

---

f. Confidence limits on population mean

1. For a sample of a population, and for 95% confidence limits on the population mean, the relative frequency with which the true population mean is actually within these

limits is 95% (i.e., 19 of 20 times the true unknown population mean will be within these calculated limits)

2. $\Pr\{1.96 \le z \le 1.96\} = 0.95$, $z = (\bar{x} - \mu)/\sigma/\sqrt{n}$

3. Therefore, $\bar{x} \pm 1.96\sigma/\sqrt{n}$ are 0.95 confidence limits on the population mean μ

4. And $\bar{x} \pm 2.58\sigma/\sqrt{n}$ are 0.99 confidence limits on the population mean μ

5. Only refers to population mean; no inference about the range of the population

g. t-distribution and t-test for statistical significance (when SD of the population, σ, is unknown)

1. Substitute an estimate of σ; use sample standard deviation, s

2. If sample n is small, then reliability of s must be determined: small sample method

3. Test of significance that population mean is μ_0

   (a) Redefine critical ratio as

$$t_{n-1} = (\bar{x} - \mu_o)/s/\sqrt{n}, \text{ where}$$
$$s = \sqrt{\Sigma (x - \bar{x})^2/(n - 1)}$$

   (b) t_{n-1} follows t-distribution with $n - 1$ df (i.e., number of independent quantities among the series), and not the standardized normal distribution (t-distribution is another theoretic probability distribution, with similar bell-shaped symmetry that changes for each df; for df > 30, same shape as normal distribution)

   (c) Calculate 95% confidence limits on population mean

$$\bar{x} \pm t_{n-1,0.05}s/\sqrt{n}$$

   (95% certainty that the mean of the population from which the sample was obtained is within this range)

4. Comparison of two sample means (compare two samples from two populations, e.g., treatment and control groups): two-sample t-test

   (a) Hypothesis: $\mu_T = \mu_C$, or $\delta \equiv \mu_T - \mu_C = 0$

   (b) Paired samples: eliminates some biologic and other variations to permit a more precise comparison

   (1) Self-paired: subject is own control; before–after comparison

   (2) Naturally paired: twins, siblings, litter mates; sequential admissions having specified criteria

   (3) Artificially paired: compared by investigator with prior knowledge of characteristics relevant to outcome(s) being studied

   (4) Calculate difference, d, for each of n paired samples; calculate mean of sample differences, $\bar{d}$

   (5) If SD of differences, σ_d, is known, then use normal distribution to test for significance

$$z = (\bar{d} - \delta)/\sigma_d/\sqrt{n} = (\bar{d} - 0)/\sigma_d/\sqrt{n}$$

   (6) If σ_d not known, then use sample SD of differences, s_d, and use t-distribution with df = (number of pairs) − 1

$$t_{n-1} = (\bar{d} - 0)/s_d/\sqrt{n}, s_d = \sqrt{\Sigma(d - \bar{d})^2/(n - 1)}$$

   (7) Confidence limits on difference between two populations

$$\bar{d} \pm t_{n-1,0.05} \sqrt{s^2}{}_d/n$$

   are 95% confidence limits of certainty that the difference, $\delta \equiv \mu_T - \mu_C$, is within this range

    (c) Independent samples: no factors known for pairing, too difficult, too many subjects or too few matches of relevant characteristics; therefore, two independent samples

        (1) Number of treatment, n_T, $\neq$ number of controls, n_C

        (2) Calculate critical ratio

$$z = (\bar{x}_T - \bar{x}_C - 0)/\sqrt{(\sigma_T^2/n_T + \sigma_C^2/n_C)}$$

        (3) If population SDs, σ_T and σ_C are unknown, use sample standard deviations, s_T and s_C, to obtain estimate of denominator, and t-test for comparison of two independent means

        (4) Assume $\sigma_T = \sigma_C = \sigma$:

           [a] $\qquad\qquad$ $SE(\bar{x}_T - \bar{x}_C) = \sqrt{[\sigma^2(1/n_T + 1/n_C)]}$

           [b] Estimate of σ^2 is weighted average of s_T^2 and s_C^2, i.e., pooled estimate of common variance

$$\text{pooled } s^2 = [\Sigma(x_T - \bar{x}_T)^2 - \Sigma(x_C - \bar{x}_C)^2]/(n_T + n_C - 2)$$

           [c] t-ratio for independent samples t-test

$$t_{nT+nC-2} = (\bar{x}_T - \bar{x}_C)/\sqrt{[\sigma^2(1/n_T + 1/n_C)]},$$
$$\text{with df} = n_T + n_C - 2$$

5. Determination of sample size: compromise between investigator and statistician

    (a) Errors that can be tolerated

        (1) α error (type I)—risk of wrongly rejecting hypothesis when it is true (e.g., 5%, 1%); conclude that difference is statistically significant when it is not

        (2) β error (type II)—risk of failing to reject hypothesis that is false; conclude that difference is not statistically significant when it is

           [a] β (%) obtained directly from table from calculated critical ratio

           [b] Operating characteristic (OC): determine a series of β for a series of μ_I; plot μ_I versus β

           [c] Always one-tailed normal curve

        (3) For test of significance on a single mean: specify α for μ_o, β for μ_I $\Rightarrow$ specify n

           [a] Upper percent cutoff point for α for normal distribution

$$z_\alpha = (\bar{x} - \mu_o)\big/\sigma/\sqrt{n}$$

lower percent cutoff point for β for normal distribution

$$z_\beta = (\bar{x} - \mu_I)\big/\sigma/\sqrt{n}$$
$$\text{where } z_\beta < 0 \text{ if } \beta < 0.5$$

           [b] $n = [(z_\alpha - z_\beta)\sigma/(\mu_I - \mu_o)]^2$

           [c] Pilot study to estimate σ

        (4) To determine sample size for comparison of two independent means:

           [a] $\sigma_T = \sigma_C = \sigma$; $n_T = n_C = n$; α error specification for no population difference (i.e., $\mu_T - \mu_C = 0$); β error specification for alternate population difference, $\mu_T - \mu_C = \delta_I$

           [b] $n = 2[(z_\alpha - z_\beta)\sigma/\delta_I]^2$

           [c] Sample size for each group is n; total sample size for entire study is 2n

        (5) To infer sample size needed to obtain desired confidence limits: 95% confidence limits on a single mean: $\bar{x} \pm 1.96\sigma/\sqrt{n}$ are 0.95 confidence limits on the population mean μ; specify range of variation that is tolerable, e.g., 20; therefore, $\pm 20 = \pm 1.96\sigma/\sqrt{n}$, $n = (1.96\sigma/20)^2$; pilot study gives σ

6. Measure a variable in three or more samples (multisample analyses), compare (test equality of) three or more means from independent samples: analysis of variance (ANOVA, ANOV, AOV)

    (a) Simple, reliable way to determine pooled s^2 (weighted estimate of σ^2, i.e., pooled estimate of common variance)

(b) F-test (F-statistic, after R.A. Fisher) of hypothesis that sample means are identical to population mean (variance ratio test for equality of means)
(c) One-way (single-factor) classification
  (1) Test for effect of one factor on variable measured (e.g., nutrient on body weight)
  (2) Assume all observations (data) distributed about common mean, μ, with variance, σ^2
  (3) Three different estimates of σ^2 from observations (i.e., mean squared deviations from the mean, or mean square)
    [a] Total

$$[\Sigma x^2 - (\Sigma\Sigma x)^2/an]/df$$

where $\Sigma\Sigma x$ is grand total of sample data, a is number of classes (groups) of sample data, n is number of samples per class, df is degrees of freedom for n data ($df = n - 1$)
    [b] Within class (among groups)

$$\Sigma x^2/\Sigma df$$

where df is for each group of n data ($\Sigma df = a(n - 1)$, a is number of classes (groups) of data)
    [c] Between class (within groups, or error)

$$[\Sigma\bar{x}^2 - (\Sigma\bar{x})^2/a]n/df$$

where a is number of classes, df is for classes of data ($df = a - 1$)
  (4) Variance ratio, F
    [a] $F = {}^{\text{mean square between classes}}/_{\text{mean square within classes}}$
      $= \{[\Sigma\bar{x}^2 - (\Sigma\bar{x})^2/a]n/df\}/\{\Sigma x^2/\Sigma df\}$
    [b] $F \sim 1$ when hypothesis is true, i.e., no difference between means of different groups
    [c] $F \gg 1$ when μ_i differs substantially
  (5) Underlying assumptions
    [a] $\sigma^2_1 = \sigma^2_2 = \sigma^2_3 = \sigma^2_i$ to test whether $\mu_1 = \mu_2 = \mu_3 = \mu_I$, and each of k samples should be from a normal population $\Rightarrow$ test for homogeneity, or use $n_1 \sim n_2 \sim n_3 \sim n_i$
    [b] ANOVA is generally "robust" (dependable) with regard to heterogeneity of variances, normality of populations
  (6) Confidence limits for any μ_I
  (7) Power and sample size, minimum difference between population means that is detectable
    [a] Calculate

$$\phi = n \sum_{I=1}^{k} (\mu_I - \mu)^2/ks^2$$

where s^2 is between class σ^2 (error mean square), k is sample group (class), μ_I is sample group mean,

$$\mu = \sum_{I=1}^{k} \mu_I/k \text{ (overall mean of all populations)}$$

    [b] Use look-up table for appropriate df for desired $\alpha = 0.05$ or 0.1
    [c] Power increases with ϕ, n, $\sum_{I=1}^{k}(\mu_I - \mu)^2$, fewer k, smaller s^2
    [d] Power $= 0.86 \Rightarrow 14\%$ chance of β error (type II)
    [e] Estimate required sample size n using successive iterations of ϕ
    [f] Minimum detectable difference between μ_I

$$\delta = \sqrt{2ks^2\phi^2/n}$$

(8) Multiple comparisons (post hoc tests): examine differences between all possible pairs of means (e.g., $\mu_1 = \mu_2 \neq \mu_I$; $\mu_1 \neq \mu_2 = \mu_I$; $\mu_1 \neq \mu_2 \neq \mu_I$)

   [a] Tukey test ("honestly significant test")—conservative

   [b] Neuman-Keuls test (Student-Neuman-Keuls test)—tends to conclude more significant differences than Tukey (more powerful)

   [c] Dunnett's test—comparison of control with other groups (i.e., $k - 1$ comparisons)

(d) Two-factor (two-way classification; factorial) ANOVA

   (1) Simultaneous analysis of effect of more than one factor on population means

      [a] Factors A, B

      [b] Levels a_i for factor A, b_i for B

      [c] N replicates of level a_i, b_i

   (2) Design study to do one experiment to suffice for the analysis

   (3) With replication: extends one-way ANOVA to include classes that have more than one sample group per class

      [a] Equal replication

      [b] Unequal replication (proportional, disproportional): delete excess data to obtain equality or proportionality; insert mean of existing data

   (4) Without replication: only one datum for each comparison; df = 0, error $\sigma^2 = 0$; ANOVA still valid

(e) Three-factor (multiway factorial) ANOVA

   (1) How do factors A, B, C affect a measured variable (e.g., temperature, FiO_2, gender on VO_2 in mechanically ventilated patients)?

   (2) Iterative calculations of F for each permutation of μ_I; compare calculated F and critical F for desired $\alpha = 0.05$ or 0.1

V. INFERENCE ON POPULATION MEANS FROM ENUMERATION (OR ATTRIBUTE) DATA (how many, how many succeeded, failed; proportions)

a. Single proportion

1. Binomial distribution: n independent trials with constant probability π

   (a) Use to calculate probability exactly, and to infer significance

   (b) $\pi = \frac{1}{2}$: equal probability of yes or no, success or failure, head or tail

   (c) Probability of x successes in n trials is

$$^nC_x\pi^x(1 - \pi)^{n-x}, \, ^nC_x \equiv n!/x!(n - x)!$$

   (d) For $n = 10$ and $\pi = \frac{1}{2}$

$$Pr(0) = (\tfrac{1}{2})^{10}$$
$$Pr(1) = 10(\tfrac{1}{2})(\tfrac{1}{2})^9$$
$$Pr(2) = (10 \times 9/2 \times 1)(\tfrac{1}{2})^2(\tfrac{1}{2})^8$$
$$Pr(0,1, or\ 2) = 56/1,024 = 0.0545$$

   (P > .05; not statistically significant, if hypothesis were that the probability of zero, one, or two heads in 10 coin-toss trials is one half)

2. Normal approximation to binomial distribution: for large n, each observation rated as success (1) or failure (0)

   (a) Mean of population, μ, corresponds to population proportion of success (i.e., $\mu = \pi$)

   (b) SD of population, $\sigma = \sqrt{\pi(1 - \pi)}$

V. Inference on population means from enumeration (or attribute) data; a. Single proportion (continued)

(c) For repeat samples of size n
  (1) Mean of sample means (proportions) from repeat samples of size n is π
  (2) SE of mean, $\sigma/\sqrt{n}$, is redefined as standard error of sample proportion, $\sqrt{\pi(1 - \pi)/n}$
  (3) Shape of frequency distribution is approximately normal, provided n is large enough (i.e., $n\pi \geq 5$ and $n(1 - \pi) \geq 5$)
  (4) Calculate critical ratios using number of successes, where $np = x$ (n is number of trials, p is proportion of success, x is number of successes)
    [a] Use to determine number of successes to achieve statistical significance
    [b] Use to obtain (95%) confidence limits on a proportion
    [c] Use to determine sample size

---

b. Comparison of two proportions (analogous to comparison of means)

1. Independent samples: test of significance, confidence limits, sample size

  (a) Hypothesis: $\pi_T = \pi_C$
  (b) Exact test: Fisher's exact test for comparison of two proportions
  (c) Approximate test: calculate critical ratio based on difference in two independent proportions, hypothesis that $\pi_T - \pi_C = 0$ and sample difference $p_T - p_C$

2. Paired samples: if paired experiments are performed, then paired data should be analyzed to avoid erroneous inference

---

c. Chi-square test

1. Approximate method of statistical inference
2. Paired or independent samples
3. Useful for comparison of several proportions; enumeration (or attribute) data
4. Does not permit calculation of confidence limits; does not (easily) permit determination of required sample size
5.
$$\chi^2(df) = \Sigma_{\text{all categories}}(O - E)^2/E$$

  where O = observed count in a category, E = expected count in that category if hypothesis is true

6. Categories correspond to table entries, i.e., fourfold table (four cells) has four quantities, or categories, in the table
7. Comparison of proportions in independent samples

  (a) From observation data, calculate expected data
    (1) Hypothesis is identical proportions (e.g., survival rates, other outcomes) for treatment and control groups
    (2) Therefore, observed proportion of total of treatment and control groups is the expected proportion
    (3) df is number of independent expected quantities
    (4) Continuity correction (for smooth normal curves, not histograms): decrease $(O - E)$ by one half
    (5) Compare two independent proportions
$$\chi_c^2(df) = \Sigma_{\text{all categories}}(|O - E| - \tfrac{1}{2})^2/E$$
$$= (|O - E| - \tfrac{1}{2})^2 \Sigma_{\text{all categories}}(1/E)$$
    where χ_c^2 is continuity correction (Yates' correction)

(6) Compare calculated χ^2_c(df) with tabulated χ^2 for appropriate df (look up χ^2 table); determine statistical significance (or insignificance)

8. Paired samples

   (a) Number of expected counts is 5 or more

   (b) Continuity correction: reduce $|O - E|$ by one half

   (c) df = 1 with 2 categories and total expected counts = total observed counts

   (d) Calculate χ^2_c(df) and compare tabulated χ^2 for appropriate df; determine statistical significance

9. Comparison of several proportions

   (a) More than two independent samples

      (1) 2 × k contingency table: two columns, k rows

      (2) Determine expected counts in each category: assume effect to be tested equally distributed (constant proportions) among each category

      (3) Proportion estimated from observed effect in the total sample (i.e., [sum of counts in row I] × [sum of counts in column I]/total counts n)

      (4) df = k − 1 (typically)

      (5) No continuity correction for df > 1

      (6) Calculate χ^2_c(k − 1 df), compare tabulated χ^2, determine statistical significance and P < (%)

      (7) Generalize

         [a] r × c contingency table (set of category or cell counts arranged in r rows and c columns)

         [b] Expected counts: $\Sigma r_i \times \Sigma c_i / n$

         [c] df = (r − 1)(c − 1)

   (b) More than two paired samples

VI. REGRESSION AND CORRELATION

a. Descriptions

1. Regression: dependent and independent variable; change of mean of dependent variable studied in response to changes in independent variable (e.g., dose–response)

2. Correlation: both variables dependent (on some other variable); quantify relationship of two variables

b. Linear regression

1. Scatter diagram—variables represented by abscissa (x) and ordinate (y) scales

2. Linear regression—fitting straight line to scatter of points

   (a) Least squares fit

      (1) Straight line placed within scatter of points such that sum of squares of deviations of points about line is minimum (i.e., minimize $\Sigma(y - Y)^2$); measured parallel to y axis

      (2) Intercept is predicted mean of dependent variable, y, when independent variable x = 0

   (b) Inference with regression lines

      (1) Sample of n observation pairs (x, y)

      (2) Determine SE of slope and intercept

      (3) For each x, each y comes from normally distributed population with means that make up the population regression line, $Y_{pop} = \alpha + \beta x$, where α and β are population slope and intercept

      (4) Least squares regression line fitted to n observed sample points, $Y = a + bx$, is an estimate

VI. Regression and correlation; b. Linear regression (continued)

(5) Assumes normal distributions of ys for each x have equal variabilities (same SD); if not, then need weighted regression analysis

(6) If σ unknown, then estimate from sample

[a] n $-$ 2 df for n deviations about line (intercept a and slope b depend on other n $-$ 2 deviations)

[b] Standard deviation from regression (or standard error of estimate)

$$s_{y.x} = \sqrt{\Sigma(y - Y)^2/(n - 2)}$$

or

$$= \sqrt{\Sigma(y - y)^2 - [\Sigma(x - \bar{x})(y - y)]^2/\Sigma(x - \bar{x})^2/(n - 2)}$$

[c] $$\text{est SE(b)} = s_{y.x}/\sqrt{\Sigma(x - \bar{x})^2}$$

and

$$\text{est SE(a)} = s_{y.x}\sqrt{[1/n + \bar{x}^2/\Sigma(x - \bar{x})^2]}$$

(7) $$\text{SE(b)} = \sigma/\sqrt{\Sigma(x - \bar{x})^2}$$

$$\text{SE(a)} = \sigma\sqrt{[1/n + \bar{x}^2/\Sigma(x - \bar{x})^2]}$$

could be obtained if σ known (rare)

(8) Test of significance and confidence on slope

[a] t-test, n $-$ 2 df, hypothesis $\beta = 0$ (i.e., no relation between x and y)

$$t_{n-2} = (b - \beta_0)/\text{est SE(b)}$$

look up $P < (?)$

[b] Confidence limits

$$b \pm t_{n-2,.05}\text{est SE(b)}$$

(i.e., chances are 19 in 20 that slope is somewhere in this range)

(9) Similar treatment for significance and confidence on intercept, predicted mean ys, and individual ys

(10) Limitations

[a] Inference applies only within experimental range of x; no extrapolation

[b] If slope $= 0$ based on linear regression analysis, there may be another (nonlinear) fit

---

c. Polynomial and multiple regression

---

d. Nonlinear regression

---

e. Correlation

1. If one or more variable, not independent

2. Coefficient of correlation (product moment correlation; Pearson's coefficient of correlation)

(a) Describes relationship between two mutually dependent variables

(b) $r = \Sigma(x - \bar{x})(y - y)/\sqrt{\Sigma(x - \bar{x})^2(y - y)^2}$

(c) $-1 < r < +1$

(1) $r = +1$ if $+$ slope and perfect correlation

(2) $r = -1$ if $-$ slope and perfect correlation

(3) $r = 0$ if no correlation

(4) $0.75 < |r| < 1$ indicates good to excellent correlation

(5) $0.95 < |r| < 1$ indicates improbably high correlation that may be artifact (e.g., one variable may be subset of the other)

(d) Inference: if no correlation among population sample of (x,y) points, what is probability of no correlation in the entire population?

    (1) Assume bivariate normal distribution (three-dimensional extension of bell-shaped normal curve; x and y plane and probability axis)

    (2) $t_{n-2} = r \sqrt{(n-2)} / \sqrt{(1-r^2)}$

        follows t-distribution with n − 2 df

        [a] Test hypothesis that population correlation is zero

        [b] Calculate t; t-table to look up P %

    (3) Correlation applies only

        [a] To linear relationship (could be a nonlinear relationship if r = 0)

        [b] Over range of (x,y)

    (4) Correlation implies that the two variables tend to be related; does not imply that one variable directly or exclusively influences the other

3. Multiple and partial correlation: compare more than two variables; compare correlation coefficients in two or more populations

VII. CLINICAL TRIALS

a. Difference between treatment and control observations

1. Sampling variation or chance: focus of statistical analysis and inference

2. Inherent differences between treatment and control groups (e.g., healthier patients with similar disease may be selected for new surgical procedure; less healthy for standard medical prescriptions)

3. Differences in handling, evaluation of treatment and control groups during investigation (e.g., more intensive care for treatment group than for control)

4. True effects of new procedure

b. Controlled clinical trial: two series, treatment and control, under simultaneous investigation; treatment and control groups maintained as alike as possible throughout the trial

1. Randomization

    (a) Patients allocated to treatment and control groups by chance, following predetermined plan designed using random number generator (or table)

    (b) Ensures no bias in allocation of treatment due to personal judgment and prejudice of investigator and patient

    (c) Sealed, serially numbered opaque envelopes containing card indicating treatment or control; as patients meet the criteria for entry into the clinical trial, the next serially numbered envelope is opened

    (d) Crossover design

        (1) Self-paired samples—the order in which patients receive treatment(s) is random (e.g., drug A followed by drug B)

        (2) Matched pairs—the two members of the pair assigned at random to treatment, control

    (e) Stratified randomization—strata formed and randomization occurs separately for subjects in each stratum (e.g., age, sex)

    (f) Random assignment—process by which subjects assigned to treatment and control groups (fundamental to controlled clinical trial); random selection refers to surveys and process of random selection of subjects from larger population

    (g) For the particular experiment: what was observed is unlikely to be explained by chance assignment into one group receiving treatment and one group not; sufficient rationale for test of significance, inference

2. Blind trials and placebos
   (a) Single blind trial—patient unaware of whether treatment or control
   (b) Double blind trial—patient and investigator unaware
   (c) Placebo (Latin: "I will please"; make-believe medicine given to please or gratify patient)—if no standard drug for use in a blind or double blind study (also, placebo procedures)

3. Ethics of controlled human clinical trial
   (a) Judgment
       (1) If hypothesis is no difference between treatment and control (i.e., do not know whether treatment is of benefit), then it is ethical for investigator to conduct controlled trial
       (2) If investigator believes the treatment is of value, then it is unethical to participate in controlled study
   (b) Can potentially beneficial drug be withheld from a (control) patient? Can placebo or sham surgery be justified?
   (c) Informed consent—requirement for all clinical studies in the United States; if not from patient, then from immediate family (parent, wife, sibling)
   (d) Design of clinical trials—investigator must show lack of bias

J. OTHER APPLIED MATHEMATICS

I. FUNCTION: correspondence between two sets of elements, domain and range, such that to each element of the domain there corresponds one, and only one, element of the range, and vice versa

a. Rule of correspondence enables determination of which element of range corresponds to each element of domain

b. Examples

1. $f(x) = c$, constant function
2. $f(x) = x$, identity function
3. $f(x) = a_0x_n + a_1x_{n-1} + \ldots + a_{n-1}x + a_n$, polynomial function
    (a) Polynomial function with degree 2: quadratic function
    (b) Quotient of two polynomial functions: rational function
4. $f(x) = \sqrt{x}$, square root function
5. Transcendental functions: not algebraic
    (a) Trigonometric
    (b) Logarithmic
    (c) Inverse trigonometric

c. Limit of function: as $x \to a$, $f(x) \to L$ for x in domain of f

$$\lim_{x \to a} f(x) = L$$

II. ASYMPTOTE

a. Line $x = a$ is vertical asymptote of curve $y = f(x)$ if

$$\lim_{x \to a} f(x) = \pm \infty$$

b. Line $y = b$ is horizontal asymptote of curve $y = f(x)$ if

$$\lim_{x \to \pm \infty} f(x) = b$$

c. General: line $y = ax + b$ is asymptote of curve $y = f(x)$ if

$$\lim_{x \to \pm \infty} [f(x) - (ax + b)] = 0$$

III. INCREMENT: if $y = f(x)$ and x_1 and $x_1 + \Delta x$ are two numbers in the domain of f, then $\Delta y = f(x_1 + \Delta x) - f(x_1)$ is the increment of the dependent variable y that corresponds to the increment Δx at x_1

IV. DERIVATIVE OF f: another function f′ with value at any point x_1 in the domain of f

$$f'(x) = \lim_{\Delta x \to 0}[f(x_1 + \Delta x) - f(x_1)/\Delta x]$$

if the limit exists, or

$$f'(a) = \lim_{x \to a}\{[f(x) - f(a)]/(x - a)\}$$

if limit exists

a. Domain of f′ is a subset of the domain of f

1. $f' \equiv D_x f \equiv dy/dx$: derivative of f with respect to x

2. Instantaneous rate of change of f(x) with respect to independent variable x when x = x_1 is limit of average rate of change

$$f'(x) = \lim_{\Delta x \to 0}[f(x_1 + \Delta x) - f(x_1)/\Delta x]$$

3. Differentials, dx and dy: for function f differentiable at x and for y = f(x), dx is arbitrary increment of x, Δx; $df = dy = f'(x)dx$ is differential of dependent variable y at x

4. Basic problems of differential calculus

   (a) Finding slope of tangent line to given curve
       (1) Tangent to graph of y = f(x) at (x_1,y_1) on the graph is the line through (x_1,y_1) with slope $f'(x_1)$
       (2) $y - y_1 = f'(x_1)(x - x_1)$
       (3) Equation of normal to graph y = f(x) at (x_1,y_1) is

$$y - y_1 = [-1/f'(x_1)](x - x_1)$$

   (b) Finding instantaneous velocity of particle moving along a straight line at varying speeds
       (1) s = f(t) is position function, instantaneous velocity of particle at time t is

$$v = f'(t) = \lim_{\Delta t \to 0} f(a + \Delta t) - f(a)/\Delta t$$

       (2) Speed of particle is $|v|$
       (3) Acceleration of a moving particle is the time-rate of change of its velocity

$$a = dv/dt = f''(t)$$

b. Partial differentiation

1. Function of two variables, z = f(x,y)

2. If y constant, partial derivative of f with respect to x

$$\delta f/\delta x = \delta f(x,y)/\delta x = \lim_{\Delta x \to 0}[f(x + \Delta x,y) - f(x,y)/\Delta x]$$

3. If x constant, partial derivative of f with respect to y

$$\delta f/\delta y = \delta f(x,y)/\delta y = \lim_{\Delta y \to 0}[f(x,y + \Delta y) - f(x,y)/\Delta y]$$

4. Geometric interpretation

   (a) Surface z = f(x,y): plane y = c intersects surface in a plane curve and $\delta f(x,c)/\delta x$ is slope of tangent to plane curve at point [x,c,f(x,c)]
   (b) Plane x = k cuts surface z = f(x,y) in plane curve and $\delta f(k,y)/\delta y$ is slope of tangent to curve at point [k,y,f(k,y)]

5. Chain rule: differentiation of functions of two or more variables, e.g., u = u(x,y) and v = v(x,y) and F = F(u,v)

   (a) $\delta F/\delta x = (\delta F/\delta u)(\delta u/\delta x) + (\delta F/\delta v)(\delta v/\delta y)$

   (b) $\delta F/\delta y = (\delta F/\delta u)(\delta u/\delta y) + (\delta F/\delta v)(\delta v/\delta x)$

   (c) Similar for three functions, e.g., u, v, w

6. Gradient; tangent plane to a surface
   (a) Vector: ordered set of numbers (x,y,z), which are the components of the vector
       (1) Magnitude $|a|$ of vector $\mathbf{a} = \sqrt{a_1^2 + a_2^2 + a_3^2}$
       (2) $\mathbf{a} + \mathbf{b} = (a_1 + b_1, a_2 + b_2, a_3 + b_3)$
   (b) Scalar (means "real number")
       (1) Quantities that can be measured with a scale
       (2) $k\mathbf{a} = k(a_1, a_2, a_3) = (ka_1, ka_2, ka_3)$
   (c) Dot product (a scalar quantity; also called scalar product)
       (1) $\mathbf{a} \cdot \mathbf{b} = (a_1, a_2, a_3) \cdot (b_1, b_2, b_3) = a_1b_1 + a_2b_2 + a_3b_3$
       (2) $\mathbf{a} \cdot \mathbf{b} = |\mathbf{a}||\mathbf{b}|\cos\theta$
   (d) Unit vectors
       (1) Any vector with length (magnitude) = 1
       (2) $\mathbf{I} = (1,0,0), \mathbf{j} = (0,1,0), \mathbf{k} = (0,0,1)$
       (3) All vectors can be expressed as linear combination of $\mathbf{I}, \mathbf{j}, \mathbf{k}$
   (e) Vector function, $\mathbf{r}$
       (1) $\mathbf{r}(t) = (f(t), g(t))$, where f and g are functions with common domain, and $(f(t), g(t))$ defines a vector for each number t in the domain
       (2) $\mathbf{r}'(t) = (f'(t), g'(t))$
   (f) Surface $F(x,y,z) = 0$, position vector $\mathbf{r}(t) = (x(t), y(t), z(t))$ that traces out curve on surface
   (g) $\nabla F = (F_x(x,y,z), F_y(x,y,z), F_z(x,y,z))$
       is gradient vector, where $F_{x,y,x}$ are partial derivatives of F; "del F"
   (h) ∇F is perpendicular to all tangents to curves that pass through a single point on surface
   (i) Tangent plane to surface $F(x,y,z) = 0$ at point $P(a,b,c) \perp \nabla F(a,b,c)$
       $$\nabla F(a,b,c) \cdot [(x - a)\mathbf{I} + (y - b)\mathbf{j} + (z - c)\mathbf{k}] = 0$$

V. DEFINITE INTEGRAL: for f defined on closed interval [a,b], and set of n subintervals (|P| is longest), if L exists such that

$$\lim_{|P| \to 0} \sum_{I=1}^{n} f(\xi i)\Delta x_i = L$$

then L is definite integral of f(x) from x = a to x = b

$$\int_a^b f(x)dx = \lim_{|P| \to 0} \sum_{I=1}^{n} f(\xi i)\Delta x_i$$

a. Trapezoid approximation of definite integral

$$\int_a^b f(x)dx \doteq (\Delta x/2)[f(x_0) + 2f(x_1) + 2f(x_2) + \ldots + 2f(x_{n-1}) + f(x_n)]$$

b. Mean value for integral: if f is continuous on interval [a,b], then μ exists between a and b such that

$$\int_a^b f(x)dx = f(\mu)(b - a)$$

c. Antiderivative of f: F, a function defined by $F(x) = \int_a^x f(t)dt$, is differentiable on closed interval [a,b] and is an antiderivative of f

$$F(x) = D_x\int_a^x f(t)dt = f(x) \,\forall\, \text{(for all) } x \text{ in } [a,b]$$

d. Fundamental theorem of integral calculus

$$\int_a^b f(x)dx = F(a) - F(b)$$

where $F'(x) = f(x)$

e. Applications

1. Plane area: $A = \int_a^b |f(x)|dx$ is area bounded by curve $y = f(x)$, x axis and vertical lines $x = a$ and $x = b$

2. Volume of solid of revolution

$$V = \pi\int_a^b [f(x)]^2 dx$$

3. Work

$$W = \int_a^b F(x)dx$$

is work done by force F (with value $F(x)$ at point x) acting along x axis as it moves from a to b

4. Liquid pressure

$$F = w\int_c^d (k - y)[f(y) - g(y)]dy$$

is force of liquid pressure on object with shape defined by $x = f(y)$ and $x = g(y)$ in liquid of depth k at depth $k - y$

VI. INDEFINITE INTEGRAL: find function F that was differentiated to give f (i.e., find the most general antiderivative of $f(x)$ such that $F'(x) = f(x)$

a. Systematic approach to inverse process of differentiation: given f, find what function was differentiated to give f

b. $\int f(x)dx = F(x) + C$

1. $\int u^n du = u^{n+1}/n + 1 + C$

2. $\int du/u = \ln|u| + C$

3. $\int e^u du = e^u + C$

4. $\int a^u du = a^u/\ln a + C$

5. $\int [f(u) + g(u)]du = \int f(u)du + \int g(u)du$

6. $\int kf(u)du = k\int f(u)du$, k constant

7. $\int u\,dv = uv - \int v\,du$

    where u and v are function of x having continuous derivatives

VII. DIFFERENTIAL EQUATION: required to relate dynamic inputs to dynamic outputs for continuous system

a. Involves one or more derivatives or differentials of an unknown function represented by a dependent variable

b. Ordinary differential equation: one dependent variable

c. Partial derivatives: partial differential equation

d. Order of differential equation: that of derivative of highest order

e. Degree of differential equation: exponent of highest power of derivative of highest order (polynomial form in dependent variable and its derivatives)

f. Solution: relation between dependent and independent variables free of derivatives and reduces differential equation to an identity

g. General solution of *n*th-order differential equation: a solution containing n independent arbitrary constants

h. Particular solution: any solution that can be obtained by assigning particular values to the arbitrary constants in the general solution

i. First order, first degree

1. $dy/dx + F(x,y) = 0$: re-expressed as: $Mdx + Ndy = 0$, where M, N contain x, y, or both, or are constants

2. Separable variables: M is function of x only and N is function of Y; only $A(x)dx + B(y)dy = 0$, with general solution: $\int A(x)dx + \int B(y)dy = C$, C constant

3. Examples

    (a) Decomposition and growth: $dS/dt = kS$, S number of bacteria in a solution, or mass of radioactive material at time t, etc.

    (1) Variables S, t separable
    $$\int dS/S = k\int dt, \ln S = kt + \ln S_0$$

    (2) For radium decay, given that 25% of original amount lost in 664 years, what is half-life? $S = 0.75S_0$ when $t = 664 \Rightarrow k = -0.00043 \Rightarrow S = \frac{1}{2}S_0$ when $t \doteq 1,600$ years

    (b) Temperature change: rate of change of temperature at time t is proportional to difference in temperature of body and surrounding medium at time t: $dB/dt = k(B - M)$, B is temperature of body, M is temperature of surrounding medium, k is proportionality constant

VII. Differential equation; i. First order, first degree (continued)

(1) Separable variables

$$dB/(B - M) = kdt$$
$$\int dB/(B - M) = k\int dt$$
$$\ln(B - 40) = kt + C$$

(2) Substitute initial conditions ($t = 0$, $B = ?$) to solve for C; substitute other data for B, t, and solve for k

(c) Linear differential equation of order n: if polynomial form of first degree in dependent variable and derivatives

(1) $d^n y/dx^n + a_1 d^{n-1}y/dx^{n-1} + \ldots + a_{n-1}dy/dx + a_n y = f(x)$

(2) Homogeneous if $f(x) = 0$

VIII. TRANSCENDENTAL FUNCTIONS

a. Natural logarithmic function

$$\ln x = \int_1^x 1/t\, dt,\ x > 0$$

1. $D_x \ln x = D_x \int_1^x 1/t\, dt = 1/x$

2. $\ln e = 1$, $e = 2.718\ldots$ (transcendental number)

3. $\ln 1 = 0$

4. $\ln ax = \ln x + c$

5. $\ln x^n = n \ln x$

6. $\ln x/a = \ln x - \ln a$

7. Logarithmic differentiation: apply logarithmic function to simplify differentiation of expressions that involve quotients, products, powers

b. Exponential function (inverse of natural logarithmic function): $y = \exp(x)$ iff (if and only if) $x = \ln y$

1. $\exp(0) = 1$

2. $\exp(1) = e$

3. $\exp(a)\exp(b) = \exp(a + b)$

4. $[\exp(a)]^r = \exp(ar)$

5. $\exp(r) = e^r$

6. $D_x e^u = e^u D_x u$, $D_u^{-1} e^u = e^u + c$

c. Trigonometric functions

1. Radian measure of angles

(a) An angle of 1 radian with its vertex at the center of a circle intercepts an arc equal in length to the radius

(b) $\theta = s/r$ is radian measure of angle with arc length s in circle of radius r (s and r same units of length)

(c) π radians in $180°$; 1 radian $\doteq 57.3°$

2. $\sin x = \sin \alpha$, $\cos x = \cos \alpha$, $\tan x = \tan \alpha$, $\cot x = \cot \alpha$, $\sec x = \sec \alpha$, $\csc x = \csc \alpha$, where α is angle with radian measure x

3. Periodic: 2π − sin, cos; π − tan, cot

4. $D_x\sin u = \cos u\, D_x u$, $D_x\cos u = -\sin u\, D_x u$, $D_x\tan u = \sec^2 u\, D_x u$, $D_x\cot u = -\csc^2 u\, D_x u$, $D_x\sec u = \sec u \tan u\, D_x u$, $D_x\csc u = -\csc u \cot u\, D_x u$

---

d. Hyperbolic functions: combinations of e^x and e^{-x} that occur frequently

1. $\sinh x = (e^x - e^{-x})/2$, $\cosh x = (e^x + e^{-x})/2$, $\tanh x = \sinh x/\cosh x$, $\coth x = \cosh x/\sinh x$, $\operatorname{sech} x = 1/\cosh x$, $\operatorname{csch} x = 1/\sinh x$

2. $D_x\sinh x = \cosh x$, $D_x\cosh x = \sinh x$, $D_x\tanh x = \operatorname{sech}^2 x$

IX. INFINITE SERIES

a. Sequence

1. Function with domain restricted to integers

2. Monotonic

   (a) Monotonically increasing: $u_1 \le u_2 \le \ldots \le u_n \le \ldots$
   (b) Monotonically decreasing: $u_1 \ge u_2 \ge \ldots \ge u_n \ge \ldots$
   (c) Convergent iff bounded, i.e., there is a number C such that $|u_n| \le C\; \forall\, n > 0$

---

b. Infinite series

1. Sequence $\{a_n\}$

2. $\displaystyle\sum_{n=1}^{\infty} a_n$ or $a_1 + a_2 + \ldots + a_n + \ldots$ is infinite series

3. $a_1, a_2, \ldots, a_n$ are terms of series

4. For $\{s_n\}$, $n = 1,2,3, \ldots$ (i.e., first n terms of $\{a_n\}$), $\{a_n\}$ is convergent if $\lim\limits_{n\to\infty} s_n = S$ (sum of infinite series); diverges if $\lim\limits_{n\to\infty} s_n$ does not exist

5. Geometric series

   (a) $\displaystyle\sum_{i=1}^{\infty} ar^{i-1} = a + ar + ar^2 + \ldots + ar^{n-1} + \ldots$
   (b) Convergent if $|r| < 1$; divergent if $|r| > 1$

6. Harmonic series

   (a) $\Sigma 1/n = 1 + 1/2 + 1/3 + \ldots + 1/n + \ldots$
   (b) Divergent

7. Power series

   (a) For $\{a_n\}$ (sequence of constants),

   $$\sum_{i=0}^{\infty} a_i x^i = a_0 + a_1 x + a_2 x^2 + \ldots a_n x^n + \ldots$$

   is power series in x

   (b) If converges for any $x_1 \ne 0$, then converges $\forall$ (for all) x such that $|x| < |x_1|$; if diverges for x_2, then diverges $\forall$ x such that $|x| > |x_2|$

   (c) Power series in $(x - b)$: $\Sigma a_n(x - b)^n$

   (1) $f(x) = a_0 + a_1(x - b) + a_2(x - b)^2 + \ldots + a_n(x - b)^n$

   (2) $f'(x) = \displaystyle\sum_{n=0}^{\infty} D_x[a_n(x - b)]^n$

   exists $\forall$ x for which power series convergent

IX. Infinite series; b. Infinite series (continued)

(3) $f''(x) = 2a_2 + (2 \times 3)a_3(x - b) + \ldots$

and

$$f^{(n)}(x) = n!a_n + (n + 1)!a_{n+1}(x - b)$$
$$+ [(n + 2)!/2!]a_{n+2}(x - b)^2 + \ldots$$

(4) $f^{(n)}(b) = n!a_n$

(5) $\int_b^x f(t)dt = \sum_{n=0}^{\infty} \int_b^x a_n(t - b)^n dt$

exists $\forall$ x for which power series convergent

(d) Taylor's series

(1) For function F defined in some way other than by a power series (e.g., F(x) = sin x) for which derivatives of every order exist at point b

$$f(x) = F(b) + F'(b)(x - b) + F''(b)(x - b)^2/2! + \ldots$$

$$+ F^{(n)}(b)(x - b)^n/n! + \ldots = \sum_{n=0}^{\infty} f^{(n)}(b)(x - b)^n/n!$$

where $b - r < x < b + r$ is interval of convergence and $0 \leq r \leq \infty$

(2) Also called Taylor's expansion of F about point b, or Taylor's series generated by the function F

(3) Whether f(x) represents F $\forall$ x

[a] $f(x) = \sum_{n=0}^{\infty} f^{(n)}(b)(x - b)^n/n! = f(b) + f'(b)(x - b)$

$$+ f''(b)(x - b)^2/2! + \ldots + f^{(n)}(b)(x - b)^n/n! + R_n(x)$$

where

$$R_n(x) = 1/n! \int_b^x (x - t)^n f^{(n+1)}(t)dt$$

[b] If $\lim_{n \to \infty} R_n(x) = 0$, f(x) represents f for all x in interval $(b - r, b + r)$

X. COMPLEX VARIABLE

a. A complex number can be put in form $a + ib$, where $i^2 = -1$ (imaginary) and a and b are real

b. Represent on x,y axes in Argand diagram similar to vector

1. $z = x + iy$, $|z| = \sqrt{x^2 + y^2}$

2. $x = r\cos\theta$, $y = r\sin\theta \Rightarrow z = r(\cos\theta + i\sin\theta)$
    is polar representation

3. $e^{x+iy} = e^x(\cos y + I \sin y)$, x,y real

XI. TRANSFORM ANALYSIS

a. Transform problem (equation) for simplified analysis using look-up table, addition, subtraction (e.g., log transform: $Y = X/Z \Rightarrow \log Y = \log X - \log Z$) followed by inverse of transform using look-up table (antilogarithm: $\log^{-1}(\log Y) = Y$)

b. Fourier transform

1. Identifies different frequency sinusoids (and their amplitudes) that combine to form a waveform

2. Decomposes waveform into sum of sinusoids of different frequencies

3. Frequency domain representation of function

4. $S(f) = \int_{-\infty}^{\infty} s(t)e^{-j2\pi ft}dt$, $s(t)$ is waveform, $S(f)$ is Fourier transform, $j = \sqrt{-1}$

5. Discrete Fourier transform for computer computation

$$S(f_k) = \sum_{I=0}^{N-1} s(t_i)e^{-j2\pi f_k t_i}(t_{i+1} - t_i), k = 0,1,\ldots,N-1$$

6. Fast Fourier transform (FFT)—algorithm to compute discrete FT more rapidly than other methods

XII. BIOLOGIC CURVES

a. Transport among body compartments

1. Single compartment: fixed compartment volume, V, one inlet, one outlet, volumetric (blood) flow rate in, Q_i, out, Q_o, inlet concentration, c_{ij}, outlet concentration, c_{oj}

   (a) $Q_o - Q_i = -dV/dt = 0, Q_o = Q_i = Q$ (constant-volume compartment)

   (b) $Q(c_{oj} - c_{ij}) = -Vd\langle c_j \rangle/dt$, $\langle c_j \rangle$

   is volume averaged concentration [$V\langle c_j \rangle = \oint c_j dV$, where V

   $= V_{blood} + V_{tissue}$; for most cases, $\langle c_j \rangle = c_j$]

   (c) At some instant, inlet (arterial) stream injected with inert material in concentration c_a; outlet (venous) concentration, c_v, will increase with time and material will accumulate in tissue volume

   $$c_v(t) = -(V/Q)dc/dt + c_a$$

   (d) Uptake (saturation): highly diffusible material (e.g., H_2) and venous outflow in equilibrium with tissue: $c_v = c\alpha$; α is solubility (partition) coefficient for inert material in blood–tissue equilibrium

   (1) $c_v = -(V/Q\alpha)dc_v/dt + c_a, c_v = c_a(1 - e^{-kt}) = \alpha c$

   where $k \equiv Q\alpha/V$

   (2) If c_v or c monitored, k can be determined and Q/V obtained

   (e) Clearance (desaturation): compartment has initial constant concentration c(0); inlet concentration c_a suddenly reduced at $t > 0$

   (1) $c_v = \alpha c(0)e^{-kt} = \alpha c$

   (2) Inert gas uptake and clearance for measurement of local blood flow

   [a] H_2 clearance from myocardium (H_2 very diffusible $\Rightarrow \alpha = 1$; V determined from tissue density and empty weight of heart)

   [b] Plot of $\ln[H_2]$ vt $\Rightarrow k \approx 0.8$ min^{-1} ($c_v/\alpha c(0) = 1 = e^{-kt}$; ln $c_v/\alpha c(0) = -kt$)

   [c] Other gases: N_2O, Kr^{85}

2. Two parallel compartments

   (a) $c_{v1} = c_1(0)e^{-k_1 t} = \alpha_1 c_1$

   $k_1 \equiv Q_1\alpha_1/V_1; c_{v2} = c_2(0)e^{-k_2 t} = \alpha_2 c_2$

   $k_2 \equiv Q_2\alpha_2/V_2$

   (b) Organ containing two distinct tissue regions (e.g., white, gray brain matter) or organ containing two distinct capillary beds (e.g., kidney)

   (c) If c_v (mix of c_{v1} and c_{v2} can be monitored

   $$Qc_v = Q_1 c_{v1} + Q_2 c_{v2}$$
   $$c_v = f_1 c_1(0)e^{-k_1 t} + f_2 c_2(0)e^{-k_2 t}$$

XII. Biologic curves; a. Transport among body compartments (continued)

(d) Plot of $\ln c_v/c_v(0)$ vt shows composite of two exponential curves; decompose with subtraction procedure (see figure)

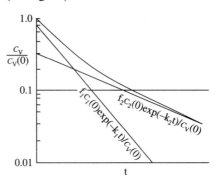

(1) Subtract long-time tail (smaller k)
(2) Determine intercepts of k_1, k_2 terms at $t = 0$: $f_1c_1(0)$, $f_2c_2(0)$
(3) Use $c_a = \alpha_1c_1(0) = \alpha_2c_2(0)$ to find f_1, f_2
(4) $Q_1/Q_2 = f_1/f_2$, $Q = Q_1 + Q_2$; measure Q, calculate V_1, V_2 with k_1, k_2; or, if know V_1, V_2, calculate Q_1, Q_2 with k_1, k_2
(5) White, gray matter perfusion, Kr^{85} in saline, scintillation detector (counts per minute versus time): composite curve decomposes into two exponentials; k_1 (gray) $\simeq 5k_2$ (white)
(6) Nondiffusible solutes; dye dilution

(e) Injected material remains in blood, no transfer to tissue

(f) $Vdc/dt = -Q(c_a - c_v)$, V $-$ blood (vascular) volume

(g) $Vc(t) = Q\int_0^t (c_a - c_v)dt$, where $c(t)$ is average concentration of

material (e.g., dye) in blood volume of organ or tissue at time t; $c(0) = 0$

(h) Finite amount of material injected, $m \Rightarrow c(t)$ increases then

decreases to 0: $0 = Q\int_0^\infty (c_a - c_v)dt$, $m = Q\int_0^\infty (c_a)dt$; therefore,

$Q = m/\int_0^\infty (c_v)dt$ (Stewart-Hamilton principle; relates Q to m and $c_v(t)$)

(i) If $c \cong c_v(t)$ (well-mixed vascular region or compartment) and $c_a(t)$ specified to be injected at constant rate for finite time, T

$$c_a(t) = c_{a0}, 0 \le t \le T; c_a(t) = 0, t > T$$

then

$$c_v(t) = c_{a0}(1 - e^{-kt}), 0 \le t \le T, c_v(t) = c_{a0}(e^{kT} - 1)e^{-kt}, t > T$$

(j) Provides typical dye-dilution or thermal-dilution curve, with peak at intersection of curves (peak is smoothed due to lack of mathematically sharp injection; dispersion in vasculature caused by molecular diffusion and eddies) (see figure)

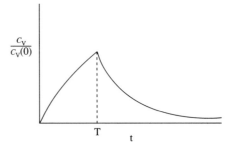

(k) Closed system—recirculation: second peak
(l) Intermittent cardiac output; thermodilution

(1) $Q = k / \int_0^{t_{30\%}} \Delta T(t) dt + A$

where $\Delta T(t)$ is temperature washout curve; A is area under $\Delta T(t)$ curve remaining after $t_{30\%}$ (exponential extrapolation); $\int_0^{t_{30\%}} \Delta T(t) dt$ is area under washout curve to $t_{30\%}$; $t_{30\%}$ is termination time for integration of $\Delta T(t)$, typically when T is 30% of peak; and $k = C_i \rho_i V_i (T_b - T_i) f / C_b \rho_b$, where $C_{i,b}$ is specific heat of injectate, blood; $\rho_{i,b}$ is density of injectate, blood; $T_{i,b}$ is temperature of injectate, blood; V_i is volume of injectate; f is correction factor for injectate temperature increase through catheter

(m) Continuous cardiac output: small heat signals (indicator) injected into blood by heater element proximal to pulmonic valve and temperature sensor in PA at catheter tip

(1) $Q = kP / \int_0^\tau R(t) dt$

where P is power delivered (watts); k is constant (periodicity of input signal, specific heat and density of blood, unit conversion factors); $R(t)$ is correlation transform function (correlates temperature response to periodic P signals with period τ); $\int_0^\tau R(t) dt$ is area under $R(t)$ versus t curve (°C/sec)

3. Solute distributes with mass transfer resistance
(a) Large extravascular volume: exchange of material from capillary bed into tissues
(1) Large, well-mixed tissue compartment
(2) Linearly distributed blood compartment
(3) Concentration of solute in blood compartment varies with length of compartment (capillaries)
(4) Over differential length dx
$$Q[c(x) - c(x + dx)] = PdA[c(x) - \alpha c_t]$$
where P is permeability (centimeters per second) of interface between two regions, $dA (= dS' dx)$ is differential interface area
(5) $Q[c(x) - c(x + dx)] = PdS' dx[c(x) - \alpha c_t]$
and, as $dx \rightarrow 0$
$$Qdc/dx = -PS'(c - \alpha c_t)$$
(6) For c_t constant (important assumption)
$$(c_v - \alpha c_t)/(c_a - \alpha c_t) = \exp(-PS'l/Q)$$
where $(c_a - \alpha c_t)$ is driving force for mass transfer, l is length of blood compartment across which concentration changes from c_a to c_v, $S'l (\equiv S)$ is interfacial area across length l
(7) Flow rate limited
$$PS/Q >> 1 \Rightarrow \exp(-PS/Q) \sim 0$$
equilibration fraction
$$E \equiv (c_v - c_v)/(c_a - \alpha c_t) \rightarrow 1 \text{ (maximum)}$$
if $(c_v - c_v) = (c_a - \alpha c_t)$, and capillary clearance
$$C \equiv QE = Q[1 - \exp(PS/Q)]$$
(8) Without very detailed anatomy, P and S not separable, but PS can be obtained from C and Q data
$$1 - C/Q = \exp(-PS/Q)$$
Semilog plot of $1 - C/Q$ versus $1/Q$, slope $= -PS$

IV Special Clinical Situations

A. PEDIATRIC ANESTHESIA

I. INTRODUCTION
II. FETAL CIRCULATION
III. NEONATAL PHYSIOLOGY

    a. Respiratory

    b. Cardiac

    c. Retinopathy

    d. Thermal regulation

    e. Hemoglobin

    f. Apnea of prematurity

IV. NEONATAL EMERGENCIES

    a. Diaphragmatic hernia

    b. Pulmonary atresia

    c. Tracheoesophageal fistula

    d. Pyloric stenosis

    e. Imperforate anus

    f. Necrotizing enterocolitis (NEC)

    g. Omphalocele/gastroschisis

    h. Myelodysplasia

    i. Pierre-Robin sequence

V. RESPIRATORY EMERGENCIES

    a. Laryngotracheobronchitis

    b. Supraglottitis

VI. RESUSCITATION OF THE NEWBORN

    a. General principles

    b. Airway

    c. Meconium aspiration

    d. Ventilation

    e. Drugs used in pediatric life support

B. OBSTETRIC ANESTHESIA

I. PHYSIOLOGY OF PREGNANCY

II. MATERNAL–FETAL PHYSIOLOGY

a. Placental transfer

b. Oxytocics

c. Tocolytics

d. Amniotic fluid

e. Physiology of labor

f. Fetal monitoring

III. COMPLICATIONS OF PREGNANCY

a. Hypertensive diseases of pregnancy

b. Endocrine

   1. Diabetes mellitus

   2. Thyroid

   3. Hypothyroidism

   4. Pheochromocytoma

c. Rh, ABO incompatibility

d. Placenta previa

e. Placenta accreta

f. Abruptio placenta

g. Amniotic fluid embolism

h. Uterine rupture

i. Postpartum bleeding

IV. ASSISTED REPRODUCTIVE TECHNOLOGIES

a. Abbreviations

b. Considerations

c. Factors influencing success

d. Steps to ART procedures

e. Ultrasound-guided transvaginal aspiration

f. Laparoscopy

V. PULMONARY ASPIRATION

a. More common in certain patients

b. Passive regurgitation required

c. Causes of increased gastric pressure

d. Types of pulmonary aspirate

e. Treatment

   1. Restore pulmonary function to normal as quickly as possible

   2. Corticosteroids not recommended

   3. Antibiotics not routinely used

   4. Antacids

   5. Metoclopramide

   6. H_2 blockers

C. CLINICAL HEMATOLOGY

I. BLOOD TRANSFUSION
II. SPECIFIC BLOOD DISORDERS
   a. Coagulation
   b. Hemoglobinopathies
   c. Erythrocyte disorders
   d. White cell disorders
   e. Platelet disorders
   f. Abnormalities of procoagulants
III. EFFECTS OF ANESTHETICS ON BLOOD SYSTEM

D. PRINCIPLES OF PAIN MANAGEMENT

I. CHRONIC PAIN THEORIES
II. CHRONIC PAIN TREATMENT
   a. Nonpharmacologic
   b. Pharmacologic

   1. Narcotic pharmacology
   2. Nonnarcotic analgesics
   3. Coanalgesics

   c. Interventional techniques
III. GENERALIZED PAIN DISORDERS
   a. Neuropathic pain
   b. Sympathetic mediated pain
   c. Multidisciplinary approach to management of chronic pain

E. MISCELLANEOUS CLINICAL ENTITIES

I. LASER SURGERY
II. OUTSIDE THE OPERATING ROOM
   a. Lithotripsy
   b. MRI
   c. CT
   d. GI
III. ELECTROCONVULSIVE THERAPY (ECT)
IV. GAMMA KNIFE
V. BURNS
VI. REGIONAL ANESTHESIA FOR OPHTHALMIC SURGERY

F. LEGAL MEDICINE

    I. **LEGAL LIABILITY**

   II. **INFORMED CONSENT**

  III. **MEDICAL NEGLIGENCE**

  IV. **LITIGATION ISSUES**

   V. **CONTRACTS AND EMPLOYMENT**

  VI. **LEGAL ISSUES RELATED TO HIV**

 VII. **ETHICAL ISSUES AT END OF LIFE**

A. PEDIATRIC ANESTHESIA

I. INTRODUCTION

a. The neonate differs in many ways from the fully developed adult. The changes that occur in the neonatal period and during infancy are continuous and significant. An important difference is a relatively greater body surface area in relation to body weight. Neonates and infants have a higher metabolic rate. The resting oxygen consumption is 6–8 ml/kg/min in the neonate, 5–6 ml/kg/min in infants, and 3–4 ml/kg/min in adults

II. FETAL CIRCULATION

a. The circulatory system is the first to become functional in early gestation. By 2 months' gestation, the human heart and major blood vessels are completely formed

b. The fetal umbilical vein is the arterial vessel that delivers oxygen and other nutrients from the placenta to the fetal heart. It has an oxygen tension of 30–35 mm Hg and an oxygen saturation of 80%

c. The liver is the first organ perfused by the umbilical vein. Essential substances, therefore, are present in high concentrations to promote protein synthesis. Most of the blood passes through the liver via the ductus venosus to the inferior vena cava, where it mixes with blood returning from the legs and abdominal viscera, and then passes to the right atrium (RA). About 60% of this blood passes through the foramen ovale to the left atrium, where it mixes with the pulmonary venous blood (small amount) and then passes to the left ventricle, ascending aorta, and coronary and cerebral vessels. The rest of the right atrial blood mixes with deoxygenated blood from the head and neck via the superior vena cava and passes to the right ventricle, pulmonary arteries, and preferentially to the descending aorta via the large ductus arteriosus that presents low resistance to blood flow. This reduces the PaO_2 below the ductus to 19–20 mm Hg (O_2 saturation 30–40%), compared with PaO_2 of 25–28 mm Hg (O_2 saturation 60%) in the ascending aorta. Thus, in the fetus there is a differential distribution of more oxygen to vital organs (head, myocardium)

---

d. In the fetus, the thicknesses of the walls of both ventricles and great vessels are similar as the resistance to blood flow from the right and left ventricles is similar. The low resistance of the placenta is largely responsible for the enormous shunt flow, representing 45% of fetal cardiac output. This allows additional oxygen supply to the fetus by the mother. The fetus has a narrow A/Vo$_2$ difference (80% − 60% = 20%), compared with (95% − 65% = 30%) in adults. The high cardiac output of the fetus is the principal mechanism that compensates for the narrow A/Vo$_2$ difference

1. Transition to postnatal circulation
    (a) At birth, the umbilical vessels are clamped, and then they close. This results in an increase in left ventricular end diastolic pressure. The lungs expand and become responsible for respiration; thus there is a decrease in pulmonary vascular resistance. The pulmonary vascular dilation is induced primarily by a rise in oxygen tension and to a lesser extent by respiratory alkalosis. The degree of response of pulmonary vascular resistance to oxygen is directly related to gestational age. Shortly after birth, the arterial PaO$_2$ is about 50–60 mm Hg. Within the first week of life, it increases to above 70 mm Hg
    (b) Pulmonary vasoconstriction is induced by hypoxemia and respiratory and/or metabolic acidosis. With the decrease in the pulmonary resistance, there is an increase in pulmonary blood flow that reduces the flow through fetal channels, which eventually close. The rise in pulmonary blood flow increases left atrial pressure and induces functional closure of the foramen ovale. The increase in PaO$_2$ constricts the ductus arteriosus, which functionally closes by the second to third day of life. By 2 months of age, the ductus becomes avascular fibrous ligament (the ligamentum arteriosum). The decrease in pulmonary vascular resistances is associated with a decrease in pulmonary vascular tone and thinning of the media of pulmonary arteries
    (c) In cases of congenital heart diseases associated with increased pulmonary flow, a state of increased pulmonary pressure occurs that may lead to irreversible narrowing of the pulmonary vessels and persistent pulmonary hypertension. Patency of the ductus arteriosis may be essential to maintain life in infants with pulmonary oligemia. Prostaglandin E$_1$ or E$_2$ infusion (0.5–1 mg/kg/min) may be administered to keep the ductus open. Administration of indomethacin, a prostaglandin synthetase inhibitor, may close the ductus
2. Persistent fetal circulation (persistent pulmonary hypertension)
    (a) Certain diseases, such as meconium aspiration, pulmonary hypoplasia, polycythemia, and idiopathic pulmonary hypertension, are associated with intense pulmonary vasoconstriction. The associated increases in right ventricular and right atrial pressures lead to shunting of blood from the right atrium to left atrium via the foramen ovale. The persistent fetal circulation may be treated by the administration of 100% oxygen, hyperventilation, correction of acidosis, and administration of a selective pulmonary vasodilator (nitric oxide)
    (b) Tolazoline, dopamine, isuprel, and PGE$_1$ are pulmonary vasodilators, but contrary to nitric oxide, they also dilate systemic vessels and decrease peripheral vascular resistance, which may not be desirable. The only available selective pulmonary vascular dilator is nitric oxide

III. NEONATAL PHYSIOLOGY

a. Respiratory

1. Prenatal development

    (a) Prenatal branching of terminal bronchioles develops by 16 weeks of fetal life

    (b) The number of airways proximal to the alveolar ducts does not increase significantly with maturation

    (c) Primitive alveoli and type II cells that produce surfactant develop by 24 weeks' gestation

    (d) Capillary proliferation surrounding saccules develops by 26–28 weeks, which makes gas exchange possible

    (e) With maturation, there is substantial growth of the alveolar portion of the lung, with a resultant increase in the number and surface area of alveolar ducts and alveolar sacs

    (f) The maturation of morphology and the surfactant system is complete by 36–40 weeks' gestation

    (g) Infants' bronchi have more cartilage and connective tissue, more glands in major bronchi, and less muscle as compared with older children. Therefore, in infants, small airway obstruction is commonly due to inflammation and edema, as opposed to muscle spasm in older children

    (h) Corticosteroids accelerate the maturation of fetal lungs

2. Surfactant

    (a) Surfactant is a complex of chemical substances present in normal mature lungs, and it maintains the physical properties of the alveoli and small airways. Surfactant alters the surface tension in the alveoli to extremely low levels and stabilizes the gas–liquid interface in the periphery of the lungs, thus preventing atelectasis

    (b) Surfactant is composed of 90% phospholipids and 10% protein. It is a phospholipid–azoprotein complex. There are at least seven phospholipids in the surfactant complex

        (1) Lecithin, a phosphatidylcholine (PC), is the main surface-active component of the surfactant. Lecithin is in a solid state at body temperature. Phosphatidylglycerol (PG) is a phospholipid that enables lecithin to become a liquid at body temperature

    (c) Surfactant is produced by alveolar type II pneumocytes. These cells function in a mature fashion by about 34 weeks of gestation

    (d) Abnormalities of surfactant, whether related to quantity or composition, lead to alveolar collapse (atelectasis)

    (e) A number of conditions are associated with surfactant deficiencies, including preterm birth, newborn respiratory distress syndrome, pulmonary edema, pneumonia, and adult respiratory distress syndrome

        (1) Premature babies who lack surfactant develop a respiratory distress syndrome (RDS) that leads to collapse of terminal alveoli and the development of hypoxia. An x-ray of the lung in RDS demonstrates a reticulogranular pattern

3. Fetal breathing

    (a) In utero, the fetus makes respiratory movements. The rate of fetal breathing is higher at 30 weeks' gestation than in a full-term fetus

    (b) Fetal breathing occurs only during rapid eye movement (REM). It is not affected by usual fluctuations in fetal PaO_2 (18–25 mm Hg) or fetal $PaCO_2$ (40–48 mm Hg)

    (c) Hypoxia abolishes fetal breathing and may induce fetal gasping. Maternal ingestion of alcohol and/or smoking also abolishes fetal breathing

    (d) Fetal $PaCO_2$ is normally 10–15 mm higher than maternal $PaCO_2$

III. Neonatal physiology; a. Respiratory (continued)

    (e) It is not clear why the fetus has to "breathe" in utero, when gas exchange is taken care of by the placenta; it might represent the prenatal practice of breathing

  4. Perinatal adaptation

    (a) At birth, the cardiovascular and respiratory systems undergo dramatic changes. During normal labor and vaginal delivery, the fetus goes through a period of considerable hypoxia, hypercarbia, and acidemia. The associated asphyxia leads to forceful fetal gasping that creates tremendous negative intrapleural pressure (up to -70 cm H_2O)

    (b) In the presence of adequate pulmonary surfactant, air is retained in the lungs, and the lung liquid is rapidly replaced by air. Gas exchange then begins in the lungs. The increase in PaO_2 and decrease in $PaCO_2$ lower the pulmonary vascular resistance; thus pulmonary blood flow increases

    (c) A relative increase in left atrial pressure leads to functional closure of the foramen ovale. These cardiovascular and pulmonary changes are delayed in premature infants

    (d) Hypoxia and/or hypercarbia can increase pulmonary vascular resistance and revert to persistent fetal circulation

    (e) Normally, the newborn ventilation is adjusted to achieve a lower $PaCO_2$ (28–29 mm Hg) than that found in older children or adults. This may be due to a poor buffering capacity of the neonate—a ventilatory compensation for metabolic acidosis

  5. Response to hypoxia

    (a) A full-term baby in a warm environment responds to hypoxia by transiently increasing ventilation

    (b) Premature infants show a biphasic response to hypoxemia—an increase in ventilation, followed by a decrease

    (c) Maturation of the respiratory system and response to hypoxic challenge may be related to postconceptual age rather than to postnatal age

  6. Response to carbon dioxide

    (a) Newborn infants respond to hypercarbia by increasing ventilation

    (b) The slope of the CO_2 response curve increases with postconceptual age as well as postnatal age, reflecting an increase in chemosensitivity

    (c) The slope of the CO_2 response curve decreases with decreasing oxygen

  7. Control of breathing

    (a) The mechanisms that control breathing are remarkably efficient. Arterial $PaCO_2$ is maintained within a very narrow range, while O_2 demand and CO_2 production vary greatly during rest and exercise

    (b) The control of breathing is accomplished by neural and chemical controls, which are closely interrelated

    (c) The rhythmic contraction of respiratory muscles is governed by the respiratory center in the brain stem, and tightly regulated with feedback systems, so as to match the level of ventilation with metabolic needs. The feedback mechanisms include central and peripheral chemoreceptors, stretch receptors in the airway and lung parenchyma via the vagal afferent, and segmental reflexes in the spinal cord provided by muscle spindles

  8. Pediatric airway

    (a) Newborn infants are obligatory nose breathers. The cephalad position of the epiglottis and close approximation of the tongue and epiglottis to the soft palate lead to increased resistance to air flow during mouth breathing. For air warming, humidification, and particle filtration, infants instinctively choose to breathe through the nose

(b) In infants, a nasogastric tube significantly increases total airway resistance and may compromise the ability to breathe. Hypertrophic adenoids may lead to partial or complete nasopharyngeal obstruction and force newborns to breathe orally. Hypertrophic tonsils may obstruct the entrance of the oropharynx. Enlarged adenoids and tonsils may lead to obstructive sleep apnea and/or postanesthesia upper airway obstruction

(c) The infant's larynx is situated at a higher level (C3–4) than the adult's (C4–5). The cricoid ring is the narrowest part of the infant's larynx. It is a circular cartilaginous ring that does not expand. Thus, the infant's larynx is funnel shaped. Trauma to the cricoid mucosa can lead to edema and upper airway obstruction (postintubation croup), and if severe enough, it may lead to fibrosis and subglottic stenosis

(d) Edema of the laryngeal mucosa increases the resistance of upper airway; its effect is seen much more often in infants than in adults

(e) Infants are particularly vulnerable to developing laryngospasm, which may become life-threatening. Laryngospasm is a sustained tight closure of the vocal cords by the contraction of the adductor muscles, and occurs most readily under light anesthesia
(1) Hypoxia and hypercarbia tend to prevent sustained laryngospasm
(2) Maintaining positive airway pressure during extubation of a child may decrease the incidence of laryngospasm

(f) The vocal cords of the neonate are slanted, such that the anterior commissure is more caudal than the posterior commissure. The epiglottis is U-shaped and protrudes over the larynx at a 45-degree angle
(1) Because of these anatomic features and the high position of the larynx, it is useful during laryngoscopy to press the larynx backwards to bring it into view. A straight laryngoscope blade may be preferred

(g) The diameter of the trachea of a newborn is 4–5 mm
(1) In a newborn infant, the distance between the carina and the vocal cords is 4–5 cm
(2) The tip of the endotracheal tube can move about 2 cm in the trachea with flexion or extension of the large head of a newborn baby
(3) The right main bronchus is less angled than the left

9. Lung volumes and elastic properties

(a) During the early postnatal years, there are rapid maturation and growth of the lungs, particularly the alveoli
(1) In infants, the lung volumes are smaller than in older children, and infants have far less reserve in the lung surface area for gas exchange
(2) The infant's thorax is extremely compliant, as the ribs are cartilaginous and horizontal and the respiratory muscles are not well developed
(3) The diaphragm and intercostal muscles of an infant have fewer type I muscle fibers, which are the slowly contracting, high-oxidative fibers adapted for sustained muscle activity. This contributes to early fatigue of an infant's respiratory muscles. Type I fibers reach the mature proportion of 55% by 8–9 months of age; in newborns, the proportion is only 25%, and in premature babies, it is only 10%

(b) The high compliance of an infant's chest wall and lungs lowers the resting lung volume and functional residual capacity (FRC)
(1) In the awake state, the inspiratory muscles have intrinsic tone that maintains the outward recoil and rigidity of the thorax. The loss of muscle tone during anesthesia would result in profound reduction of FRC, airway closure, and ventilation–perfusion imbalance, even in healthy infants
(2) The marked reduction of FRC secondary to airway closure results in a marked increase in the alveolar–arterial gradient of PO_2. In infants, postoperative

hypoxemia occurs frequently. A low level of positive end-expiratory pressure can minimize airway closure, increase FRC, and may improve PaO_2

(c) Persistent airway closure under anesthesia may lead to resorption atelectasis. Because adequate ventilation depends on diaphragmatic movement, anything that inhibits diaphragmatic descent will cause hypoventilation. Abdominal distension with gas can seriously impair inspiration

10. Respiratory function

(a) When calculated according to body weight, respiratory parameters in the newborn, including tidal volume, dead space, vital capacity, and specific compliance, are rather similar to those in the adult

(1) The respiratory rate and alveolar ventilation in an infant are much higher (30–40 per minute) than in an adult (10–15 per minute), due to the infant's higher metabolic rate

(2) The lungs of infants have less oxygen reserve

(3) An infant can become hypoxic much faster than an adult

(4) In infants, inspired anesthetic gases equilibrate with pulmonary blood much faster than in adults secondary to high alveolar ventilation and decreased functional residual capacity

11. Periodic breathing and apnea

(a) In full-term babies, normally there are brief apneic pauses during REM sleep that usually disappear by 3 months of age

(b) Periodic breathing occurs in all preterm infants during REM sleep. It decreases with increasing postconceptual age

(c) Premature babies hypoventilate during periodic breathing

(d) Oxygen administration to premature babies decreases periodic breathing; on the other hand, hypoxia increases the incidence of periodic breathing and lengthens the duration of apneic spells

b. Cardiac

1. The newborn heart: at birth, the size of the right ventricle equals that of the left ventricle and they are closely interrelated. There is increased work of the left ventricle and decreased work of the right ventricle, secondary to an increase in the peripheral vascular resistance and a decrease in the pulmonary vascular resistance. The size of the left ventricle continues to increase. By 6 months of age, the left ventricle has twice the muscle of the right ventricle. The newborn myocytes are smaller, more rounded, and more primitive, and have relatively more noncontractile elements. They cannot generate as much force as adult myocytes. The fetal myocardium is less compliant. The right ventricular compliance exceeds the left ventricular compliance. In the newborn, the Frank-Starling phenomenon is more limited as compared with an adult. There is relatively less sarcoplasmic reticulum in the fetal myocardium. With increasing maturity, voltage-dependent calcium channels regulating calcium entry into the cell increase in number. Calcium is a useful inotropic agent in the neonatal period

(a) Autonomic regulation

(1) At birth, there is decreased sympathetic innervation to the heart, and a significant postnatal development of sympathetic innervation occurs

[a] There are decreased catecholamine stores in the myocardium. Sympathetic stimulation provides both chronotropic and inotropic effects; however, the chronotropic effect predominates

[b] The control of vascular tone and myocardial contractility depends on adrenal function and circulating catecholamines

[c] There are an intact parasympathetic innervation and function similar to those of adults. Newborns respond to such stimuli as hypoxia and airway instrumentation by bradycardia and hypotension

[d] The β-receptor's sensitivity to catecholamines, such as isoproterenol, is well developed in the immature myocardium

(b) Heart rate: The normal heart rate in newborns is much higher than in adults. As the newborn ventricle is rigid and has fixed stroke volume, the cardiac output of newborns depends on the heart rate. The heart rate decreases substantially during the first few months of life and then decreases gradually until adulthood

(1) Bradycardia may occur during anesthesia due to hypoxia, laryngoscopy, intubation, endotracheal suction, traction of eye muscles, and the administration of certain drugs, such as halothane, suxamethonium, or neostigmine. The prophylactic administration of atropine may be indicated

(c) Electrocardiogram: At birth, right ventricular dominance occurs, and as the infant grows, the ECG reflects increasing dominance of the left ventricle. Normal sinus rhythm is the norm, but sinus arrhythmias and sinoatrial blocks may occur

(d) Blood pressure is directly related to cardiac output and peripheral resistance. The blood pressure gradually increases. In premature infants, the pressures are lower than in full-term babies. Systolic blood pressure at birth varies between 70 and 90 mm Hg, is about 100 between 1 and 6 years of age, and reaches adult values by 18 years of age

(e) Cardiac output in neonates is high, 2–5 L/min/m^2, or 200 ml/kg/min as compared with 100 ml/kg/min in adults. Cardiac output increases with age, but the cardiac index varies little, 2.5–4 L/min/m^2. Stroke volume of an infant is 4 ml per beat. Only 30% of neonatal myocardium has contractile elements compared to 60% in adults. Immature myocardium generates less force than adult myocardium

(1) The neonatal ventricles function at a plateau. The myocardium is less responsive to preload and less tolerant of an increase in afterload

(2) Neonates and infants have a relatively fixed stroke volume. The cardiac output of newborns depends on the heart rate

(3) The ventricles have reduced compliance

(4) Oxygen consumption increases from 4–6 ml/kg/min in the full-term newborn to about 8 ml/kg/min by 4 weeks of age, and then gradually decreases to 3.3 ml/kg/min in adults

(5) Pulmonary artery pressure decreases dramatically at birth and reaches adult levels by 6–8 weeks of age

[a] Pulmonary hypertensive crisis may result from hypoxia, hypercartria, acidosis, bronchospasm, and/or sympathetic stimulation

(6) Mean right atrial pressure is 1–5 mm Hg. Extremely large volumes cause small changes in right atrial pressure in newborns and infants as the atrium is very compliant. A rise of CVP in newborns is mainly caused by right atrial outflow obstruction

c. Retinopathy: retinopathy of prematurity (ROP) occurs as a result of an injury, and it starts as retinal vascular narrowing, followed by obliteration of retinal vessels, development of new vessels (neovascularization), retinal hemorrhage, retinal detachment, and blindness

1. ROP occurs during maturation of infant retina. During gestation, the nasal edge of the retina matures earlier than the temporal edge. ROP occurs mostly in the temporal region, which matures by 42 to 44 weeks of gestation

2. The role of intraoperative oxygen administration has been questioned
   (a) In premature babies, intraoperative oxygen saturation should be maintained between 93% and 95% to avoid hyperoxia. However, ROP has been reported in full-term babies who had never been exposed to more than room air. It has been also reported in infants with congenital cyanotic heart disease
   (b) Spontaneous regression of ROP occurs in 85% of cases. Treatment is directed at preventing the progression of ROP and repairing retinal defects. As the immature avascular retina secretes an angiogenic factor that stimulates vasoproliferation, ablation of the avascular retina (cryotherapy) should inhibit the release of angiogenic factor and thus minimize the neovascularization
3. In case of retinal detachment, a scleral buckling procedure is recommended
   (a) If neovascularization has progressed into the vitreous, vitrectomy may be indicated, via either a "closed" or an "open-sky" approach

d. Thermal regulation

1. Thermostasis
   (a) Body temperature is the result of the balance among the factors leading to heat loss, gain, and the distribution of heat within the body
   (b) An increase in heat loss or a decrease in heat gain may lead to hypothermia
   (c) To increase heat production, the body increases metabolic rate, and vasoconstricts to decrease heat loss
   (d) The CNS receives multiple sensory inputs about the state of thermal balance throughout the body
   (e) Temperature receptors are located in the hypothalamus, skin, respiratory tract, gastrointestinal tract, and spinal cord
2. Thermal regulation in neonates
   (a) Neonates have an intact central temperature control mechanism, which is limited
       (1) An infant can readily lose heat because an infant has a relatively large surface area, thin skin, and less subcutaneous fat
       (2) In an infant, if the head is exposed, a significant heat loss can occur
   (b) The important mechanisms to increase heat production are activity, shivering, and nonshivering thermogenesis
       (1) Infants do not shiver
       (2) In an anesthetized infant, nonshivering thermogenesis (heat production by brown fat metabolism) is the only mechanism for heat production
       (3) Brown fat composes 2–3% of body weight. It is located between the scapulae, in the neck, in the mediastinum, and around the kidneys and adrenals
       (4) Brown fat is a specialized tissue with rich blood supply, a high mitochondrial content, and a rich sympathetic nerve supply
       (5) When an infant gets cold, there is an increase in norepinephrine production, an increase in metabolism of brown fat, and an increase in heat production
       (6) The increase in brown fat metabolism is associated with a larger proportion of cardiac output diverted through the brown fat
   (c) The increase in norepinephrine production may lead to pulmonary vasoconstriction and an increase in pulmonary artery pressure, and may predispose to increased right-to-left shunting
       (1) The associated peripheral vasoconstriction may lead to hypoperfusion, acidosis, and apnea, particularly in premature babies
       (2) Hypoxia, infection, and birth injury can adversely affect a neonate's thermal stability

3. Heat exchange can take place by conduction, convection, radiation, and evaporation
    (a) Conduction
        (1) In a cold environment, heat can be lost from an infant's skin to the immediately adjacent environment, which could be surrounding air, clothing, or a blanket
        (2) The large surface area of an infant allows for the rapid loss of heat via conduction
        (3) The rate of heat transfer depends on the gradient of heat between the skin and the adjacent environment
        (4) Heat loss by conduction can be decreased
            [a] By warming the adjacent environment (surrounding air, blanket, irrigating solution)
            [b] By thermal insulation: an effective thermal insulator poorly conducts heat from its surface that is in contact with the infant's body. By warming the surface of the insulator that is in contact with the infant's body, the rate of heat loss by conduction is decreased
        (5) Blankets, drapes, and head covering can be effective thermal insulators
    (b) Convection
        (1) In the operating room, air is able to move freely. This movement of air results in an effective loss of heat as it maintains a temperature gradient between the body's surface and its immediate adjacent environment
        (2) Heat loss by convection can be decreased by keeping an infant in a warm incubator, covering the infant with a blanket, covering the head, and using surgical drapes
    (c) Radiation: the infant's body, the walls and other objects around the body emit infrared radiation
        (1) If the temperature of these objects is less than the temperature of the infant's body, then the rate of heat radiated from the body to the surrounding objects is more than the rate of radiation from the objects to the infant's body
        (2) Radiation is the major mechanism of heat loss under normal conditions
        (3) Radiation heat loss can be reduced by monitoring the temperature of the room and using a radiant heat lamp and/or a blanket
        (4) Reflecting the emitted radiation back to the skin also decreases the rate of heat loss by radiation (using aluminized plastic)
    (d) Evaporation: 20% of total body heat loss is due to evaporation
        (1) The rate of heat loss by evaporation can be increased by sweating
        (2) The driving force for evaporation is the difference between the vapor pressure of the skin and that of the environment
            [a] Heat exchange by evaporation happens at the skin and the lungs
            [b] The rate of respiratory evaporative heat loss is increased by breathing cool dry gases as they have a low vapor pressure
        (3) An infant spends 8–10% of total caloric expenditure to warm and humidify respiratory gases
        (4) Using a heated humidifier (active heating and humidification) can minimize calories lost through the respiratory system and maintain the integrity of respiratory mucosa
        (5) The temperature of heated gases should be monitored close to a patient's airway to guard against overheating
        (6) The heat and moisture exchanges help to humidify respiratory gases and to decrease heat loss. In children, they are less effective in maintaining body temperature as compared with active humidification and warming (using a heated humidifier)

III. Neonatal physiology (continued)

---

e. Hemoglobin

1. Oxygen transport
    (a) The hemoglobin content of newborn blood is about 19 g/100 ml, and consists of mostly fetal hemoglobin (HbF)
    (b) Fetal hemoglobin has a greater affinity for oxygen than does adult Hb (HbA). Oxygen is more strongly attached to fetal Hb.
    (c) The P_{50} (the partial pressure of oxygen at which 50% of Hb is saturated with oxygen) of HbF is 19 mm Hg as compared with 27 mm Hg in HbA
    (d) As the infant grows, HbF is replaced by HbA, and P_{50} increases to the adult value, enhancing oxygen unloading. This compensates for the physiologic anemia that occurs at 3 months of age. In premature infants and those with respiratory distress syndrome 2,3-DPG levels and P_{50} values are lower than for full-term babies
    (e) At birth, erythropoiesis activity stops, but in cases of severe anemia or congenital heart disease, an increase in plasma erythropoiesis is seen

2. Blood volume

Premature infants	95–100 ml/kg
Full-term infants	85–90 ml/kg
Children	70–80 ml/kg
Adults	65–70 ml/kg

    (a) The cardiac output/blood volume ratio is higher in infants than in adults, and thus blood flow and oxygen carriage are relatively greater
    (b) Hemoglobin (Hb) at birth ranges from 18 to 20 g/100 ml of blood. The level drops until 2–3 months of age, and then gradually rises again toward adult values
    (c) Erythropoietin regulates red cell production in response to oxygen availability
        (1) Erythropoietin is present in fetal plasma, disappears shortly after birth, and rises at about 3 months of age secondary to physiologic anemia. An associated increase in reticulocyte count is noted. The effect of physiologic anemia is partially offset by increasing HbA content of the cells
    (d) Chronic hypoxemia increases erythropoietin and erythrocyte production from the normal daily 1% rate to 2% (slow process)
    (e) Adult hemoglobin (HbA) has two alpha and two beta chains in its molecule, in contrast to fetal hemoglobin (HbF), which has two alpha and two gamma chains
    (f) HbF is about 90–95% until 36 weeks' gestation, when it begins to be replaced by HbA, and the blood concentration of 2,3-DPG increases
        (1) At birth, HbF is 70–80%, but gradually decreases until by 6 months of age, only a small amount of HbF persists
        (2) HbF has a greater affinity for oxygen than HbA, due to the reduced binding of 2,3-DPG to HbF
        (3) In the fetus, the hemoglobin–oxygen dissociation curve is shifted to the left
        (4) The P_{50} of HbF is only 18–20 mm Hg compared with the adult Hb of 27 mm Hg

3. Oxygen unloading capacity of HbF and HbA
    (a) The umbilical venous blood is 65% saturated in the mother and 80% saturated in the fetus due to
        (1) Beneficial leftward shift of the oxygen dissociation curve
        (2) Its low affinity to 2,3-DPG
        (3) Low concentration of 2,3-DPG in the fetus. Oxygen binds more tightly to HbF than to HbA leading to higher O_2 saturation in fetal arterial circulation as compared with the adult's

(b) In addition

(1) The fetus delivers O_2 preferentially to the most vital organs, extracts more O_2 from blood, and has a relatively high cardiac output leading to adequate O_2 transport with relatively low PaO_2

(2) Unloading the oxygen to tissues occurs at the steep part of the O_2 dissociation curve

(3) As the O_2 dissociation curve of HbF is left shifted its curve is steeper than the curve of HbA. Therefore, HbF unloads O_2 to fetal tissues better than does HbA. This is a good example of the efficiency of fetal circulation

(4) The advantage of a low P_{50} in the fetus is that O_2 is taken up more readily in the placenta, and it is less readily released in the tissues

(5) Most of the fetal iron stores are built up in the last trimester of pregnancy; premature babies have less iron and less Hb

4. Oxygen transport

(a) If increased oxygen is demanded, it is mainly met by an increase in cardiac output, while alveolar ventilation is increased to maintain proper levels of alveolar PO_2 and PCO_2

(b) The amount of oxygen carried by the plasma is small (0.3 ml/dl per 100 mm Hg)

(c) Most oxygen molecules in blood combine reversibly with Hb to form oxyhemoglobin. Each molecule of Hb combines with four molecules of oxygen; 1 g of oxyhemoglobin combines with 1.34 ml of oxygen

(d) As blood circulates through the lungs, O_2 tension increases from the mixed level of about 40 mm Hg to 100 mm Hg, and Hb is saturated to about 97%. A further increase in PO_2 results in a very small increase in O_2 saturation. As blood circulates through the capillaries, oxygen is taken up by the tissues, and both PO_2 and O_2 saturation decrease

(e) The P_{50}, which is the PO_2 of whole blood at 50% saturation, indicates the affinity of Hb for oxygen

(1) The blood of normal adults has an SO_2 of 50% when PO_2 is 27 mm Hg at 37°C and pH is 7.4

(2) An increase in blood pH increases oxygen affinity of Hb (Bohr effect)

(3) A decrease in temperature increases the oxygen affinity and shifts the oxygen–Hb dissociation curve to the left

(4) An increase in red cell 2,3-DPG decreases the oxygen affinity of Hb, increases P_{50}, and increases the unloading of O_2 at the tissue level

(f) In the newborn, blood oxygen affinity is extremely high and P_{50} is low (19 mm Hg) because HbF reacts poorly with 2,3-DPG; thus, oxygen delivery at the tissue level is low, despite higher red blood cell mass and Hb level

(1) After birth, the total Hb level decreases P_{50} increase rapidly. This is associated with increased levels of ATP and 2,3-DPG

(2) The 2,3-DPG level is high in infants and decreases toward adult levels by age 10

f. Apnea of prematurity is an unexplained cessation of breathing for 20 seconds or longer, or a shorter respiratory pause associated with bradycardia, cyanosis, or pallor, and it occurs most commonly during REM sleep

1. Apnea of prematurity is of two types

(a) Central apnea is neuronal in origin and is associated with no respiratory movement. It may be related to an immature respiratory control mechanism

(b) Obstructive apnea is attributable to upper airway obstruction while respiratory effort continues

III. Neonatal physiology; f. Apnea of prematurity (continued)

      (1) Excessive relaxation of the genioglossus muscle during sleep or anesthesia may lead to obstructive apnea in premature babies, particularly in those with poor pulmonary compliance

      (2) Fatigue of immature respiratory muscles may contribute to apnea in preterm infants

      (3) In some preterm infants (less than 2 kg), apnea continues without apparent effort to breathe until cardiorespiratory arrest occurs (sudden infant death syndrome)

2. Postoperative apnea and bradycardia in former premature babies

   (a) Factors that increase the risks of postoperative apnea and bradycardia are postconceptual age less than 52 weeks, necrotizing enterocolitis, neurologic problems, and anemia

   (b) Regional anesthesia may be associated with a lower incidence of postoperative apnea and bradycardia

      (1) The administration of sedatives or hypnotics during regional anesthesia increases the risk of postoperative apnea and bradycardia

   (c) Postoperative apnea and bradycardia usually occur within the first 12 hours postoperatively

      (1) To detect postoperative apnea and bradycardia, it is important to adopt multiple methods of apnea monitoring simultaneously, including pneumocardiogram (tranthoracic impedance to measure chest wall movement), pulse oximetry, and nursing staff observation

   (d) Caffeine (5–10 mg IV) decreases the incidence of postoperative apnea and bradycardia. Theophylline has also been effective. The mechanism of its action could be both central and peripheral, as it prevents respiratory muscle fatigue

IV. NEONATAL EMERGENCIES

a. Diaphragmatic hernia

1. Incidence is one to two in 5,000 live births

2. Herniation of abdominal contents into the thorax at 8 weeks of gestation with resultant ipsilateral lung hypoplasia

3. 90% are on the left side (foramen of Bochdalek)

4. 25% have associated cardiac anomalies

5. Presentation: scaphoid abdomen, respiratory distress

   (a) Awake intubation is recommended

   (b) Avoid mask ventilation if possible

   (c) Pass OG tube to evacuate stomach after an airway is secured

   (d) Preductal arterial line is helpful (right hand)

6. Be aware of potential for contralateral PTX (pressure necessary to expand hypoplastic area is higher than the pressure required to rupture a normal lung, i.e., use low inflation pressures, rapid rate)

7. Hyperventilation to arterial CO_2 levels 25–30 is recommended to decrease PVR and minimize right-to-left shunting

8. Honeymoon period postoperatively with deterioration secondary to persistent pulmonary hypertension and hypoxia

9. Surgical approach is via abdominal incision with either primary closure or closure with a synthetic patch

10. ECMO used now to support infants for a few days prior to correction; 30–60% mortality

b. Pulmonary atresia with intact intraventricular septum

1. Prevalence
   (a) 1% of congenital heart disease
2. Etiology
   (a) Fusion of pulmonary valve cusps
       (1) 80% of patients
   (b) Combined infundibular and valvular atresia
       (1) 20% of patients
3. Obligate anatomic features
   (a) Atrial septal defect or patent foramen ovale
   (b) Patent ductus arteriosus
       (1) Maintained with prostaglandins or surgical systemic to pulmonary shunt
4. Common features
   (a) Hypoplastic pulmonary valve and main pulmonary trunk
   (b) Tricuspid regurgitation
5. Occasional features
   (a) Right and left main pulmonary artery stenosis
6. Pathophysiology
   (a) Blood returning from the venae cavae enters the right atrium, crosses the atrial septum to the left atrium (common mixing chamber), and then flows to the left ventricle, out the aorta through the ductus arteriosus to the pulmonary artery
7. Clinical presentation
   (a) Tachypnea and cyanosis at birth
   (b) Hypoxemia with metabolic acidosis
       (1) Secondary to obstruction to pulmonary blood flow
   (c) Congestive heart failure
   (d) Heart murmur
   (e) ECG abnormalities
       (1) Right atrial enlargement and right axis deviation
8. Chest x-ray abnormalities
   (a) Prominent right atrium and left ventricle
   (b) Decreased pulmonary vascular markings
9. Diagnosis
   (a) Two-dimensional echocardiogram
   (b) Cardiac catheterization to explicitly define anatomy
10. Palliative treatment
    (a) Prostaglandin E (PO or IV)
    (b) Balloon atrial septostomy
    (c) Surgical palliation
        (1) Pulmonary valvotomy
            [a] Open or closed
            [b] For patients with a normal right ventricle
        (2) Traditional systemic to pulmonary shunts
            [a] Blalock-Taussig shunt—subclavian artery to pulmonary artery
            [b] Potts shunt—descending aorta to pulmonary artery
            [c] Waterston shunt—ascending aorta to pulmonary artery
        (3) Current shunts
            [a] Modified Blalock-Taussig shunt
                i) Gortex graft is used to connect the subclavian artery to the pulmonary artery

IV. Neonatal emergencies; b. Pulmonary atresia (continued)

        ii) Placed on opposite side of aortic arch

        iii) Goal is to obtain arterial O_2 saturation of 75% with pulmonary to systemic flow ratio of 2:1 (higher saturations with higher pulmonary flow result in pulmonary edema and left ventricular failure)

11. Definitive surgical treatment

    (a) Rastelli procedure (anastomosis of right ventricle to pulmonary artery later in life)

12. Anesthetic implications

    (a) Primary hemodynamic goal

        (1) Preservation of pulmonary blood flow by preventing increases in PVR and decreases in systemic vascular resistance (SVR)

    (b) Avoid airway obstruction, acidosis, dehydration, hypovolemia, and high airway pressures

    (c) High alveolar concentrations of inhalation anesthetics are poorly tolerated secondary to hypotension and impaired contractility (especially in the infant with a fixed stroke volume)

    (d) Continue all measures to maintain ductal patency

    (e) Right-to-left shunts theoretically increase the speed of induction with IV agents and slow inhalation inductions (secondary to decrease in pulmonary blood flow)

c. Tracheoesophageal fistula (TEF)

1. 90% of cases with esophageal atresia are associated with TEF

2. Incidence is one in 3,000 live births

3. Type C esophageal atresia with a distal fistula most common

4. Associated with VATER syndrome: V—vertebral; A—anal; T—TEF; E—esophageal atresia; R—radial or renal anomalies. TEF presentation, usually after first feeding, with respiratory distress

5. Preoperative management

    (a) Discontinue oral feeds

    (b) Semiupright position

    (c) Continuous suction on a proximal pouch

6. Anesthetic management

    (a) Warm room

    (b) Premedicate with atropine 10–20 μg/kg

    (c) Awake intubation or Rapid Sequence Induction

    (d) Tube positioned distal to a fistula; above carina (bevel anterior intubate right mainstream and pull back until you hear bilateral BS)

    (e) Spontaneous ventilation with halothane

    (f) If needed, gentle positive pressure ventilation—avoid gastric distention

    (g) Left lateral decubitus position for right thoracotomy, ligation of fistula, and esophageal anastomosis

    (h) Gastrostomy performed in critically ill infant under local anesthesia to decompress the stomach

    (i) Careful attention to secretions in endotracheal tubes

    (j) Extubation in vigorous healthy infants

    (k) Postoperative management determined by degree of prematurity, associated lesions, and degree of pulmonary dysfunction

    (l) Most frequent complication is atelectasis and pneumonitis

7. Mortality

    (a) Overall survival is 65–75%

8. Outcome for survivors

   (a) Asymptomatic 15 to 20 years later
   (b) Always at risk for recurrent URI
   (c) Esophageal stricture, which may require dilation
   (d) Congenital lobar emphysema
       (1) Awake intubation or intubation with an inhalation induction followed by maintenance of spontaneous ventilation
       (2) Avoid N_2O
       (3) Most commonly affects left upper lobe but may involve entire lung

d. Pyloric stenosis

1. Incidence is one in 500 live births

2. More frequent in males than in females

3. Presents during second to sixth week of life with projectile nonbilious vomiting

4. Palpable "olive"

5. Medical, not surgical, emergency

6. Hypokalemic hypochloremic metabolic alkalosis

7. Volume resuscitation required—LR, full-strength salt solution

8. Correction of electrolytes: Na^+ over 130 mEq/L; Cl^- over 85 and increasing

9. Anesthetic management

   (a) Full stomach
   (b) OG suction three times to evacuate stomach
   (c) Pre O_2, atropine, rapid-sequence induction
   (d) Narcotics not usually needed
   (e) Extubate at end of procedure

e. Imperforate anus

1. Incidence is one per 5,000 live births

2. R/O associated lesions; VATER syndrome

3. Anesthetic concerns

   (a) Risk of aspiration
   (b) Avoid N_2O
   (c) Volume replacement—may have increased third-space fluid requirements
       (1) 10 ml/kg/hr of crystalloid or colloid may be needed if surgery is extensive
       (2) Follow urine output, vital signs, skin turgor
       (3) Invasive monitors for moribund infants
   (d) Potential for sepsis

f. Necrotizing enterocolitis (NEC)

1. Predominantly in preterm infants

   (a) 5–15% infants under 1,500 g
   (b) Mortality 10–30%

2. Present with thrombocytopenia, anemia, coagulopathy, hyperglycemia

   (a) Severe cases—metabolic acidosis and hypotension

3. Narcotic/muscle relaxant technique, avoid N_2O

IV. Neonatal emergencies; f. Necrotizing enterocolitis (continued)

4. Blood products available

(a) Massive volume requirements—1–2 blood volumes

(b) Etiology uncertain but secondary to inadequate blood supply to gut

---

g. Omphalocele/gastroschisis: intestinal obstruction; major intravascular fluid deficits

1. Omphalocele

(a) One in 10,000 live births

(b) 20% have associated cardiac lesions

(c) Epigastric omphalocele—high incidence of congenital heart disease; hypogastric omphalocele—exstrophy of bladder

(d) Occurs around 12th week of gestation

2. Gastroschisis

(a) Incidence is one in 15,000 live births

(b) Herniated viscera and intestine

(c) Usually to the right of the umbilicus

(d) Lack of membranous sac

(e) Problems

(1) Fluid loss, metabolic acidosis

(2) Hypothermia

(3) Sepsis

(f) Preoperative management

(1) Massive volume replacement 20 cc/kg LR and 5% albumin or more may be needed

(2) Herniated viscera protected with Saran wrap or moist sterile dressing

(3) Arterial line (UAC or radial) helpful

(g) Anesthetic management

(1) Gastric decompression

(2) Monitors—pulse oximeter on lower extremity

(3) Pre O_2, atropine 10–20 µg/kg, rapid-sequence induction or awake intubation if infant has difficult airway or is severely hypotensive

(4) Adequate muscle relaxation needed

(5) Anesthesia consists of volatile agents or narcotics or combination. Decision to close primarily or with silon chimney depends on

[a] Inspiratory peak pressures (if over 30–35, respiratory compromise may follow)

[b] Perfusion to lower extremities—increased intra-abdominal pressure reduces venous return and organ perfusion

(6) Extubation depends on size of repair and ventilatory status. Usually, transported intubated and sedated to ICU

---

h. Myelodysplasia: abnormality in fusion of the embryologic neural groove during the first month of gestation. Failure of neural tube closure results in meningocele (herniation of meninges) or myelomeningocele (herniation of neural elements)

1. Myelomeningocele

(a) Commonly occurs in lumbosacral region (75%)

(b) Associated with Arnold-Chiari type II malformation and hydrocephalus. Rarely exhibits increased ICP

(c) Surgical emergency—high risk of infection and death

(d) Infection risk less than 7% if defect is repaired within 48 hours of birth

(e) Anesthetic considerations

    (1) Coexisting disease

        [a] Arnold-Chiari

        [b] Hydrocephalus

    (2) Airway management may be difficult

    (3) Positioning—protection of neuroplaque

    (4) Volume status—potential for large third-space losses

    (5) Potential for hypothermia

(f) Induction

    (1) Either in left lateral position

    (2) Or supine with the sac protected by a cushioned ring

    (3) Either a nondepolarizing muscle relaxant or succinylcholine can be used safely

(g) Positioning: after intubation, the patient is turned prone. Chest and hip rolls are used to

    (1) Facilitate ventilation

    (2) Ensure that the abdomen is free

    (3) Reduce intra-abdominal pressure

    (4) Decrease bleeding from epidural plexus

        [a] Avoid excessive rotation of the neck

i. Pierre-Robin sequence

1. Early mandibular retrognathia is the primary defect with secondary failure of the tongue to descend from between palatal shelves

2. Characterized by glossoptosis, retrognathia, and cleft palate

3. Anesthetic concerns: difficult airway—have backup plans available, surgeon available, tracheostomy set available, and a variety of tubes and blades and a fiberoptic bronchoscope

4. Intubation

    (a) Awake look; perform direct laryngoscopy after topical anesthesia, premedication with atropine (20 μg/kg), and appropriate sedation. (Avoid deep sedation.) Neonates—no sedation. Always maintain spontaneous ventilation. If unable, then

    (b) Maintain spontaneous ventilation with halothane and 100% O_2

        (1) Provides margin of safety

        (2) CPAP 10 cm H_2O to prevent upper airway obstruction

        (3) Nasopharyngeal airway, "jaw thrust" when the patient is sufficiently anesthetized to tolerate it

            [a] Laryngoscopy performed with traction on the tongue via a suture, forceps, or retractor

            [b] Jackson anterior commissure laryngoscope

            [c] Laryngeal mask airway

            [d] Fiberoptic bronchoscopy—needs appropriate equipment and experience

    (c) Elective tracheostomy

        (1) Problems associated with pediatric tracheostomies

            [a] Accidental decannulation

            [b] Obstruction

            [c] Hemorrhage

            [d] Air leaks

V. RESPIRATORY EMERGENCIES

a. Laryngotracheobronchitis: also called croup, a common cause of upper airway obstruction in children

1. Viral etiology usually parainfluenza 3
2. Gradual onset associated with an upper respiratory infection
3. Edema present from pharynx down into the small airways
   (a) Most significant edema is in the subglottic region
4. Characteristics
   (a) Biphasic stridor
   (b) Retractions
   (c) Hoarseness
   (d) Barking cough
   (e) Age 6 months to 3 years
5. Treatment
   (a) Self-limiting process
   (b) Humidified air ± supplemental O_2 if needed
   (c) Corticosteroids
   (d) With severe distress may need racemic epinephrine treatments
   (1)

Racemic epinephrine dosages	
0–1 year	0.2 ml of 2.25% solution
1–3 years	0.3 ml of 2.25% solution
3–6 years	0.4 ml of 2.25% solution
>6 years	0.4 ml of 2.25% solution

   All doses are mixed with 2 cc of NS and delivered by a nebulizer
   (2) Watch for "rebound" effect. Racemic epinephrine has a short duration of action and symptoms may recur
   (e) Endotracheal intubation indicated for treatment of hypoxia and CO_2 retention
   (1) Tube 0.5 to 1.0 mm smaller in diameter than predicted
   (2) Usually wait 72 hours before extubation
   (3) Look for sign of air leak around ETT prior to extubation
   (4) Antibiotics not needed unless there are signs of bacterial superinfection

b. Supraglottitis (epiglottitis): acute, life-threatening cause of upper airway obstruction; *Hemophilus influenza* infection of supraglottic structures

1. Characteristics
   (a) Sudden onset
   (b) Drooling
   (c) Dysphagia
   (d) Sitting forward
   (e) Appear toxic, high fevers
   (f) Ages 2 to 6 years most common; cases have been reported in adults
2. Diagnosis—based on clinical grounds
   (a) X-rays are not necessary to confirm the diagnosis
   (b) Patients should be placed on O_2 by face mask and accompanied by a physician capable of providing an airway (intubation or tracheostomy)

    (c) If the patient is not in severe respiratory distress, a lateral radiograph of the neck may aid in diagnosis

    (d) Avoid examining oropharynx or IV placement

3. Treatment

    (a) Airway

        (1) Intubation performed under general anesthesia with ENT specialist in room available to perform emergency tracheostomy

        (2) Assortment of laryngoscope blades, tubes (smaller size than expected), and tracheostomy set open

        (3) Induction performed, with child in sitting position, gradually with halothane and 100% O_2

            [a] Parental presence at discretion of anesthesiologists

        (4) 10-cm CPAP may be necessary to treat upper airway obstruction

            [a] All attempts must be made to keep the child calm

                i) Avoid examining oropharynx

                ii) Avoid IV placement while awake

        (5) Laryngoscopy performed under deep anesthesia after an IV is started and the patient is pretreated with 20 μg/kg of atropine

        (6) Visualization of classic "cherry red" epiglottis confirms the diagnosis

        (7) Edema of the lingual surface of the epiglottis, uvula, arytenoids, aryepiglottic folds, and false vocal cords can cause severe obstruction. In order to visualize the vocal cords, a forceful manual chest compression may open up the airway or produce bubbles that serve as a guide for intubation

        (8) Cultures are taken prior to antibiotic therapy

        (9) Some authors advocate electively changing the orotracheal tube to a nasotracheal tube

    (b) Complications

        (1) Accidental or self-extubation can be disastrous

            [a] Minimal sedation, elbow restraints, close observation in intensive care setting with spontaneous ventilation using humidified air

            [b] Alternative protocols include mechanical ventilation, full sedation, and muscle relaxation to prevent extubation and laryngeal trauma

        (2) Pulmonary edema

            [a] Negative pressure pulmonary edema has been reported after severe cases

            [b] Benign course

    (c) Antibiotic therapy

        (1) Ampicillin

        (2) Chloramphenicol

        (3) Cefuroxime (100 to 200 mg/kg per day)

    (d) Extubation

        (1) Average duration of intubation is 36 hours

        (2) Resolution of fever and development of air leak are good indicators of success

        (3) Some advocate repeat examination of the epiglottis via fiberoptic route or direct laryngoscopy prior to extubation

VI. RESUSCITATION OF THE NEWBORN

a. General principles

1. Rapid initiation of basic life support (CPR) is essential

2. In infants, the major cause of cardiac arrest is hypoxemia due to airway obstruction and respiratory depression

VI. Resuscitation of the newborn; a. General principles (continued)

(a) Establishing a clear airway and ventilation with 100% O_2 is the first step
(b) Cardiac compression
(c) IV access
(d) Drug administration
(e) Direct-current countershock when appropriate

3. Efficient organization of the resuscitation effort is of great importance for optimal outcome

(a) A single experienced individual should be in charge of coordinating the resuscitation effort
(b) At least three individuals are needed to resuscitate a newborn—the first to establish an airway and ventilate (bag, mask, mouth to mouth), the second to perform cardiac compression, and the third to establish an IV and administer necessary drugs

4. Fetal monitoring can help to predict which neonate may require resuscitation and be prepared for it

b. Airway

1. The upper airway should be immediately suctioned using a bulb syringe to remove blood, mucus, or meconium from oropharynx. Then each nostril should be suctioned, as most neonates are obligate nose breathers

2. Suctioning should be limited to 10-second intervals

3. While suctioning, monitoring of the heart rate is necessary as suctioning may lead to severe bradycardia secondary to vagal stimulation and/or hypoxia

4. If airway obstruction is below the vocal cords, intubation and suctioning should be performed

c. Meconium aspiration probably occurred if thick meconium-stained amniotic fluid is found

1. Suctioning should begin immediately after delivery of the head by the obstetrician

2. Intubation and suctioning are repeated until no significant amount of meconium is suctioned

3. Heart rate should be monitored during suctioning

4. Positive airway pressure is avoided, if possible, before meconium suctioning so as not to drive the meconium into the periphery of the tracheobrachial tree. But if the newborn develops cyanosis and/or bradycardia, gentle positive-pressure ventilation with 100% oxygen should be started immediately

d. Ventilation

1. If a newborn does not breathe adequately, ventilation via a bag and mask should be indicated

2. A peak inflation pressure of 25–50 cm H_2O may be required to establish ventilation

3. Adequacy of ventilation should be assessed

e. Drugs used in pediatric advanced life support

Drugs	Dosage (Pediatric)	Remarks
Adenosine	0.1–0.2 mg/kg Maximum single dose: 12 mg	Rapid IV bolus
Atropine sulfate	0.02 mg/kg	Minimum dose: 0.1 mg Maximum single dose: 0.5 mg in child, 1.0 mg in adolescent
Bretylium	5 mg/kg; may be increased to 10 mg/kg	Rapid IV
Calcium chloride 10%	20 mg/kg	Give slowly
Dopamine hydrochloride	2–20 μg/kg/min	Alpha-adrenergic action dominates at ≥15–20 μg/kg/min
Dobutamine hydrochloride	2–20 μg/kg/min	Titrate to desired effect
Epinephrine for bradycardia	IV/IO: 0.01 mg/kg (1:10,000, 0.1 ml/kg) ET: 0.1 mg/kg (1:1,000, 0.1 ml/kg)	Be aware of total dose of preservative administered (if preservatives are present in epinephrine preparation) when high doses are used
Epinephrine for asystolic or pulseless arrest	First dose IV/IO: 0.01 mg/kg (1:10,000, 0.1 ml/kg) ET: 0.1 mg/kg (1:1,000, 0.1 ml/kg) IV/IO doses as high as 0.2 mg/kg of 1:1,000 may be effective Subsequent doses IV/IO/ET: 0.1 mg/kg (1:1,000, 0.1 ml/kg) • Repeat every 3–5 minutes IV/IO doses as high as 0.2 mg/kg of 1:1,000 may be effective	Be aware of total dose of preservative administered (if preservatives are present in epinephrine preparation) when high doses are used
Epinephrine infusion	Initial at 0.1 μg/kg/min Higher infusion dose used if asytole present	Titrate to desired effect (0.1–10 μg/kg/min)
Lidocaine	1 mg/kg	
Lidocaine infusion	20–50 μg/kg/min	
Sodium bicarbonate	1 mEq/kg per dose or 0.3 × kg × base deficit	Infuse slowly and only if ventilation is adequate

B. OBSTETRIC ANESTHESIA

I. PHYSIOLOGY OF PREGNANCY—all organs affected during pregnancy

a. Cardiovascular system

1. Cardiac output increases by 50%
   (a) Peaks at 32 weeks' gestation
   (b) 60% increase in cardiac output due to augmented stroke volume
2. In the immediate postpartum period, cardiac output increases maximally
   (a) Can rise 80% above control values
3. Peripheral resistance, the diastolic BP, and MABP decrease during pregnancy; any rise in BP during pregnancy is pathologic
4. Aortocaval compression in supine position
   (a) Leads to decrease in cardiac output and decreases in uterine blood flow
   (b) Left uterine displacement essential

b. Blood

1. Physiologic anemia of pregnancy due to increase of blood volume more than to increase of red blood corpuscles (1 liter of plasma versus 0.5 liter of RBC)
2. Pregnancy considered a hypercoagulable state
   (a) Due to increase in blood coagulation factors
   (b) Increased incidence of thrombosis, embolism, and DIC during pregnancy
3. 2-3–Diphosphoglycerate (DPG) increases, which allows easy release of O_2 at the placenta to fetus
4. Plasma pseudocholinesterase concentration decreases
   (a) Probably due to dilution
   (b) No significant clinical effects occur

c. Respiratory system

1. Minute ventilation increased mainly due to increased tidal volume
2. Blood gas: $PaCO_2$ reduced (32 torr); pH maintained by renal compensatory effect
3. Inspiratory capacity (IV and IRV) increases
4. FRC (ERV and RV) decreases and approaches closing volume, leading to increased possibility of shunting in supine position
5. Total lung volume not changed
6. Pregnancy and asthmatics
   (a) Mild to moderate asthmatics—effect of pregnancy on asthma variable
   (b) Adverse effect on patient's respiration in severe asthmatics during pregnancy
       (1) Diaphragmatic elevation
       (2) Increased O_2 demand
           [a] Due to pregnancy
           [b] Due to increased work of respiration
   (c) Pregnancy increases O_2 demand
       (1) O_2 reserve reduced by decreased FRC
       (2) Parturient rapidly becomes hypoxic when deprived of O_2

d. Renal system—GFR (glomerular filtration rate) increased during pregnancy

1. Due to increased renal plasma flow
2. BUN and creatine concentration decrease about 40–50%

e. Gastrointestinal system

1. GI motility, food absorption, and lower sphincter pressure decreased during pregnancy due to level of plasma progesterone
2. Increased gastric acid secretion due to increased secretion of hormone gastrin

f. Central nervous system and peripheral nervous systems

1. Increased progesterone and endorphin concentrations during pregnancy implicated as cause of decrease in MAC of inhalational agents
2. Wider dermatomal spread of sensory anesthesia
    (a) Observed in parturients following use of epidural anesthesia
    (b) Reduced epidural space volume caused by engorged venous plexus due to aortocaval compression
3. Enhanced sensitivity of peripheral nerve to local anesthetic documented in humans

II. MATERNAL–FETAL PHYSIOLOGY

a. Placental transfer

1. No continuity between maternal and fetal circulation
2. Barrier called blood–placental barrier (B-P-B). Transmission of drugs across membrane depends on
    (a) Lipid solubility: thiopental easier to penetrate than muscle relaxant
    (b) Gradient across the membrane
    (c) Electrical charge, i.e., ionized versus un-ionized
        (1) Pk_a very important
        (2) Fetal acidosis can cause ion trapping of local anesthetics
    (d) Molecular size
        (1) Quaternary ammonium compounds do not cross easily
            [a] Glycopyrrolate and muscle relaxant versus atropine
            [b] Insulin and heparin do not cross placenta due to large molecular weight
    (e) Protein binding
        (1) Drug with high protein maternal binding capacity—bupivacaine
            [a] Less transmitted than that having low protein binding (lidocaine)
        (2) Fetal/maternal ratios 0.3 and 0.5, respectively

b. Oxytocics

1. Stimulate uterine muscles to contract
2. Indication
    (a) Induce labor
    (b) Augment labor
    (c) Treat uterine atony
    (d) Induce abortion

3. Synthetic oxytocin (Pitocin)
   (a) Fetal monitoring required—potential severe bradycardia
   (b) Direct vasodilator—hypotension in hypovolemic patient
4. Prostaglandins
   (a) Prostaglandin E_2 (PGE_2) in gel form. Placed vaginally to induce "ripening" of cervix before inducing labor
   (b) Prostaglandin $F_{2\alpha}$ by intramuscular or intrauterine injection
      (1) Very effective for postpartum hemorrhage
      (2) Contraindicated for asthmatics
5. Ergot preparations cause severe vasoconstriction
   (a) Methergine (methylergonovine) minimal vasoconstrictive effect if used IM
   (b) IV injection can cause severe hypertension

c. Tocolytics

1. Inhibit uterine contractions
2. Indications
   (a) Treat preterm labor
   (b) Stop excessive uterine contractions
   (c) Help in reversing uterine inversion
   (d) Facilitate manual removal of retained placenta
3. Beta-adrenergic agonists
   (a) Ritodrine
   (b) Terbutaline
   (c) Actions
      (1) Relaxation of uterus
      (2) Bronchial tree due to β_2 stimulation
4. Magnesium sulfate
   (a) Inhibits uterine contraction by antagonizing Ca^{2+}
   (b) Dosage 2–4 g IV over 20 minutes followed by 1–2 g/hr
   (c) Therapeutic level 4–8 mg/dl
   (d) $MgSO_4$ toxic can cause
      (1) Hemodynamic collapse
      (2) Respiratory paralysis
   (e) $MgSO_4$ potentiates action of muscle relaxants, especially nondepolarizing type

d. Amniotic fluid

1. Total volume 0.5–2 liters
2. Product of
   (a) Transudate from placenta
   (b) Fetal membrane plus urine excretion
   (c) Respiratory tract fluid secretion
3. Amniotic fluid replaced daily caused by
   (a) Fetal swallowing
   (b) Reabsorption by intestines and transfer across placenta
4. Amniotic fluid blood gas not correlated with fetal condition
   (a) Amniotic fluid low PO_2
   (b) High PcO_2

(c) Low pH (6.0–7.15)

5. L-S ratio (lecithin–sphingomyelin ratio) obtained by amniocentesis. Fetal lungs considered mature when L-S ratio 2.0 or greater

e. Physiology of labor

1. Onset of labor—unknown mechanism; strong, regular rhythmic contractions
2. Stages of labor
3. First stage of labor
    (a) Latent phase
        (1) Cervical dilation slow
        (2) Usually ends at about 3 cm cervical dilations
    (b) Active phase
        (1) Rapid cervical dilation follows latent phase
        (2) Ends by full dilation and complete effacement
    (c) First stage of labor pain caused by
        (1) Uterine contractions
        (2) Cervical dilation
    (d) Spinal segments involved are T_{10}–L_1
4. Second phase of labor

    (a) Extends from full cervical dilation to delivery of fetus
    (b) Spinal segments involved are S_2, S_3, S_4
5. Third phase of labor

    (a) Delivery of placenta and fetal membranes
    (b) This stage of delivery usually painless
    (c) Manual removal can be very painful, requiring segmental block or general anesthesia
    (d) Recently, nitroglycerine (sublingual spray or IV), amyl nitrate, or terbutaline has been used to allow relaxation of uterus

f. Fetal monitoring

1. Fetal heart rate

    (a) Normal 120–160 bpm with good baseline variability
    (b) Abnormal heart rate
        (1) Fetal tachycardia > 160 bpm; caused by
            [a] Early hypoxia
            [b] Maternal disease—fever, hyperthyroidism
            [c] Exogenous drugs—atropine, ephedrine, β-sympathomimetic drugs
            [d] Fetal tachyarrhythmias
        (2) Fetal bradycardia < 100 bpm; caused by
            [a] Fetal hypoxis
            [b] Head compression or cord compression
            [c] Blockers
    (c) Fetal deceleration patterns (three types—early, late, variable)
        (1) Early decelerations—benign, caused by fetal head compression during contractions
        (2) Late decelerations indicate utero placental insufficiency
        (3) Variable decelerations, usually benign, caused by cord compression
2. Fetal scalp blood sampling

    (a) Normal scalp pH 7.30–7.25
    (b) pH of 7.25–7.20 required repeated determination

(c) pH less than 7.20, especially with loss of beat to beat variability and fetal decelerations, indicates immediate delivery

III. COMPLICATIONS OF PREGNANCY

a. Hypertensive diseases of pregnancy: several categories are recognized by the American College of Obstetricians and Gynecologists (ACOG) and may overlap—chronic hypertension; transient/gestational hypertension of third trimester; preeclampsia superimposed on chronic hypertension; preeclampsia/eclampsia/PIH

1. Chronic hypertension
   (a) Occurs before 20th week
   (b) Endures beyond sixth week postpartum

2. Gestational hypertension
   (a) Not accompanied by proteinuria or generalized edema
   (b) Develops in last weeks of pregnancy or immediately after delivery
   (c) Dissipates within 2 weeks

3. Pregnancy-induced hypertension (PIH)—hypertension after 20th week of gestation and lasting up to sixth week postpartum
   (a) ACOG definition
      (1) Hypertension
         [a] An increase in systolic blood pressure of at least 30 mm Hg and/or an increase in diastolic blood pressure of at least 15 mm Hg above prepregnancy values, or
         [b] Two consecutive measurements of 140/90 mm Hg or over taken at least 6 hours apart
      (2) Proteinuria
         [a] Urinary excretion of 100 mg/dl or more of protein in two random urine specimens collected at least 6 hours apart
         [b] Urinary excretion of 300 mg or more protein in a 24-hour urine specimen
      (3) Edema
         [a] Clinically evident swelling
         [b] Rapid weight gain (indicating extensive fluid retention)
   (b) Severe PIH exists when any of the following findings are present
      (1) Sustained increase in blood pressure to 160/110 mm Hg or more
      (2) Urinary excretion of 5 g or more of protein in 24 hours
      (3) Oliguria, defined as the production of 500 ml or less of urine in 24 hours
      (4) Pulmonary edema
      (5) Cerebral and/or visual disturbances
      (6) Epigastric pain
      (7) Coagulopathy (or, in some cases, the HELLP syndrome: Hemolysis, Elevated Liver enzymes, Low Platelet count)
      (8) Fetal growth retardation
   (c) The condition is termed eclampsia when seizure occurs, independent of the severity of PIH, and in the absence of other causes of seizure
   (d) Incidence
      (1) 5–7% of all pregnancies
      (2) Second leading cause of maternal mortality, implicated in 20% of maternal deaths and 6–10% of perinatal deaths

(e) Etiology
  (1) Unknown, investigation ongoing—probable imbalance of vasoconstrictors (thromboxane and angiotensin) and vasodilator (prostacyclin)
  (2) May be secondary to widespread endothelial damage
  (3) Initiating factor may be immunologic, genetic, or an initial decrease in uterine blood flow by abnormal placental implantation or growth
  (4) For whatever reason, generalized arteriolar vasoreactivity with salt and water retention develops
(f) Risk factors
  (1) Primarily young primigravidas
  (2) Previous PIH
  (3) Extremes of childbearing age
  (4) Family history
  (5) Multiple gestation
  (6) Other complications of pregnancy
  (7) Erythroblastosis fetalis
  (8) Polyhydramnios
  (9) Molar pregnancy
  (10) Diabetes mellitus
  (11) Lupus erythematosus
  (12) Chronic hypertension
  (13) Other vascular disorders
(g) Pathophysiology: Generalized endothelial damage with vasoconstriction involves every organ system
  (1) CNS—areas of focal ischemia exist and are probably a secondary result of vasospasm. Ischemia responsible for seizures and reports of cortical blindness
    [a] Hyperreflexia, hyperirritability
    [b] Increased incidence of seizures (eclampsia), 30% are postpartum
    [c] Cerebral edema rare unless eclamptic
    [d] Monitor symptoms of headache, visual disturbances, and irritability
    [e] Cerebral hemorrhage leading cause of maternal death
  (2) Airway
    [a] Edema of face, larynx
    [b] Intubation, airway management may be difficult
    [c] Coagulopathies make nasal intubation attempts prone to causing hemorrhage
    [d] Small-diameter endotracheal tubes down to 5.5 mm should be available
    [e] Awake fiberoptic may be advisable
  (3) Respiratory
    [a] Normal respiratory changes of pregnancy occur in mild PIH
    [b] Pulmonary edema tendency increased
      i) Leaky capillaries, hypoalbuminemia
      ii) LV failure
    [c] Some treatments for PIH: narcotics, sedatives may predispose to weakness or decreased respiratory drive
  (4) Cardiovascular/hemodynamic/volume
    [a] Classical presentation
      i) High CO—may precede the HTN
      ii) High SVR
      iii) Decreased circulating volume
      iv) Increased LV work
    [b] In severe preeclampsia, no reliable correlation between CVP and PCWP. However, a CVP of 6 mm Hg or less is usually not associated with a high PCWP or pulmonary edema and may indicate decreased intravascular volume

III. Complications of pregnancy; a. Hypertensive diseases of pregnancy (continued)

      [c] PCWP does not always correlate with development of pulmonary edema
      [d] High PCWP should suggest LV dysfunction
      [e] Plasma volume reduced
          i) Total plasma albumin decreased
          ii) Total red cell mass usually unaffected
   (5) Renal
      [a] Decreased renal blood flow
      [b] Increased renin, angiotensin, and catecholamines
      [c] Increased atrial natriuretic factor
      [d] Decreased GFR and creatinine clearance
      [e] Increased uric acid
      [f] May progress to renal failure
          i) Function deteriorates with severity of PIH
          ii) Fibrin deposits in glomerular tufts
          iii) Glomeruli leak albumin, lose protein, retain sodium
      [g] Etiologies of oliguria and treatments
          i) Hypovolemia—fluid
          ii) Renal artery vasospasm—vasodilators (may be intrinsic renal disease)
          iii) Fluid overload with cardiac dysfunction—dopamine
      [h] Initially treat with judicious fluid bolus if no response—will require invasive monitoring for appropriate management
      [i] Acute renal failure reported, although rare
   (6) Uteroplacental unit
      [a] Increased blood viscosity
      [b] Uteroplacental blood flow decreased 50–70%
      [c] IUGR common
      [d] Marginal placental function with little reserve
          i) Placenta frequently aged with infarcts and fibrin deposit
          ii) Increased incidence of abruption
   (7) Uterus
      [a] Hyperactive
      [b] Marked increased sensitivity to oxytocin
      [c] Preterm labor common
   (8) Coagulation
      [a] Platelet dysfunction
      [b] Coagulation activation
      [c] Thrombocytopenia
          i) Increased consumption
          ii) Decreased platelet life span
          iii) Immune mechanism
      [d] Bleeding time controversial
      [e] Thromboelastograph may have role in future
   (9) Hepatic
      [a] Mild to moderate preeclampsia—minimal hepatic involvement
      [b] Severe preeclampsia and HELLP; periportal hemorrhages, increased LFTs, ischemia, generalized swelling, subcapsular hematoma, hepatic rupture
      [c] Symptom: epigastric pain
      [d] If hepatic involvement is suspected
          i) Obtain large-bore IV access
          ii) Blood products should be available
          iii) Invasive hemodynamic monitoring

        iv) Lab: hepatocellular enzymes, CBC with platelets, coagulation profile
- (10) HELLP
  - [a] Hemolysis elevated liver enzymes low platelets
  - [b] High fetal and maternal mortality
  - [c] Usually occurs before 36 weeks
  - [d] Malaise 90%
    - i) Epigastric pain 90%
    - ii) Nausea/vomiting 50%
    - iii) Nonspecific viral syndrome
  - [e] No correlation with severity of PIH
  - [f] Rapidly progresses to DIC and fulminant liver and renal failure
  - [g] Treatment—immediate delivery, supportive care
- (h) Mortality
  - (1) Intracranial hemorrhage
  - (2) CHF with pulmonary edema
  - (3) Acid aspiration
  - (4) Postpartum hemorrhage
  - (5) DIC
  - (6) Acute renal failure
  - (7) Ruptured liver
  - (8) Septic shock
- (i) Management goals
  - (1) Optimize hemodynamic status
  - (2) Prevent convulsions
  - (3) Balance fetal outcome against maternal mortality
  - (4) Definitive therapy of PIH is delivery
- (j) Obstetric management
  - (1) Bed rest
  - (2) Left lateral decubitus position
  - (3) Antihypertensives
  - (4) Anticonvulsants
  - (5) Fetal assessment and monitoring
  - (6) Lab: CBC with platelet, LFTs, coagulation profile, creatinine, BUN
  - (7) Severe PIH frequently requires pulmonary artery catheterization for appropriate management. Indications include pulmonary edema or oliguria unresponsive to judicious fluid challenge. Vasodilator, fluid, and inotropic support may be required based on individualized treatment for filling pressures, cardiac function, and SVR. Obstetric decisions will be made regarding timing and mode of delivery. Preterm deliveries are sometimes necessary for maternal safety. Vaginal delivery is preferred, although cesarean section is frequently required
- (k) Antihypertensives
  - (1) Goal of therapy
    - [a] Prevent life-threatening increases in maternal MAP
    - [b] Do not lower MAP more than 25%—may decrease placental perfusion
  - (2) Hydralazine
    - [a] Direct arteriolar vasodilator
    - [b] Reflex tachycardia
    - [c] Increased renal blood flow
    - [d] Dose: 5–10 mg IV—blood pressure reduction occurs in 10–15 minutes; incremental dosing until desired effect
  - (3) Labetalol
    - [a] α- and β-blocker
    - [b] Acute crisis or prior to induction of general anesthesia
    - [c] Dose: incremental to 1 mg/kg

III. Complications of pregnancy; a. Hypertensive diseases of pregnancy (continued)

            i) 5–10 mg IV titrated every 5–10 minutes
            ii) Cumulative dose 300 mg or less
            iii) May preserve uterine blood flow
        (4) Esmolol
           [a] β-blocker
           [b] Fetal bradycardia may occur
           [c] Small doses have been ineffective at blunting pressor response to intubation
           [d] Caution with β-blocker if myocardial depression or pulmonary congestion is present
    (l) Magnesium
        (1) Therapeutic effects
           [a] Anticonvulsant
           [b] Vasodilation (transient decrease in blood pressure)
        (2) Dose 2–4 g over 15–20 minutes
        (3) Followed by infusion 1–2 g/hr
        (4) Therapeutic range 4–6 mEq/L
        (5) Mechanism of action
           [a] Inhibits acetylcholine release
           [b] Competes with calcium entry into cardiac and smooth muscle
           [c] Decreased end-plate sensitivity to acetylcholine
           [d] Decreased muscle membrane excitability
           [e] Decreased central nervous system irritability
           [f] Uterine inhibitory effect—may require labor augmentation
        (6) Neonatal hypotension postdelivery if blood levels high. Monitor blood levels to maintain therapeutic range
        (7) Follow DTRs
        (8) Reduce dose if oliguria develops
        (9) Overdose—apnea or inadequate respiration may develop
        (10)Cardiac failure (over 10 mEq/L)
        (11)Treatment of toxicity
           [a] Calcium
           [b] Airway control
         (12)Drug interactions
           [a] Increased sensitivity to muscle relaxants: overdose → weakness → apnea or inadequate respiration may develop
           [b] Calcium channel blocker
              i) Hypotension
              ii) Respiratory compromise
              iii) Cardiac toxicity may develop with combination of calcium channel blockers and magnesium
    (m) Anesthetic management
        (1) Epidural
           [a] Effective analgesia/anesthesia for vaginal and surgical delivery
           [b] Hemodynamic stability. Avoids hemodynamic stimulus of laryngoscopy and awake extubation should cesarean section become necessary
           [c] Maintenance or improvement of tissue perfusion, specifically uteroplacental blood flow. May increase intervillous blood flow by decreasing maternal catecholamine levels with the sympathetic blockade
           [d] Avoidance of pharmacologic depression
        (2) Special considerations with PIH
           [a] Coagulopathy. Most guidelines use platelet count of 100,000 as cutoff for safety for regional anesthetic. Anecdotal evidence—safe with platelet

count less than 100,000. Bleeding time is not a useful predictor by recent evidence. Prolongation of coagulation profile or decreased fibrinogen may herald development of DIC. Coagulation profile should be obtained at least every 8 hours in severe PIH—more often, if worsening

- [b] Hemodynamics
    - i) Volume status must be assessed
    - ii) Individualize fluid therapy
        - a) IV access separate from magnesium IV line
        - b) Patients frequently on fluid restriction, calculate fluid balance
        - c) Urine output must be adequate
- (3) Mild PIH
    - [a] Noninvasive blood pressure monitoring
    - [b] Fluid bolus 5–10 ml/kg nondextrose-containing fluid
- (4) Severe or accelerating PIH: invasive monitoring as guide for rehydration. If severe hypoalbuminemia, colloid may be indicated
- (5) Epidural anesthetic management in PIH
    - [a] Avoid aortocaval compression—maintain LUD
    - [b] Avoid maternal hypotension
    - [c] Avoid decreasing uterine blood flow
    - [d] Avoid epinephrine-containing solutions
    - [e] Slow segmental titration of local anesthetic
    - [f] Slower-onset agents will minimize hemodynamic changes
    - [g] Patients may have exaggerated response to vasopressors
        - i) Ephedrine—reduce dose
        - ii) Phenylephrine—may further decrease uteroplacental blood flow
- (6) Subarachnoid block
    - [a] Coagulation restrictions of any regional block
    - [b] May precipitate severe hypotension if attempted for cesarean section although low block may be safely used for vaginal delivery. Some studies claim PIH patients are actually less sensitive to sympathetic blockade
    - [c] Same management precepts as epidural
- (7) General anesthesia
    - [a] May be required if there is fetal distress or some contraindication to regional
    - [b] Evaluate airway
        - i) PIH patients frequently have laryngeal edema
        - ii) Awake fiberoptic may be necessary
    - [c] Clear antacid within 30 minutes of induction
    - [d] Maintain LUD
    - [e] Preoxygenation
    - [f] Monitors appropriate for hemodynamic stability
    - [g] Rapid-sequence induction
        - i) Some degree of hemodynamic control prior to induction is desirable, preferably a diastolic less than 100 mm Hg
        - ii) Maternal cerebral hemorrhage is a leading cause of maternal mortality. Abrupt increases in systemic and pulmonary artery pressures may cause pulmonary edema
    - [h] Blunt hemodynamic response to laryngoscopy
        - i) Labetalol
        - ii) Lidocaine
        - iii) Nitroprusside
        - iv) Nitroglycerin
        - v) Trimethaphan
        - vi) Narcotics

III. Complications of pregnancy; a. Hypertensive diseases of pregnancy (continued)

     [i] Muscle relaxants
         i) Decreased plasma pseudocholinesterase even beyond the normal decrease of pregnancy
         ii) Magnesium—no defasciculation required
         iii) Muscle relaxants will have a prolonged duration of action and a decreased dose may be required
         iv) Monitor dosages with peripheral nerve stimulator—titrate to effect

b. Endocrine

1. Diabetes mellitus
    (a) Normal physiologic changes of pregnancy
        (1) Insulin resistance
        (2) Increased lipolysis
        (3) Ketogenesis
        (4) One in 700–1,000 pregnancies develops diabetes
    (b) Gestational diabetes
        (1) Definitions and management goals
            [a] Glucose intolerance during pregnancy
            [b] Diagnose and control prior to 30 weeks to prevent macrosomia
            [c] Diet control may be possible
            [d] Goal—fasting glucose less than 105 mg/dl
        (2) Classification of pregnant diabetic patients
            [a] Class A: Diabetic prior to pregnancy; diet control; any age at onset
            [b] Class B: Insulin required before pregnancy; onset 20 years of age or older; duration less than 10 years; obese women tend to be insulin resistant
            [c] Class C: Onset 10–20 years of age; duration 10–20 years
            [d] Class D: Onset less than 10 years of age; duration over 20 years or chronic hypertension (not PIH) or benign retinopathy; fetal macrosomia or intrauterine growth retardation possible; maternal retinal microaneurysms may progress during pregnancy
            [e] Class F: Diabetic nephropathy; anemia and hypertension common; intrauterine growth retardation common; perinatal survival 85%
            [f] Class R: Malignant proliferative retinopathy; risk of vitreous hemorrhage or retinal detachment; route of delivery controversial
            [g] Class H: Coronary artery disease; grave maternal risk
        (3) Fetal complications associated with maternal DM
            [a] Increased major congenital anomalies (threefold), especially if poor control during early development
            [b] Macrosomia
            [c] Intrauterine fetal distress
            [d] Prematurity
            [e] Respiratory distress syndrome
            [f] Neonatal hypoglycemia and hyperglycemia
            [g] Neonatal hyperbilirubinemia
            [h] Decreased buffering capacity—more prone to intrauterine hypoxia and acidosis
        (4) Maternal complication associated with maternal DM
            [a] Increased incidence of hypertension
            [b] Stiff joint syndrome
            [c] Diabetic ketoacidosis
                i) Fetal death rate 90%

     ii) Dehydration, hyponatremia, hypokalemia common
    [d] Uteroplacental perfusion
     i) Compromised, even with mild, well-controlled gestational diabetes
     ii) Hemoglobin A_{1c} increased—impaired oxygen transport and release
   (5) Drug interactions
    [a] Beta-adrenergic drugs
     i) May be given for preterm labor
     ii) Hyperglycemia a common side effect
     iii) Metabolic acidosis may result
    [b] Corticosteroids
     i) Given to accelerate lung maturation
     ii) Potent hyperglycemic effect—monitor insulin requirements
   (6) Anesthetic management
    [a] Collaborative effort with obstetricians
    [b] Tight control of maternal blood glucose
    [c] Regardless of technique, diabetic parturients require
     i) Meticulous attention to maintenance of placental perfusion pressure
     ii) Aggressive, rapid treatment of hypotension
     iii) Monitoring of serum glucose levels
     iv) Equipment and personnel for neonatal resuscitation and monitoring; neonatal glucose levels may fall
     v) Postpartum monitoring; maternal insulin requirements drop dramatically
    [d] Epidural
     i) Decreased maternal catecholamine release during labor may benefit placental perfusion
     ii) Decreased maternal lactic acid production (decreased fetal acidosis)
    [e] Subarachnoid
     i) Safe with prevention of hypotension and adequate hydration with nonglucose-containing fluid
     ii) In advanced disease, epidural may be preferable as these patients may be more prone to hemodynamic compromise following subarachnoid block
    [f] General endotracheal
     i) May be intubation problems secondary to stiff joint syndrome
     ii) Unable to monitor central nervous system of mother for hypoglycemia when asleep—follow serial glucoses hourly

 2. Thyroid
  (a) Normal pregnancy
   (1) Mild thyroid gland hypertrophy
   (2) Free thyroxine and triiodothyronine levels normal although absolute levels may be increased
  (b) Hyperthyroidism
   (1) Etiologies
    [a] Graves' disease 80%
    [b] Nontoxic goiter
     i) May increase in size with pregnancy
     ii) Dyspnea, dysphagia, changes in phonation
     iii) Potential for airway obstruction
    [c] Subacute thyroiditis
    [d] Chronic thyroiditis
    [e] Hyperemesis gravidarum
     i) Most have elevated thyroid tests
     ii) Possibly high human chorionic gonadotropin (hCG) thyroid stimulating properties

III. Complications of pregnancy; b. Endocrine (continued)

   iii) Resolves spontaneously
  [f] Hydatidiform mole
   i) One in 2,000 pregnancies
   ii) Trophoblastic tissue produces hCG
   iii) Surgical removal of mole indicated
 (2) Clinical presentation of Graves' disease
  [a] Mild
   i) Course benign
   ii) Minimal drug therapy
  [b] Severe
   i) Disease present long term causes large goiters, weight loss, visual changes
   ii) May present with
    a) Nausea/vomiting
    b) Heat intolerance
    c) Excessive sweating
    d) Easy fatigability
    e) Arrhythmias and dyspnea
    f) Pulmonary edema
    g) Congestive heart failure
    h) Reversible cardiomyopathy
   iii) Cardiac manifestation usually seen in long-standing disease with poor control, but may be associated with severely compromised left ventricular function. Thyroid hormones appear to have a direct effect on the heart
 (3) Obstetric complications
  [a] Pregnancy-induced hypertension
  [b] Anemia
  [c] Sepsis
  [d] Preterm delivery
  [e] Intrauterine death
  [f] Neonatal hyperthyroidism
  [g] Severity of complication closely related to degree of control with antithyroid medications
 (4) Obstetric management
  [a] Hospitalization for stabilization may be required
  [b] Antithyroid drugs
   i) Propylthiouracil (PTU)
   ii) Methimazole (Tapazole)
  [c] β-blockers—propranolol
  [d] Antiarrythmics
   i) Digoxin for atrial tachyarrythmias
   ii) Lidocaine for ventricular arrhythmias
  [e] Anticoagulation—patients with sustained atrial fibrillation
 (5) Anesthetic management
  [a] No elective surgery until euthyroid
  [b] Avoid medications that stimulate sympathetic nervous system
   i) Anticholinergics
   ii) Ketamine
   iii) Pancuronium
  [c] Adequate depth of anesthesia prior to surgical stimulation
  [d] Regional anesthesia
   i) Avoids hemodynamic changes of intubation/extubation

        ii) Avoids instrumenting airway, which may be compromised by enlarged thyroid gland

        iii) Sympathetic blockade may be desirable

        iv) *Caution*: may have exaggerated response to vasopressors

     [e] General anesthesia

        i) Increased basal metabolic rate and O_2 consumption

        ii) Routine general endotracheal monitoring and precautions

        iii) Cooling blanket, ice available for hyperthermia

  (6) Thyroid storm

     [a] Rare, only 2% of pregnancies with thyrotoxicosis

     [b] Precipitating factors

        i) Labor

        ii) Cesarean delivery

        iii) Infection

     [c] Manifestation

        i) Tachyarrhythmias, atrial fibrillation

        ii) Fever

        iii) Agitation, disorientation

        iv) Tremor

        v) Abdominal pain

        vi) Vomiting/diarrhea

        vii) May progress to congestive heart failure

     [d] Laboratory

        i) Leukocytosis

        ii) Elevated liver enzymes

        iii) Thyroid tests

        iv) Hypercalcemia

     [e] Management—as in thyrotoxicosis

3. Hypothyroidism

  (a) Associated with spontaneous abortion

  (b) Uncommon in term pregnancy

    (1) Mild symptoms: May be difficult to distinguish from normal symptoms of pregnancy

     [a] Fatigue

     [b] Cold intolerance

     [c] Cool dry skin

     [d] Coarse hair

     [e] Hoarseness

     [f] Constipation

    (2) Severe symptoms

     [a] Decreased deep tendon reflex

     [b] Edema

     [c] Cardiomegaly

     [d] Decreased myocardial contractility

     [e] Congestive heart failure

     [f] Pleural and/or pericardial effusions

  (c) Anesthetic management

    (1) Increased sensitivity to narcotics, sedatives, and general anesthesia

    (2) Decreased intravascular fluid volume

    (3) Prolonged response to muscle relaxants

    (4) Prone to hyponatremia, hypoglycemia, and hypothermia

  (d) Recommendation

    (1) Careful hydration

    (2) Warm fluids/blankets

    (3) Monitored titration of drugs for both regional and general anesthesia

III. Complications of pregnancy; b. Endocrine (continued)

4. Pheochromocytoma
    (a) Rare—high fetal/maternal mortality
    (b) Symptoms
        (1) Anxiety
        (2) Headache
        (3) Paroxysmal hypertension not associated with proteinuria
        (4) Diaphoresis
        (5) Palpitations, arrhythmias
        (6) Episodic attacks promoted by
            [a] Fetal movement
            [b] Uterine contractions
            [c] Changes in posture
    (c) Pathophysiology
        (1) Paroxysmal catecholamine excess
        (2) Decreased plasma volume
        (3) Falsely elevated hematocrit
        (4) Orthostatic hypotension
    (d) Medical management
        (1) Chemical control with adrenergic blocking drugs
            [a] α-blockers
                i) Phenoxybenzamine
                ii) Prazosin—required prior to instituting beta-blockade
            [b] β-blockers
                i) Propranolol
                ii) Labetalol (α and β)
                iii) Esmolol. *Caution*—may induce fetal bradycardia and increase uterine tone
        (2) These drugs are of unproven safety in pregnancy but fetal well-being can only follow maternal hemodynamic stability
    (e) Anesthetic management
        (1) Same as for nonpregnant patients with pheochromocytoma
            [a] Chemical control of adrenergic responses and synthesis
            [b] Avoidance of sympathomimetics
            [c] Invasive monitoring
                i) A-line
                ii) CVP
                iii) Foley catheter
            [d] Adequate preoperative medication
            [e] Avoid halothane due to increased sensitivity to catecholamines
            [f] Adequate depth for laryngoscopy to prevent sympathetic stimulation
            [g] Vasodilators readily available to treat persistent hypertension
        (2) Avoid all drugs or situations that promote catecholamine release or arrhythmias
            [a] Drugs
                i) Anticholinergics
                ii) Histamine-releasing drugs
                iii) Pancuronium
                iv) Halothane
                v) Droperidol
                vi) Ephedrine
            [b] Situations
                i) Fear
                ii) Anxiety

    iii) Pain
    iv) Labor
     v) Hypoxia
    vi) Hypercardia
   vii) Hypotension
  (3) Additional concerns related to pregnancy
    [a] Rapid sequence induction after first trimester
    [b] Maintain left uterine displacement
    [c] Fetal monitoring as long as possible and for 24 hours postop following surgery other than cesarean
    [d] Tocolysis with caution
  (4) Regional anesthesia is acceptable and may be advantageous as combined technique for nonobstetric surgery
    [a] Careful adequate hydration
    [b] Slow titration of level
    [c] Epidural may be preferable to subarachnoid to avoid precipitous drop in blood pressure
    [d] Treat hypotension with direct-acting vasopressors
    [e] Vasodilators available for hypertensive crisis

c. Rh, ABO incompatibility

1. Hemolytic disease of newborn

  (a) Transplacental passage of fetal erythrocytes with antigen foreign to mother
  (b) Maternal immunologic response
    (1) Early—high-molecular-weight IgM; does not cross placenta
    (2) Late—low-molecular-weight IgG; crosses placenta; binds to fetal RBC, induces their destruction

2. Erythroblastosis fetalis

  (a) Classically Rh-D negative mother with Rh-D positive fetus
  (b) 1.5 per 1,000 births
  (c) Attempts at prevention with Rh immune globulin
    (1) 8% failure rate
    (2) 50% mildly affected
    (3) 25% moderately affected
      [a] Anemia
      [b] Hyperbilirubinemia
    (4) 25% severely affected—hydrops fetalis

3. Pathophysiology

  (a) Hemolytic anemia
  (b) Immature nucleated RBCs (erythroblasts) released
  (c) Hyperbilirubinemia
  (d) Hepatosplenomegaly
  (e) Severe hemolysis (20–25%)
    (1) Generalized edema
    (2) Extreme ascites (hydrops fetalis)
    (3) Hypoalbunimia
    (4) Pulmonary edema—hypoplasia
    (5) Petechial hemorrhages

4. Antenatal management of RH-sensitized woman

  (a) Early delivery
  (b) Intrauterine fetal transfusion at 30–32 weeks' gestation

5. Anesthetic management
   (a) Fetus at increased risk for distress
   (b) Will not tolerate further insults
   (c) Diligently maintain placental perfusion
   (d) Maintain oxygenation
   (e) Prevent and/or aggressively treat hypotension
   (f) No clear drug preferences as long as titrated slowly
   (g) Epidural less likely than spinal to cause rapid shifts in blood pressure
   (h) Prehydration
   (i) Preoxygenate and maintain O_2 supplementation

6. General anesthesia
   (a) Standard precaution for cesarean section remembering that the premature hydropic fetus is at significant increased risk
   (b) Preoxygenate
   (c) Maintain placental perfusion pressure
   (d) Left uterine displacement
   (e) 100% Fio_2 until delivery
   (f) Avoid hyperventilation
   (g) Neonatologist available for neonatal resuscitation

d. Placenta previa

1. Incidence: One in 200–250 pregnancies
   (a) Twice normal incidence in a pregnancy immediately following a cesarean section
   (b) Previous previa—recurrence 5%
   (c) Increasing maternal age
   (d) Previous cesarean section or uterine surgery
   (e) 10% incidence with four or more previous cesareans

2. Symptoms
   (a) Painless vaginal bleeding
   (b) Spotting—severe hemorrhage
   (c) May or may not stop spontaneously

3. Diagnosis
   (a) Ultrasound 95% accuracy
   (b) Different types fairly even distribution
       (1) Complete partial
       (2) Low-lying anterior
       (3) Low-lying posterior
   (c) Following diagnosis, several management options
       (1) 60–90% at least one antepartum hemorrhage, expectant management if bleeding resolves
       (2) Maintain IV access
       (3) Type and screen current
       (4) Bed rest until fetal maturity, distress, or bleeding

4. Double setup
   (a) Patient prepped and draped for cesarean section—in lithotomy position
   (b) Two IVs—16–18 gauge
   (c) Blood in room at least two units
   (d) Blood warmer
   (e) If patient has bled, restore volume ($\pm$ CVP)
   (f) Oral antacid

(g) All necessary equipment for general endotracheal anesthesia

(h) Preoxygenate

(i) Left uterine displacement

e. Placenta accreta: general incidence one in 2,500 to one in 4,300

1. Placenta accreta—placenta attached onto myometrium

2. Placenta increta—placenta attached into myometrium

3. Placenta percreta—placenta penetrates through the myometrium into surrounding tissues

   (a) Bowel
   (b) Bladder
   (c) Large vessels

4. Also classified as total, partial, or focal

5. Predisposing factors for placenta accreta

   (a) Prior cesarean section—incidence rises with number of prior cesarean sections
   (b) Placenta previa
   (c) Prior uterine manipulation (D&C, myomectomy)
   (d) Congenital malformation of uterus
   (e) Daughter of mother on DES
   (f) Uterine tumors (fibroids)
   (g) Multiparity
   (h) (?) smoking

6. Complications of placenta accreta

   (a) Massive hemorrhage
   (b) Preterm labor due to myometrial stimulation
   (c) Uterine rupture second trimester—delivery
   (d) Uterine inversion

7. Massive intraoperative blood loss is common

   (a) 2,000–15,000 ml (normally at least 3–4 liters)
   (b) 30–70% require emergency cesarean section
   (c) 20% develop intraoperative coagulopathies
   (d) Earlier mortality 34%, more recently down to 3%

8. Anesthetic management

   (a) Placenta previa, no accreta on ultrasound, no predisposing factors for accreta: SAB or epidural
   (b) Placenta previa, no accreta on ultrasound, one to three previous cesarean sections: epidural or GETA
   (c) Placenta previa, four or more previous cesarean sections, placenta accreta: GETA (epidural)

f. Abruptio placenta

1. Separation of a previously normally implanted placenta after 20 weeks' gestation and before the birth of the fetus—10–15% are severe, 85–90% are marginal separation

   (a) Incidence overall
       (1) 0.2–2.4%
       (2) 33% of all antepartum hemorrhages
   (b) Maternal mortality: 1.8–2.8%
   (c) Fetal mortality: up to 50%

III. Complications of pregnancy; f. Abruptio placenta (continued)

2. Etiology
   (a) Hypertensive diseases
   (b) High parity
   (c) Uterine abnormalities
   (d) Prior abruptio (0.1% recurrence rate)
   (e) Drugs: especially cocaine abuse
   (f) Spontaneous preterm rupture of membranes

3. Symptoms
   (a) Abdominal pain
   (b) Vaginal bleeding
   (c) May be concealed—retroplacental hemorrhage of up to 4,000 ml sequestered in uterus reported
   (d) Uterine irritability or hypertonicity
   (e) Maternal hypotension
   (f) Fetal distress or death
   (g) Coagulopathy

4. Diagnosis
   (a) Clinical
   (b) Ultrasound
   (c) Laboratory
       (1) Hgb/Hct
       (2) PT/PTT
       (3) Fibrinogen (normal in pregnancy 400–600 mg %)
       (4) FSP
       (5) Platelets

5. Management considerations
   (a) Degree of abruption
   (b) Gestational age
   (c) Maternal hemodynamic and hematologic stability
       (1) Hypotension
       (2) Hemorrhagic shock
       (3) DIC (20–40%)
       (4) Acute renal failure (1–4%)
       (5) Postpartum hemorrhage
       (6) Ischemic organ necrosis
   (d) Fetal well-being

6. Anesthetic management
   (a) Mild–moderate (85–90%)
       (1) Stable mother and fetus
       (2) Labor may be induced
       (3) Two large-bore IVs
       (4) Blood available
       (5) Clotting studies and hematologic profile
       (6) Continuous fetal monitoring
       (7) Regional anesthesia is acceptable if
           [a] No evidence of hypovolemia
           [b] Uteroplacental perfusion appears adequate
           [c] Clotting parameters normal
           [d] Careful titration following adequate preload to prevent hypotension
   (b) Severe (10–15%)
       (1) Emergency cesarean section if fetus viable

(2) Vigorous volume resuscitation of mother

(3) Regional anesthesia contraindicated

(4) Induction and maintenance of general anesthesia

    [a] Select agents appropriate to degree of maternal hemodynamic compromise

    [b] Ketamine controversial

(5) DIC is common

(6) Blood products—large quantities may be required

(7) Clotting factors—FFP, platelets, cryoprecipitate

(8) Uterine atony may occur

(9) Emergency hysterectomy

g. Amniotic fluid embolism

1. Rare: one in 8,000 to one in 80,000: mortality 80% +

    (a) Amniotic fluid and thromboembolism constitute the leading cause of maternal mortality in the United States. Some amniotic fluid probably routinely enters the maternal circulation

    (b) Associated with entire range of pregnancy: first-trimester abortions to 48 hours postpartum

    (c) May be a long delay between entrance of fluid into circulation and onset of symptoms

2. Symptoms

    (a) Seizures (10–20%)

    (b) Severe respiratory distress

    (c) Pulmonary edema (70%)

    (d) Cardiovascular collapse

    (e) Disseminated intravascular coagulation (40%)

    (f) Uterine atony—myometrial depressant effect of amniotic fluids

    (g) Classically

        (1) Sudden dyspnea

        (2) Severe hypotension

        (3) Cardiovascular arrest

    (h) Fetal distress

3. Hemodynamic consequences

    (a) Many patients do not survive the initial phase and are not invasively monitored

    (b) Animal data contradictory and of questionable relevance to human patients

    (c) Monitored human patients

        (1) Mild–moderate increase in pulmonary artery pressures

        (2) Variable increase in CVP

        (3) Increased PCWP

        (4) Left ventricular dysfunction

4. Coagulopathy

    (a) 40% of patients who survive initial event develop coagulopathy

        (1) Inconclusive etiology

        (2) Trophoblast has potent thromboplastinlike effects

        (3) Decreased fibrinogen

        (4) Increased PT

        (5) Increased PTT

        (6) Increased FSP

        (7) Thrombocytopenia

    (b) Proposition that it is not the amount or route of amniotic fluid entering the circulation but rather an abnormal amniotic fluid makeup

5. Predisposing factors
   (a) Advanced maternal age
   (b) Placental abnormalities
       (1) Abruptio
       (2) Placenta accreta
       (3) Placenta previa
   (c) Multiparity
   (d) Rapid hard labor (no valid data to support)
   (e) First-trimester abortion
   (f) Abdominal trauma
   (g) Amniocentesis
   (h) Normal term delivery
   (i) Cesarean section
   (j) Intrauterine fetal death

6. Diagnosis
   (a) Central venous aspirate or at autopsy pulmonary artery contains squamous cells or debris of fetal origin
   (b) Now questioning if these are incidental findings common to all pregnant patients
   (c) Diagnosis is by clinical presentation with supportive laboratory studies

7. Differential
   (a) Septic shock
   (b) Aspiration pneumonia
   (c) Acute myocardial infarction
   (d) Pulmonary thromboembolism
   (e) Placental abruptio
   (f) Eclampsia
   (g) Local anesthetic toxicity
   (h) Cerebrovascular accident

8. Treatment
   (a) Oxygenation
       (1) Hypoxia often profound
       (2) Intubate
       (3) 100% FiO_2
   (b) Support cardiac output
       (1) Heart failure predominates
       (2) CPR
       (3) Inotropes, afterload reduction
       (4) Fluids
       (5) Invasive monitoring to guide therapy
   (c) Correct coagulopathy
   (d) Consider operative delivery of fetus; many facets involved in decision to operate on patient with cardiovascular collapse and DIC

h. Uterine rupture

1. Significance
   (a) One in 1,000 to one in 15,000 in United States
   (b) 0.5% of all maternal mortality
   (c) Accounts for 50% of deaths due to uterine hemorrhage
   (d) Fetal mortality up to 80%
   (e) Bleeding more significant in complete rupture of unscarred uterus

2. Symptoms

   (a) Severe abdominal pain—may be referred shoulder pain
   (b) Change of abdominal contour
   (c) Severe fetal distress or death
   (d) Vaginal bleeding
   (e) Hemodynamic compromise
   (f) Hemorrhagic shock
   (g) Actually wide presentation depending on etiology and completeness of rupture

3. Etiology/risk factors

   (a) Previous cesarean section or uterine surgery
   (b) Previous curettage or infection
   (c) Uterine abnormalities, thinning
   (d) Trophoblastic invasion of myometrium—placenta percreta
   (e) Multigravida, especially with cephalopelvic disproportion
   (f) Trauma
   (g) Use of prostaglandins to induce labor, reports of rupture as early as 15 weeks
   (h) Spontaneous (80%)

4. Management

   (a) Recognition
       (1) Up to 65% recognized only after vaginal delivery or upon cesarean section
       (2) Ultrasound—very helpful in diagnosis
   (b) Definitive management dictated by maternal hemodynamic stability
       (1) Emergency laparotomy and delivery
       (2) Repair of dehiscence of scar may be possible
       (3) Unscarred rupture almost always requires hysterectomy
   (c) Hemorrhage—leading cause of maternal mortality
   (d) Surgery may need to proceed to gain control of bleeding even before full fluid resuscitation: blood loss may be extreme (over 15,000 ml reported)
   (e) Regional anesthesia—contraindicated in presence of hemorrhage: emergency general anesthetic usually required. If functioning epidural in place and patient is hemodynamically stable *and* without ongoing bleeding, then epidural anesthesia for laparotomy may be utilized

5. Controversy

   (a) Should epidural anesthesia be withheld for women at risk for uterine rupture?
   (b) No evidence to support lack of ability to properly diagnose uterine rupture after epidural placement. Some suggest keeping block lower than T10 and a slightly less dense (i.e., lower-concentration) solution than might normally be used. However, the pain is severe and appears to be appreciable, even with an epidural

i. Postpartum bleeding

1. Causes

   (a) Retained placenta
   (b) Placenta percreta
   (c) Uterine atony
   (d) Cervical laceration or tear
   (e) Uterine inversion

2. Uterine atony

   (a) 2–5% all vaginal deliveries
   (b) Up to 2,000 ml blood loss in 5 minutes

3. Associated factors

   (a) High parity

III. Complications of pregnancy; i. Postpartum bleeding (continued)

    (b) Polyhydramnios
    (c) Multiple births
    (d) Retained placenta
    (e) Large fetuses (seven times normal risk if fetus weighs over 4,500 g)
    (f) Excessive oxytocic use
    (g) Precipitous or prolonged labor
    (h) Chorioaminonitis (especially resistant to treatment)
    (i) Prior history of postpartum hemorrhage
    (j) Tocolytics
        (1) Beta sympathomimetics
        (2) Ritodrine
        (3) Terbutaline
        (4) Magnesium sulfate
    (k) Inhalational agents
        (1) 1 MAC—interferes with spontaneous uterine activity
        (2) 2 MAC—blocks oxytocin-induced contractions

4. Symptoms

    (a) Painless vaginal bleeding postpartum
    (b) Rising fundus if cervical os occluded
    (c) Maternal hemodynamic instability
        (1) Decreased blood pressure
        (2) Increased heart rate

5. Management

    (a) Vigorous volume resuscitation
    (b) Stimulate uterine contraction
        (1) Pharmacologic
        (2) External massage
    (c) Operative control of bleeding
        (1) Interruption of uterine blood supply
        (2) Emergency hysterectomy
    (d) Pharmacology
        (1) Withdraw any agents that interfere with uterine contraction
        (2) Oxytocin
            [a] 20 units/1,000 ml balanced salt solution
           [b] No IV bolus
               i) Does not produce better contraction
               ii) Profound vasodilation and hypotension possible
        (3) Calcium chloride, especially effective after magnesium sulfate
        (4) Ergot alkaloids
            [a] 0.2 mg methylergonovine intramuscularly
           [b] Hypertension may be severe, especially in vasospastic patient or one receiving vasopressors
           [c] Do not use in hypertensive patient; coronary-spasm–induced myocardial infarction reported
        (5) Postaglandins: prostaglandin $F_2\alpha$
           [a] 0.25–0.5 µg 15 methyl prostaglandin $F_2\alpha$
           [b] Intramuscular or intramyometrial
           [c] Side effects
               i) Nausea, vomiting, diarrhea
               ii) Slightly elevated temperature
    (e) Surgical
        (1) Pitressin infusion into bleeding vessel

      (2) Embolization of pelvic arteries

      (3) Ligation of uterine arterial supply

      (4) Hysterectomy, expected blood loss up to 15,000 ml

  6. Anesthetic options

    (a) Dictated by bleeding and maternal hemodynamic stability

    (b) General endotracheal anesthesia generally required for laparotomy

    (c) Vigorous fluid resuscitation early in course

IV. ASSISTED REPRODUCTIVE TECHNOLOGIES (ART) — differences based on timing and placement of products

a. Abbreviations. IVF: in vitro fertilization—egg and sperm combined in laboratory, fertilized egg transferred to uterus; GIFT: gamete intrafallopian transfer—direct transfer of sperm/egg mixture into fallopian tube; ZIFT: zygote intrafallopian transfer—egg and sperm combined in laboratory, zygote transferred to fallopian tube

b. Considerations

1. Maternal safety

2. Fetal safety

3. Maternal comfort

4. Cost

5. Rapid recovery

6. Risks—management

c. Factors influencing success

1. Stress

2. Hormonal milieu

3. Endometrium

4. Uterine contractions

5. N_2O/CO_2 pneumoperitoneum

6. Maternal age

7. Maturity of egg at harvest

8. Ovarian or fallopian tube trauma

9. Male factors

10. Timing

11. pH

12. Anesthetic agents—N_2O controversial

d. Steps to ART procedures

1. Ovulation enhancement

(a) Chemically induced
(b) Monitored
    (1) Ultrasound
    (2) Blood-hormone levels
(c) Induced ovulation. Ovulation occurs in 36 hours—*timing critical*

2. Oocyte harvest

    (a) Ultrasound-guided transvaginal aspiration
    (b) Abdominal laparoscopy—traditional method of harvest

3. Transfer

    (a) IVF—no anesthetic required, relatively painless
    (b) GIFT—laparoscopic or minilaparotomy
    (c) ZIFT—laparoscopic or minilaparotomy

e. Ultrasound-guided transvaginal aspiration

1. Steps

    (a) Ultrasound probe
    (b) Visualization of follicles
    (c) Needle aspiration—may be up to 30 insertions of needle through the back of vaginal wall, brief but intense repetitive painful stimulation

2. Anesthetic goals

    (a) Pain relief
    (b) Stress hormone reduction
    (c) Minimize drug exposure
    (d) Safety
    (e) Quick recovery

3. Anesthetic management

    (a) IV sedation
        (1) Propofol
        (2) Propofol with alfentanil
        (3) Midazolam
        (4) All have records of safety alone or in combination with monitored care to titrate to drowsy but arousable level of consciousness; patients frequently require rather heavy sedation, which may prolong recovery
    (b) Paracervical block
        (1) Usually used with IV sedation
        (2) Concern over findings of lidocaine in follicular fluid; possible ill effects on cleavage rate
    (c) Regional-subarachnoid or epidural
        (1) Subarachnoid
            [a] Pro: rapid onset, predictable duration, dense blockade, minimal drug exposure, T6 level required
            [b] Con: outpatient procedure, risk of PDPH—decreased incidence with small gauge needles, nausea—multi- factorial
        (2) Epidural
            [a] Pro: can adjust for duration of procedure; ideally less chance of PDPH, although "wet tap" with 18-gauge Tuohy virtually assures a PDPH
            [b] Con: requires more drug exposure than SAB; usually takes longer for onset; higher failure rate—secondary to "thick" sarval nerve sheaths; sensory blockade may not be as dense; epidural narcotics may help to

intensify sensory blockade; if used, use a short-acting narcotic such as 50 µg fentanyl to minimize chance of postoperative respiratory depression
   i) Risks
      a) Respiratory depression
      b) Pruritus
      c) Urinary retention
      d) Nausea/vomiting

f. Laparoscopy

1. Anesthetic considerations

  (a) Routine hemodynamic alterations
    (1) Increased intra-abdominal pressure
    (2) Decreased venous return
    (3) Decreased CVP, blood pressure, CO, circulating blood volume
  (b) Potential catastrophic event—air embolism

2. Anesthetic management

  (a) Routine monitoring
  (b) Augmented local
    (1) Reported acceptable
    (2) Simplicity
    (3) Low cost
    (4) Patient safety
    (5) Poor patient acceptance
  (c) Regional—success limited by
    (1) Steep Trendelenburg position
    (2) Pneumoperitoneum
    (3) Manipulation of fallopian tubes
  (d) General endotracheal
    (1) Numerous studies to evaluate effects of drugs on cleavage rates inconclusive
    (2) Clear benefits to reduction of stress hormones
    (3) N_2O controversial
    (4) Propofol appears to be a very satisfactory option: no teratogenicity, antiemetic, rapid recovery
    (5) Standard setup
      [a] Preop sedation
      [b] Oral bicarbonate
      [c] Routine monitoring
      [d] OG tube to decompress stomach
        i) Help minimize surgical injury to bowel
        ii) Decreased nausea and vomiting

V. PULMONARY ASPIRATION

a. More common in certain patients

1. Obtunded patients

2. Unconscious patients

3. Patients with full stomachs

4. Patients with depressed protective laryngeal reflexes

5. Patients in the third trimester of pregnancy or in labor

b. Passive regurgitation required

1. Increased gastric pressure
2. Incompetence of gastroesophageal valvular mechanisms

c. Causes of increased gastric pressure

1. Delayed gastric emptying due to pain
2. Anxiety
3. Trauma
4. Obstetric labor
5. Pyloric and intestinal obstruction
6. Narcotic analgesia

d. Types of pulmonary aspirates

1. Particulate matter
   (a) May result in airway obstruction
   (b) Airways affected depend on size of particles
   (c) Acute asphyxia if large airways obstructed
   (d) If distal airways obstructed, atelectasis, and ventilation/perfusion mismatched, right to left shunting
       (1) Hypoxemia common
       (2) Lung abscess may result
2. Liquid gastric contents
   (a) Lung injury depends on
       (1) Amount aspirated
       (2) pH of aspirate
       (3) Whether or not bacteria present in aspirate
   (b) Aspiration more severe if pH of aspirate is less than 2.5 and volume is 25 cc or greater
   (c) Aspiration of blood does not cause chemical burn of tracheobronchial tree

e. Treatment

1. Restore pulmonary function to normal as quickly as possible
   (a) First, clear airway
   (b) Mouth, pharynx, and trachea should be suctioned
   (c) Administration of high concentrations of O_2
   (d) Bronchoscopy if aspirated materials suspected solid
   (e) No need to bronchial lavage to neutralize acid of aspirate
       (1) Mucosal damage occurs within seconds of aspiration
       (2) Bronchial secretion neutralizes acid within minutes
   (f) Large aspiration may require
       (1) Intubation
       (2) Mechanical ventilation
       (3) Positive end-expiratory pressure
2. Corticosteriods not recommended
3. Antibiotics not routinely used unless pulmonary infection occurs

4. Antacids
    (a) Objectives
        (1) Neutralize acid in gastric contents
        (2) Should always avoid particulate antacids—aspiration of gastric fluids containing particulate antacids may cause significant and persistent pulmonary damage despite increase in gastric fluid pH
    (b) Antacids given before induction of anesthesia almost 100% effective in increasing gastric fluid pH above 2.5
    (c) Nonparticulate or soluble antacids offer certain advantages
        (1) Mix with gastric contents easily
        (2) Aspiration of soluble antacids associated with faster recovery
        (3) Less likely to cause a foreign body reaction
        (4) Available preparations
            [a] Sodium citrate
            [b] Bicitria, which contains sodium citrate and citric acid

5. Metoclopramide
    (a) Metoclopramide dopamine antagonist useful for
        (1) Reducing gastric fluid volume by increasing lower esophageal sphincter tone
        (2) Speeding gastric emptying time
        (3) Acting as an antiemetic—no known effect on gastric pH
            [a] Selective peripheral cholinergic agonist
            [b] Facilitates the action of acetylcholine on proximal GI tract
            [c] Its gastrokinetics effect opposed by atropine and opioids
        (4) Its gastrokinetic effect could be useful prior to induction of anesthesia in these patients
            [a] Outpatients
            [b] Obese patients
            [c] Trauma patients
            [d] Parturients
            [e] Patients with full stomachs
    (b) Reglan (metoclopramide) may be given orally or parenterally
        (1) After oral dose of 10 mg, onset of action is 30–60 minutes
        (2) Peak plasma concentration: 40–120 minutes
        (3) If given IV, onset of action: 1–3 minutes
    (c) Side effects of Reglan
        (1) Possibility of extrapyramidal symptoms
        (2) Sedation
        (3) Dysphoria
        (4) Rash
        (5) Dry mouth
    (d) Should be avoided in these situations
        (1) Patient with pheochromocytoma
        (2) GI obstruction (debatable)
        (3) Patients taking monoamine oxidase inhibitors, tricyclic antidepressants, or other drugs that may cause extrapyramidal symptoms

6. H_2 Blockers
    (a) H_2 receptor antagonists block histamine-induced secretion of acid by gastric parietal cells
        (1) Blockers reduce risks of aspiration by increasing gastric pH
        (2) Reduce risks by decreasing volume of gastric contents
    (b) Cimetidine (Tagamet)
        (1) Should be given 45–60 minutes prior to surgery
        (2) Produces large number of side effects
            [a] Inhibits p450 cytochrome

V. Pulmonary aspiration; e. Treatment (continued)

        [b] Reduces hepatic blood flow
     (3) Cimetidine reduces clearance of many drugs that require oxidative degradation
        [a] Lidocaine
        [b] Propranolol
        [c] Diazepam
        [d] Theophylline
        [e] Warfarin
        [f] Phenobarbital
        [g] Phenytoin and others
     (4) Crosses blood–brain barrier
        [a] Can produce CNS dysfunction
           i) Agitation
           ii) Confusion
           iii) Delayed awakening from anesthesia
        [b] May predispose to bronchoconstriction in asthmatic patient
  (c) Other H_2 blockers highly effective with fewer side effects than cimetidine
     (1) Zantac
     (2) Ranitidine
     (3) Famotidine

C. CLINICAL HEMATOLOGY

I. BLOOD TRANSFUSION

a. Blood storage

1. One unit whole blood, 450 ml blood, 63 ml preservative, hematocrit (HCT) 36–40%
2. Packed cells—200–250 ml blood + CPD (citrate phosphate dextrose) HCT 70–80%
3. Packed cells + CPD adenine + mannitol + glucose, HCT 55%
4. Shelf life at 1–6°C—CPD blood 21 days—CPD adsol blood 42 days
5. Survival of over 70% RBCs at 24 hours posttransfusion
6. All stable clotting factors present
7. Labile factor VIII—25% left after 24 hours
8. Labile factor V—50% left after 14 days
9. Platelets—nonviable after 24–48 hours

b. Filters

1. Microfilters (20–40 μm) for cardiopulmonary bypass and thrombocytopenia patient
2. Standard (170 μm) for all other transfusions

c. Blood warming

1. Rapid transfusions in adults over 100 ml/min
2. Exchange transfusions in infants
3. Transfusions in children over 5 ml/kg/hr
4. Cold agglutinins active in vitro at 37°C
5. Transfusions via central venous line

d. Medication into blood units: avoid because

1. May cause hemolysis if drug has high pH
2. Difficult to differentiate drug or transfusion reaction
3. If blood reaction, stop transfusion; full dose of drug not given
4. Risk of introduction of infection

e. Blood products—dangers

1. Infection
   (a) Viruses
      (1) Hepatitis C—majority of transfusion-related hepatitis cases. Anti-HCV now used. Screening has reduced the risk to less than 1 in 3,000 units of blood or components transfused
      (2) Hepatitis B—7–17% transfusion-related hepatitis. Tests may not detect low-level viremia
      (3) HIV—window period: no antibodies, but blood infective. Risk of transmission one in 225,000 units

I. Blood transfusion; e. Blood products—dangers (continued)

  (4) HTLVI—T-cell leukemia/lymphoma, tropical spastic paraparesis—not tested for, risk is very low
  (5) HTLVII—not tested for, hairy cell leukemia, risk is very low
  (6) Cytomegalovirus/Epstein-Barr virus—both not tested for and have been transfused with subsequent infection
 (b) Bacteria
  (1) Syphilis—*Treponema pallidium* not viable more than 72 hours at 4°C. Test inexpensive, may indicate "high risk" donor
 (c) Protozoa: malaria, toxoplasmosis, babesiosis
2. Immunological suppression
 (a) Renal transplant survival—statistically improved survival, however, immune suppression drugs better
 (b) Malignancy—reports mixed regarding patients with existing malignancy; survival may be shortened
 (c) Postoperative infections—may be increased
3. Alloimmunization—reactions vary from mild fever, chills, urticaria to fatal hemolysis (ABO incompatibility)
4. Anaphylaxis—may be due to antibodies against proteins, white cells, or platelets
5. Transfusion-related acute lung injury (TRALI): noncardiogenic pulmonary edema within 2–4 hours of transfusion, possibly due to leuko-agglutinin reactions. Edema clears within 48 hours. High risk: obstructive airway disease; multiple transfusions; multiparous patients
6. Adverse transfusion reactions: treatment
 (a) All reactions—stop transfusion, check blood tag, blood bank forms, patient identification. Untoward reaction reports completed by nurse and doctor
 (b) Mild reactions—IV open with crystalloid, give antihistamines, resume transfusion at slower rate. No improvement, stop transfusion
 (c) Acute hemolysis—may need epinephrine, corticosteroid, or forced diuresis. Notify attending physician and blood bank. Collect 10–15 ml urine and blood in anticoagulated and clotted tubes—send with administration set and all unused blood back to blood bank. Baseline urea, electrolytes, coagulation screen
7. Massive transfusions (more than one blood volume in less than 24 hours) problems
 (a) Hyperkalemia: high K+ levels in old blood, may be problem if transfusion more than 1.5 ml/kg/min. ECG: peaked T, wide PR and QRS, progress to loss of P, raised ST, ventricular fibrillation or cardiac standstill in diastole. Treat with IV calcium. Posttransfusion, with rewarming, K+ goes into red cells—serum levels may drop to subnormal
 (b) Hypocalcemia: citrate chelates ionized calcium. Clinically, usually not important, transient ± 10 minutes occurs with transfusion more than 1.5–2 ml/kg/min. ECG: prolonged QT; wide QRS; flat T with decreased blood pressure. Treat with IV calcium. Risk greatest in neonates with low calcium stores
 (c) Acid-base derangements: initial acidosis becomes alkalosis as citrate metabolized to bicarbonate; routine bicarbonate not required
 (d) Hypothermia
  (1) Oxygen dissociation: oxygen-carrying capacity (2.3 DPG) in CPDA stored blood normalizes in a few hours
  (2) Microembolism: microfilters (20–40 μm) slow transfusion and do not decrease clinically important microemboli formation
  (3) Hyperglycemia: dextrose in CPD may cause problems in children
  (4) Dilutional thrombocytopenia: only occurs above two blood volume

replacements unless abnormal functioning or low initial platelet count. One blood volume replacement lowers platelet count 30–40%

(5) Dilutional coagulopathy: after 1.5 blood volume replacement with stored old blood there are still enough factors V and VIII to initiate clotting. With packed cells, frozen plasma supplementation needed after one blood volume

8. Perioperative anemia: transfusion guidelines

   (a) Acceptable hemoglobin requirement: estimated for each patient based on
       (1) Cause and chronicity of anemia
           [a] Concomitant diseases, e.g., thyroid, liver
           [b] Chronic anemia is hemodynamically stable—with normal blood volume, vasodilation, capillary recruitment, increased oxygen extraction ratio, increased 2:3 DPG (diphosphoglycerate)
           [c] Acute anemia—hemodynamically unstable, i.e., acute blood loss
       (2) Symptoms of anemia—dyspnea on effort, excessive tiredness, weakness, tachycardia at rest. Correct prior to surgery
       (3) Smokers—smoking causes mild carbon monoxide poisoning and hemoconcentration. Stop 24 hours presurgery
       (4) Proposed operation and surgeon—expected blood loss, skill of surgeon
       (5) Cytotoxic antibody risk—transfusion in patient with chronic renal failure creates cytotoxic antibodies. Harder to find compatible organ donor

9. Acute blood loss

   (a) Clinical signs

% Blood Volume Lost	Clinical Signs
10	None
20–30	Orthostatic hypotension Tachycardia
40	Tachycardia Hypotension Tachypnea Sweating

   (b) Treatment
       (1) Correct cause of hemorrhage
       (2) Restore intravascular volume with crystalloids, colloids, blood, or a combination of these

10. Treatment of anemia

    (a) Preop: hemoglobin 8 g/ml or less—if no evidence of acute blood loss
    (b) Nonurgent surgery
        (1) Investigate nutritional causes for anemia
        (2) Postpone operation
        (3) Iron/nutrition supplements
        (4) Hemoglobin rises 1 g per week after 7–10-day delay
    (c) If surgery can be delayed temporarily
        (1) Packed red blood cells
        (2) Transfusion 4 hours per unit
        (3) 1–2 days prior to surgery
        (4) Furosemide if cardiopulmonary overload
    (d) Urgent surgery
        (1) Chronic anemia—commence infusion slowly
        (2) Acute anemia (blood loss) with signs of shock—rapid replacement with blood if Hb 9 g/ml or less
        (3) CVP or pulmonary artery pressure monitoring
    (e) Volume of blood to transfuse: to increase Hb 1 gm/ml—4 ml/kg packed cells, 6 ml/kg whole blood

    (f) Optimum blood ordering

        (1) Hospital policy should include a regularly revised and readily available maximum blood ordering schedule (MBOS)

        (2) Type and screen (group and screen) if unsure of blood required

        (3) Negative antibody screen—99.94% compatibility

        (4) Full cross-match—99.95% compatibility

    (g) Blood loss during surgery: Measurement

        (1) Weigh swabs

        (2) Visual assessment of blood on drapes, swabs, and floor

        (3) Volume in suction bottles

        (4) Serial hemoglobin or hematocrit

f. Platelets

1. Normal values: adult—300,000 mm^3; full-term or preterm newborn—250,000 mm^3

2. Recommended value presurgery more than 50,000 mm^3

3. Collection, storage, and transfusion

    (a) Random donor: one unit has 5,500 mm^3 platelets plus 50–70 ml plasma

    (b) Single donor (platelet phoresis): 50–70,000 platelets

    (c) Storage: 20–24°C with continuous agitation

    (d) "Shelf" life: 5 days

    (e) Transfusion: via half-size 170-μm filter with minimal tubing

4. Dosage

    (a) Adults—one random unit increases platelet count 5,000–8,000 mm^3

    (b) Children—0.1 to 0.2 unit/kg increases platelet count 30–50,000 mm^3

    (c) Lower platelet increase if sepsis, splenomegaly, platelet auto- or alloantibodies, or if chemotherapy

    (d) Use ABO and rhesus specific

    (e) Operate within 12 hours

    (f) Hemolytic uremic syndrome and autoimmune thrombocytopenia—platelets ineffective

    (g) Hereditary functional platelet disorders, e.g., von Willebrand's disease—treat with desmopressin acetate, cryoprecipitate

5. Drug effects on platelets

    (a) Aspirin permanently inhibits cyclooxygenase—platelet aggregation function affected for effective life (7–10 days)

    (b) NSAIDs temporarily inhibit platelet aggregation

    (c) Codeine, opiates, acetaminophen—no effect on platelets

6. Surgical contraindications—need a careful drug history of analgesics, with potential platelet aggregation effects, over the week prior to neurosurgery or middle ear surgery

g. Frozen plasma

1. Collection, storage, and transfusion

    (a) 200–250 ml plasma from whole blood within 6 hours of donation

    (b) Stored at − 18°C up to 1 year

    (c) Loss of labile factors V and VIII less than 30%

    (d) Thaw at 30–37°C with constant agitation

    (e) Use within 6 hours of thawing (FDA rule)

    (f) Use ABO compatible

     (g) Use standard 170-μm filter

2. Indications

     (a) Multiple coagulation defects (liver, renal disease)
     (b) Replacement of proved factor deficiencies
     (c) Reversal of coumadin, succinylcholine effects
     (d) Massive blood transfusion (over 1.5–2 blood volumes)

3. Not recommended

     (a) To reconstitute packed cells routinely
     (b) As a plasma volume expander
     (c) As a source of protein
     (d) As a routine postcardiopulmonary bypass
     (e) For small blood transfusions (less than 1.5 blood volumes)

4. Dosage: dilutional coagulopathy—10–30 ml/kg over 90–120 minutes

h. Cryoprecipitate

1. Collection, storage, and transfusion

     (a) 200 antihemophilic units (AHU) of factor VIII plus 250 mg fibrinogen from single donor pack
     (b) Store at $-18°C$
     (c) Thaw at $37°C$
     (d) Use standard 170-μm filter

2. Indications

     (a) Massive rapid blood transfusion over 1.5–2 blood volumes
     (b) Preexisting intravascular coagulopathy due to prolonged shock

i. Autologous transfusion

1. Conditions

     (a) Healthy patient, HCT over 34%, donates a unit of blood every 4–7 days, and up to four units preoperation
     (b) Last donation, 3 days preoperation
     (c) Piggyback technique: transfuse one unit "old" blood, remove two units "fresh" blood
     (d) Possible to have four units of less than 10-day-old autologous blood preoperation
     (e) Recombinant erythropoietin can be used if initial low HCT

2. Advantages of autologous transfusion

     (a) Infection risk only during collection and storage
     (b) No risk: incompatibility reactions, host-versus-graft reaction isoimmunization
     (c) Patient's blood dynamics: improved rheology, increased 2:3-DPG, bone marrow primed to increase RBC production postoperation
     (d) Leukocyte production increased—immune system enhanced
     (e) May enhance patient's self-esteem and confidence

3. Contraindications: relative and absolute

     (a) Technical difficulty: poor venous access, severe vasovagal reaction to phlebotomy, patient unable to give consent (pediatrics)
     (b) Concomitant disease: preexisting anemia, infection, severe heart or lung disease, hypertension (unless well controlled), epilepsy, insulin-dependent diabetes, cerebrovascular disease
     (c) Patient has hepatitis B or C or is HIV positive: fear by blood bank of accidental crossover contamination or transfusion
     (d) Urgent surgery: no time to collect blood

I. Blood transfusion; i. Autologous transfusion (continued)

j. Intraoperative blood salvage

1. Possible where no bowel soiling, tumor cell, or bacteria contamination
2. Simple scavengers: anticoagulate, filter (170 μm), and retransfuse
3. Cell savers: anticoagulate, wash, filter, spin, retransfuse—usually require dedicated technician; red cell survival only mildly reduced

k. Preoperative hemodilution

1. Postanesthesia induction—presurgery, an equivalent volume of colloid or crystalloid transfused as blood is withdrawn (two to three units)
2. 1 ml colloid is equivalent to 1 ml blood
3. 3 ml crystalloid is equivalent to 1 ml blood
4. Drop patient's HCT to 27–33%
5. Reinfuse first with last unit (freshest) removed
6. Time taken, 7–10 minutes per unit removed
7. Central venous line may be required

l. Preoperative assessment of patient with a bleeding problem

1. Specific questions should include
   (a) Do you or any of your family bleed a lot from small cuts, or bruise easily?
   (b) Have you had teeth extracted or had nosebleeds? If so, for how long did you bleed and did you bleed again the next day?
   (c) What medicines, including OTCs, do you take for pain or headaches?
   (d) When did you last take aspirin?
2. Specific examination and tests
   (a) Look for bruising, petechiae, signs of liver failure
   (b) Coagulation screen—extrinsic function—prothrombin time. Intrinsic function—activated partial thromboplastin time. Fibrinogen (2–4 g/L), D-dimer for fibrin degradation products (less than 200 pg/ml)
   (c) Thromboelastogram—platelet function, fibrin deficiency, fibrinolysis
   (d) Platelet function—aggregation tests, bleeding time (less than 10 minutes)
   (e) Hematologist's opinion if history of genetic bleeding disorder, liver disease, disseminated intravascular coagulation, or fibrinolysis

II. SPECIFIC BLOOD DISORDERS

a. Coagulation

1. Physiology
   (a) Vascular phase
       (1) Vasoconstriction
       (2) Most intense in traumatized, crushed blood vessels
       (3) Less if blood vessels sharply transected
       (4) For small cuts, can provide hemostasis
   (b) Platelet phase
       (1) Subendothelial exposure—initiates platelet aggregation

   (2) Platelets release serotonin—causes localized vasoconstriction

   (3) Release of thromboxane A_2 causes secondary aggregation of more platelets

   (4) Hemostatic plug of platelets

   (5) Activation of circulating procoagulants

  (c) Procoagulant phase

   (1) Intrinsic and extrinsic pathways form active factor X, initiate formation of fibrin

   (2) Clot retraction with fibrin requires platelets

   (3) Plasmin splits fibrin into fibrin degradation products (FDP)

   (4) High concentrations of FDP inhibit fibrin cross-linking and produce platelet dysfunction; inhibit further clot formation

 2. Disseminated intravascular coagulation—bleeding due to uncontrolled activation of the coagulation system; thrombi formation causes consumption of platelets and procoagulants

  (a) Causes include

   (1) Low cardiac output due to hemorrhagic shock, sepsis, or burns

   (2) Retained placenta

   (3) Central nervous system trauma

   (4) Prolonged extracorporeal circulation

  (b) Diagnosis

   (1) Bleeding from wound sites, IV placements

    [a] Platelet count less than 100,000

    [b] Prothrombin time and partial thromboplastin time increased

    [c] Fibrinogen under 150 mg/ml

    [d] Increased fibrin degradation products

  (c) Treatment

   (1) Correct underlying disorder

    [a] Fresh frozen plasma

    [b] Cryoprecipitate

    [c] Platelets

b. Hemoglobinopathies

 1. General physiology

  (a) Hemoglobin

   (1) Four globin chains complexed with a heme group

   (2) Normal adult has two alpha and two beta globin chains

   (3) Heme—tetrapyrrole ring with hexavalent iron atom at center

   (4) Four valencies combine iron to the pyrrole ring; one valency combines to one globin chain

   (5) One valency combines reversibly with oxygen

  (b) Oxygen carriage

   (1) Each hemoglobin molecule combines reversibly with four oxygen molecules

   (2) Steep sigmoidal oxyhemoglobin dissociation curve affected by partial pressure oxygen and carbon dioxide, pH, temperature, 2,3-DPG, and electrolyte concentrations

   (3) Shift curve to left: alkalosis (acute), cold, decreased 2,3-DPG, hemoglobin variants

   (4) Decreased 2,3-DPG: stored blood, hypophosphatemia (diabetes, burns), septic shock, acidosis (chronic), hyperthyroidism

   (5) Shift curve to right: acidosis (acute), hyperthermia, increased 2,3-DPG

   (6) High 2,3-DPG: hypoxia (chronic), anemia (chronic), uremia, hepatic failure, alkalosis (chronic), hyperthyroidism

  (c) Erythropoiesis—controlled by erythropoietin

   (1) Erythropoietin

II. Specific blood disorders; b. Hemoglobinopathies (continued)

        [a] Glycoprotein
        [b] Stimulates stem cells into red cell precursors
        [c] Kidneys main site of production
        [d] Minor sites include liver, macrophage system
        [e] Increased by
           i) Hypoxia—within 10–30 hours
           ii) Anemia
           iii) Poor cardiopulmonary function
           iv) Kidney disorders, hypernephroma, renal infarcts, hydronephrosis, renal cysts
        [f] Decreased by renal failure
    (d) Human recombinant erythropoietin
      (1) Problems include
        [a] Hypertension
        [b] Thrombosis of AV fistulae
        [c] Increased blood viscosity

2. Sickle cell disease

    (a) Hemoglobin S due to substitution valine for glutamic acid at sixth position on beta hemoglobin chain. Electrophoretic confirmation
    (b) Sickle cell trait—heterozygous with hemoglobin genotype AS
      (1) 20–40% hemoglobin S
      (2) 10% U.S. black population
      (3) Sickling occurs if PaO_2 is less than 20 mm Hg
      (4) Usually asymptomatic
    (c) Sickle cell anemia—homozygous genotype SS
      (1) 70–90% hemoglobin S
      (2) 0.3–1% U.S. black population
      (3) Sickling if PaO_2 less than 40 mm Hg
      (4) Severe hemolytic anemia and crises
    (d) Anesthetic management
      (1) Maintain adequate hydration
      (2) Maintain normal body temperature
      (3) Avoid hypoxia and respiratory depression
      (4) Avoid acidosis
      (5) Prevent circulatory stasis by improper body positioning
      (6) Increase inspired FiO_2
      (7) Transfusion of erythrocytes may depress bone marrow and increase blood viscosity
      (8) Treat postoperative pain adequately

3. Thalassemias—hereditary disorders in certain ethnic groups

    (a) Alpha thalassemia: alpha globin chain abnormal (four genes on chromosome 16)
      (1) Oriental and black populations
      (2) Alpha$_2$
        [a] Single nonfunctioning gene
        [b] Asymptomatic or mild microcytosis
      (3) Alpha$_1$ (minor)
        [a] Two nonfunctioning genes
        [b] Mild microcytic anemia, basophilic stippling reticulocytosis
      (4) Alpha major (HbH)
        [a] Three nonfunctioning genes
        [b] Sensitive to oxidant drugs
        [c] Severe macrocytic anemia

                 [d] Still has some normal hemoglobin

        (5) Hydrops fetalis

            [a] Four nonfunctioning genes

            [b] Incompatible with life

    (b) Beta thalassemia (Cooley's anemia): Beta globin chain abnormal (two genes on chromosome 6)

        (1) Mediterranean Europeans, Arabs, black population

        (2) Several varieties

        (3) More severe disease than alpha

        (4) Major form (homozygous) ultimately fatal

    (c) Anesthetic implications

        (1) High-output congestive cardiac failure common

        (2) Hyperplastic bone marrow may cause facial bone deformity, making intubation difficult

    (d) Gaucher's disease

        (1) Inborn error of glycolipid metabolism

        (2) Ashkenazi Jews

        (3) Hepatosplenomegaly

        (4) Long bone erosions

        (5) Anemia, leukopenia, thrombocytopenia

        (6) Brownish skin pigmentation

    (e) Anesthetic implications

        (1) Fragile long bones—gentle patient handling

        (2) Hepatosplenomegaly—take full-stomach precautions

        (3) Platelets may be required presurgery

c. Erythrocyte disorders

  1. Anemia—hemoglobin concentration less than the norm for age and sex

    (a) Causes of chronic anemia: normal platelets and leukocytes

        (1) Chronic blood loss: normochromic, normocytic anemia

        (2) Iron deficiency: hypochromic microcytic anemia

            [a] Decreased red blood cell volume

            [b] Increased iron-binding capacity

            [c] Decreased serum ferritin

            [d] Decreased iron in bone marrow aspirate

        (3) Vitamin B_{12} deficiency (pernicious anemia): normochromic macrocytic anemia plus hypersegmented neutrophils

            [a] Increase serum iron, lactic dehydrogenase, bilirubin

            [b] Causes

                i) Malabsorption

                    a) Lack of intrinsic factor (gastric parietal cells)

                    b) Crohn's disease (regional enteritis)

                      • Ileal bypass or resection

                      • Sprue

                      • Radiation-induced ileitis

                      • Ileal tuberculosis

                      • Lymphoma

        (4) Folate deficiency: usually nutritional causes

            [a] Increased requirement

                i) Infancy

                ii) Pregnancy

                iii) Hemolytic anemia

                iv) Hyperthyroidism

            [b] Dietary

II. Specific blood disorders; c. Erythrocyte disorders (continued)

                                i) Alcoholism

                              ii) Fad diets or other malabsorption

                            iii) Hyperalimentation (incomplete)

                    [c] Malabsorption

                              i) Alcoholism

                              ii) Small-intestine disease

                                a) Regional enteritis

                                b) Sprue

                            iii) Small bowel resection

                            iv) Lymphoma

                            v) Congenital folate malabsorption

                              a) Drug induced

                              b) Folate reductase inhibitors

                              c) Antiepileptic drugs

                              d) Oral contraceptives and estrogens

                              e) Sulfasalazine

                            vi) Biochemical

                              a) Congenital errors of folate metabolism

    (b) Anesthetic implications—iron deficiency or megaloblastic anemia

        (1) General

            [a] Try to correct nutritionally prior to surgery

            [b] If symptomatic and urgent surgery, may need transfusion

            [c] Chronic anemia usually well compensated

        (2) Megaloblastic anemias

            [a] Atrophic glossitis—careful lip care

            [b] Hepatic dysfunction

            [c] Neurologic manifestations in 50%—document carefully before anesthesia, avoid regional anesthesia

            [d] Avoid nitrous oxide because of effect on methionine synthase

            [e] Avoid succinylcholine if myelopathy present

    (c) Hemolytic anemia—red cell survival less than 120 days

        (1) Signs

            [a] Reticulocytes, frequent schistocytes, and cell fragments

            [b] Heinz bodies in G6PD

            [c] Splenic hypertrophy (reticuloendothelial breakdown)

                 i) Jaundice

                 ii) Cholelithiasis

        (2) Cause of hemolytic anemia

            [a] Congenital types—skeletal abnormalities

                 i) Increased bilirubin (indirect)

                 ii) Decreased serum haptoglobin

                iii) Increased LDH (iso-enzymes 1 and 2)

                iv) Methemoglobinemia

                 v) Hemosiderinuria

            [b] Injury to red cell membrane

                 i) Immune hemolytic disease

                 ii) Autoimmune hemolytic anemia

                iii) Hereditary spherocytosis

                iv) Paroxysmal nocturnal hemoglobinuria

                 v) Toxins and venoms

                vi) Traumatic mechanical injury and infection, e.g., malaria

               vii) Spur cell anemias

            [c] Defective red cell membrane

        i) Unstable hemoglobins
       ii) Thalassemias
     iii) Erythropoietic porphyria
     iv) Glucose-6-phosphate dehydrogenase (G6PD) deficiency
      v) Pyruvate kinase deficiency
     vi) Hemoglobinopathies

  (3) Anesthetic implications
     [a] Depends on cause of anemia
     [b] Certain drugs may need to be avoided, e.g., barbiturates in erythropoietic porphyria. Aspirin, phenacetin, sulfonamides in G6PD
       i) Avoid nitrous oxide (bone marrow depression)
      ii) May have to give corticosteroids
     iii) Patient may be on immunosuppressives
     iv) Other organ system may be affected, e.g., liver, kidneys

(d) Aplastic anemia: usually pancytopenia
  (1) Causes
    [a] Chemotherapy
    [b] Solvents
    [c] Radiation
    [d] Viral infection
    [e] Immunologic disorders
    [f] Chloramphenicol
    [g] Fanconi's syndrome
    [h] Diamond-Blackfan syndrome
  (2) Anesthetic implications
    [a] Corticosteroids may be needed perioperatively
    [b] Careful asepsis practiced
    [c] Correct platelets and hemoglobin preoperation
    [d] Gentle intubation as risk of hemorrhage
    [e] Maintain high PaO_2 and cardiac output to ensure adequate tissue oxygenation

d. White cell disorders

1. Agranulocytosis
  (a) Causes
    (1) Drug induced—phenothiazines, antiepileptics, various antibiotics, including chloramphenicol, gold, phenylbutazone, procainamide, amphetamines, cancer chemotherapeutic agents
    (2) Toxins—benzone derivatives
    (3) Radiation
    (4) Infection: bacteria, viruses, protozoa and rickettsia
    (5) Immunologic: Felty's syndrome, systemic lupus erythematosus
  (b) Symptoms
    (1) Sore throat, fever
    (2) High mortality despite antibiotics
  (c) Anesthetic implications
    (1) Strict aseptic techniques
    (2) Avoid prolonged nasal intubation because of sinusitis risk
    (3) Anesthesia may lower immunity further

2. Myeloproliferative diseases
  (a) Leukemia
    (1) Acute—myelogenous
    (2) Acute—lymphocytic

        (3) Chronic—myelogenous

        (4) Hairy cell leukemia

        (5) Anesthetic implications

            [a] Strict aseptic techniques

            [b] Splenomegaly creates full-stomach potential

            [c] Anemia and thrombocytopenia may be present secondary to therapy—may need correction

            [d] Multiple drug regimens, including steroids, may interfere with anesthetic agents

            [e] Swelling of gums may make intubation difficult

    (b) Multiple myeloma

        (1) Monoclonal cell population, usually IgG

        (2) Bence Jones proteins in urine

        (3) Plasma levels immunoglobulin over 2 g/dl

        (4) Anesthetic implications

            [a] Hyperviscosity syndrome if plasma protein concentrations over 5–7 g/dl. May cause angina, congestive cardiac failure, neurologic deficits. May need plasmapheresis presurgery

            [b] Coagulopathy from abnormal platelets or inhibition of Factors I, II, and XI may need correcting

            [c] Hypercalcemia—correct if possible presurgery

            [d] Renal failure—maintain adequate hydration

            [e] Lytic lesions render bones fragile. Neck may be unstable—care when ventilating

            [f] Multiple drug therapy, including steroids, may interfere with anesthetic agents

            [g] Avoid cooling—cryoglobin precipitation may occur

            [h] Avoid regional techniques because of coagulopathy risk

e. Platelet disorders

    1. Von Willebrand's disease

    (a) Most common inherited platelet disorder

    (b) Autosomal dominant

    (c) Severity of disease variable

    (d) Von Willebrand's factor necessary for platelet aggregation

    (e) Factor VIII levels often decreased

    (f) Capillary fragility common

    (g) Laboratory: history of bleeding after minor cuts or surgery

        (1) Prolonged bleeding time

        (2) Decreased factor VIII and von Willebrand's antigen levels

        (3) Abnormal ristocetin aggregation

        (4) Anesthetic implications: correct prior to surgery with desmopressin (arginine vasopressin, DDAVP) in types I and IIa, not in Type IIb or cryoprecipitate

f. Abnormalities of procoagulants

    1. Tests

    (a) Prothrombin time (PT)

        (1) Factor VII (extrinsic system and common pathway)

        (2) Add calcium and tissue thromboplastin to citrated blood

        (3) Normal 60% of control

- (b) Activated partial thromboplastin time (aPTT)
    - (1) Intrinsic system and common pathway
    - (2) Add kaolin + calcium + negatively charged activator to citrated blood
    - (3) Less than 50 seconds (neonates, 65–150 seconds)
- (c) Thrombin time (TT)
    - (1) Common pathway
    - (2) Add thrombin to activate fibrinogen
    - (3) Less than 12 seconds (neonates, 13–20 seconds)

2. Hemophilia A

- (a) Hereditary deficiency factor VIII
- (b) X-linked recessive with variable expression
- (c) Incidence one in 10,000 to 25,000
- (d) Continued bleeding from damaged large vessels
- (e) Less than 1% factor VIII—high risk of spontaneous hemorrhage into large joints, nose, soft tissues, urinary tract
- (f) 10–15% factor VIII—asymptomatic until trauma or surgery
- (g) Prolonged PTT
- (h) Normal PT, bleeding time, platelet count
- (i) Treat with factor VIII concentrates
- (j) May develop antibodies to infused factor VIII
- (k) DDAVP (arginine vasopressin analogue) increases factor VIII

3. Anesthetic implications

- (a) Factor VIII levels to 100% for surgery
- (b) Maintain factor VIII at over 50% 10–14 days post major operation
- (c) 12 hourly factor VIII infusions required
- (d) Avoid intramuscular injections
- (e) Careful intubation
- (f) Avoid nasal intubation if possible because of risk of mucosal tear
- (g) Careful extremity positioning to avoid hemarthroses or hematomas
- (h) Use of DDAVP alone may be adequate for dental extractions

4. Hemophilia B (Christmas disease)

- (a) Factor IX lack
- (b) Hereditary X-linked
- (c) Incidence one in 200,000
- (d) Prolonged PTT
- (e) Bleeding problems as severe as hemophilia A
- (f) Treat with factor IX concentrates
- (g) Half-life of factor IX—24 hours

5. Anesthetic implications: as for hemophilia A

III. EFFECTS OF ANESTHETICS ON BLOOD SYSTEM

a. Hemopoiesis—nitrous oxide (for days) may depress bone marrow

1. Halothane depresses cultured murine bone marrow cells

b. Immune function

1. Volatile agents depress neutrophil chemotaxis and lymphocyte transformation

c. Coagulation

1. Regional anesthesia may increase platelet aggregation less than general anesthesia. Less deep vein thrombosis with regional techniques

D. PRINCIPLES OF PAIN MANAGEMENT

I. CHRONIC PAIN THEORIES

a. Restrictive—mind–body dualism

1. Psychological
2. Radical operant-behavioral
3. Radical cognitive

b. Neurophysiologically based

1. Peripheral sensitization
2. Central sensitization
3. Gene induction
4. Pain "memory"—wind-up phenomenon of wide dynamic range neurons
5. Destruction of inhibitory pathways
6. Damage to control processing

c. Comprehensive

1. Gate control theory
2. Nonradical operant-behavioral
3. Cognitive-behavioral
4. International Association for the Study of Pain: "Pain is an unpleasant sensory and emotional experience associated with actual or potential tissue damage, or described in terms of such damage"

II. CHRONIC PAIN TREATMENT

a. Nonpharmacologic

1. Education
   (a) Generalized and specific
   (b) Didactic lectures, information sheets, and books are useful
2. Psychotherapy
   (a) To improve patients' function, by enabling patients to work toward specific and realistic goals, long- and short-term, in their chosen activities
   (b) To reduce patients' intake of analgesic and psychotropic medications, insofar as their action is not consistent with the aims of treatment and with goal attainment. This is achieved by changing pain-contingent (p.r.n.) drug regimens to time-contingent (i.e., around-the-clock regularly scheduled) drug use, and reducing the dose gradually
   (c) To reduce patients' maladaptive behavior by not reinforcing it, and teaching more direct and appropriate methods of communication
   (d) To increase patients' "well behavior" by reinforcing efforts toward increased activity and goal attainment, or toward following the agreed-upon treatment program
   (e) To teach patients the skills of monitoring thoughts and feelings, and of challenging and changing dysfunctional thoughts and distorted beliefs

II. Effects of anesthetics on ; a. Nonpharmacologic (continued)

   (f) To give the patients coping skills to return to vocational and avocational pursuits
   (g) To interact and support the family and significant others to decrease secondary reinforcement patterns and improve coping skills
   (h) Individual psychotherapy and group psychotherapy are used

3. Physical therapy: to increase patients' activity level. Exercise is incompatible with pain behavior and is necessary to develop fitness, flexibility, and range of movement. Achievable goals should be set

   (a) Electrical modalities usually not useful—ultrasound interferential, galvanic stimulation
   (b) Mobilization and manipulation
   (c) Generalized exercise program
   (d) Specific exercise and stretching programs
   (e) Spray or cold and stretch techniques
   (f) Trigger-point desensitization
   (g) Heat or cold
   (h) Gait analysis and retraining

4. Occupational therapy

   (a) Activities of daily-living assessment and retraining
   (b) Job task analysis and specific related exercises
   (c) Job modification

5. Transcutaneous nerve stimulator (TENS)

   (a) A device to produce nonpainful electrical paresthesia in area of pain
   (b) Neuromodulation occurs at central-level, low-frequency pulse width at high repetitions; "close the gate." High-frequency pulse width at low repetition; increase endorphins
   (c) Analgesia during period of stimulation only or for hours afterward
   (d) Need to individualize therapy
   (e) Main side effect—skin rash from pads
   (f) Patient uses unit at home, encourages self-reliance
   (g) Contraindication: "on demand" cardiac pacemaker, over the carotid sinus

6. Acupuncture

   (a) Classic—to stimulate "energy flow" through channels or meridians, localized, well-defined points of access
   (b) Trigger point therapy—tender or trigger points "needled" to decrease pain or spasm
   (c) Mechanisms—probably involves neuromodulation of transmitters, including endorphins, substance P, calcitonin gene-related peptide, cholecystokinin, and C fos expression

7. Biofeedback

   (a) Electronic devices detect, amplify, and convert various biologic responses into easily processed information
   (b) Documented efficacy in many chronic pain conditions, including
       (1) Myofascial syndromes
       (2) Raynaud's phenomenon
       (3) Headaches, chronic tension, migraine, cluster
       (4) Temporomandibular joint dysfunction
       (5) Sympathetic mediated pain
       (6) Restless leg syndrome

b. Pharmacologic

1. Narcotic pharmacology
   - (a) Pharmacodynamics
     - (1) Definition—the effect of the drug on the body
     - (2) Five groups of opioid receptors
       - [a] Mu
         - i) Mu_1—mediates both spinal (mu_1 accounts for 40% of the opioid receptors in spinal cord) and supraspinal analgesia; euphoria; dependence; miosis; nausea/vomiting; urinary retention; pruritus; temperature increase, tolerance
         - ii) Mu_2—respiratory depression; constipation; sedation; no analgesia
       - [b] Kappa
         - i) Mediates spinal analgesia (kappa accounts for 50% of the opioid receptors in spinal cord); dysphoria; sedation; miosis; respiratory depression (ceiling effect); diuresis
       - [c] Sigma
         - i) No analgesic effect; slight stimulation of respiration; dysphoria; mydriasis; muscle rigidity; hyperthermia
         - ii) Not a true opioid receptor as other drugs, such as the antipsychotics and antihistamines, bind to this receptor
       - [d] Delta
         - i) Augments mu receptor (delta accounts for 10% of the opioid receptors in spinal cord); apnea; nausea/vomiting, pruritus
       - [e] Epsilon
         - i) Pharmacodynamic action unknown
     - (3) Opioid receptor location
       - [a] Brain—periaqueductal gray (PAG), limbic system, medial thalamic nuclei, area postrema
       - [b] Spinal cord—substantia gelatinosa (lamina II)
       - [c] Peripheral nerves and ganglia
       - [d] Adrenal medulla
       - [e] Gut
     - (4) Mechanism of action
       - [a] Supraspinal receptors
         - i) Most of the supraspinal receptors mediating analgesia are found in the PAG. Stimulation of these receptors activates descending fibers, which modulate C-fiber input into lamina II of the spinal cord. The modulating neurotransmitters released are norepinephrine and serotonin
       - [b] Spinal cord receptors
         - i) Stimulation of the opioid receptors in lamina II of the spinal cord results in the inhibition of substance P release from the presynaptic terminal and increased potassium conductance in the postsynaptic terminal
       - [c] Peripheral opioid receptors
         - i) Controversy exists as to the role of peripheral receptors in analgesia; however, stimulation of these receptors on nerve terminals results in inhibition of substance P release from these terminals
     - (5) Agonists
       - [a] Mu
         - i) Naturally occurring opium derivatives—morphine, codeine
         - ii) Partially synthetic derivatives of morphine—hydromorphone, oxymorphone, heroin, oxycodone

II. Effects of anesthetics on ; b. Pharmacologic (continued)

           iii) Synthetic compounds—levorphanol, methadone, propoxyphene, meperidine, fentanyl, sufentanil, alfentanil

      [b] Kappa

           i) Pentazocine, butorphanol, nalorphine (partial), nalbuphine (partial)

      [c] Sigma

           i) Pentazocine, butorphanol, nalorphine, nalbuphine

      [d] Delta

           i) Dezocine

      [e] Epsilon

           i) None

(6) Antagonists

    [a] Mu

          i) Pentazocine, butorphanol, nalorphine, nalbuphine, naloxone, naltrexone

(7) Equianalgesic doses

Drug	Equianalgesic Dose (mg)		Parenteral:Oral Dose Ratio
	IM	PO	
Morphine	10	60	0.17
Alfentanil	0.4	—	—
Codeine	120	200	0.60
Fentanyl	0.1	—	—
Hydrocodone	—	30	—
Hydromorphone	1.5	7.5	0.20
Levorphanol	2	4	0.50
Meperidine	75	300	0.25
Methadone	10	20	0.50
Oxycodone	—	30	—
Oxymorphone	—	10	0.10
Propoxyphene	—	130	—
Sufentanil	0.02	—	—
Buprenorphine	0.3	—	—
Butorphanol	2	—	—
Dezocine	10	—	—
Nalbuphine	10	—	—
Pentazocine	30	150	0.20

(8) Tolerance

    [a] Defined as decreased effect following repeated administration of opioids or increasingly greater doses required to achieve the desired effect

    [b] Commonly see tolerance to supraspinal effects of the drug, such as analgesia, respiratory depression, euphoria, dysphoria, sedation, nausea/vomiting. Tolerance does not occur with constipation and miosis

    [c] More likely to develop tolerance with rapidly increasing doses or large doses with short dosing intervals

    [d] Occurs after about 2–3 weeks of continuous administration

    [e] Can be reversed after about a 2-week drug-free interval (drug holiday)

(9) Dependence

    [a] Physical dependence

         i) A pharmacologic property of all opioid drugs. It means that withdrawal symptoms will occur if the opioid is abruptly discontinued or if an antagonist is administered

ii) Signs and symptoms of opioid withdrawal

Hours After Last Dose	Signs and Symptoms
8–12	Lacrimation, rhinorrhea, yawning, sweating
18–20	Dilated pupils, anorexia, gooseflesh, tremors, restlessness, irritability, anxiety
48–72	Increased irritability, insomnia, marked anorexia, violent yawning, severe sneezing, muscle spasms, generalized body aches, nausea/vomiting, diarrhea, abdominal cramping, increased heart rate, increased blood pressure, chills and hyperthermia, flushing, low back pain, hyperpnea

iii) Because of the long half-life of methadone, the withdrawal symptoms progress more slowly

iv) Withdrawal can be prevented with a slow taper over 10–14 days

[b] Psychological dependence (addiction)

i) A psychological and behavioral syndrome characterized by compulsive drug use, overwhelming interest in securing a supply, and return to drug use after drug detoxification. Addicted persons may exhibit drug hoarding, acquisition of drugs from multiple sources, increasing drug dosage on their own, and drug sales

ii) There is considerable evidence that addiction is a rare outcome of opioid use by patients, at least among those with no prior history of drug abuse. Causes of addiction lie more in the psychology of the patient and in the environment than in the qualities of the medically administered drugs

(10) Side effects

[a] Respiratory depression

i) Produced by stimulation of opioid receptors located in the brain stem

ii) Treatment is titration (not bolusing) of naloxone, 0.04 mg every 1 minute

[b] Nausea and vomiting

i) Vomiting center stimulated by three areas

a) Chemoreceptor trigger zone

• Directly stimulated by opioids

• Stimulated by dopamine and serotonin, therefore, inhibited by the antidopaminergics and antiserotonergics

b) Vestibular system

• Opioids sensitize the vestibular apparatus to movement

• Stimulated by cholinergics and histamine, therefore, inhibited by the anticholinergics and antihistamines

c) GI tract

• Opioids decrease gut motility

• Stimulated by cholinergics, therefore, inhibited by the anticholinergics

[c] Constipation

i) Results from mu_2 receptor stimulation in the GI tract

[d] Pruritus

i) Results from mu_1 receptor stimulation in spinal cord

ii) More common with intraspinal opioids (72–85%) than IV morphine (38–60%)

iii) Treat with nalbuphine or naloxone

(b) Pharmacokinetics

(1) Definition—the effect of the body on the drug

    (2) Absorption
        [a] Oral administration
            i) Readily absorbed in the GI tract, but due to the first-pass effect through the liver, the bioavailability of the various opioids will differ (see "Parenteral: oral ratios" above)
        [b] IM/IV
            i) Rapid absorption and bypasses the first-pass effect
            ii) No significant difference between SC/IM, however, the rate is related to blood flow through muscle (deltoid more than vastus lateralis more than gluteus maximus)
        [c] Rectal
            i) Rapid but erratic absorption; also bypasses first-pass effect
        [d] Transdermal
            i) New form of administering fentanyl
            ii) Slow onset
            iii) Drugs delivered by this route must have
                a) High lipid solubility
                b) High potency
                c) Low molecular weight
            iv) System composed of four functional layers
                a) Occlusive backing—prevents loss of drug and entry of water into drug system
                b) Drug reservoir mixed with alcohol—alcohol increases permeability of skin to fentanyl and enhances rate of drug flow
                c) Release membrane adhesive—controls rate of drug release from reservoir; fentanyl-saturated silicone layer holds system in place and effectively administers a bolus of fentanyl after application
                d) Protective peel strip
            v) Absorption
                a) Free base penetrates better than ionized form
                b) Penetration can vary 46–66%; variations in drug penetration between skin regions can vary 20–40%
                c) Fentanyl concentration undetected for about 2 hours due to formation of skin depot
                d) Appreciable plasma levels 8–12 hours after application
                e) Factors increasing absorption: vigorous exercise, excessive hydration, occlusion of skin surface, skin damage, hyperfunction of sweat glands, hyperthermia, increased vascular perfusion
    (3) Volume of distribution (Vd)
        [a] Apparent volume of a drug must be distributed if the concentration everywhere is equal to that in the plasma
        [b] Dependent on lipid solubility, protein binding, and ionization
        [c] The higher the Vd at steady state, the longer is the $T_{1/2 \text{ life}}$
        [d] Vd over 1 liter/kg suggests the drug has a greater affinity for tissue than for plasma
        [e] With the exception of alfentanil, all of the opioids have Vd over 1 liter/kg
        [f] Because of differences in lipid solubility, protein binding, and ionization, all of the opioids have similar Vds. This stresses the fact that no one property will determine Vd; one must look at all of the factors to predict Vd
    (4) Metabolism/elimination
        [a] Clearance (Cl) (ml/min)
            i) Rate at which a given proportion of Vd is rendered drug-free

    ii) The higher the plasma clearance, the shorter is the $T_{1/2\text{ life}}$ (however, if the drug has a very low Vd steady state, it has a slow $T_{1/2}$ in spite of the low plasma clearance because more drug is available for clearance, i.e., alfentanil)

[b] Hepatic metabolism
    i) Opioids are hepatically metabolized
    ii) Opioid metabolism depends more on plasma concen- tration and hepatic blood flow than on intrinsic microsomal activity, therefore, liver dysfunction has little effect on opioid metabolism unless it is severe
    iii) Opioids are high-extraction drugs, therefore, they are avidly removed by the liver and their kinetics depend on blood flow (as opposed to low-extraction drugs, which are dependent on the intrinsic capacity of the liver)
    iv) Morphine and meperidine have active metabolites
       a) Morphine → morphine-6-glucuronide
       b) Meperidine → normeperidine

[c] Renal elimination
    i) The kidneys excrete the metabolites that can accumulate in renal disease
       a) Normeperidine has half the potency of meperidine as an analgesic but twice its potency as a convulsant
       b) Morphine-6-glucuronide—potent analgesic effect but also serves as a reservoir for the parent drug, which can be released by plasma hydrolysis and made available to cross the blood–brain barrier

Average Pharmacokinetic Data for Four Opiates

	Morphine	Meperidine	Fentanyl	Methadone
pKa	8.0	8.5	8.4	9.3
Percent un-ion at ph 7.4	23	< 10	< 10	< 10
Lipid solubility	1.4	39	813	116
Protein binding (%)	30	70	84	89
$T_{1/2}$ elimination (hours)	2–4	3–5	2–4	24–48
Vd steady state (L/kg)	3–5	3–5	3–5	3.2–4.4
Clearance (ml/min/kg)	10–20	8–18	10–20	0.9–1.9
Oral availability (%)	20–30	52	—	90

(c) Agonist opiates
  (1) Morphine
    [a] Reference standard for all opioids
    [b] Available in a controlled-release preparation
      i) The morphine is embedded in a wax base that slowly releases the morphine
      ii) Analgesia peaks in 90–120 minutes (compared with 30–90 minutes for the immediate release)
      iii) Tablet cannot be broken in half as this will release a large quantity of the morphine
  (2) Codeine
    [a] Weak opioid with low incidence of physical dependence
    [b] Side effects less intense
    [c] Higher lipid solubility than morphine
    [d] Higher oral bioavailability than morphine
    [e] Effective antitussive agent (agent of choice because of low dependence risk)

II. Effects of anesthetics on ; b. Pharmacologic (continued)

      [f] Greater histamine release than morphine
- (3) Hydrocodone
  - [a] Pharmacologic activity similar to codeine
  - [b] Used to be used as an antitussive only, but now commonly used as an analgesic
- (4) Hydromorphone
  - [a] Is six to eight times more potent than morphine
  - [b] Easily absorbed in GI tract
  - [c] Fewer side effects than morphine
  - [d] More likely to produce psychological dependence
  - [e] More water-soluble than morphine, therefore, it can be used in relatively large IM doses
  - [f] Very effective antitussive agent
- (5) Oxymorphone
  - [a] Seven to 10 times more potent than morphine
  - [b] Comes in 5-mg rectal suppositories
  - [c] Derivative of hydromorphone
- (6) Oxycodone
  - [a] Qualitatively similar to morphine in all respects
- (7) Levorphanol
  - [a] Four times more potent than morphine
  - [b] Incidence of nausea and vomiting and constipation less than other agents
  - [c] Duration is somewhat longer than morphine
- (8) Methadone
  - [a] Slightly more potent than morphine
  - [b] Less dependence-producing than morphine
  - [c] Less euphoria and less sedation
  - [d] Well absorbed orally
  - [e] Long half-life (therefore, good for addiction programs)
  - [f] Takes a while to reach steady state
- (9) Propoxyphene
  - [a] A derivative of methadone
  - [b] Less effective an analgesic than codeine
  - [c] 60 mg no more effective than 600 mg of aspirin
  - [d] 32 mg no more effective than placebo
  - [e] Alleged lower dependence potential
  - [f] Higher cost than codeine
  - [g] Bioavailability 50%
  - [h] Large Vd (10–20 L/kg), which accounts for its long half-life of approximately 10 hours
- (10) Meperidine
  - [a] Less smooth-muscle contraction than morphine and less constipation
  - [b] Normeperidine may accumulate and precipitate seizures
    - i) Significant at large doses (over 1 g/day) or in renal failure
    - ii) Half-life of normeperidine is 10–20 hours
  - [c] Dose-dependent cardiodepressant effect may change pharmacokinetics
  - [d] Toxic interaction with MAO inhibitors
  - [e] Has local anesthetic properties
  - [f] Has an atropinelike activity (may cause tachycardia)
  - [g] Little effect on cough reflex
- (11) Fentanyl
  - [a] 80 to 100 times more potent than morphine
  - [b] Transdermal patch becoming popular

(12) Sufentanil
- [a] 500 to 1,000 times more potent than morphine

(13) Alfentanil
- [a] 40 times more potent than morphine

(14) Dezocine
- [a] Used only by the IM or IV route
- [b] Analgesic potency and pharmacokinetics similar to morphine
- [c] Ceiling effect on respiratory depression
- [d] Low potential for abuse

(d) Agonists–antagonists

(1) Butorphanol
- [a] Kappa and sigma agonist
- [b] Partial mu antagonist
- [c] Produces significant sedation
- [d] 50% less nausea/vomiting than morphine and other side effects are less common
- [e] Ceiling effect on respiratory depression

(2) Nalbuphine
- [a] Chemically related to oxymorphone
- [b] Pharmacologic effects similar to morphine but has a ceiling effect on respiratory depression
- [c] Kappa and sigma agonist
- [d] Potent mu antagonist
- [e] Sedation similar to butorphanol

(3) Pentazocine
- [a] Kappa and sigma agonist
- [b] Mu and epsilon antagonist
- [c] High doses cause an increase in heart rate and blood pressure
- [d] Higher incidence of psychomimetic effects (anxiety, dysphoria, nightmares, and hallucinations)
- [e] Bioavailability 20%

(4) Buprenorphine
- [a] Partial mu agonist
   - i) It has both agonist and antagonist activity, depending on the dose
- [b] Dissociates from receptors very slowly, therefore, once effects have been produced, not easily reversed by opioid antagonists
- [c] Shows antagonist activity at high doses

(e) Antagonists

(1) Naloxone
- [a] Short acting (30–45 minutes)
- [b] Has been associated with tachycardia, hypertension, pulmonary edema, and cardiac dysrhythmia (attributed to sudden increase in sympathetic nervous system activity)

(2) Naltrexone
- [a] Similar to naloxone
- [b] Active in oral form

(f) General guidelines for narcotic treatment in chronic pain

(1) Because of the many problems with opioids, such as the side effects, tolerance, dependence, potential misuse, and legal issues, the chronic use of opioids must be done cautiously. Unfortunately, many patients are denied the potential benefits of narcotics because of misconceptions

(2) Opioids are not appropriate for all pain syndromes. They tend to work well in nociceptive pain, which is pain with no coexisting nervous system pathology (such as peripheral nerve injury or spinal cord injury). Narcotics tend not to work well in neuropathic pain, which is pain secondary to nervous

system pathology. This is a general response but does not apply to all patients as some patients with neuropathic pain respond to opioids but usually require a larger dose

(3) Watch for and treat all side effects

(4) Be cautious in starting chronic opioid therapy in

[a] The young patient

[b] Severe psychological pathology (personality disorders, schizophrenia, depression); chaotic family; or social environment chaos

[c] Prior history of chemical dependency

(5) Patients with a low risk of abuse potential are

[a] Middle aged or older with no prior drug or alcohol abuse and with a stable family and social history

2. Nonopioid analgesics

(a) Nonsteroidal anti-inflammatory drugs (NSAIDs)

(1) The NSAIDs are a class of nonopioid analgesics that have antiinflammatory, antipyretic, and analgesic properties

(2) Mechanism of action

[a] The breakdown of arachidonic acid by the enzyme cyclooxygenase results in the production of prostaglandins. These prostaglandins induce inflammation and directly sensitize the peripheral terminals of C fibers to thermal, mechanical, and chemical stimuli. Because of this sensitization, the chemical mediators, such as bradykinin, histamine, and substance P, exert a greater effect on the pain receptors. The NSAIDs inhibit cyclooxygenase by acetylating this enzyme and preventing this cascade

(3) Classification of NSAIDs commonly used for analgesia

[a] Salicylic acid derivatives—aspirin, diflunisal, salsalate, choline magnesium salicylate, magnesium salicylate, sodium salicylate

[b] Anthranilic acid derivatives—mefenamic acid, meclofenamate sodium

[c] Propionic acid derivatives—fenoprofen calcium, flurbiprofen, ibuprofen, ketoprofen, naproxen

[d] Pyrrole derivatives—ketorolac

(4) Side effects

[a] Gastrointestinal

i) Cause localized irritation of the gastric mucosa from a direct effect of the NSAIDs

ii) Higher doses may cause erosive gastritis and gastric hemorrhage secondary to a decrease in PGE_2 and PGI_2. These prostaglandins both inhibit gastric acid secretion and stimulate cytoprotective intestinal mucus

iii) Aspirin and the more potent antiinflammatory NSAIDs have the highest GI irritation while the propionic acid derivatives have the lowest

[b] Hematologic system

i) With the exception of aspirin, all of the NSAIDs reversibly inhibit platelet aggregation. Aspirin irreversibly inhibits platelet aggregation and thus lasts for the life of the platelets

ii) Use NSAIDs with caution in patients with underlying bleeding problems (i.e., on anticoagulant therapy)

[c] Renal system

i) Sodium and water retention is possible but rare

ii) Nephrotoxicity is rare and becomes manifest by hematuria, proteinuria, and nephrotic syndrome

(5) Pharmacokinetics

[a] Absorption

   i) All of the above-mentioned NSAIDs have a high oral bioavailability (80–100%). Ketorolac is the only NSAID approved for IM injection

[b] Volume of distribution

   i) All NSAIDs have a low volume of distribution (less than 1 L/kg). This low volume of distribution is attributable to the high protein binding (80–99%)

[c] Metabolism

   i) All NSAIDs are metabolized by the liver by oxidation and conjugation

   ii) Because the enzymes involved in the biotransformation of the NSAIDs are saturable, the elimination half-life will increase with increased dose

[d] Elimination

   i) The conjugated and oxidized products of the NSAIDs are eliminated by the kidney

(6) General considerations for NSAIDs

[a] The NSAIDs are recommended for the relief of mild to moderate pain; however, depending on the mechanism behind the pain, the NSAIDs can be quite effective. If there is a strong inflammatory component to the pain, the NSAIDs can provide potent pain relief (e.g., bone pain)

[b] The analgesic actions of the NSAIDs are very similar across drugs but they can differ greatly in duration of action

[c] For moderate to severe pain, the NSAIDs are commonly combined with opioids

(b) Acetaminophen

(1) Acetaminophen is a para-aminophenol derivative that differs from the NSAIDs because of its lack of antiinflammatory properties

(2) Mechanism of action

[a] The mechanism of action of acetaminophen is unknown. It may produce its analgesia by nitric oxide synthase inhibition in the spinal cord

[b] Acetaminophen does inhibit brain cyclooxygenase, which may account for its antipyretic activity

(3) Pharmacokinetics

[a] The pharmacokinetics of acetaminophen is very similar to the NSAIDs with the exception of a larger volume of distribution due to its low protein binding (20%)

[b] Acetaminophen is metabolized by the liver and eliminated by the kidney

(4) Side effects

[a] The side effects of acetaminophen are minimal. It does not have the GI irritation or the platelet inhibition that the NSAIDs have

[b] The major serious side effect is hepatic necrosis, which can occur with large doses (10–15 g). This hepatic necrosis results from the formation of *N*-acetyl-benzoquinoneimine, which reacts to glutathione and sulfhydryl groups of proteins. The treatment of this toxicity is acetylcysteine, which binds to *N*-acetyl-benzoquinoneimine and inactivates it

(5) General considerations

[a] Acetaminophen is appropriate for mild to moderate pain relief when an anti-inflammatory effect is not necessary

[b] It is commonly used in combination with opioids

3. Coanalgesics

(a) The coanalgesics are drugs used in pain management that may or may not have intrinsic analgesic properties but may provide pain relief in certain pain syndromes or potentiate the common analgesics, such as opioids

II. Effects of anesthetics on ; b. Pharmacologic (continued)

(b) Antidepressants

(1) The antidepressants are commonly used in chronic pain syndromes for pain relief. The analgesic doses are lower than the antidepressant doses. Whether the antidepressants actually treat underlying depression (which is known to exacerbate chronic pain) with a corresponding decrease in pain is unknown. However, it appears that these drugs have a direct effect on certain painful conditions

(2) Mechanism of action

[a] Inhibition of reuptake of biogenic amines (norepinephrine and serotonin) into the nerve terminals results in an increase in the concentration and duration of action of these neurotransmitters at the synapse

[b] Both serotonergic and noradrenergic neurons in the brain stem project to and inhibit C-fiber input into the spinal cord. The antidepressants are thought to activate these descending inhibitory neurons

[c] As discussed in the opioid pharmacology section, the opioids also activate these brain-stem inhibitory neurons and the antidepressants potentiate the action of the serotonin and norepinephrine released by the opioids

(3) Classes of antidepressants

[a] Tertiary amines—imipramine, amitriptyline, doxepin

[b] Secondary amines—desipramine, nortriptyline

[c] Atypical—trazadone

(4) Pharmacokinetics

[a] The antidepressants have a long half-life and thus can be given in a single daily dose. These drugs are metabolized by the liver and the tertiary amines, imipramine and amitriptyline, are demethylated to desipramine and nortriptyline, respectively

(5) Side effects

[a] The antidepressants have anticholinergic, antihistaminic, antidopaminergic, and alpha$_1$ blocking activity. Because of this activity, the following side effects may occur

i) Anticholinergic side effects—dry mouth, constipation, urinary retention, sedation

ii) Antihistaminic side effects—sedation

iii) Alpha$_1$ blockade—orthostatic hypotension

[b] The sedation may be advantageous as many chronic pain patients suffer from insomnia. Also because of this side effect, the drug is usually given at bedtime. The antidepressants with fewer anticholinergic effects (i.e., trazadone) are less sedating

[c] The antidepressants cause depression of cardiac excitability and, therefore, may result in cardiac conduction defects

(6) Pain syndromes that have been shown to respond to antidepressants

[a] Postherpetic neuralgia

[b] Diabetic neuropathy

[c] Tension headache

[d] Migraine headache

[e] Atypical facial pain

(7) General considerations

[a] The antidepressants are most effective for diffuse, burning, and dysesthetic pain

[b] In patients over 65, start with 10 mg at night and increase by 10 mg as tolerated

[c] In patients under 65, start with 25 mg and increase by 25 mg as tolerated (if these patients are extremely sensitive, drop to 10 mg)

[d] Most patients can be managed at below antidepressant dosages. However, some patients may require antidepressant levels, in which case, blood levels should be monitored

(c) Anticonvulsants

  (1) The anticonvulsant drugs have been demonstrated to be effective in pain syndromes with an intermittent lancinating quality

  (2) Mechanism of action

    [a] The mechanism of action is unclear, however, the anticonvulsants appear to affect the peripheral nerves in much the same way that they affect the brain. Whereas the anticonvulsants suppress ectopic foci in the brain, thus preventing seizures, they also reduce the discharges from sites of ectopic foci in damaged peripheral nerves, which are thought to be responsible for intermittent lancinating pain. They most likely suppress this abnormal activity by blocking the sodium channel

  (3) Anticonvulsants used in chronic pain management

    [a] Gabapentin—agent of choice

    [b] Carbamazepine—agent of choice

    [c] Phenytoin

    [d] Valproic acid—least used

  (4) Side effects

    [a] Unlike the tricyclic antidepressants, the anticonvulsants are chemically unrelated and, therefore, have different side effects

    [b] Liver toxicity

      i) Although all of the anticonvulsants possess the potential for liver toxicity, valproic acid and tegretol have the highest incidence. In fact, because of the high risk of liver toxicity seen with valproic acid, this drug is rarely used in chronic pain management. Carbamazepine has a slightly increased risk of liver toxicity, therefore, LFTs should be monitored. Gabapentin—no risk liver damage.

    [c] Aplastic anemia

      i) Carbamazepine is the only anticonvulsant with the potential to cause aplastic anemia. The CBC must be monitored when prescribing this drug

    [d] Gingival hyperplasia

      i) Phenytoin may cause gingival hyperplasia, and if this occurs, the drug must be discontinued

  (5) Conditions responsive to the anticonvulsants

    [a] Trigeminal neuralgia

    [b] Glossopharyngeal neuralgia

    [c] Paroxysmal pains of multiple sclerosis

    [d] Miscellaneous lancinating pains

      i) Postlaminectomy

      ii) Postamputation

      iii) Postherpetic neuralgia

    [e] Diabetic neuropathy

  (6) General considerations

    [a] In patients with a seizure disorder acute withdrawal is manifested as seizures. Therefore, the anticonvulsants must be weaned slowly. In patients without a history of seizures, withdrawal rarely occurs. However, if these patients are receiving high doses, it is wise to taper the drug

(d) Antiarrhythmics

  (1) Some of the antiarrhythmics have been shown to affect certain chronic pain syndromes. These drugs work much the same way as the anticonvulsants in that they are effective in treating pain that is intermittent and lancinating. They also are effective in pain that has an allodynic and dysesthetic

II. Effects of anesthetics on ; b. Pharmacologic (continued)

component. Bretylium and guanethidine are used in the treatment of sympathetically maintained pain

(2) Antiarrhythmics used in chronic pain management
   [a] Bretylium—used in IV regional blocks only
   [b] Guanethidine—used in IV regional blocks only, not approved for use in the United States
   [c] Lidocaine—used for diagnostic purposes only, although may act therapeutically
   [d] Mexiletine—most commonly used; lidocaine derivative
   [e] Tocainide—uncommonly used; lidocaine derivative

(3) Mechanism of action
   [a] Bretylium and guanethidine
      i) Both of these drugs act by inhibiting the release of norepinephrine from the postganglionic adrenergic neurons. Because of this action, they produce a chemical sympathectomy. Bretylium lasts 12–24 hours whereas guanethidine lasts 24–72 hours. The chemical sympathectomy produced by these drugs decreases the pain associated with sympathetically maintained pain. They are also diagnostic for this syndrome
   [b] Lidocaine and derivatives
      i) Appear to act on ectopic foci in damaged nerves much the same way as the anticonvulsants. They suppress the abnormal activity in peripheral nerves through sodium channel blockade

(4) Side effects
   [a] Nausea and vomiting
      i) Nausea and vomiting may occur with all of the antiarrhythmics. They are commonly seen in IV regional blockade with bretylium after the tourniquet is deflated. They are also common with mexiletine if the dose of this drug is increased too rapidly. A slow increase over a few days to weeks will prevent this side effect
   [b] Tremors/irritability
      i) Mexiletine may cause tremors and irritability, especially in older patients. This side effect usually disappears if the dose is decreased
   [c] Seizures
      i) Lidocaine and the derivatives may cause seizures if given in high-enough doses. However, this is extremely rare in the dosage range used for chronic pain management

(5) Conditions responsive to the antiarrhythmics
   [a] Bretylium and guanethidine—sympathetically maintained pain
   [b] Lidocaine and derivatives—see Anticonvulsants

(6) General considerations
   [a] A lidocaine infusion is commonly performed as a diagnostic test to determine if mexiletine will be effective in the treatment of the pain syndrome. Usually, 5 mg/kg of lidocaine is administered IV over 30 minutes. One tries to push the blood level of the lidocaine up until lightheadedness and sedation are present. These symptoms correspond to a plasma level of approximately 2–3 μg/ml and should be adequate to provide pain relief. If no pain relief is present at this blood level, then the decision is made that mexiletine will be ineffective. If pain relief occurs, then it is worthwhile to give a trial of the mexiletine

(e) Alpha$_1$ blockers and alpha$_2$ agonists
   (1) The sympathetic nervous system (SNS) is involved in many chronic pain syndromes. If it is determined that the SNS is involved in the pain problem,

then medications can be administered to alter the SNS. The alpha blockers and alpha$_2$ agonists are used for this purpose

(2) Mechanism of action

[a] Peripheral nerve terminals possess alpha receptors that may become active in neuropathic pain conditions. The SNS releases norepinephrine, which stimulates these receptors and leads to pain. The alpha blockers block the action of NE on these receptors and the alpha$_2$ agonists inhibit the release of NE from the postganglionic sympathetic nerve terminals. In this way, these drugs produce a chemical sympathectomy

(3) Alpha$_1$ blockers used in chronic pain management

[a] Phentolamine—IV administration only

[b] Prazosin

[c] Phenoxybenzamine

(4) Alpha$_2$ agonists used in chronic pain management

[a] Clonidine

(5) Side effects

[a] Orthostatic hypotension

i) This is the most common side effect. The alpha receptors are also located on blood vessels where they increase vascular tone, therefore, if this response is inhibited, orthostasis results

ii) As the body fluids shift to compensate for the change in vascular tone, this side effect usually disappears with time

[b] Sedation

i) Clonidine may cause sedation due to its central effect

(6) General considerations

[a] A phentolamine infusion is commonly performed prior to starting oral prazosin, phenoxybenzamine, or clonidine therapy. Routinely, 0.5–1 mg/kg of phentolamine is infused IV over 30 minutes until pain relief occurs or unacceptable tachycardia or hypotension occurs. The hypotension can be prevented with prehydration and the tachycardia can be treated with β-blockers. If this infusion is successful, a trial of prazosin, phenoxybenzamine, or clonidine is warranted

(f) Miscellaneous drugs

(1) Antihistamines

[a] Hydroxyzine is the only antihistamine that has been proven to have intrinsic analgesic activity of its own

[b] Hydroxyzine potentiates the effects of narcotics, and because of this, it is commonly used in conjunction with them

[c] Histamine activates C-fiber afferents leading to pain. This may explain the analgesic activity of hydroxyzine

(2) Skeletal muscle relaxants

[a] The use of muscle relaxants is usually a part of a therapeutic regimen and they are rarely given alone. In conjunction with opioids, NSAIDs, and physical therapy, they can be quite effective in pain management

[b] Antispasmodic agents—Valium, baclofen, dantrolene

[c] Centrally acting skeletal muscle relaxants—carisoprodol, chlorphenesin carbamate, chlorzoxazone, cyclobenzaprine hydrochloride, methocarbamol, orphenadrine citrate

(3) Sedatives, hypnotics, and tranquilizers

[a] These medications have little place in the management of chronic pain syndromes. Benzodiazepines often cause significant disturbances of REM sleep, tolerance and habituation can be a problem, and these drugs can be extremely difficult to withdraw

II. Effects of anesthetics on (continued)

---

c. Interventional techniques

1. Diagnostic blocks

    (a) Zygapophyseal (facet) joint
    (b) Sacroiliac joint
    (c) Selective nerve root block
    (d) Dorsal primary ramus nerve block
    (e) Costovertebral
    (f) Peripheral nerve block
    (g) Differential spinal

2. Diagnostic infusion

    (a) Lidocaine
    (b) Phentolamine
    (c) Fentanyl
    (d) Pentothal

3. Diagnostic and therapeutic procedures

    (a) Stellate ganglion block
    (b) Lumbar sympathetic block
    (c) Thoracic sympathetic block
    (d) Celiac plexus block
    (e) Superior hypogastric block
    (f) Ganglion impar block
    (g) Sacroiliac joint block
    (h) Epidural blood patch
    (i) Epidural steroids
    (j) Transforaminal steroids
    (k) Interlaminar steroids
    (l) Neurolytic procedures
        (1) Chemolysis
        (2) Cryotherapy
        (3) Radiofrequency ablation
    (m) Motor point block
        (1) Phenol
        (2) Alcohol
        (3) *Botulinus* toxin
    (n) Indwelling epidural catheter
    (o) Intrathecal catheter
    (p) Indwelling interpleural catheter
    (q) Spinal cord stimulator

III. GENERALIZED PAIN DISORDERS

a. Neuropathic pain

1. Characteristics of pain

    (a) Continuous burning (causalgia)
    (b) Episodic, spontaneous shocklike paroxysms
    (c) Allodynia (light touch causes pain)
    (d) Hyperalgesia (mild noxious stimulus causes severe pain)
    (e) Foci of hypersensitivity may trigger pain

  2. Associated with

  (a) Nerve damage: trauma, surgery, diabetes mellitus, herpes zoster, phantom limb pain
  (b) No obvious nerve damage
  (c) Central nervous system damage: central dysesthetic pains
  (d) Nerve damage
    (1) Microneuromas: regenerating nerves are sensitive to ion fluxes, cold, mechanical stimulation, norepinephrine
  (e) No obvious nerve damage
    (1) Up-regulation of alpha$_1$ receptors on C fibers causes sensitivity to norepinephrine
    (2) Stimulation of central wide dynamic range neurons cause radiation to neighboring WDRs creating somatoform pain distribution, secondary hyperalgesia, early immediate gene induction, pain memory, and possibly damage to inhibitory interneurons

  3. Treatment of neuropathic pain

  (a) Peripheral nerve or neuroma blocks—local anesthetic or neurolytic
  (b) TENS
  (c) Oral
    (1) Gabapentin (Neurontin)
    (2) Mexilitine
    (3) Carbamazepine (Tegretol)
    (4) Sodium valproate (valproic acid)
    (5) Phenytoin (Dilantin)
    (6) Clonazepam (Klonopin)
    (7) Opioids
  (d) Dermal—capsaicin (Zostrix), aspirin, in ether suspension, EMLA cream
  (e) Epidural/intrathecal—opioids ± local anesthetic
  (f) Spinal cord stimulation
  (g) Psychotherapy—coping strategies, biofeedback

  4. Possible future treatment of neuropathic pain

  (a) NMDA (*N*-methyl-*D*-aspartate) and non-NMDA antagonists
  (b) Gangliosides
  (c) Long-acting local anesthetics
  (d) Nitric oxide synthase inhibitors
  (e) Systemic substance P depletors or antagonists
  (f) Metabotropic or glutamate receptor antagonists

---

b. Sympathetic mediated pain (SMP). (New terminology: Complex regional pain syndrome Type I.) Unknown prevalence, probably higher than commonly believed, higher incidence in females, often mid-30. Older terminology includes reflex sympathetic dystrophy, Sudeck's atrophy, minor or major causalgia, posttraumatic dystrophy, shoulder–hand syndrome

  1. Proposed mechanisms of cause

  (a) Up-regulation of alpha$_1$ receptors on pain nerve terminals
  (b) Excitation of wide-dynamic-range neurons in the central nervous system
  (c) Central misinterpretation of A beta fiber input as pain

  2. Clinical features

  (a) Pain—severe constant burning, often in glove or stocking distribution
  (b) Swelling—often present, pitting or nonpitting edema
  (c) Motor function—diminished, progresses to atrophy

      (d) Tremor—difficulty initiating movement, muscle spasms

      (e) Skin changes—skin and tissue atrophy, dryness, scaling, hair loss, nail changes

      (f) Vasomotor instability—Raynaud's phenomenon, cool, cyanosed or red or hot, hyperhidrosis (increased sweating)

      (g) Joint changes—swelling and tenderness, synovial abnormalities

      (h) Bone changes—patchy osteoporosis, increased vascularity, increased osteoclastic activity

      (i) Bilateral involvement—18–50% of cases

      (j) If foot affected—plantar fasciitis prominent

3. Stages of SMP

    (a) Stage I

      (1) Onset pain near site of injury

      (2) Hyperesthesia

      (3) Localized edema

      (4) Muscle spasm

      (5) Stiffness and limited mobility

      (6) Temperature changes—initially warm, red, and dry; later cyanotic, cold, and sweaty

      (7) Average duration—1–3 months, may resolve spontaneously or respond rapidly to treatment

      (8) Hyperhidrosis (increased sweating)

    (b) Stage II

      (1) Pain more severe and diffuse

      (2) Edema spreads, becomes brawny in nature

      (3) Hair scant, nails brittle, cracked, heavily grooved

      (4) Spotty osteoporosis—becoming more diffuse

      (5) Thickening of joints

      (6) Muscle wasting

      (7) Average duration—3–6 months

    (c) Stage III

      (1) Marked, irreversible trophic changes

      (2) Intractable pain involving entire limb

      (3) Joints may become ankylosed

      (4) Contractions of flexor tendons, occasionally subluxations

      (5) Bone deossification, marked and diffuse

4. Etiology

    (a) Trauma (usually minor)—most frequent

    (b) Surgery

    (c) Ischemic heart disease with myocardial infarction

    (d) Cervical spine or spinal cord disorders

    (e) Cerebral lesions

    (f) Infections

    (g) Repetitive motion disorder

    (h) Unknown

5. Diagnosis

    (a) Clinical presentation

    (b) Cold stressor test—severe pain with cold

    (c) Radiology

      (1) Fine-detail x-ray

      (2) Bone absorptimetry

      (3) Three-phase radionuclide bone scan

    (d) Galvanic skin test (cutaneous pain threshold)
    (e) Histologic changes of synovium and synovial fluid
    (f) Thermographic studies
    (g) Sympathetic blockade significantly decreases pain
        (1) Sympathetic ganglia
        (2) Regional—Bier's block
        (3) Systemic—phentolamine

6. Treatment of sympathetic mediated pain

    (a) Decreasing peripheral input
        (1) Lysis of nerve adhesions (surgical removal of noxious input)
        (2) Local anesthetic blockade
        (3) TENS
    (b) Physical therapy—scrub-and-carry technique
    (c) Psychotherapy—coping techniques, biofeedback, family therapy
    (d) Blocks—nerve blocks
        (1) Sympathetic blockade
        (2) IV regional blocks
    (e) Sympathectomy
        (1) Surgical
        (2) Chemical
        (3) Radiofrequency
    (f) Drugs
        (1) Alpha-adrenergic blockers
        (2) NSAIDs
        (3) Analgesics, including opioids
        (4) Tricyclics and related compounds
        (5) Gabapentin
    (g) Dermal—clonidine patch, useful over small localized area SMP
    (h) Implantable devices
        (1) Spinal cord stimulator
        (2) Peripheral nerve stimulator
        (3) Morphine pump

7. Response to treatment

    (a) Correlated to early diagnosis and treatment
    (b) 50% continue to have significant pain and disability

---

c. Multidisciplinary approach to management of chronic pain

1. Staffing

    (a) Core
        (1) Physician trained in pain management
        (2) Pain psychiatrist/psychologist
            [a] Physical therapist
            [b] Occupational therapist
            [c] Nurses trained in pain management
    (b) Consulting
        (1) Neurologist
        (2) Psychiatrist
        (3) Neurosurgeon
        (4) Neuropsychologist
        (5) Family practitioners
        (6) Vocational counselor
        (7) Job placement counselor

III. Generalized pain disorders; c. Multidisciplinary approach to management of chronic pain (continued)

2. Treatment plan
   (a) Psychometric testing
   (b) Patient examined by physician and psychologist
   (c) Patient's significant other present when possible
   (d) Physician and psychologist discuss the patient
   (e) The treatment plan is discussed with the patient and significant other, if present
3. Multidisciplinary chronic pain management program
   (a) Goals should include
       (1) Education: lecture and handouts
       (2) Psychotherapy: group and individual
       (3) Relaxation training: biofeedback, hypnosis, group relaxation
       (4) Exercise: generalized (aerobic) and specific (stretching)
       (5) Occupational therapy: activities of daily living, task analysis
       (6) Report back: individual review with patient
       (7) Medication rationalization: planned withdrawal or trialing of medication
       (8) Vocational guidance

E. MISCELLANEOUS CLINICAL ENTITIES

I. LASER SURGERY

a. **Approach to airway—breathing spontaneously, ET tube, jet ventilation**

b. **Evaluation of airway—neck mobility, mouth opening, chest size, Mallampatti airway classification**

c. **Choice of jet ventilation versus ET intubation**

d. **ET tube choice—metal-impregnated tube, plastic tube wrapped with metal tape**

e. **Risk factors: fire or combustion, perforation of cuff on ET tube, inability to ventilate, laryngospasm**

f. **Anesthetic agents of choice—IV agents, short-acting muscle relaxants versus spontaneous ventilation, reduced oxygen concentration if possible**

g. **Laser excision produces less edema than blunt dissection or electrocautery, postoperative laryngeal edema is lessened**

II. OUTSIDE THE OPERATING ROOM:
location of facility—proximity to support service, such as PACU, anesthesia equipment; should meet same standards as operating room; anesthesia requirements—airway, pain control, nonmovement

a. Lithotripsy

1. Advertised as "painless" procedure
2. A need for some sedation and adequate pain control
3. Stone disruption dependent on number of impulses and amplitude
4. Impulses are synchronized with heart rate
5. Adequate airway access—patient in supine position

b. MRI

1. Usually diagnostic with no pain
2. Limited airway accessibility

3. Nonmovement determines success of final "film" or image
4. Electrical and metal conductive limitations, need MRI compatibility of all machines and monitors
5. Patient is far from anesthetist
6. Induction and emergence in location other than MRI unit

c. CT

1. Diagnostic, no pain
2. Limited airway accessibility
3. Nonmovement
4. Less limiting facility, does not require special machinery or monitors

d. GI

1. Diagnostic but very stimulating
2. Competition for the airway in upper GI endoscopy
3. Patient positional changes that may alter approaches to airway
4. Bleeding is possible

III. ELECTROCONVULSIVE THERAPY (ECT)

a. Introduction

1. Central nervous system (CNS) seizure activity is responsible for the beneficial effect of ECT, although the exact mechanism of therapeutic effects is not understood
2. In the United States, ECT is performed on approximately 100,000 psychiatric patients per year
3. Aim of anesthesiologist: to provide safe and effective anesthesia without interfering with the beneficial effects of ECT

b. ECT administration

1. Electroconvulsive shock is applied to one or both cerebral hemispheres to induce a seizure
2. Goal: to produce a therapeutic generalized seizure 30–60 seconds in duration. A good therapeutic effect is generally not achieved until a total of 400–700 seizure-seconds have been induced
3. Only one treatment is given per day. Therefore, patients are usually scheduled for a series of treatments, usually two or three per week
4. EEG monitoring is a necessity and provides a guideline for achieving optimal therapeutic effects. The goal is to apply the minimum electric current necessary to produce adequate seizure activity in the brain, as documented by EEG changes

c. Physiologic effects of ECT-induced seizures

1. Seizure activity is characteristically associated with an initial parasympathetic discharge followed by a more sustained sympathetic discharge

2. The initial phase is characterized by bradycardia and increased secretions. Marked bradycardia (less than 30 beats per minute) and even transient asystole (up to 6 seconds) may occur. Anticholinergic agents can be useful in both the prevention and treatment of these vagal effects, although their routine use is controversial

3. Hypertension, tachycardia and cardiac dysrhythmias often accompany the seizure and may last for several minutes. To minimize these side effects, pretreatment with a short-acting antihypertensive drug may be indicated, such as alpha-adrenergic or beta-adrenergic blockers or nitroglycerin

4. There is also a transient increase in CBF, ICP, IOP, and intragastric pressure

d. Clinical indications

1. Primary

    (a) Major depressive disorders
    (b) Recurrent depressive states
    (c) Acute schizophrenia
    (d) Acute manic states

2. Secondary

    (a) Chronic schizophrenia
    (b) Psychosomatic disorders
    (c) Failure of pharmacologic therapy
    (d) Chronic pain syndromes

e. Contraindications to ECT

1. Absolute

    (a) Recent MI (less than 3 months)
    (b) Recent stroke (less than 1 month)
    (c) Intracranial mass or increased ICP
    (d) Unstable aneurysm of a major vessel
    (e) MAOI therapy

2. Relative

    (a) Angina pectoris
    (b) Congestive heart failure
    (c) Significant pulmonary disease
    (d) Recent bone fractures
    (e) Severe osteoporosis
    (f) Pregnancy
    (g) Glaucoma
    (h) Retinal detachment
    (i) Thyroid disease
    (j) Thrombophlebitis

f. Preanesthetic assessment

1. Patients scheduled for ECT should undergo the same thorough preoperative evaluation as would any other patient who is to receive GA

III. Electroconvulsive therapy; f. Preanesthetic assessment (continued)

2. PE should pay particular attention to cardiopulmonary and neurologic functions. The condition of the patient's teeth should be noted

3. Minimum labs include CBC, UA, lytes, glucose, BUN, Cr, and liver enzymes. An ECG is also indicated, and in an older patient, cervical and thoracic spine x-rays should be reviewed

4. Although patients undergoing ECT are often anxious, pretreatment sedation is usually not required and may unnecessarily prolong the recovery period

g. Anesthetic protocol for ECT

1. Apply routine monitors, including ECG, BPC, and pulse oximeter

2. Establish IV access

3. Place an oral airway

4. Administer an IV anesthetic (barbiturates, etomidate, or propofol). Since these induction agents have anticonvulsant properties, small doses must be used. Seizure threshold is increased and seizure duration is decreased by all of these agents. Alfentanil can be a useful adjunct in patients with a high seizure threshold, in an effort to minimize the induction dose

5. Ventilate lungs with oxygen by mask. In fact, hyperventilation (approximately 90 seconds) can increase seizure duration and is routinely employed in most centers

6. Inflate a tourniquet on the arm opposite the IV catheter (permits seizure visualization as the arm is isolated from the muscle relaxant)

7. Administer a short-acting muscle relaxant (usually succinylcholine)

8. Induce seizure

9. Monitor blood pressure every minute to assess the degree of hypertensive response and guide antihypertensive therapy, if necessary

10. Allow the patient to recover. Controlled or assisted mask ventilation using a self-inflating bag device or an anesthesia circle system is required until spontaneous respirations resume

h. Post-ECT recovery room care

1. Monitor vitals for 30–60 minutes

2. Patient may exhibit confusion and memory loss, which rarely last more than 24 hours

3. Once awake and stable, the patient may be discharged to the psychiatric floor or home (in the care of a friend or relative)

i. Complications

1. Prior to modified ECT and the use of muscle relaxants, fracture of thoracic vertebrae or long bones was the most common complication

2. Currently, patients most often complain of HA, muscle aches, pretreatment anxiety, and memory disturbance

3. Skin burns, lacerations of the tongue and oral mucosa, as well as damage to the eyes and teeth, are rare complications

IV. GAMMA KNIFE

a. Functional mechanism

1. Used for certain tumors and arteriovenous malformations
2. Gamma knife focuses multiple radiation beams at central target; CNS lesion
3. Thick metal helmet with radial columnar openings focuses radiation emitted from cobalt dome
4. Patient's head, in helmet, moves into cobalt radiation source
5. Beams intersect at target, create radiolesion at site of CNS pathology

b. Procedure

1. Stereotactic frame is attached to patient's head
2. Radiographic studies performed for stereotactic analysis
   - (a) MRI—special equipment and consideration due to magnet
   - (b) CT
   - (c) Angiography
3. Treatment plan constructed using stereotactic studies
   - (a) Multiple spherical radiolesions to be produced
   - (b) Combined make up shape of CNS lesion
   - (c) Pan construction facilitated by computer, but takes time
4. Patient positioned on gamma knife, outside closed radiation source
5. Columnator helmet applied to stereotactic frame
   - (a) One or several helmets may be utilized according to treatment plan
   - (b) Head precisely positioned within helmet according to x, y, z axis
6. All personnel exit gamma-knife room
   - (a) Patient monitored by video camera
   - (b) Communication by intercom if awake
7. Radiation source opens and patient moved on motorized cart until head is within radiation source
   - (a) Mechanized movement by operator remote control
   - (b) Opportunity for disconnections or tension on lines/tubes
   - (c) Time in knife according to treatment time
8. Multiple exposures to create total radiolesion
   - (a) Patient moved from radiation source, which then closes
   - (b) Personnel reenter gamma-knife room
   - (c) Patient's head repositioned within columnator helmet
   - (d) Personnel exit and next exposure initiated

c. Anesthesia needs

1. Adult patients usually treated with IV sedation; remain awake
2. Pediatric patients often require general anesthesia
   - (a) Induction at time stereotactic frame applied
   - (b) Anesthetic continues through radiographic studies
   - (c) Transported under anesthesia to different locations for studies and treatment
3. Anesthetic planned according to underlying CNS pathology and level of stimulation
   - (a) Consider ICP and BP factors

IV. Gamma knife; c. Anesthesia needs (continued)

      (b) Little stimulation once stereotactic frame in place

      (c) CNS pathology is factor in anesthetic selection; none incompatible with gamma knife itself

    4. Special areas for management planning

      (a) Transport under general anesthesia; monitoring, emergency equipment

      (b) Remote monitoring; ascertain visual contact with patient and monitors on video screen

      (c) Patient movement by remote control is potential disconnect time; position tubes and lines over patient with sufficient slack, and observe on video during move

      (d) Standard considerations for pediatric patient under long general anesthetic, away from operating room; temperature, fluid administration, urine output, etc.

      (e) Extubation; at end of procedure in gamma-knife suite versus transport to PACU prior to extubation

V. BURNS

a. Pathophysiology

1. Skin is the largest organ of the body, protecting against infection, fluid loss, and loss of body temperature

2. Accurate assessment of burn injury based on burn size or body surface area (BSA)

3. Rule of "9's" is used for adult burn assessment: head, each upper extremity—9%; anterior trunk, posterior trunk, each lower limb—18%; perineum—1%; all totaling 100%

4. Depth of burn—1 degree, 2 degree, 3 degree, major burns 2 degree and 3 degree

5. Morbidity/mortality increases and correlates with greater BSA area and age, e.g., 80-year-old patient with 35% BSA burn equals 115% probable mortality

6. Cardiovascular response—early burn period, CO down to 50% of normal

    (a) Decreased preload, decreased afterward, and myocardial depression

7. Alteration of cell permeability to Na^+ ion $\rightarrow$ increase in Na^+ and water influx into the cell

8. Release of vasoactive substances and toxins may cause further microvascular injury

9. Edema occurs not only in burned tissue, but in nonburned tissue, especially soft tissue or mucosa

10. Hypovolemic shock, hypoproteinemia, occur early in burn injury

11. Hyperkalemia may occur from as early as 6 hours to 6 months following burn injury

12. Stress of burn injury causes increase in catecholamine release, ADH, renin, and angiotensin, all of which can cause renal vasoconstriction, which can lead to decrease in renal blood flow

13. Inhalation burns can cause damage to trachea or pulmonary tree

    (a) Steam causes greater heat injury to lower respiratory tract

    (b) Inhalation of gases divided into pulmonary irritants (phosgene, HCL, ammonia) and nonpulmonary irritants (CO_2 and CO)

    (c) Increased CO levels lead to formation of carboxy hemoglobin, which reduces oxygen delivery to tissues

14. Sepsis—skin breakdown leading to massive infection, CV instability, and pressor support

b. Preoperative preparation

1. Fluid resuscitation—according to formula, e.g., Parkland, 4 cc/% burn/kg body weight, one half of 24-hour requirement in the first eight hours. Second 24 hours, same total with special attention to urine and serum Na^+, K^+, and osmolarity

2. Attention to CV stability, temperature, and Hg

3. Airway assessment—in high-degree burn, prophylactic securing of the airway is indicated since edema formation is extensive in head and neck region

4. Chronic burn eschar, contractures to face, mouth, and neck may prohibit routine airway management. There is a need for alternate airway access, e.g., fiberoptic intubation or use of LMA

5. Need for T&C RBCs since blood loss is extensive in the excision of burn tissue

6. Tracheostomy through burn tissue increases morbidity greatly; patient is susceptible to *Pseudomonas* infection to cartilaginous tracheal rings

7. Stability of concomitant medical problems, e.g., heart failure, pulm edema, renal failure, sepsis, pulmonary insufficiency

8. Adequacy of oxygenation checked

c. Intraoperative management

1. Airway: can airway be safely accessed while the patient is asleep or must airway be approached with the patient awake

2. Muscle relaxants

   (a) Succinyl choline–induced hyperkalemia is greatly increased; may begin as early as 6 hours and peak at about 7 days postinjury; maximal increase in serum K^+ following succinyl choline may take place at 3 weeks following initial injury

   (b) Avoid succinyl choline where possible, even in early burn injury, deferring to nondepolarizing muscle relaxants

   (c) Nondepolarizing muscle relaxants—patient may develop increased need for repeated doses due to rapid metabolization; may still have minor accumulative effects

3. Narcotics

   (a) Dose requirements may be significantly increased due to increase in metabolic rate and drug metabolism; care for histamine release and blood pressure alteration in the hypovolemic patient

   (b) Drug and dose examples: fentanyl, 10–20 μg/kg; sufentanil, 1 1/2–3 μg/kg; morphine, 0.2-0.5 mg/kg

4. Monitors

   (a) ECG leads may be difficult to place; may select staples or short metal needles to skin to access ECG lead

   (b) Blood pressure monitor—accurate blood pressure assessment through noninvasive routes on various extremities; if stability or accurate measurement is a problem, intra-arterial monitoring may be necessary

   (c) Temperature—core temperature probe necessary; use of warming devices to prevent heat loss; patient may lose an average of 1–3°F even in warm room; most acceptable temperature is 100°F to prevent breakdown of proteins and glucose

   (d) Invasive monitors—use where necessary to obtain accurate measurement of vitals; however, there is an increased incidence of septicemia with indwelling lines that pass through contaminated or burned tissue. Remove soon as stability improves

        (e) Foley catheter—as assessment of U/o and early renal function; try to maintain more than 1 cc/kg/hr

    5. Fluids

        (a) Check previous albumin/protein levels—replace albumin instead of crystalloid if low or BP/CVP are low

        (b) Check preop H/H—if low, begin transfusion of RBCs early to prevent CV instability during major excision of burn eschar

        (c) Transfuse warmed RBCs 0.5–1 cc RBC/% area excised

        (d) Transfuse FFP with suspected/documented coagulopathy, following PT/PTT or TEG

        (e) Platelets not usually a problem

        (f) Crystalloid volume replaced at reasonable amount according to blood pressure, U/o, CVP

    6. Inhalation anesthetic agents

        (a) Care for high percent and blood pressure instability, especially where there is hypovolemia

        (b) Ease of use by concentration/titration to adjunct narcotics

        (c) May be useful to control bronchospasm, especially in pulmonary burns

        (d) Fairly quick awakening leading to extubation and recovery

        (e) May want to avoid halothane due to sequential or many repeated anesthetics in this injury

        (f) Anesthetic requirement may be high due to increased metabolic rate

    7. Ketamine

        (a) May be useful for burn scrub alone or as induction agent, due to its analgesia and maintenance of blood pressure and heart rate

d. Recovery period

    1. Extubation or ventilation: since large fluid resuscitation is often required and pulmonary compromise may occur with inhalation burns, ventilation and ET tube may be the choice for the end of the procedure. Extubate only when adequate assessment has been made to extent of tracheal mucosal edema, respiratory status, recovery from muscle relaxant, and adequate respiratory recovery following high-dose narcotics

    2. Analgesia

        (a) Pain control necessary following excision and grafting; titrate narcotics to pain control and respiratory response

    3. Bleeding

        (a) Postoperative bleeding may occur due to larger surface areas excised; care for volume and blood replacement that is not readily visible due to extensive dressing; monitor H/H, CVP, and replace where necessary

VI. REGIONAL ANESTHESIA FOR OPHTHALMIC SURGERY

a. Innervation of the eye

    1. Sensory

        (a) Ophthalmic nerve—branch of trigeminal (CN V); sensory to cornea, ciliary body, iris, lacrimal gland, conjunctiva, eyelid, and eyebrow

  (b) Ciliary ganglion—branch of oculomotor (CN III); autonomic and sensory innervation of cornea, iris, and choroid

 2. Motor

  (a) Oculomotor (CN III): all extraocular muscles except superior oblique and lateral rectus

  (b) Trochlear (CN IV): supplies superior oblique

  (c) Abducens (CN VI): supplies lateral rectus

  (d) Facial (CN VII): orbicularis muscle of upper and lower lid. Optic nerve (CN II) not necessary to block for anesthesia of eye

b. Candidates for regional anesthesia

 1. Most eye procedures (including cataract, PKP, trabeculectomy, retinal and vitreous surgery, lid surgery)

 2. Patient capable of communicating/understanding

 3. Patient capable of lying flat for 2 or more hours

c. Monitoring

 1. Blood pressure (usually NIBP)

 2. ECG

 3. Pulse oximeter

 4. Respirations (usually plethysmography; CO_2 monitoring difficult)

d. Setup for block

 1. IV access mandatory

 2. Airway equipment, oxygen source, ambu bag (or anesthesia circuit) for emergency airway management

 3. Suction

 4. Resuscitative drugs

e. Techniques

 1. Retrobulbar

  (a) Local anesthetic injected into muscle cone; sharp or blunt needle, 25 gauge or smaller; eye in neutral position; 4 cc local anesthetic injected through lower lid along inferior orbital rim between lateral one third and medial two thirds; needle is directed straight down to depth of about 25 mm, then angled up medially toward apex of orbit to a depth of 35 mm

  (b) Facial nerve supplementation: frequently required for akinesia; after retrobulbar injection, needle is withdrawn to just beneath skin and redirected laterally toward the corner of the eye; 3 cc local anesthetic is injected for subcutaneous wheal in temporal region

  (c) Advantages: single injection, smaller volume of local anesthetic, rapid onset

  (d) Disadvantages: potential for damage to globe, optic nerve, vascular structures

 2. Peribulbar

  (a) Local anesthetic injected outside muscle cone; sharp 27–30-gauge needle; eye in neutral position; two injections necessary: (1) 4 cc injected through lower lid along lower orbital rim between lateral one third and medial two thirds at a needle depth of 25 mm; (2) 3 cc superiomedial injection through the upper lid midway between medial canthus and supraorbital notch; needle—20 mm. Facial nerve supplementation often necessary

    (b) Advantages: decreased incidence of trauma to globe, optic nerve, or vessels; good anesthesia of lid

    (c) Disadvantages: two injections—more painful to patient, larger volume of local anesthetic, slower onset

---

f. Local anesthetics: usually an equal mixture of 2% lidocaine and 0.75% bupivacaine. 7.5–15 µ/ml hyaluronidase added to soften globe and improve spread of local anesthetic

---

g. Sedation: given prior to block for pain relief and amnesia. Very little additional sedation usually needed during procedure. Avoid oversedation; surgeon needs alert, cooperative patient

---

h. Complications: overall incidence of complications (including minor)—one in 500

    1. Minor hemodynamic changes—hypotension, bradycardia, diaphoresis, nausea, probably vagally mediated, secondary to pain of injection

    2. Oculocardiac reflex—afferent limb via trigeminal nerve, efferent limb via vagus; induced by eye manipulation during block; usually resolves spontaneously

    3. Retrobulbar hemorrhage—incidence one in 700; signs—proptosis, eye becomes hard, visible blood; apply pressure immediately for 20 minutes; surgical intervention (lateral canthotomy) may be necessary

    4. Eye trauma—perforation of globe, optic nerve damage

    5. Brain-stem anesthesia—manifested as apnea or cardiac disturbances; secondary to communication of optic nerve sheath and subarachnoid space; not reported with peribulbar technique

    6. Seizures—secondary to intravascular injection, probably arterial since very small volume of local anesthesia can cause seizure

F. LEGAL MEDICINE

I. LEGAL LIABILITY

a. Criminal liability

1. Violation of state penal code or federal statute
2. Applies to controlled substances and fraud
3. Penalties are fines and incarceration

b. Civil liability

1. Violation of civil statutes and/or common law
2. Tort law: medical negligence, informed consent/battery
3. Penalty is award of monetary damages

c. Vicarious liability

1. One party held liable for the acts/omissions of another party
2. Master–servant relationship
   (a) One party has right to control acts of the other party
   (b) Doctor–CRNA relationship
   (c) Doctor held liable for negligence of CRNA
3. Independent contractor (IC)
   (a) Employer does not have right to control acts of IC
   (b) May exist when one physician hires other physicians
   (c) Employer physician *may* not be held liable for negligence of physicians employed
4. Ostensible agency; apparent agency; agency by estoppel
   (a) Entity may be held liable for negligence of nonemployees
   (b) May apply when services of physicians are provided by hospital operation
   (c) Patient does not select physician, i.e., anesthesiologist

I. INFORMED CONSENT

a. Consent required for touching of another person's body

1. Right to privacy includes self-determination
   (a) Right to determine what will be done to one's body
   (b) Right to be left alone
   (c) Right to be touched only by choice
2. Battery exists when nonconsensual touching occurs
   (a) Intentional tort, not negligence; touching was intended
   (b) Compensatory and punitive damages are possible

b. Consent and disclosure of risks

1. Implied consent is possible

      (a) Patient who gets on stretcher knowing he or she is going to the operating room implicitly consents to surgery

      (b) Knowledge of risks of surgery will influence decision to consent

      (c) Consent is presumed when life-saving procedure required on incompetent patient

  2. Expressed consent involves exchange of information

      (a) May be given by patient or surrogate

      (b) May be verbal or written

      (c) Written provides evidence of level of discussion, understanding, and agreement by consenting patient

  3. Informed consent involves disclosure of risks

      (a) Disclose material risks; those that would influence a reasonable person in making a decision

      (b) Incidence and severity of known risks, e.g., sore throat (high incidence/low severity), death (low incidence/high severity)

      (c) Extent of required disclosure varies among states according to statute and lay versus professional standards as to reasonable person making decision

c. Limited consent

1. Patients may consent to therapy with specific restrictions or limitations

2. Administration of blood or blood components may be refused

3. May restrict resuscitative efforts: do not resuscitate (DNR)

4. Patients must be aware of risks due to limitations imposed on treatment

d. Litigation involving consent

1. Lack of consent as a solitary charge is a difficult case to make

2. Plaintiff must prove case by preponderance of evidence

      (a) Specific risks were not disclosed

      (b) The nondisclosed risk(s) occurred

      (c) Had risk(s) been disclosed, no consent would have been given

3. Lack-of-consent issues often accompany cases that are based on negligence

III. MEDICAL NEGLIGENCE

a. Four elements must exist: duty, breach of duty, causation, damages

1. Each must be proved by plaintiff

2. Burden of proof is preponderance of evidence

      (a) More likely than not

      (b) In all medical probability (not mere possibility)

      (c) With reasonable certainty

      (d) 51% of the time

3. Defense prevails if any one element can be defeated

b. Duty

1. Based on doctor–patient relationship
2. Requires performance in compliance with standards of care
   (a) What would be done by a reasonably prudent person in the same or similar circumstances
   (b) Physicians of similar training and experience
   (c) Standards of care are broad-based due to board certification and policies of specialty societies
3. Medical expert used to establish standards of care
   (a) The reasonably prudent person
   (b) Physician of similar training and experience
   (c) Responds to factual issues and hypothetical situations

c. Breach of duty

1. Failure to act within standards of care; violation of standard
2. Medical record and testimony establish course of care
3. Opinion(s) of expert(s) establish compliance or noncompliance with standards of care

d. Causation

1. Connection between breach of duty and injury to plaintiff
2. Violation of standard must be a contributing cause
3. "But for" the breach of duty the damages (injury) would not have occurred

e. Damages

1. Money sought to compensate the plaintiff for injury suffered due to defendant's negligence
2. Actual damages; compensate plaintiff for
   (a) Medical expenses; current and future
   (b) Lost income
   (c) Loss of earning capacity
   (d) Loss ot consortium
   (e) Pain and suffering
3. Punitive damages
   (a) Available for gross negligence
   (b) Punishment for defendant's wanton and willful disregard for welfare of others

IV. LITIGATION ISSUES

a. Medical malpractice = medical negligence = professional negligence

1. Violations of standards of care are very common
2. Rarely do violations of standards of care result in injury to patient or damages
3. Seldom do acts of negligence result in lawsuit; often triggered by poor interpersonal interactions
4. Doctors win nearly all malpractice cases that go to trial

5. A relationship of trust—good rapport—with patients and their families is the best insurance against malpractice litigation

---

b. Statute of limitations

1. As a rule, the plaintiff has 2 years after his or her injury to file a negligence suit
2. For minors, 2 years after reaching the age of majority is usually allowed
3. There is some variation among the states as to the application of limitation statutes

---

c. Medical records

1. Will be part of any medical lawsuit
2. Should be accurate and complete when made
3. Appropriate correction of errors is acceptable in medical records
4. Correction or modification of medical records in anticipation of litigation traditionally backfires

---

d. Skeleton of a lawsuit

1. Parties
   (a) Plaintiff: party initiating lawsuit; usually the (angered) injured patient, but others, such as family members, may join as coplaintiffs or file on behalf of an incompetent or deceased patient
   (b) Defendant: the party being sued; usually there are multiple defendants, which include physicians, nurses, the hospital, equipment manufacturers and maintenance agencies, drug manufacturers
2. Filing a lawsuit is accomplished according to procedural rules, which vary among the states
   (a) Prior to filing a lawsuit, notice to potential defendants may be required
   (b) Legal action is initiated by filing a complaint or petition with the court that sets forth allegations against the defendant, who is served at the time suit is filed
   (c) The defendant, through his or her attorney, files a responsive pleading, which may deny allegations set forth by the plaintiff
   (d) Pleadings may be amended and/or supplemented as the lawsuit progresses
3. Discovery phase of litigation begins after lawsuit is initiated
   (a) Parties must exchange information according to discovery rules
   (b) Interrogatories between parties require written responses to questions
   (c) "Requires for production" means that certain identified documents in the hands of adverse parties are to be provided to or accessed by the opposing party
   (d) Deposition is a means of obtaining sworn testimony of witnesses and parties
   (e) Subpoena duces tecum and requests for admissions are among other discovery tools
4. Settlement offers
   (a) May be made by either side and quickly resolve case if accepted
   (b) Best negotiations are made when discovery process has allowed distillation of liabilities and damages
5. Trial
   (a) Plaintiff has burden of proof, requiring each element of the case be proved by a preponderance of the evidence

    (b) War of experts testifying on behalf of each party

    (c) Emotional appeal of plaintiff's case and sincerity/credibility of defendants are key issues for jury

    (d) Fact issues for jury are usually liability of any of the defendants, and then damages attributable to the defendants found liable

e. Insurance and defense

1. Liability insurance (almost) always provides legal defense

2. Attorney is to protect his or her client, not insurer who is paying the bill

3. With multiple defendants insured by a single insurer, each defendant may require a separate attorney; defense of one may incriminate another

4. Attorney's goal is defeat one or more elements of plaintiff's case

    (a) This defendant's duty to plaintiff was unrelated to injury suffered

    (b) Any wrongdoing on the part of this defendant was a mere error in judgment and not a violation of any standard of care

    (c) What this defendant did wrong had nothing to do with the plaintiff's injury

    (d) The plaintiff's injury, if any, is insignificant

5. Separate counsel, in addition to insurance defense, may be appropriate

    (a) When damages sought exceed insurance coverage

    (b) Insurer disclaims liability to the case, or suggests quick, cheap settlement

    (c) Insurance attorney not doing his or her job and insurer refuses to assign another

V. CONTRACTS AND EMPLOYMENT

a. Group practices have a variety of characteristics according to structure

1. Partnerships allow exposure of personal assets of one partner to cover liabilities of others

2. Corporations are desirable for numerous reasons, including asset protection, benefit packages, taxation strategy

b. Understanding of working relationship is important

1. Structure and function of employing entity

    (a) Number of shareholders, partners, and employees

    (b) Existing contracts with hospitals, HMOs, PPOs, other managed care plans

    (c) Utilization and role of CRNAs

    (d) Benefit package; insurance, vacation, retirement plan

    (e) Future employment prospects

2. Restrictions in the event of termination

    (a) Noncompete clause commonly present in employment contract

    (b) Usually enforceable if reasonable in time and geographic constraint

    (c) Restriction can have limitations built into agreement

VI. LEGAL ISSUES RELATED TO HIV

a. Nondiscriminatory medical care

1. Medical care of HIV-infected patients should be similar to that of other patients with communicable diseases
2. As a private individual a physician can choose whether or not to enter a doctor–patient relationship
3. Once in a doctor–patient relationship, a physician may not abandon a patient, but may terminate the relationship provided the patient is afforded time and opportunity to find another physician to care for him or her
4. Federal law (Americans With Disabilities Act) prohibits discrimination against disabled individuals; applies widely, including hospitals and medical practices; includes HIV-infected patients within penumbra of disability definition

b. Occupational Safety and Health Administration (OSHA) requirements

1. All patients should be treated using universal precautions; presumption of infection
2. Specific as to handling of contaminated sharp objects
3. Requires utilization of personal protective equipment; gloves, goggles
4. Severe penalties for violation by employer or employee

c. HIV testing

1. Government can require HIV testing in the name of public interest
2. Currently routine testing for HIV antibody is performed according to local policies
3. Some states specify the conditions under which a patient can be required to have HIV testing; usually related to concerns for the health and welfare of others

d. Disclosure of HIV status

1. A patient's positive HIV status is private information
2. The law will only protect individuals who disclose this information appropriately—spouse, perhaps other parties at known risk from the infected patient
3. A physician who is HIV positive has a duty to disclose that status to patients if the physician performs procedure with high exposure risk; considered a material risk that would influence patient in consenting to procedure

VII. ETHICAL ISSUES AT END OF LIFE

a. Autonomy and self-determination

1. Patients have a right to refuse treatment, even when treatment will sustain life
2. Decisions may be made by others on behalf of incompetent patients
   - (a) Spouse
   - (b) Adult children
   - (c) Parents

(d) Nearest living relative
3. Patient's desire is fundamental question
    (a) May be set forth in living will or similar document; seldom used
    (b) Surrogate decision maker may be identified by power of attorney
    (c) States vary in level of evidence required to establish patient's desire

b. Living will statutes and natural death acts
1. Legislative enactments that protect physicians in allowing patient to die
2. Mechanisms through which life support can be withheld/withdrawn

Index

A-bands, 87
Abdominal arteries, intra-, 87
Abdominal muscles
  expiration by, 13
  regional anesthesia in obese patients
    and, 146
Abdominal pain, in cirrhosis, 248
Abducens (VI) nerve, 571
ABG, *see* Arterial blood gas
Ablation, cardiovascular, 103–104
Abortion
  oxytocics in, 501–502
  spontaneous, hypothyroidism
    associated with, 513
Abruptio placenta, 517–519
Abscess of lung
  computed tomography of, 10
Absence seizures, 167
Absolute pressure, 101, 412
Abuse
  of benzodiazepines, 340
  obesity and, 67
Accelerography, 384–385
Accessory muscles, inspiration and, 12
Accessory (XI) nerve
  laryngeal innervation, 4–5
Acebutolol
  as beta₂ antagonist, 289
  as vasodilatory beta antagonist, 95
Acetaminophen
  for chronic pain, 553
  platelet transfusions and, 532
Acetaminophen, as exogenous toxin, 170
Acetazolamide, kidney failure affecting,
    234
Acetylcholine (ACh), 162–163, 282
  binding sites, 353
  as cholinergic agonist, 289
  nerves using, 282
  renal blood flow affected by, 200
  sympathetic chain ganglia, 280
  synthesis and hydrolysis, **354**
  as vasoactive compound, 30, 282
Acetylcholine (ACh) receptors,
    162–163, 283, 353

Boldface page numbers denote tables or illustrations.

glycoproteins, 162
location, 162–163
muscarinic, *see* Muscarinic receptors
nicotinic, *see* Nicotinic receptors
Acetylcholinesterase, 282
  edrophonium, break down of, 379
ACh, *see* Acetylcholine (ACh)
Acid-base, 20–21
  carbon dioxide (CO₂), 20–21
Acid-base balance
  neuromuscular blockage affected by,
    356
  renal, 211–213
Acidemia, perinatal, 482
Acidosis
  as diabetic ketoacidosis complication,
    271
  hyperchloremic, 216, 271
  lactic, 271
  local tissue, local anesthetics causing,
    349
  metabolic, *see* Metabolic acidosis
  and pulmonary atresia, 492
  respiratory, *see* Respiratory acidosis
Acini, 253
Acromegaly, 256–257
ACTH, 275
  secondary adrenocortical
    insufficiency and, 265
  secretion, drugs to suppress, 262
Activated clotting time (ACT), 243
Activated partial prothrombin time
    (aPTT), 541
Activation energy, 429
Active transport, 306
Activity metabolism flow coupling, 156
Actual damages, 575
Acupuncture, 544
Acute adrenocortical insufficiency,
    265–266
Acute anaphylaxis, 390–392
  clinical manifestations, 391
  definition, 390
  diagnosis, 391–392
  epinephrine for, 33
  mechanism, 390
  mediators, types of, 391
  prophylaxis, 392

treatment, 392
Acute asthma
  management in pregnancy, 56
  symptoms, 56
Acute autonomic hyperreflexia, 299
Acute blood loss, transfusions for, 531
Acute cholecystitis, 247
Acute hemolytic transfusion reaction,
    250
Acute hypocalcemia, 261, 262
Acute intermittent porphyria
  thiopentone causing, 318
Acute kidney failure, 228–232
  acute tubule necrosis causing,
    229–230
  in cardiopulmonary bypass, 239
  etiology, 228–232
  in heat stroke, 147
  immunological factors, 228, 232
  ischemic disorders causing, 229–230
  metabolic factors, 232
  obstructive disorders causing, 228
  pyelonephritis causing, 232
  sepsis causing, 230
  toxic causes, 230–232
  traumatic factors, 232
Acute liver failure, in heat stroke, 148
Acute lupus pneumonitis, 57
Acute lymphocytic leukemia
  doxorubicin as treatment, 388
Acute mountain sickness, 63
Acute myocardial infarction
  amniotic fluid embolism
    differentiated, 520
  hyperosmolar nonketonic coma,
    concurrent with, 272
Acute tubule necrosis
  acute kidney failure caused by,
    229–230
  mortality, 229
Acyclovir, kidney failure affecting, 233
Addiction, to opioid drugs, 547
Addisonian crisis, 265–266
Addison's disease, 264
Additive law, 450
Adenoids, hypertrophic, 483
Adenosine
  as antidysrhythmic, 96

Adenosine, *continued*
  in pediatric life support, **499**
  renal vascular resistance and, 199–200
  urologic effects of, 238
Adenosine deaminase binding protein
  tubule damage and excretion of, 223
Adenosine triphosphate, 88
  as antidysrhythmic, 96
  in malignant hyperthermia, 297
ADH, *see* Antidiuretic hormone
Adjusted rates, 448
Adrenal cortex, 253
  secretion of, 264
Adrenalectomy, bilateral
  for glucocorticoid excess, 262
  supplement cortisol during, 262
Adrenal gland
  anatomy, 252–253
  arterial supply, 253
  cortex, 253, 264
  hemorrhage of, 265
  hypothyroidism affecting function, 259, 260
  innervation, 253
  medulla, *see* Adrenal medulla
  regulation, 253
  tumors of, Cushing's syndrome caused by, 262
  venous drainage, 253
  weight, 253
Adrenal glucocorticoids, *see* Glucocorticoids
Adrenal medulla, 280
  pheochromocytomas arising from, 266
  using epinephrine, 283
  using norepinephrine, 283
Adrenal mineralocorticoids, *see* Mineralocorticoids
Adrenergic agents, 55
Adrenergic fibers, 160
Adrenergic receptors, 283–284
  activities, 90–91
  alpha, *see* Alpha adrenoreceptors
  beta, *see* Beta adrenoreceptors
  dopamine, 284
Adrenergic system
  and renal vascular resistance, 197
Adrenocortical response
  insufficiency of, 264–266
  opioids affecting, 332
Adriamycin, *see* Doxorubicin
Adult hemoglobin (HbA), 488
  oxygen unloading capacity of, 488–489
Adult respiratory distress syndrome (ARDS)
  in Guillain-Barré syndrome, 60
  during labor, 57
  surfactant deficiencies associated

  with, 481
Advanced life support
  drugs used in pediatric, **499**
Aerodynamic navigation, limit of, 62
Afferent fibers, 279
Afferent neurons, 279
Afferent pain pathways, 159, 279
Afterdepolarization, 85–86
Afterload
  dobutamine decreasing, 92
  intra-aortic balloon counterpulsation reducing, 104
Agency by estoppel, 573
Aging, 139–143
  see also Elderly persons
  anesthetic requirements, decrease in, 141
  arginine vasopressin and, 209–210
  diseases related to, 139
  increased risk, disease associated with, 139
  kidney anatomy and, 195
  pancuronium and, 367
  pathophysiology of, 140–143
  pipecuronium and, 368
  postoperative attention, 143
  and protein binding, 142, 307
  rocuronium and, **369**
Agonists
  alpha, *see* Alpha agonists
  beta, *see* Beta agonists
  cholinergic, 289–291
  opioid, 333–336, 545–546, 549–551
Agranulocytosis, 539
Air embolism, 174–177
  anesthetic technique, 177
  arterial, *see* Arterial air embolism
  capnography, 176
  clinical practice, 176–177
  definition, 174
  hemodynamics in, 176
  hyperbaric oxygen therapy for, 71–72, 75, 177
  hypercarbia due to, 51
  iatrogenic causes, 71
  monitoring, 175–176
  murmur in, 176
  paradoxical, 175
  procedures with incidence of, 174–175
  transcutaneous CO_2 detection, 176
  treatment, 177
  venous, 174, 175
Air evacuation
  environmental considerations during, 64
  medical considerations during, 64
  supplemental O_2 during, 64
Airway
  as fire risk zone, 430

  in neonatal resuscitation, 498
  in obese patients, 67, 144, 145
    regional anesthesia and, 146
  pediatric, 482–483
  pregnancy-induced hypertension affecting, 505
  reflexes, aging and, 141–142
Airway assessment, 569
Airway maintenance
  in acromegaly, 257
  as anaphylaxis treatment, 392
  in heat stroke, 148
  in local anesthetics-induced seizure treatment, 350
Airway obstruction
  in Arnold-Chiari malformation, 187
  and pulmonary atresia, 492
  of small airway, in infants, 481
  supraglottitis as, 496
Airway pressure release ventilation, 53
Airway resistance, 15–16
Akinesia, in neuroleptic malignant syndrome, 299
Alanine transaminase, tests of, 243
Albumin
  and plasma oncotic pressure, 242
  as plasma protein, binding of, 306
  tests of, 243
Albuterol, 32, 288
  associated with uterine hemorrhage, 55
Alcohol
  as combustible fuel, 429
  enzyme induction caused by, 244
  as exogenous toxin, 170
  fetal breathing affected by, 481
Aldosterone, 204–205, 264, 275–276
  adrenal suppression of, etomidate causing, 322
  adrenocortical insufficiency and, 264
  in ascites therapy, 248
  blood pressure and, 90
  drug effects on, 205
  interactions, 204–205
  regulation of, 276
  renal effects, 204
    acid-base balance, 212
    magnesium excretion and, 216
    potassium balance, 214
    tubular function and, 204–205
  spironolactone and, 227
Aldosteronism, 263
Alfentanil, 335
  central nervous system affected by, 163
  as opiate agonist, 551
  as opioid agonist, 335
Alkaline-manganese-zinc batteries, 444
Alkaline phosphatase
  pseudohyperparathyroidism and levels of, 261

tests of, 243
Alkaloid, ergot, 286
Alkalosis, respiratory, 21
Allergic interstitial nephritis, 223
Allergic reactions, 393–394
    to diprivan, 320
    to local anesthetics, 351–352
    to thiopentone, 318
    to transfusion, 250
Allograft rejection, steroid use during, 387
Alloimmunization, transfusion-related, 530
Allopurinol, kidney failure affecting, 233
Alloxan, pulmonary vascular resistance influenced by, 18
Alopecia, doxorubicin causing, 388
Alpha-adrenergics, tubular function and, 205
Alpha adrenoreceptors, 283–284
    see also specific adrenoreceptors
    agonists, see Alpha agonists
    antagonists, see Alpha antagonists
Alpha$_1$ adrenoreceptors, 283–284
    see also specific adrenoreceptors
    agonists, 285
    antagonists, 286–287, 556–557
    postsynaptic, 90
Alpha$_2$ adrenoreceptors, 284
    see also specific adrenoreceptors
    agonists, 285–286
        for chronic pain, 556–557
        and renal acid-base balance, 212
    antagonists, 287
    postsynaptic, 284
    presynaptic, 90–91, 284
Alpha agonists, 284–286
    see also specific alpha agonists
    alpha$_1$, 285
    alpha$_2$, 212, 285–286, 556–557
Alpha antagonists, 286–287
    see also specific alpha antagonists
    alpha$_1$, 286–287
        for chronic pain, 556–557
    alpha$_2$, 287
    nonselective blockade, 286
    for pheochromocytoma in pregnancy, 514
Alpha thalassemia, 536–537
Altered consciousness, in neuroleptic malignant syndrome, 299
Alternating current, 431
Altitude, 61–64
    disorders associated with, 62–64
    gas laws, 61–62
    hypoxia and, 17, 62–63
    physical factors, 64
    physiology of, 61–64
    respiration and, 26

respiratory gas pressures at increasing, **65**
Altitude sickness, 63
Alupent, see Metaproterenol
Alveolar brush cells, 6
Alveolar concentrations, 46–47
    blood uptake and, 47
    distribution and, 308
    hyperventilation and, 48
    inspired concentrations, less than, 46–47
    uptake and ventilation associated with, 47
Alveolar ducts, 6
    prenatal development of, 481
Alveolar edema, lung compliance reduced with, 13
Alveolar epithelial cells, 6
Alveolar hypoventilation, hypercarbia due to, 51
Alveolar macrophages, 6
Alveolar sacs, 6
    prenatal development of, 481
Alveolar type II pneumocytes
    surfactant produced by, 481
Alveolar ventilation (VA)
    delivery of gas to alveoli and, 47
    in infants, 484, 489
Alveoli, 6
    collapse, see Atelectasis
    fibrosis of, see Pulmonary fibrosis
    gas diffusion to capillaries from, 22
    prenatal, 481
    septa, 6
        protease transport and, 29
    surface tension and, 14
Amantidine
    kidney failure affecting, 233
    in neuroleptic malignant syndrome treatment, 300
American College of Obstetricians and Gynecologists, 504
American National Standards Institute, 427–428
American Society for Testing and Materials (ASTM), 37
Americans with Disabilities Act, 578
Amiloride, kidney failure affecting, 234
Amino acids
    deamination of, 242
    excitatory, 178
    proximal tubule, reabsorption by, 217
Aminoglycosides
    acute kidney failure caused by, 231
    kidney failure affecting, 233
Aminophylline
    for acute asthma in pregnancy, 56
    in anaphylaxis treatment, 392
Aminotransferase tests, 243
Amiodarone, 95

Ammonia regulation, 242
Amniocentesis, 503
Amniotic fluid, 502–503
    blood gas, 502–503
    embolism of, 519–520
Ampere-hours, 444
Amphotericin B, 231
Amplifiers, single processing, 436
Amplitude levels, 445
Amplitude scan, 420
Amrinone, 92
Amylase excretion, 223
Anaerobic metabolism, cerebral, 177–178
Anaeroid pressure gauge, 101
Analeptics, 166
Analgesia
    in burn injuries, 569
    in obese patients, 147
Analog-digital converters, 434
Analog mobile phone service, 443
Anaphylactic reactions
    anaphylactoid reactions compared, 393
    to muscle relaxants, 393
    promethazine causing, 344
    thiopental causing, 393
Anaphylactoid reactions, 392–393
    anaphylactic reactions compared, 393
    atracurium causing, 359
    bleomycin causing, 389
    to radiocontrast media, 394
    thiopental causing, 393
    vecuronium causing, 372
Anaphylaxis
    acute, 33, 390–392
    diprivan causing, 320
    transfusion-related, 530
Anastomotic circle, 151
Androgenic steroids, 276
Anectine, see Succinylcholine
Anemia, 537–539
    aplastic, 539
    chronic, 537–538
    Cooley's, 537
    hemolytic, 538–539
    as hypercalcemia sign, 260
    and hypothyroidism, 260
    as induced hypotension contraindication, 293
    as kidney failure complication, 232
    and neonatal erythropoiesis activity, 260
    perioperative, transfusions in, 531
    in pregnancy, 500
    in premature infants, 490
    pseudohyperparathyroidism accompanied by, 261
    treatment, 531–532
Anemia coagulopathy, 493

Anephric state, 237
Anesthesia machines
    cylinders, *see* Cylinders
    as fire risk zone, 430
    perioperative hypoxemia and
        disorders of, 51
    pressure gauges on, 37
    proper connections, ensuring, 38
    scavenger system at same level as, 40
Anesthetic agents
    see also specific anesthetics
    assisted reproductive technologies
        affected by, 523
    as cerebral protection, 178–179
    depth and adequacy of, 158–159
    distribution, *see* Distribution; Uptake
        and distribution
    enzyme induction caused by, 244
    naloxone causing reversal of, 330
    uptake, *see* Uptake and distribution
Aneurysm(s)
    of abdominal aorta, 120
    as electroconvulsant therapy
        contraindication, 565
    of internal carotid artery, 255
    intracranial, 179–182
Angina, 99
    as electroconvulsant therapy
        contraindication, 565
    therapy for, 99
Angiography
    cerebral, *see* Cerebral angiography
    percutaneous transhepatic
        cholangiography, 247
    pulmonary, 115
Angiotensin, 30
Angiotensin-converting enzyme (ACE),
    30
Angiotensin-converting enzyme
        inhibitors (ACEI)
    in cardiopulmonary bypass, 239
    kidney failure affecting, 233
Angiotensin II, 30
    effects of, 205–206
    renal acid-base balance and, 212
    and renal vascular resistance, 197–198
    tubular function and, 205–206
Ankylosing spondylitis, 12
Annulus fibrosus, 152
Anorexia
    in cirrhosis, 248
    as diabetic ketoacidosis sign, 269
ANP, *see* Atrial natriuretic peptide
ANQ 9040, 372
Antacids
    as premedication in obese patients, 146
    for pulmonary aspiration, 527
Antagonists
    alpha adrenoreceptors, *see* Alpha
        antagonists

benzodiazepine, 343
beta, *see* Beta antagonists
muscarinic, *see* Muscarinic
    antagonists
nicotinic, 291–292
opioid, 329–330, 336–338, 546
serotonin, 268
Anterior cord syndrome, 171
Anterior longitudinal ligament, 153
Anterior pituitary hormones, 274
Anterior serrati muscles, 12
Anthranilic acid derivatives, 552
Antianginal agents, 99
Antiarrhythmics
    see also Antidysrhythmics; specific
        antiarrhythmics
    for chronic pain, 555–556
    in pregnancy, 131
Antibiotics
    allergic reactions to, 394
    atracurium interacting with, 359
    cistracurium interacting with, 361
    for congenital heart disease, 128
    muscle relaxants interacting with, 355
    for supraglottitis, 497
Antibody production, 390
Anticholinergic agents, 33–34, **380**–381
    see also specific anticholinergics
    age-related effects, 141
    for asthma in pregnancy, 55
    mechanism of action, 33
    structure, 380
Anticholinesterases, 289–291
    see also specific anticholinesterases
    muscle relaxants interacting with, 355
    pharmacology, **378**–380
    therapeutic uses, 290
Anticoagulants
    as cardiac drug in pregnancy,
        130–131
    coumarin, in pregnancy, 130–131
    heparin, *see* Heparin
Anticonvulsant agents
    for chronic pain, 554–555
    enzyme induction caused by, 244
    hypoparathyroidism and, 261
    thiopentone as, 317
Antidepressants
    central nervous system affected by,
        166
    for chronic pain, 554–555
Antiderivative of f, 465
Antidiuretic hormone (ADH), 90
    ascites associated with secretion of,
        247
    in diabetes insipidus management,
        255–256
    urine output and, 318
Antidiuretics, 332
Antidromic conduction, 161–162

Antidysrhythmics, 92–96, 121
    see also Antiarrhythmics; specific
        antidysrhythmics
    classes of, 92–96
    restoration of normal physiology
        prior to, 121
    side effects, 121
Antiemetics, 343–345
Antihistamines
    for asthma in pregnancy, 55
    for chronic pain, 557
Antihypertensive drugs, 106
    for pregnancy-induced hypertension,
        507–508
Anti-inflammatory agents
    see also specific anti-inflammatory
        agents
    as bronchodilators, 34
    nonsteroidal, *see* Nonsteroidal
        anti-inflammatory drugs
Antimineralocorticoid therapy, 263
Antiparkinsonian medications, 166
Antipruritic agents, 320
Antipsychotic therapy
    central nervous system affected by,
        166
    neuroleptic malignant syndrome as
        complication, 299–300
Antipyretic effects, NSAIDs causing,
    338
Antirejection drugs, 386–389
Antisialagogues, 99
Anus, imperforate, 493
Aorta, 84
    abdominal aneurysm rupture, 120
    chest x-ray of, 8, 10
    insufficiency, in pregnancy, 133
    supply to lower extremities, 87
Aortic arch, 84
    afferents in, 279
    baro-control receptors in, 90
Aortic cross-clamping, 238
Aorticorenal ganglia, 280
Aortic regurgitation (AR), 107–108
Aortic stenosis, 106–107
    pathophysiology, 106–107, 134
    in pregnancy, 107, 133–134
Aortic valve, 84
    replacement of, 106
Aortocaval compression, 500
Apert's syndrome, 191
Aplastic anemia, 539
Apnea
    Arnold-Chiari malformation and, 187
    diving reflex induced by, 77
    in infants, 484
    local anesthetics causing, 350
    of prematurity, 489–490
    transient, thiopentone causing, 318
Apparent agency, 573

Apprehension, in pulmonary embolism, 115
Aqueduct stenosis, *see* Arnold-Chiari malformation
Arachnoid, spinal, 154
Arachnoiditis, 172
Arc discharge, 435
ARDS, *see* Adult respiratory distress syndrome (ARDS)
Arduan, **367**–368
Argand diagram, 470
Arginine vasopressin, 209–210, 274
    effects, 209
    elderly persons, fluid balance in, 218
    interactions, 209–210
    polyuria and, 237
    renal acid-base balance affected by, 213
Ar-Hg mix, 435
Armstrong line, 62
Arnold-Chiari malformation, 187–189
    and pediatric meningomyelocele, 186, 494
Arousal, in coma assessment, 169
Arrhythmias
    see also specific types
    anaphylaxis causing, 391
    cardiac, 78
    hypercarbia resulting in, 51
    junctional, 375
    naloxone causing, 330
    succinylcholine causing, 375
Arterial air embolism
    cerebral, *see* Cerebral arterial gas embolism (CAGE)
    hyperbaric oxygen therapy, 75
    mechanism, 174
    pathophysiology, 175
Arterial blood
    obese patients, access in, 69, 146
    pulmonary, *see* Pulmonary arteries
    and respiratory control, 26
Arterial blood gas
    in anaphylaxis treatment, 392
    continuous in vivo arterial blood gas monitors, 405
    ex vivo monitor, 405
    in obese patients, 146
    preoperative evaluation, 50
Arterial blood pressure
    enflurane decreasing, 311
    halothane decreasing, 310
    measurement of, 413–416
    methohexitone decreasing, 319
    thiopentone decreasing, 318
Arterial hypertension, obesity and, 66
Arterial line
    in induced hypotension, 293
    in neonatal diaphragmatic hernia, 490
Arterial O_2 saturation (SpO_2), 409–410

Arterial system, myocardial, 86
Arterial thrombosis, 271
Arterial-venous blood, 409
Arterial waveform, 415
Arteriogram, of urologic system, 196
Arterioles, 7
    blood flow resistance, site of, 18
    vasoconstriction, 280
Arteriosclerosis, 105–106
Arteriovenous graft, 48
Arteriovenous malformations
    cerebral, 182
    fluid balance in elderly as factor, 218
    gamma knife used on, 567
Artificial hearts, total, 105
Arytenoid cartilage, 4
A scan, 420
Ascending aorta, 84
Ascites, 247–248
    in cirrhosis, 248
    lung compliance reduced with, 13
Aspartate transaminase tests, 243
Asphyxia, 76
Aspiration
    as anesthetic emergency, 391
    neonatal meconium, 498
    prophylaxis induction, hypothyroidism and, 260
    pulmonary, 60
    ultrasound-guided transvaginal, 524–525
Aspiration pneumonia, 520
Aspiration pneumonitis, 60
Aspirin, platelet transfusions and, 532
Assist-controlled ventilation, 53
Assisted reproductive technologies, 523–525
Association for the Advancement of Medical Instrumentation, 427–428
Asthma, 49–50
    chronic, vital capacity (VC) and, 12
    clinical manifestations, 50
    epinephrine for, 33
    ipratropium bromide for, 33
    pathology, 49–50
    in pregnancy, 54–57, 500
    preoperative preparation, 50
    promethazine causing, 344
    pulmonary embolus differentiated, 115
    theophylline for pregnant patients, 55
Asymptote, 463
Atelectasis
    in infants, 484
    lung compliance reduced with, 13
    as postoperative complication, 52
    surfactant abnormalities causing, 481
    as transesophageal fistula complication, 492

Atenolol, 94, 289
Atheroembolic disease, 223
Atmosphere and space, line between, 63
Atonic seizures, 167
ATP, *see* Adenosine triphosphate
Atracurium
    histamine release from, 393
    as nicotinic antagonist, 291–292
    as nondepolarizing muscle relaxant, **357**–359
Atresia
    esophageal, 492
    pulmonary, 491–492
Atrial fibrillation, 123
    mitral stenosis in pregnancy and, 132
    therapy, 123
Atrial flutter, 123
Atrial natriuretic factor (ANF), 90
Atrial natriuretic peptide, 30
    cardiovascular effects, 208
    effects of, 207–208
    glomerular filtration rate and, 202
    interactions, 208–209
    receptors, 206–207
    regulation of, 207
    renal effects, 207–208
        acid-base balance, 213
        renal vascular resistance, 200
        tubular function, 206–209
Atrial premature beats, 123
Atrial septal defect
    in pregnancy, 134
    in pulmonary atresia, 491
Atrioventricular heart block, 121
Atrioventricular junctional area and node, 85
Atropine, **380**
    as muscarinic antagonist, 291
    as organophosphate treatment, 290
    to reverse neuromuscular blockade, **380**–381
    in transesophageal fistula premedication, 492
Atropine sulfate, **499**
Atrovent, 33
Augmented ventilation, 49
Autoimmune states
    rheumatoid disease, 4, 58
    sarcoidosis, 50, 58–59
    systemic lupus erythematosus, 57–58
    thrombocytopenia, platelet transfusions in, 532
Autologous transfusion, 533
Automaticity changes in rhythm disorders, 120
Autonomic hyperreflexia, 160, 298–299
Autonomic nervous system
    anatomy, 279
    and blood flow control, 90

Autonomic nervous system, *continued*
  bodily functions controlled by, 279
  centers of function, 279
  disorders of, *see* specific nervous
      system disorders
  feedback to, 279
  information transmission in, 282–284
  and neonatal heart regulation,
      484–485
  neurotransmitters, *see*
      Neurotransmitters
  pharmacology, 284–292
  receptors, 283
    see also specific receptors
Autonomy, at end of life, 578–579
Autoregulation of blood flow, 89
  cerebral, 157
  metabolic products as basis for, 89
  renal vascular resistance, 197
Averages, in statistics, 449
AVMs, *see* Arteriovenous
      malformations
AVP, *see* Arginine vasopressin
Awake intubation
  in congenital lobar emphysema, 493
  fiberoptic, 51, 257, 490
  in Pierre-Robin sequence, 495
  in transesophageal fistula, 492
Awareness
  in coma assessment, 169
  and depth of anesthesia, 159
Axillary artery, 87
Axonal transmission, 161, 280
Azathioprine, 355
Aztreonam, 233
Azygous vein, 8

Bacteria
  as exogenous toxin, 171
  transfusion-transmitted, 529–530
Bainbridge reflex, 27
Bain modification of Malpeson D
      system, 44, **45**
Balloon atrial septostomy, 491
Band gap, 432, 433
Bandwidth limits, of internet, 442
Baralyme, 315–316
Barbiturates
  central nervous system affected by,
      164
  as cerebral protection, 178
  in elderly persons, 142
  enzyme induction caused by, 244
  as hyperthyroidism premedication,
      258
  kidney failure affecting, 233–234
Barium hydroxide, 46
Barking cough, in
      laryngotracheobronchitis, 496
Baro-control, 90

Baroreceptor-mediated reflex
      tachycardia, 310
Baroreceptors
  aging and, 140
  hypothyroidism and response of, 259,
      260
  pulmonary artery, 27
Basal ganglia, 151
  calcification of, 261
Basal metabolic rate
  aging and, 141
  in hypothyroidism, 259
Basal small airways, in obesity, 66
Baseband LAN, 438
Basilar arteries, 86
Batteries, 444–445
  equipment powered by, 427
Battery, 573
Bayes' theorem, 451
Bean effect, 75
Becker's muscular dystrophy, 60
Beclomethasone inhaler, 55
Belladonna alkaloids, 99
Bellows classification, 52
Bench top analyzers, 402–404
Benzodiazepine antagonists, 343
Benzodiazepine receptors, 339
Benzodiazepines, 163, 339–342
  see also specific benzodiazepines
  abuse potential of, 340
  central nervous system affected by,
      163, 340
  characteristics, 339–340
  in elderly persons, 142
  elimination of, 340
  fentanyl and, adverse effects, 328
  flumazenil and, 326
  as hyperthyroidism premedication,
      258
  intraoperative awareness and, 159
  as ketamine premedication, 323
  kidney failure affecting, 234
  metabolism, 340
  metabolites, 339
  as methohexitone pretreatment, 319
  side effects, 340
  for status epilepticus, 168
  urologic system affected by, 228
Beta-adrenergics
  for acute asthma in pregnancy, 56
  in gestational diabetes, 511
Beta adrenoreceptors, 283, 284
  agonists, *see* Beta agonists
  antagonists, *see* Beta antagonists
  in neonates, 485
Beta$_1$ adrenoreceptors, 284
  antagonists, 289
  postsynaptic, 91
Beta$_2$ adrenoreceptors, 284
  agonists, 32–33, 212, 288

  postsynaptic, 91
Beta$_3$ adrenoreceptors, 284
Beta agonists
  see also specific beta agonists
  beta$_2$, 32–33, 212, 288
  as bronchodilators, 31–33
  central nervous system affected by, 165
  nonselective, 32, 287–288
  renal potassium balance and, 214
  and renal vascular resistance, 197
  as tocolytics, 502
Beta antagonists, 94–95, 288–289
  see also specific antagonists
  as angina therapy, 99
  beta$_1$, 289
  cardioselective, 94–95
  kidney failure affecting, 234
  nonselective, 94, 288–289
  for pheochromocytoma in pregnancy,
      514
  in pregnancy, 131
  for prolonged QT syndrome, 125
  vasodilatory, 95
Beta blockers, *see* Beta antagonists
Betamethasone, **277**
Beta$_2$-microglobulin excretion
  proximal tubule damage, 223
Beta-sympathominetics, *see* Beta
      adrenergics
Beta thalassemia, 537
Bicarbonate ion, CO_2 transport as, 24
Bifascicular heart block, 122
Bilateral hilar lymphadenopathy
      (BHL), 59
Bile ducts, dilated
  in choledocholithiasis, 247
  in chronic cholelithiasis, 247
Biliary excretion, 245
  of bilirubin, 242, 243
  obesity affecting, 67, 145
  of urobilinogen, 243
Bilirubin
  excretion of, 242, 243
  tests of, 244
Binomial distribution, 451, 457–458
Biofeedback, 544
Biologic curves, 471–473
Biotransformation of drugs
  enflurane, 312
  halothane, 310–311
  isoflurane, 313
  in lungs, 29
  obesity affecting, 67, 145
  sevoflurane, 315–316
Biphasic stridor, 496
Bladder, 195
  infections, preoperative evaluation
      of, 239
  rupture, as prostatic resection
      complication, 238

Bladder neck obstruction, 344
Blalock-Taussig shunt, 491
Blanking time, 445
Bleeding
    in burn injuries, 569
    induced hypotension, to control, 292
    preoperative assessment of, 534
Bleeding time (BT), 243
Bleomycin, 389
Blind trials, 462
Blood
    arterial, *see* Arterial blood
    lungs as filter, 28
    lungs as reservoir, 27
    in pregnancy, 500
    units of, *see* Blood units
    venous, 28, 69
Blood flow
    autoregulation of, *see* Autoregulation
        of blood flow
    cerebral, *see* Cerebral blood flow
        (CBF)
    coronary blood flow, 86, 89
    in liver, 87, 91, 141, 244
    measurement of, 398–401
    parasympathetic nervous system, and
        control of, 90
    protein binding in elderly and, 307
    regional
        anesthetic distribution and, 308
        protein binding in elderly and, 307
    renal, *see* Renal blood flow
    right ventricle requirements, 89
    sympathetic nervous system and, 90
    during systole, 89
    and thyroid hormone, 90
    ventilation-perfusion, 16–18
Blood gas, 20
    amniotic fluid, 502–503
    anesthetic gas transfer, 47
    arterial, *see* Arterial blood gas
    measurement of, 20, 402–405
    oxygen, *see* Oxygen in blood gas
    in pregnancy, 500
    and ventilation/perfusion ratio, 20
Blood:gas partition coefficient, 41, **42**
    rate of recovery and, 308
Blood-placental barrier (B-P-B), 501
Blood pressure
    aging and regulation of, 140
    arterial, *see* Arterial blood pressure
    components of, 89
    control of, 89
    in kidney failure therapy, 236
    neonatal, 485
    norepinephrine increasing, 91
    perfusion pressure, 89
    in pregnancy, 500
Blood pressure monitor
    in burn injuries, 569

    in ophthalmic surgery, 571
Blood transfusion, 529–534
    autologous, 533
    massive, 530–531
    reaction to, 249–250, 530
    transfusion-transmitted diseases,
        249–250, 529–530
Blood units, 529
Blood volume
    cerebral, 156
    circulating, obesity and increased,
        66
    hypothyroidism affecting, 259
    loss of, transfusions in, **531**
    neonatal, **488**
"Blue bloater", 49
BMR, 141, 259
Bodily fluids, boiling point of, 62
Body mass index (BMI), 66, 143
Body surface area, 568
Bohr effect, 23
Bone
    catabolism, parathyroid hormone
        affecting, 275
    chest x-ray of, 9
    kidney failure affecting, 233
Bone marrow, transient suppression of,
    389
Bone resorption
    hyperparathyroidism causing, 260
    parathyroid hormone affecting, 275
Botulism, 171
Bourdon pressure gauge, **38,** 101
Bowel gas, 429
Boyle's law, 35
    altitude physiology, 61, 64
    and hyperbaric oxygen therapy, 76
BP, *see* Blood pressure
Brachial artery, 87
Bradycardia
    belladonna alkaloids causing, 99
    as cisatracurium side effect, 360
    diving reflex causing, 77
    d-tubocurarine causing, 370
    in former premature babies, 490
    as hypothyroidism symptom, 259
    in neonates, 485
    as parasympathetic nervous system
        response, 281
    sinus, 122–123, 375
    succinylcholine causing, 375
Bradycardia-tachycardia syndrome, 123
Bradykinin
    renal blood flow affected by, 200
    as vasoactive nonapeptide, 30
Brain, 151–152
    craniosynostosis location in, 189
    norepinephrine reducing blood flow
        to, 91
    swelling, 180

    tumors, hypertension caused by, 183
    volumes, 157
Brain death, 185
Brain edema
    acute intracranial hypertension
        caused by, 183
    as intracranial aneurysm
        complication, 180
Brain levels of anesthetic, 47
Brain resuscitation, 79–80
Brain stem, 151
    Arnold-Chiari malformation and,
        187–188
    hemorrhage of, 269
    respiratory regulation affected by
        injury, 27
    spinal cord as continuation of, 153
Brain-stem anesthesia, 572
Brain-stem auditory evoked potentials
    (BAEP), 156
Breach of duty, 574–575
Breast cancer, metastatic, 254
Breath flow rate measurement, 400–401
Breathing
    see also Respiration
    decreased efficiency, and obesity, 66
    fetal, 481–482
    neonatal control of, 482
    periodic, in infants, 484
Breathing systems, 43–46
    as fire risk zone, 430
Brethaire, *see* Terbutaline
Bretylium, 95
    for chronic pain, 556
    kidney failure affecting, 234
    in pediatric life support, **499**
Bridge circuits, **436**
Brightness modulation, in ultrasound,
    421
Broadband LAN, 438
Bromide
    as halothane metabolite, 310–311
    toxicity of, 311
Bromocriptine, 300
Bronchi, 5–6
    in infants, 481
Bronchial arteries, 87
Bronchial blocker, 51
Bronchioles, 6
Bronchitis, chronic, 49
    vital capacity (VC) and, 12
Bronchoconstriction
    anaphylaxis causing, 391
    carcinoid presenting with, 268
    cromolyn sodium for prevention of,
        34
    5-Hydroxytryptamine affecting, 30
    from leukotrienes, 31
    as parasympathetic nervous system
        response, 281

Bronchoconstriction, *continued*
  from prostaglandins, 31
  from thromboxanes, 31
Bronchodilation
  belladonna alkaloids causing, 99
  in pregnant patients, 55
  sympathetic nervous system affecting, 281
Bronchodilators
  see also specific bronchodilators
  anticholinergic agents, 33–34
  anti-inflammatory agents, 34
  beta-adrenergic agonists, 31–33
  enflurane as, 311
  halothane as, 310
  methylxanthine agents, 34
  nitric oxide (NO) as, 29
  prostaglandins as, 31
  relaxation of uterine muscles with, 57
Bronchoscopy
  with endobronchial fiberoptic intubation, 51
  in near-drowning, 79
Bronchospasm
  as cistracurium side effect, 360
  lung compliance reduced with, 13
  postpartum hemorrhage therapy associated with, 56
  preoperative preparation of, 50
Bronkosol, 32–33
Brown-Sequard syndrome, 173
B scan, in ultrasound, 421
Bubbler water humidifiers, 54
Bulletin boards, on internet, 441
Bullous emphysema, 49
Bumetanide, 226
  compatabilities, **225**
  kidney failure affecting, 234
BUN, in diabetic ketoacidosis, 270
Bunsen solubility coefficient, 41
Bupivacaine, 352
  cardiac effects of, 347, 351
  pregnancy and, 351
Buprenorphine, 336, 551
Burns, 568–570
  atracurium use following, 359
  electrical, 426
  hyperbaric oxygen therapy for, 74, 75
  intraoperative management, 569–570
  neuromuscular blockade affected by, 357
  pathophysiology, 568
  preoperative preparation, 569
  recovery period, 569–570
Bus, 437, 438
Butorphanol, 336, 551
Butyrophenones, 299
Bypass, *see* Cardiopulmonary bypass

CABG, 52

CAD, *see* Coronary artery disease (CAD)
Caffeine
  neonatal bradycardia risk reduced with, 490
  neonatal postoperative apnea risk reduced with, 490
CAGE, *see* Cerebral arterial gas embolism (CAGE)
Calcitonin, 275
  calcium balance affected by, 215
  in hyperparathyroidism therapy, 260
  synthetic, for hypercalcemia, 275
Calcium
  in neonates, 484
  parathyroid regulating, 252
Calcium, ionized (Ca^{2+})
  balance in urologic system, 215
  in malignant hyperthermia, 297
  parathyroid hormone and, 275
  point-of-care analyzers, 404
  renal excretion, calcitonin and, 275
  serum, in hyperparathyroidism, 260
Calcium blockers, 99
Calcium chloride, **499**
Calcium metabolism, 252
Calculi, 260
Cancer
  breast, metastatic, 254
  carcinomas, *See* Carcinoma(s)
  intrathoracic, pulmonary embolus differentiated, 115
  lung, 12, 254
  metastatic disease, *see* Metastatic disease
  obesity and, 65
  sarcomas, doxorubicin as treatment of, 388
Capacative transducers, 101
Capacitance, 431, 432
Capillaries, 7
  diffusion of gas from alveolus to, 22
  prenatal, 481
Capnography, 176
Carbachol, 289
Carbamazepine, 167–168
Carbaminohemoglobin, 24
Carbidopa, 300
Carbohydrate enzymes, pancreas and, 254
Carbohydrate metabolism, 242
Carbon dioxide
  carbaminohemoglobin, 24
Carbon dioxide (CO_2)
  absorbers of, 46
  as acid base, 20–21
  circle breathing system, absorption in, 46
  concentration in blood, 24
  neonatal response to, 482

Rotameter measurement of, 398
  transport of, 24
Carbon dioxide tension (P_{CO_2}), 157
  bench top analyzers, 402–404
  continuous in vivo arterial blood gas monitor, 405
  point-of-care analyzers, 404
Carbonic anhydrase inhibitors, 224
Carbon monoxide, 170
  poisoning
    hyperbaric oxygen therapy for, 73, 75
    mechanism of injury, 73
  retention, in laryngotracheobronchitis, 496
Carbon-zinc batteries, 444
Carcinoids, 267–268
Carcinoid syndrome, 267
Carcinoma(s)
  hepatocellular, 249
  squamous cell, 389
  treatment of, 388
Cardiac arrest, *see* Ventricular fibrillation
Cardiac catheterization, 491
Cardiac cycle, 88
Cardiac function monitoring, 420–422
Cardiac impulse conduction disturbances, 121–122
Cardiac myocytes, 87
Cardiac output, 88
  aging and, 140
  in amniotic fluid embolism, 520
  anesthetic gas transfer proportional to, 47
  and blood volume ratio, 488
  decreased
    enflurane, 311
    halothane, 310
    methohexitone, 319
    as parasympathetic nervous system response, 281
    thiopentone, 318
  diprivan and, 320, 321
  factors in, 88
  fetal, 480
  hypothyroidism affecting, 259, 260
  neonatal, 485, 489
  obesity and, 66, 144
  in pregnancy, 500
Cardiac reserves, 260
Cardiac veins, anterior, 86
Cardiomyopathy, 110–113
  peripartum, 137
  ventricular function and, 89
Cardiopulmonary bypass, 116–118
  atrial natriuretic peptides and, 209
  coagulopathies in, 119–120
  in congenital heart disease, 128
  pancuronium used in, 367
  urologic effects of, 239

Cardiopulmonary resuscitation, neonatal, 497
Cardiorespiratory arrest, in preterm infants, 490
Cardiorespiratory evaluation, of obese patients, 68, 145
Cardioselective beta antagonists, 94–95
Cardiovascular collapse, 391
Cardiovascular depression, 328
Cardiovascular drugs, interactions with, 355
Cardiovascular implants, 428
Cardiovascular system, 83–87
  see also specific structures
  aging, 140
  anaphylaxis affecting, 391
  angiotensin II affecting, 206
  arginine vasopressin affecting, 209
  atracurium affecting, 359
  atrial natriuretic peptide affecting, 208
  benzodiazepines affecting, 340
  burn response of, 568
  cirrhosis affecting, 248
  desflurane affecting, 314
  diazepam affecting, 324
  diprivan affecting, 320
  disorders of
    see also specific disorders
    obesity and, 66–67
    theophylline causing, 34
  Doppler ultrasound, 102, 421–422
  droperidol affecting, 345
  d-tubocurarine affecting, 370
  echocardiogram, *see* Echocardiography
  electrical activity and conduction, 85–86
  electrophysiology, 103–104
  enflurane affecting, 311
  etomidate affecting, 321
  fentanyl affecting, 327
  flow and resistance, 100–101
  halothane affecting, 310
  hypothermia affecting, 295
  hypothyroidism affecting, 259
  isoflurane affecting, 312–313
  ketamine affecting, 323
  local anesthetics affecting, 351
  malignant hyperthermia affecting, 297
  methohexitone affecting, 319
  metocurine affecting, 364
  midazolam affecting, 325
  mivacurium affecting, 365
  myocardial innervation, 86
  obesity and, 66–67, 144
  in obstetrics, 129–139, 500
  pacemaker, permanent, 103
  pancuronium affecting, 366–367

  pathophysiology of aging, 140
  perinatal adaptation, 482
  pharmacology, 90–99
  physics of, 100–105
  physiology, 87–90
  pipecuronium affecting, 368
  pregnancy-induced hypertension affecting, 505–506
  reversal agents affecting, 380
  rocuronium and, 369
  scintigraphic imaging, 102–103
  succinylcholine affecting, 375
  systemic circulation, 86–87
Cardioversion, electrical, 103, 121
Carotid arteries, 86
  internal, 151, 255
Carotid sinus
  afferents in, 279
  baro-control receptors in, 90
Carotid surgery, 155
Cascade water humidifiers, 54
Catecholamines
  in induced hypotension, 293
  in neonates, 484
  pheochromocytoma and, 266
  production of, 253
Catheterization, cardiac, 491
Catheters
  central venous, 293
  Foley, in burn injuries, 569
  indwelling bladder, 293
  pulmonary artery, **416**
  pulmonary artery flotation, 69
  right arterial, positioning of, 177
  thermodilution, 220
Cauda equina syndrome, 173
Caudate lobe, 241
Causation, 574–575
CBF, *see* Cerebral blood flow (CBF)
CCr, 220, 259
Celiac artery, 87
Celiac ganglia, 280
Cells
  oxygen diffusion into, 24
  urinalysis of, 219
  in wireless telecommunications, 443
Cellular casts, 223
Cellular phones, 443
Central apnea, in infants, 489–490
Central channel, 353–354
Central cord syndrome, 171–172
Central line, in obese patients, 69
Central nervous system, 151–154
  see also specific structures
  aging and, 141
  belladonna alkaloids affecting, 99
  benzodiazepines affecting, 163, 340
  diazepam affecting, 324
  diprivan affecting, 320
  disorders of, 166–185

  see also Specific diseases and disorders
  pediatric, 185–191
  droperidol affecting, 345
  electrophysiology, 154–156
  etomidate affecting, 164, 321
  fentanyl affecting, 327
  histamine production and, 391
  ketamine affecting, 164, 323
  local anesthetics affecting, 350–351
  malignant hyperthermia affecting, 297
  methohexitone affecting, 319
  midazolam affecting, 325
  opioids affecting, 332
  physiology, 154–163
  in pregnancy, 501
  pregnancy-induced hypertension affecting, 505
  seizure activity, and electroconvulsant therapy, 564
  theophylline affecting, 34
  thiopentone affecting, 318–319
Central nervous system oxygen toxicity, 75
Central processor unit, 436–437
Central venous catheter, 293
Central venous line, 534
Central venous pressure lines, 416
  air embolism associated with, 174, 176
  sites for, 416
Cephalosporins, 234
Cerebellum, 151
Cerebral angiography
  in aneurysms, 179
  in brain death, 185
  for coma, 169
Cerebral arterial gas embolism (CAGE)
  causes, 71
  hyperbaric oxygen therapy for, 71, 75
Cerebral arteries, 151
Cerebral blood flow (CBF), 86–87, 156–157
  anesthetics effecting, **158**
  brain death and, 185
  control of, 157
  enflurane affecting, 311
  hypercarbia increasing, 51
  hypnotics affecting, 163
  hypocarbia decreasing, 51
  hypothermia affecting, 295
  sedatives affecting, 163
  thiopentone decreasing, 317
  vs function, 156–157
Cerebral blood volume (CBV), 156
Cerebral edema
  as diabetic ketoacidosis complication, 271

Cerebral edema, *continued*
high-altitude, 63
in near-drowning, 77
respiratory regulation affected by,
26–27
Cerebral hypoxia, 297
Cerebral ischemia, 297
Cerebral metabolic rate, 317
Cerebral metabolic requirements,
177–178
Cerebral perfusion pressure (CPP), 318
Cerebral protection, 177–179
Cerebral radionuclide scan, 169
Cerebral system
desflurane affecting, 314
disorders
see also specific disorders
in near-drowning, 77–78
positron emission tomography of,
446
enflurane affecting, 311–312
halothane affecting, 310
isoflurane affecting, 312–313
sevoflurane affecting, 315
Cerebral vasculature, 151–152
Arnold-Chiari malformation and, 187
Cerebral veins, 152
Cerebrospinal fluid (CSF), 157–158
absorption of, 157
anesthetic agents affecting, 158
drainage
as fiberoptic pressure probe
problem, 419
as subarachnoid bolt complication,
418
normal volume, 157
pediatric meningomyelocele, leakage
in, 186
production of, 157–158
Cerebrovascular accident
amniotic fluid embolism
differentiated, 520
diabetic ketoacidosis differentiated,
269
as electroconvulsant therapy
contraindication, 565
Cerebrovascular system
respiratory control affected by, 26
surgery of, electroencephalogram
used in, 155
Cerebrum, 151
Cervical laceration or tear, 521
Cervical spine
obesity and flexion of, 67, 145
vertebrae, 152
x-rays, 169
Cesarean section, 57
aortic stenosis and, 134
mitral regurgitation and, 133
mitral stenosis and, 132

peripartum cardiomyopathy and, 137
primary pulmonary hypertension and,
139
Tetralogy of Fallot and, 136–137
Channel, 442
Charged-couple device, 445
Chemical control of respiration, 25, 26
Chemicals, PVR influenced by, 18
Chemical urinalysis, 219
Chemotherapy
and cytotoxins, 387
kidney failure affecting, 234
Chest pain, 115
Chest wall rigidity, 332
Chest x-rays, 7–10
preoperative evaluation, 50
in pulmonary atresia, 491
in pulmonary embolism, 115
Cheyne-Stokes breathing, 26–27
Children
see also Infants; Neonates; Premature
infants
Apert's syndrome, 191
Arnold-Chiari malformation in, *see*
Arnold-Chiari malformation
cerebral arteriovenous malformations
in, 182
craniofacial reconstruction in, 191
craniosynostosis in, 189–191
Crouzon's disease, 191
diving reflex in, 77
Duchenne type muscular dystrophy
in, 60
meningomyelocele in, 185–187
mivacurium use in, 365
phenobarbital as seizure treatment
in, 167
pipecuronium in, 368
thiopentone dose in, 317
vecuronium in, 372
Chips, 433–434
Chi-square test, 458–459
Chloride
balance in urologic system, 216
as halothane metabolite, 310–311
pseudohyperparathyroidism and
levels of, 261
serum, in hyperparathyroidism, 260
Chloroform, 170
Chloroprocaine, 352
neurotoxicity of, 351
Chlorpromazine, 31
Cholangitis, 246–247
Choledocholithiasis, 247
Cholelithiasis, obesity and, 65
biliary excretion altered by, 67
Cholesterol
hypercholesterolemia, 105
hypothyroidism affecting, 259
smoking and, 105

Cholinergic receptors, 353
agonists, 289–291
muscarinic antagonists, *see*
Muscarinic antagonists
nicotinic antagonists, 291–292
succinylcholine stimulating, 375
Cholinesterase, 374–375
Chorionic tissue, 257
Christmas disease, 541
Chronic anemia, 537–538
Chronic asthma, VC and, 12
Chronic bronchitis, 49
vital capacity (VC) and, 12
Chronic cholelithiasis, 247
Chronic hypertension
as induced hypotension
contraindication, 293
in pregnancy, 504
Chronic hypocalcemia, 261
Chronic kidney failure, 232
Chronic obstructive pulmonary disease
(COPD), 49
atrial natriuretic peptides and, 209
ipratropium bromide for, 33
pulmonary embolus differentiated,
115
spirometry in, 12
Chronic pain
electroconvulsant therapy for, 565
intervention techniques, 558
multidisciplinary approach to,
561–562
theories on, 543
treatment, 543–558, 565
Chronic pain syndromes, 565
Chronologic age, 139
Chronotropy, 89
Cigarette smoking, 105
Ciliary ganglia, 281, 571
Cimetidine, 527–528
Cine computed tomography, 446
Circle breathing system, **45–46**
Circle of Willis, 86–87, 151
Circuit, 432
Circuit elements, 432
Circulation
cerebral, *see* Cerebral blood flow
(CBF)
collateral, in acromegaly, 257
coronary
microanatomy, 89
venous drainage, 86
fetal, 126, 479–480
in heat stroke, 147
mechanical circulatory assist devices,
104
persistent fetal, 480, 482
postnatal, transition to, 480
pulmonary, *see* Pulmonary circulation
sevoflurane affecting, 315

systemic, 86–87
Cirrhosis
  chronic, 247
  clinical features, 248
  death rates, 248
  liver transplantation for, 249
  signs and symptoms, 248
Cisatracurium, **360**–361
Cisplatin, 232
Civil liability, 573
Clark polarographic electrode, 410
Clearance
  defined, 305
  of local anesthetic, 349
Cleft palate, 495
Clinical data, 450
Clinical trials, 461–462
Clocks, in microprocessors, 437
Clonic seizures, 167
Clonidine, 98, 285–286
  kidney failure affecting, 234
  naloxone antagonism of, 330
Closed breathing system, 43
  circle system as, 45–46
Closing capacity, obesity and, 144
Clostridial myonecrosis
  hyperbaric oxygen therapy for, 73–74,
    75
  mechanism of injury, 73
Clotting factors
  dysfunction of, coagulation defects
    and, 119
  synthesis of, 242
CO, *see* Cardiac output
Coagulation, 534–535
  anesthetics affecting, 542
  pregnancy-induced hypertension
    affecting, 506
  tests of, 242–243
Coagulopathies, 118–120
  in abdominal aorta aneurysm, 120
  in amniotic fluid embolism, 519
  anemia, necrotizing enterocolitis and,
    493
  dilutional, 531
  homeostasis, 119
  liver disease and, 242
  as liver transplantation complication,
    249
  pathophysiology, 119
  physiology, 118
  pulmonary embolus and, 114
  as ventriculostomy contraindication,
    418
  Von Willebrand factor, 119
Coanalgesics, 553–555
Coaxial cable, 439–440
Coccygeal vertebrae, 152
Cockcroft equation, 202
Code division multiple access, 443

Codeine
  as opiate agonist, 549–550
  platelet transfusions and, 532
Coefficient of correlation, 460–461
Coefficient of variation (CV), 449
Cold intolerance, 259
Collecting duct, 212
Colored microspheres, 220
Color flow Doppler (CFD), 422
Columnator helmet, 567
Coma, 169
  barbiturates for induction of, 164
  hyperosmolar nonketonic coma,
    271–273
  myxedema, 259
Compartmental approach, 304–305
Complex partial convulsion, 167
Complex variable, 470
Compliance, respiratory, 13
  in infants, 483–484
  left ventricular, obesity and, 67
Compressed air, breathing, 71–72
Compressed gas, 52
Compressed Gas Association, 428
Compression stockings, 115
Compressive spondylosis, 172
Computed tomography, 446
  of chest, 10
  for coma, 169
  contrast, of urologic system, 196
  of craniosynostosis, 189
  dynamic, in renal blood flow
    measurement, 220
  emission, 446
  in intracranial aneurysms, 179
  outside operating room, 564
Computer networks, 438–442
Concentration effect, 48–49
Conditional probability, 450
Conduction, neonatal heat exchange
    via, 487
Conductive floors, 429
Conductors, 431
Congenital defects
  chronic intracranial hypertension
    caused by, 184
  heart disease, *see* Congenital heart
    disease
Congenital heart disease, 125–128
  cyanosis in, 127
    retinopathy of prematurity and, 486
  and neonatal erythropoiesis activity,
    260
  postnatal, 480
  in pregnancy, 129, 134–137
  and pulmonary atresia, 491
Congenital lobar emphysema, 493
Congestive heart failure
  as electroconvulsant therapy
    contraindication, 565

  in pulmonary atresia, 491
  pulmonary embolus differentiated,
    115
Conjugation, in hepatic drug
    metabolism, 241
  opioids, 332
Consciousness, level of, 169
Constipation
  as hypothyroidism symptom, 259
  from opioid drugs, 547
Constrictive chest wall lesions, 12
Continuous hemodialysis, 236
Continuous in vivo arterial blood gas
    monitors, 405
Continuous positive airway pressure,
    413
Continuous probability distribution,
    452
Continuous-wave Doppler ultrasound,
    421
Contractility, increased
  as fight-or flight response, 280
  sympathetic nervous system causing,
    280
Contracts, 577
Contrast CT, of urologic system, 196
Controlled clinical trial, 461–462
Controlled ventilation
  with critical care ventilators, 53
  in induced hypotension, 293
Contusion, central cord syndrome
    caused by, 171
Conus medullaris syndrome, 173
Convection, neonatal heat exchange
    via, 487
Convulsions, 166–169
  see also Seizures
Cooley's anemia, 537
Copper kettle vaporizers, 35–36
Core body temperature measurement,
    295
Coronary arteries, 86
Coronary artery disease (CAD)
  aging and, 140
  obesity and, 65
  in pregnancy, 137–138
  risk factors, 137
Coronary blood flow
  microanatomy, 89
  venous drainage, 86
Coronary heart disease, in pregnancy,
    129
Coronary sinus, 83, 86
Corporations, 577
Correlation, 459, 460–461
Cortical necrosis, 229
Corticospinal tract, 160
Corticosteroids, **277**
  for asthma in pregnancy, 55
  as bronchodilators, 34, 55

Corticosteroids, *continued*
  and fetal lung maturation, 481
  in gestational diabetes, 511
  as laryngotracheobronchitis
      treatment, 496
  in pregnancy, 55, 481, 511
Corticotropin-related peptides, 274
Cortisol, 264
  see also Hydrocortisone
  adrenal suppression of, 322
  adrenocortical insufficiency and, 264
  blood pressure and, 90
  excess, 262
  mineralocortical insufficiency and,
      264
  phosphate reabsorption and, 216
  release during surgery, 262
  stress and, 275
Cortisone, **277**
Cough
  in elderly patients, 141–142
  in high-altitude pulmonary edema, 63
  in laryngotracheobronchitis, 496
  as pulmonary embolism symptom,
      115
Coumadin, 115
Coumarin, 130–131
Cranial nerves
  dysfunctions of
    Arnold-Chiari malformation and,
        187–188
    trismus, 297–298
    facial (VII) nerve, 571
    glossopharyngeal nerve (IX), 279
    oculomotor (III) nerve, 571
    trigeminal nerve, 297–298
    vagus, *see* Vagus (X) nerve
Cranial vault, 183
Craniectomy, strip, 189
Craniofacial reconstruction, in
      children, 191
Craniosynostosis, 189–191
Craniotomy
  electroencephalogram used in, 155
  epidural ICP monitor insertion via,
      419
Creatinine
  in diabetic ketoacidosis, 270
  plasma, 220
  in pregnancy, 501
  preoperative evaluation of, 239
  production, and muscle mass,
      220–221
  serum, 221
Creatinine clearance, 220
  hypothyroidism affecting, 259
Cricoid cartilage, 4
Cricoid mucosa, 483
Cricoid ring, in infants, 483
Criminal liability, 573

Critical care ventilators, 52–53
Critical hypoxia, 62
Critical pressure, 43
Critical temperature, 42–43
Cromolyn, 55
Cromolyn sodium, 34
Croup, 496
Crouzon's disease, 191
Cryoprecipitate transfusion, 533
Crystalline solids, 432–433
Curare, 291
Current, 431
  source of, 432
Cushing's disease, 262
Cushing's syndrome, 262
Cutaneous flushing, 268
CXR, 127–128
Cyanocobalamin, 220
Cyanosis
  anaphylaxis causing, 391
  in congenital heart disease, 126, 127,
      486
  in high-altitude pulmonary edema, 63
  methemoglobinemia causing, 351
  in pulmonary atresia, 491
  as pulmonary embolism sign, 115
  retinopathy of prematurity and, 486
  Tetralogy of Fallot in pregnancy and,
      137
Cyclosporin, 386–387, 387
Cylinders
  E cylinders, 37, 38, **39**
  ensuring proper connections, 38
  oxygen, 37
  Pin Index Safety System, 38, **39**
Cystic duct obstruction, 247
Cystoscopy, transurethral, 238
Cysts, central cord syndrome caused by,
      172
Cytochrome P-450, 243
  enzyme induction, 244
  foreign substances in lung and, 31
  halothane and, 310–311
  lungs as site for oxidation by, 28–29
  sevoflurane and, 316
Cytotoxins
  see also specific cytotoxins
  classification, 387–388
  indications, 387
  neoplastic disease, use in, 387

Dalton's law, 35, 61
Damages, 574–575
Dantrolene, 300
Data acquisition
  by computed tomography, 446
  by microprocessor, 436–437
Dead space, in newborns, 484
Death
  brain death, 185

  local anesthetics causing, 350
  natural death acts, 579
  sudden, *see* Sudden death
  sudden infant death syndrome, 490
  transfusion-related, 249
Death rates
  cirrhosis, 248
  ischemic heart disease, 105
Decamethonium, 296
Decompression sickness
  etiology, 72–73
  hyperbaric oxygen therapy for, 72–73,
      75
Deep femoral arteries, 87
Deep venous thrombosis, 114
Defense Advanced Research Project
      Agency, 441
Defensive mechanism, of lungs, 28
Defibrillation, 103
Defibrillators, 428
Definite integral, 465–466
Degeneration, of intervertebral disk, 152
Degreasing agents, as fuel, 429
Degree of freedom (df), 449
Dehydration, 492
Dental air drills, 174
Department of Health and Human
      Services, 423
Department of Transportation (DOT)
      regulations, 37
Dependence, on opioid drugs, 546–547
Depolarization, 162, 373
Depolarizing muscle relaxants, 354,
      373–378
  characteristics, 373
  hypothermia affecting, 356
Depressant drugs, 260
Depth and adequacy of anesthesia
  awareness and, 159
  central nervous system and, 158–159
  history, 158–159
  monitoring, 159
Descending inhibitory pathways,
      159–160
Desflurane
  central nervous system affected by,
      164, 314
  effect on organ systems, 314
  physical properties, 314
  urinary system, effects on, 228
  vaporizers used with, 36
Detector, in gas chromatography, 407
Deutscher Normenauschuss, 428
Dexamethasone, **277**
Dexamethasone suppression test, 262
Dexmedetomidine, 285
  as cerebral protection, 178
Dextran, 115
Dextromethorphan, 178
Dezocine, 551

Diabetes
    arytenoid cartilage affected by, 4
    obesity and, 65, 67
Diabetes insipidus, 255–256
Diabetes mellitus, 268–273
    as arteriosclerosis risk factor, 105
    gestational, 510–511
    hyperosmolar nonketonic coma,
        271–273
Diabetes mellitus, continued
    ketoacidosis associated with, 269–271
    obesity and, 67, 144
    perioperative management, 268
    in pregnancy, 510–511
Diabetic ketoacidosis, 269–271
    absent in hyperosmolar nonketonic
        coma, 272
Dialysis
    as hyperparathyroidism therapy, 260
    in kidney failure therapy, 236
Diaphragmatic hernia, neonatal, 490
Diaphragmatic muscles, 12
    left ventricle and, 83
Diaphragm pressure gauge, 101
Diarrhea, 268
Diastole, 88, 89
Diastolic coronary perfusion, 104
Diastolic filling, 88
Diastolic function, 89
Diastolic pressure, 89
Diatrizoate, 220
Diazepam, 340–341
    as IV induction agent, 323–324
    as seizure treatment, 167
    local anesthetics-induced seizure, 350
Dielectrics, 431
Diet, see Nutrition
Diethyl ether, 158–159
Differential equations, 467–468
Digital data compression, 443
Digital integrated circuits, 434
Digitalis, in pregnancy, 130
Digital mobile phone service, 443
Digoxin, 234
Dilated cardiomyopathy, 110–111
Diltiazem, 96
Dilutional coagulopathy, 531
DINAMAP, 414
2-3-Diphosphoglycerate (DPG), 500
Diprivan, 319–321
Dipyridamole perfusion scintigraphy,
        102
Disclosure
    of HIV status, 578
    of treatment risks, 573–574
Discovery in litigation, 576
Disk degeneration, 152
Disk herniation, 152
Disopyramide, 93
Dispersion chamber, 406

Disposable devices, 429
Disseminated intravascular
        coagulation, 535
Dissolved gas, 64
Distal tubule, 194, 203
Distribution, 304–305
    see also Uptake and distribution
    Fa/Fi ratio, 308
    regional blood flow and, 308
Diuresis
    in ascites therapy, 248
    solute, polyuria differentiated, 256
Diuretics
    for cardiac/hydrostatic pulmonary
        edema, 54
    central nervous system affected by,
        165
    in hyperparathyroidism therapy, 260
    kidney failure affecting, 234
    osmotic, 227
    potassium-sparing, 227–228
    thiazide, 227, 262
    urinary system, 224–228
Diving, scuba, see Scuba diving
Diving reflex, 77
Dizocilipine, 178
Dobutamine, 92, 287
Dobutamine hydrochloride, **499**
Doctor-patient relationship, 575, 578
Domain Name System (DNS), 441
Domain of f', 464
Dopamine, 282
    as beta agonist, 287–288
    as inotrope, 91–92
    renal effects, 92
        acid-base balance, 212
        in cardiopulmonary bypass, 239
        renal vascular resistance, 197
        tubular function, 206
    as vasodilator, 480
    as vasopressor, 165
Dopamine adrenoreceptors, 91–92,
        283, 284, 299
Dopamine agonists, 300
Dopamine hydrochloride, **499**
Dopexamine, 288
Doppler effect, 421
Doppler ultrasound, 421–422
    of air embolism, 176
    of blood flow rate, 220, 399–400
    cardiovascular measurement, 102,
        421–422
    continuous-wave Doppler ultrasound,
        102, 421–422
    duplex scanners, 422
    pulse wave, 102
    renal blood flow, 220
    transcranial, 185
Dorsal respiratory group, 25
Double blind trials, 462

Double-burst stimulation, 383
Double lumen tube, 51
Doxacurium, **361**–362
Doxorubicin, 388–389
Dp/dt, 89
D-Penicillamine, 355
Dreams, ketamine causing, 323
Dromotropy, 89
Drop attacks, 167
Droperidol, 344–345
Drowning, near-, 76–80
Drug absorption, 306
Drug displacement, in aging, 142
Drug-induced hepatitis, 246
Drug interactions
    with atracurium, 359
    with atrial natriuretic peptide,
        208–209
    with cardiovascular drugs, 355
    with cistracurium, 361
    with exogenous steroids, 265
    in gestational diabetes, 511
    with muscle relaxants, 355
    neuromuscular blockade affected by,
        355–356
Drug metabolism
    benzodiazepines, 339, 340
    bromide as halothane metabolite,
        310–311
    and cytochrome P-450, 243
    halothane metabolites, 310–311
    in hepatic system, 241
    hypothyroidism affecting, 260
    liver failure and, 248
Drug reactions, 390–394
Drugs
    excretion of, see Excretion of drugs
    as exogenous toxins, 170
    hyperosmolar nonketonic coma,
        associated with, 272
Drug transport, 306
    pulmonary circulation for, 87
Dry skin, 259
D-tubocurarine, **369**–371
Duchenne's muscular dystrophy, 60
    malignant hyperthermia associated
        with, 298
    pulmonary manifestations, 60
Ductus arteriosus, 480
    in pulmonary atresia, 491
Duodenum, phosphate absorbed at,
        216
Duplex scanners, 422
Dura mater, spinal, 154
Duty, 574–575
Dysphagia
    Arnold-Chiari malformation and, 187
    supraglottitis, associated with, 496
Dyspnea
    anaphylaxis causing, 391

Dyspnea, *continued*
  as diabetic ketoacidosis sign, 269
  in high-altitude pulmonary edema, 63
  as pulmonary embolism symptom,
      115
Dysrhythmias, 120–125
  see also specific dysrhythmias
  antidysrhythmics, *see*
      Antidysrhythmics
  cardiac, 122–124
  cardiac impulse conduction
      disturbances, 121–122
  diagnosis, 120–121
  pathogenesis, 120
  preexcitation syndromes, 124–125
  prolonged QT syndrome, 125, 261
  treatment, 120
Dystrophies, 60–61
  Becker's muscular dystrophy, 60
  Duchenne type muscular dystrophy,
      60, 298
  myotonic dystrophy, 60–61, 359
  posttraumatic, 559
  reflex sympathetic, 160, 559
Dysuria, 239

Earth orbit communication systems, 444
ECG, *see* Electrocardiogram
Echocardiography, 102
  in air embolism, 175
  generation of image, 102
  in pericardial effusion, 113
  in pulmonary atresia, 491
  in pulmonary embolism, 115
Eclampsia, 504
  acute kidney failure caused by, 230
  amniotic fluid embolism
      differentiated, 520
Ecothiopate, 290
Edema
  alveolar, 13
  American College of Obstetricians
      and Gynecologists definition, 504
  anaphylaxis causing, 391
  as anesthetic emergency, 391
  in burn injuries, 568
  cerebral, *see* Cerebral edema
  of cricoid mucosa, in infants, 483
  with laryngotracheobronchitis, 496
  periorbital, 259
  pulmonary, *see* Pulmonary edema
  small airway obstruction in infants
      caused by, 481
  transcutaneous P_{O_2} monitoring
      affected by, 410
EDHF, 198
EDRF, 197
Edrophonium
  acetylcholinesterase and break down
      of, 379

  as anticholinesterase, 290
EDTA, 220
Education, in chronic pain treatment,
      543
EEG, *see* Electroencephalogram
Effective renal plasma flow (eRPF),
      219–220
Effusion
  pericardial, *see* Pericardial effusion
  pleural, *see* Pleural effusion
Eicosanoids, 31
Eisenmenger's complex, 126
Eisenmenger's syndrome, in pregnancy,
      135–136
Ejection fraction, 89
Ejection phase of cardiac cycle, 88
  hypothyroidism affecting, 259
EKG, *see* Electrocardiogram
Elastase transport, 29
Elderly persons
  cough in, 141–142
  d-tubocurarine in, 370
  endotracheal tube removal in, 141
  exaggerated anesthetic effects in, 142
  fluid balance in, 218
  glomerular filtration rate in, 202
  muscle relaxants in, 142, 357
  pipecuronium in, 368
  protein binding in, 307
  pyelonephritis causing acute kidney
      failure, 232
  regional anesthesia in, 143
  renal acid-base balance in, 213
  sodium balance in, 213
Elective vs emergency surgery, 140
Electrical cardioversion, 103, 121
Electrical charge, 431
  blood-placental barrier and, 501
Electrical left ventricle assist system,
      104
Electricity, 426, 431–432
Electric power
  distribution in hospitals, 425–426
  patient safety, 425–428
  for ventilators, 52
Electrocardiogram
  ambulatory, safety standards, 428
  in burn injuries, 569
  neonatal, 485
  in obese patients, 69, 146
  in ophthalmic surgery, 571
  in pericardial effusion, 113
  in pericarditis, 113
  in pulmonary atresia, 491
  in rhythm disorders, 120
Electroconvulsant therapy (ECT),
      564–566
Electroencephalogram, 154–155
  as anesthetic depth monitor, 159
  in brain death, 185

  in complex partial convulsion, 167
  during electroconvulsant therapy, 564
  in induced hypotension, 293
  scalp, 154
  in seizures, 167
  thiopentone affecting, 317
Electrolytes
  electric charge of, 431
  imbalances, in near-drowning and
      arrhythmias, 78
  in kidney failure therapy, 235–236
  neuromuscular blockage affected by,
      356
  regulation, in hepatic system, 242
  urinalysis, 219
Electromagnetic blood flow monitor,
      399
Electromedical apparatus, 434–438
  risk categories, 427
  safe current limits for, 427–428
  transducers, *see* Transducers
Electromyography, 384
Electronic mail (e-mail), 441
Electrosurgical devices
  safety standards, 428
  spark from, 429
Elevated anion gap metabolic acidosis,
      269
Elimination, 304–305
  of benzodiazepines, 340
  Hofmann, of atracurium, 358
  of naloxone, 337
  of narcotics, 548–549
  renal, *see* Renal drug elimination
ELISA, 392
Embolectomy, pulmonary, 115
Embolism
  air, *see* Air embolism
  amniotic fluid, 519–520
  pulmonary, *see* Pulmonary embolism
  reflex response by respiratory system,
      28
Emergence delirium, 323
Emergency vs elective surgery, 140
Emission computed tomography, 446
Emotionally demanding, obese persons
      as, 67, 145
Emphysema, 49
  bullous, 49
  congenital lobar, 493
  pulmonary vascular resistance and,
      19
Employment, 577
Empyema, 10
Encainide, 94
Encephalopathy, hepatic, 248
Enclosure, of electromedical apparatus,
      427
Endarteritis, 19
Endobronchial fiberoptic intubation, 51

Endocardial fibrosis, 268
Endocardial viability ratio, 104
Endocrine system, 252
    see also specific structures and
        disorders
    hypothermia affecting, 295
    kidney failure affecting, 233
    obesity and, 66, 67, 144
    pharmacology, 274–277
    pregnancy complications, 510–515
Endogenous vasoactive compounds,
        29–30
    see also specific compounds
Endometrium, 523
Endorphins, 331
    concentrations, in pregnancy, 501
Endoscope
    GI endoscopy, 175, 564
    optic fibers in, 435
Endothelial derived hyperpolarizing
        factor, 198
Endothelial derived relaxing factor, 197
Endothelin, 198–199
Endotracheal intubation
    chest x-ray of position of, 8
    in gestational diabetes, 511
    in laryngotracheobronchitis, 496
    removal in eldcrly patients, 141
    secretions in tube, 492
    size of tube, in acromegaly, 257
Endotracheal suction, 485
End-tidal CO_2, in obese patients, 69,
        146
Energy band model, 432–433
Energy density, 444
Enflurane, 311–312
    central nervous system affected by,
        164
    seizures and, 168
Enterochromaffin cells, 267
Enzymes
    induction, 244
    thiopentone affecting, 318
Eosinophil chemotactic factor, 391
Eosinophilic granuloma, 254
Eosinophiluria, 223
Ephedrine, 98
    in pregnancy, 130
Epidural anesthesia
    in gestational diabetes, 511
    in pregnancy, 56
        atrial septal defect and, 134
        primary pulmonary hypertension
            and, 138–139
        ventricular septal defect and, 135
    in pregnancy-induced hypertension,
        508
    in transvaginal aspiration, 524–525
Epidural blockade, 299
Epidural ICP monitoring, 419

Epidural tumor, 173
Epigastric omphalocele, neonatal, 494
Epiglottis
    innervation, 4
    neonatal, 482
Epilepsy
    psychomotor, 319
    temporal lobe, 166
Epinephrine, 282, 287
    adrenal medulla releasing, 280
    in anaphylaxis treatment, 392
    atracurium, drug interactions with,
        359
    as beta agonist, 33
    enflurane and, 311
    halothane and, 310
    as inotrope, 91
    in pediatric life support, **499**
    racemic, **496**
    renal blood flow affected by, 201
    as vasoconstrictor, 349, 350
    as vasopressors, 165
EPO, *see* Erythropoietin
Equianalgesic doses, **546**
Ergot alkaloid, 286
Ergot preparations, 502
Erythroblastosis fetalis, 515
Erythrocyte(s)
    chronic hypoxemia affecting
        production of, 488
    disorders of, 537–539
    sympathetic nervous system affecting,
        281
Erythropoiesis, 535–536
Erythropoietin, 210, 535–536
    at birth, 488
    chronic hypoxemia affecting
        production of, 488
    disease interactions, 210
    effects, 210
    kinetics, 210
    production, 210, 223–224
    release, 210, 223–224
    therapy, 224
Escherichia coli endotoxin, 18
Esmolol, 95, 289
    in pregnancy, 131
    for pregnancy-induced hypertension,
        508
Ester-allergic reactions, 393
Ester local anesthetics, 351
Ethanol, 170
Ether, 170
Ethical issues
    controlled human clinical trials, 462
    at end of life, 578–579
Ethmoid sinus, 3
Ethmozine, 94
Ethosuxamide, 167
Ethylene glycol, 170

Etidocaine, 352
Etomidate
    central nervous system affected by,
        164, 321
    as IV induction agent, 321–322
    seizures and, 168
Eustachian (pharyngotypamic) tube, 3
Evaporation, neonatal heat exchange
        via, 487
Evoked potentials, 155–156
Evoked response, 381
Excitatory amino acids, 178
Excretion
    of adenosine deaminase binding
        protein, 223
    of amylase, 223
    of beta$_2$-microglobulin, 223
    biliary, *see* Biliary excretion
    by liver, 243
    of potassium, 263, 275
    renal, *see* Renal excretion
    sodium, 90, 238
    tubule damage and, 223
    as tubules injury indication, 223
Excretion of drugs
    aging and, 141
    etomidate, 321
    fentanyl, 327
    ketamine, 322
    midazolam, 325
    molecular weight affecting, 245
    polarity affecting, 245
    renal, *see* Renal excretion
    sufentanil, 328
    thiopentone, 317
    in urine, 245
Exercise
    as ischemic heart disease risk factor,
        105
    oxygen transport and, 23
    respiration regulation and, 26
Exogenous iodine, 275
Exogenous steroids, 265
Exogenous toxins, 170–171
Expiration, 13
    and airway resistance, 16
    forced expiratory flow rate, 15
    peak expiratory flow rate, 15, 50
    positive end expiratory pressure, 53,
        413
Expiratory pressures, 413
Expiratory reserve volume (ERV),
        10–11
Explicit awareness, 159
Explosion and fire hazards, 428–430
Exponential function, 468
Express consent, 574
External centrifugal pumps, 104
External intercostal muscles, 12
External pulsatile assist devices, 104

Extracellular fluid volume(s)
  hypothyroidism affecting, 259
  increased by kidney failure, 233
  in lungs, 27
Extracorporeal membrane oxygenation
      (ECMO), 104
  in neonatal diaphragmatic hernia, 490
Extramedullary tumor, dorsal, 173
Extrapulmonary problems, lung
      compliance and, 13
Extravascular transducer, 415
Extubation
  in burn injuries, 569
  in supraglottitis, 497
  in transesophageal fistula, 492
Ex vivo monitors, 405
Eye
  innervation of, 571
  muscles traction, neonatal
      bradycardia due to, 485
  ophthalmic surgery, 570–572
Eyebrow, lateral thinning of, 259

Facial fractures, 3
Facial (VII) nerve, 571
Facilitated diffusion, 306
F-actin, 87
Fa/Fi ratio, 308
Fallopian tube trauma, 523
Famotidine, 527–528
Fat compartment, obesity affecting, 67,
      145
Fatigue
  electricity causing, 426
  as hypothyroidism symptom, 259
Fatty acids, 14
FDA Policy Board, 423
Febrile convulsions, 167
Federal Food Drug and Cosmetic Act,
      423–424
Femoral arteries, 87
Fentanyl
  body weight and, 145
  central nervous system affected by,
      163
  as IV induction agent, 326–328
  as opiate agonist, 550
  as opioid agonist, 333–334
  sufentanil compared, 329
Fetal channels, 480
Fetal deceleration patterns, 503
Fetal gasping, 481, 482
Fetal hemoglobin (HbF), 488
  oxygen unloading capacity of,
      488–489
Fetal monitoring, 503–504
  predicting need for neonatal
      resuscitation, 498
Fetal scalp blood sampling, 503–504
Fetal ultrasound sonography, 186

Fetal umbilical vein, 479
  hemoglobin in blood, 488
Fetus
  beta-blockers affecting, 131
  circulation of, 127, 479–480
  development of, surfactant formed
      late in, 14, 481
  gestational diabetes affecting, 510
  heart rate, 503
Fever(s)
  bleomycin causing, 389
  as induced hypotension
      contraindication, 293
  as pulmonary embolism sign, 115
  supraglottitis, associated with, 496
Fiberoptic intubation, 50–51
  awake, 51
    in acromegaly, 257
    in neonatal diaphragmatic hernia,
      490
Fiberoptic pressure probe, 418–419
Fibrillation
  atrial, 123, 132
  defibrillation, 103
  defibrillators, 428
  ventricular, see Ventricular
      fibrillation
Fibrin degradation products (FDP),
      242
Fibrinolysis, 119
Fibrosis
  bleomycin causing, 389
  endocardial, 268
  pulmonary, see Pulmonary fibrosis
Fibrotic pleurisy, 12
Fight-or-flight system, 279
File service, 440
Filing a lawsuit, 576
Filtration
  glomerular, see Glomerular filtration
  lungs providing defensive, 28
  particulate, 28
  pulmonary circulation for, 87
Fire hazards, 428–430
First-degree atrioventricular heart
      block, 121
First order, first degree, 467–468
Fistula, neonatal tracheoesophageal,
      492–493
5-HIAA, 267
5-HT, 30
  see also Serotonin
5-Hydroxyindoleacetic acid
  carcinoid syndrome and, 267
  as metabolite of serotonin, 267
5-Hydroxytryptamine, 30
  see also Serotonin
51W89, **373**
Fixed cardiac output syndromes
  and methohexitone, 319

and thiopentone, 318
Flammability limits, 429
Flammable anesthetic agents, 428, 430
Flank pain, 239
Flecainide, 94
Flow
  through orifice, 100–101
  through tube, 100–101
Flowmeter, gas Rotameter, 100–101,
      398
Fluid exchange in lungs, 27
Fluid overload, 238
Fluid resuscitation, 569
Fluids replacement
  see also Hydration
  in burn injuries, 569
  as hyperosmolar nonketonic coma
      therapy, 273
  as hyperparathyroidism therapy, 260
Fluid wave, in ascites, 248
Flumazenil, 163
  as benzodiazepine antagonist, 343
  as IV induction agent, 325–326
Fluoride
  acute kidney failure caused by, 231
  as enflurane metabolite, 312
  ion release, in obese persons, 145
  sevoflurane, and concentration of,
      316
Flushing
  anaphylaxis causing, 391
  as cistracurium side effect, 360
Focal neurologic exam, 169
Folate deficiency, 537–538
Foley catheter, 569
Folic acid, 185
Follicle, thyroid hormone stored in, 274
Foramen ovale, 480
  closure of, 482
  in pulmonary atresia, 491
Foramina, 152
Forced expiratory flow rate between 25
      and 75% exhaled volume
      (FEF$_{25-75}$), 15
Foreign substances, 31
Formoterenol, 33
Fourier transform, 471
Fractional secretion of any substance,
      221–222
Fractures
  chest x-rays for, 8
  as electroconvulsant therapy
      contraindication, 565
  facial, 3
  of mandible, 3
  pathologic, as hypercalcemia sign,
      260
  of zygomatic arch, 3
Frank-Starling curve
  cardiac output and, 88

in neonates, 484

FRC, see Functional residual capacity (FRC)

Free plasma drugs, 306

Free-water clearance, 223
  diabetes insipidus and, 256
  hypothyroidism affecting, 260

Frequency-dependent blockade, 347

Frequency distribution, 449

Frequency hopping, 443

Fresh-water aspiration, 77

Friedreich's ataxia, 173

Frontal sinus, 3

Frozen plasma transfusion, 532–533

Fulminant hepatic failure, 249

Function (f), 463
  derivative of, 464–465
  domain of, 464

Functionalization, in hepatic drug metabolism, 241

Functional residual capacity (FRC), 11
  anesthetic diluted in, 47
  gas uptake into, 47
  in infants, 483–484
  obesity affecting, 66

Furosemide
  central nervous system affected by, 165
  compatabilities, **225**
  effects, 224–226
  interactions, 226
  kidney failure affecting, 234
  kinetics, 224

GaAs, 433

Gadolinium-DTPA, 220

Gallbladder, 241

Gallstones, 247

Gamete intrafallopian transfer (GIFT), 523

Gamma-glutamyl transaminase tests, 243

Gamma knife, 567–658

Ganglia
  see specific ganglia
  basal, 151, 261
  ciliary, 281, 571
  parasympathetic, 281–282
  stellate, 86, 280
  sympathetic, 280

Ganglion blocking agents
  stellate, 125
  trimethaphan, see Trimethaphan

Gas(es)
  dissolved, 64
  inspired and expired, measurement of, 406–408

Gas chromatography, 407–408

Gaseous oxygen, see Oxygen, compressed

Gas evacuation (scavenging), 38–40

Gas exchange
  aging and, 140
  perinatal, 482
  perioperative changes in, 52
  prenatal development of, 481
  pulmonary circulation and, 87

Gas flow rate measurement, 398–401

Gas gangrene, hyperbaric oxygen therapy for, 73–74, 75

Gas laws
  Boyle's law, see Boyle's law
  Dalton's law, 35, 61
  Henry's law, see Henry's law
  Pascal's law, 35, 61

Gas transfer, 47

Gas transport
  barriers to, 22
  concentration of gas, 21
  diffusion of, 21–22

Gastric emptying, 260

Gastric pH, obesity and, 67, 144

Gastric pressure, 526

Gastric volume in fasting state, obesity and, 67, 144

Gastrointestinal mucosa, 267

Gastrointestinal system
  amrinone affecting, 92
  doxorubicin affecting, 389
  fentanyl affecting, 327
  hypothermia affecting, 295
  kidney failure affecting, 233
  NSAIDs affecting, 338, 552
  obesity and, 66, 67, 144
  in pregnancy, 501

Gastrokinetic agents, in obese patients, 68, 146

Gastroparesis, 259

Gastroschisis, neonatal, 494

Gastrotomy, 492

Gas volume measurement, 401

Gaucher's disease, 537

Gauge pressure, 101

Ge, 433

Gender
  as arteriosclerosis risk factor, 105
  hyperthyroidism and, 257
  and lung capacities, 11

General anesthesia
  age-related effects, 141, 143
  in autonomic hyperreflexia prevention, 299
  central nervous system and, 158
  lung compliance reduced with, 13
  malignant hyperthermia during, 296
  in obese patients, 69, 147
  perioperative changes in gas exchange, 52
  in pregnant patients
    during Cesarean section, 57, 137
    Eisenmenger's syndrome, 136

gestational diabetes, 511
induction, 129
peripartum cardiomyopathy, 137
pregnancy-induced hypertension, 509–510
primary pulmonary hypertension, 138
regional combined with, 69, 147
for status epilepticus, 168
urologic system affected by, 228
vs regional anesthesia, 143

Generalized pain disorders, 558–562

Generalized seizures, 167

Genetic factors
  in craniosynostosis, 189
  in malignant hyperthermia, 296
  in obesity, 145

Genitourinary system
  see specific structures and disorders
  benzodiazepines affecting, 340
  fentanyl affecting, 328

Geometric series, 469

Gestational diabetes, 510–511

Gestational hypertension, 504

GFR, see Glomerular filtration rate

Giant-cell granuloma, 254

GI endoscopy
  and incidence of air embolism, 175
  outside operating room, 564

Glandular dysfunction
  see also specific types of dysfunctions
  Addison's disease causing destruction, 264
  hypoparathyroidism and, 261

Glasgow coma scale, 169

Glaucoma
  as electroconvulsant therapy contraindication, 565
  promethazine and, 344

Global hypoxia, 17

Glomerular filtration, 194
  aging and, 195
  obesity affecting, 67
  phosphate filtration, 216

Glomerular filtration rate, 201–202
  carbonic anhydrase inhibitors and, 224
  elderly persons and, 202
  hypothyroidism affecting, 259
  induced hypotension affecting, 238
  infrarenal clamping affecting, 238
  markers of filtration, 220
  measurement of, 220–221
  mechanical ventilation affecting, 238
  modified Starling equation, 201
  in neonates, 218
  oliguria and, 219, 237
  perinatal age and, 202
  regulation of, 201–202
  suprarenal clamping affecting, 238
  urine flow rate and, 219

Glomerulonephritis
acute kidney failure caused by, 228, 232
eosinophiluria and, 223
preoperative evaluation, 239
Glossopharyngeal nerve (IX), 279
Glossoptosis, 495
Glucagon, 276
phosphate reabsorption and, 216
renal acid-base balance and, 213
Glucocorticoid excess, 262
Glucocorticoids, 264, 275
cortisol, see Cortisol
functions of, 275
glomerular filtration rate and, 202
regulation of, 275
Gluconeogenesis, 242
sympathetic nervous system increasing, 281
Glucose
buffer function, 242
calculation of reabsorption, 221
in diabetic ketoacidosis, 270
intolerance, obesity and, 67, 144
point-of-care analyzers, 404
proximal tubule, reabsorption by, 217
urinalysis, 219
Glucosuria, incidence of, 221
Glutamate, 178
Glutethimide, 244
Glycogenolysis, 281
Glycolysis, 242
Glycoprotein hormones, 274
Glycoproteins
as acetylcholine (ACh) receptors, 162
alpha, binding of, 306
Glycopyrrolates, 99, 291, **380**
as ketamine premedication, 323
to reverse neuromuscular blockade, 381
Goose bumps, 280
Grafts
allograft rejection, steroid use during, 387
arteriovenous, 48
protection of, 236
skin, therapy for compromised, 74, 75
Grand mal seizures, 167, 350
Granular casts, 223
Graphic user interface (GUI), 441
Graves' disease, 257
clinical presentation, 512
and hyperthyroidism, 511
Gravity, PBF influenced by, 16
Gray matter, 151
midbrain periaqueductal, 159
Griseofulvin, 244
Ground fault circuit interrupter (GFCI), 426
Group practices, 577

Growth hormone, hypersecretion of, see Acromegaly
Guanethidine, 556
Guillain-Barré syndrome, 60
Gynecology, and air embolism, 174

Hair loss, 259
Half-life, 305
Halothane, 309–311
biotransformation, 310–311
blood-gas coefficient of, 41
central nervous system affected by, 164
effect on organ systems, 310
and hemopoiesis, 541
neonatal bradycardia due to, 485
as nonflammable, 429
in obese patients, 309–311
physical properties, 309–310
in Pierre-Robin sequence, 495
toxicity, 310–311
in transesophageal fistula, 492
Halothane hepatitis, 246, 311
Hansel's stain, 223
Hard palate, 3–4
Harmonic series, 469
Hb, see Hemoglobin
H$_2$ blockers, 527–528
HbO$_2$, 409
HCO$_3$$_-$, 270
Headache, in diabetic ketoacidosis, 269
Head and neck surgery, 174
Heart, 83–85
aging affecting, 140
blood supply, 86
chest x-ray of, 8
disorders of
see also specific cardiac disorders
hyperthyroidism causing, 258
impaired conduction, 351
as kidney failure complication, 232
failure of, 12
innervation, 86
neonatal, 484–485
vagus nerve, 86, 282
local anesthetics affecting, 347, 351
of neonate, 127, 484–485
and diaphragmatic hernia, 490
parasympathetic nervous system affecting, 282
sympathetic nervous system affecting, 280
Heart blocks, 121–122
Heart murmur, 491
Heart rate
aging and, 140
and diastolic time for myocardial perfusion, 89
enflurane increasing, 311
fetal, 503

intra-aortic balloon counterpulsation slowing, 104
neonatal, 485
parasympathetic nervous system decreasing, 282
sympathetic nervous system increasing, 280
thiopentone increasing, 318
Heat conservation, 296
Heat exchange, in neonates, 487
Heat loss, 294
minimizing, 296
in neonates, 486
Heat production, 294
in neonates, 486
Heat stroke, 147–148
HEELP, pregnancy-induced hypertension and, 507
Hemachromatosis, 254
Hematologic system
hyperthyroidism affecting, 258
hypothermia affecting, 295
NSAIDs affecting, 552
Hematoma(s)
acute intracranial hypertension caused by, 183
central cord syndrome caused by, 171
chronic intracranial hypertension caused by, 183
intracerebral, as induced hypotension contraindication, 293
Hematopoietic system, 297
Hematuria, 239
Hemisection, spinal cord, see Brown-Sequard syndrome
Hemoconcentration, 270
Hemodialysis, 236
Hemodilution, preoperative, 534
Hemodynamic monitoring, 392
Hemodynamics
in air embolism, 176
in amniotic fluid embolism, 519
in kidney failure therapy, 236
in ophthalmic surgery, 572
in pregnancy-induced hypertension, 505–506, 509
Hemoglobin, 535
adult, (HbA), 488–489
anemia, Hb requirements in, 531
carbaminohemoglobin, 24
fetal, 488–489
metabolism, in hepatic system, 242
methemoglobinemia, 351
neonatal, 488–489
oxygen bound to, see Oxyhemoglobin
point-of-care analyzers, 404
Hemoglobinopathies, 535–537
Hemolysis
in newborn, 515
transfusion-related deaths from, 249

Hemolysis elevated liver enzymes low platelets, 507
Hemolytic anemia, 538–539
Hemolytic transfusion reaction, 249, 250
Hemolytic uremic syndrome, 532
Hemoperfusion, 236
Hemophilia A, 541
Hemophilia B, 541
Hemophilus influenza infection, 496
Hemopoiesis, 541
Hemoptysis, 115
Hemorrhage
    adrenal, 265
    brain-stem, 269
    in heat stroke, 147
    as liver transplantation complication, 249
    postpartum, treatment of, 56
    as prostatic resection complication, 238
    retinal, 63–64
    retrobulbar, 572
    uterine, 55
Hemostasis
    in congenital heart disease, 127
    nonsteroidal anti-inflammatory drugs causing, 339
Henry's law, 35, **41**
    altitude physiology, 61, 64
Heparin
    in pregnancy, 130–131
    as pulmonary embolism therapy, 115
    subcutaneous, postoperative use in obese patients, 70, 147
Hepatic artery, 87, 241
Hepatic encephalopathy, 248
Hepatic fatty infiltration, obesity and, 67, 144
Hepatic lobes, 241
Hepatic metabolism
    of drugs, 241
    of narcotics, 549
    of thiopentone, 317
Hepatic system, 241
    blood supply, 241
    coagulation function, 242
    disorders of
        see also specific hepatic disorders
        atracurium, use in, 359
        mivacurium use in, 365
        neuromuscular blockade affected by, 356
    drug metabolism, 241
    enflurane affecting, 312
    halothane affecting, 310
    histology, 241
    isoflurane affecting, 312–313
    methohexitone affecting, 319
    parathyroid hormone and, 275

pharmacokinetics, 244
pharmacology, 244–245
physiology, 241–244
pregnancy-induced hypertension affecting, 506–507
synthetic function, 242
Hepatitis, 245–246
Hepatitis A, 245
Hepatitis B, 245
    transfusion-transmitted, 249, 529–530
Hepatitis C, 245
    transfusion-transmitted, 529–530
Hepatobiliary system, 328
Hepatocellular carcinomas, 249
Hepatocytes, zone of, 241
Hepatorenal syndrome, 230
Hepatotoxicity, 387
Hering-Breuer inflation reflex, 25
Hernia(s)
    hiatal, obesity and, 67, 144
    neonatal diaphragmatic, 490
Herniation
    of intervertebral disk, 152
    of posterior cranial fossa, 183
Hexamethonium, 291
Hg biliverdin bilirubin, 242
Hiatal hernia, obesity and, 67, 144
High airway pressures, 492
High-altitude cerebral edema, 63
High-altitude pulmonary edema, 63
High-frequency jet ventilation, 53
High-frequency oscillation, 53
High-frequency positive pressure ventilation, 53
High-frequency ventilation, 53
High radio frequency (RF), 442
Hip arthrography, 175
Histamine, 30, 391
Histamine antagonists, 234
Histamine release
    atracurium and, 359
    d-tubocurarine causing, 370
    muscle relaxants causing, 393
    succinylcholine causing, 375
    vecuronium causing, 372
Histotoxic hypoxia, 62
HIV
    legal issues regarding, 578
    testing for, 578
    transfusion-transmitted, 529–530
HNKC, 271–273
Hoarseness
    as hypothyroidism symptom, 259
    in laryngotracheobronchitis, 496
Hodgkin's disease, 388
Hofmann elimination, 358
Homeostasis, 119
Hormone-replacement therapy
    for hypopituitarism, 255
    hypothyroidism from inadequate, 259

insulin therapy, 271, 273
Hormones, 274–276
    see also specific hormones
    assisted reproductive technologies affected by, 523
    blood flow control via, 90
    blood pressure control via, 89
    lungs processing, 29
Hospitals, electric power distribution in, 425–426
H$_1$ receptor antagonists, 392
H$_2$ receptor antagonists
    in anaphylaxis treatment, 392
    as premedication for obese patients, 68
    as premedication in obese patients, 146
HRS, 230
HTML, 442
HTTL, 442
Human recombinant erythropoietin, 536
Humidifiers, 53–54
Humidity, 41–**42**
Humoral influences, on PVR, 18
Hyaline membrane disease, 14
Hydralazine, 98
    central nervous system affected by, 165
    for pregnancy-induced hypertension, 507
Hydration
    see also Fluids replacement
    and hyperparathyroidism, 261
    intravenous, in congenital heart disease, 128
Hydrocephalus
    Arnold-Chiari malformation causing, see Arnold-Chiari malformation
    chronic intracranial hypertension caused by, 184
    as intracranial aneurysm complication, 180
    in pediatric meningomyelocele, 186
Hydrocodone, 550
Hydrocortisone, **277**
    for acute asthma in pregnancy, 56
Hydrogen, renal potassium balance and, 214
Hydrogen ion concentration (H+)
    and acid base, 21
    in primary aldosteronism, 263
Hydrogen peroxide wound irrigation, 174
Hydromorphone, 550
Hydrophilic drugs, obesity and, 145
Hydrostatic pressure
    and pulmonary blood flow, 17
    pulmonary edema and, 54
Hyoid, 4

Hyperaldosteronism, 205
Hyperbaric oxygen therapy, 70–76
  for air embolism, 71–72, 75, 177
  transcutaneous Po$_2$ monitoring, 411
Hyperbolic functions, 469
Hypercalcemia
  acute tubule necrosis and, 229
  hyperparathyroidism causing, 260
  signs and symptoms of, 260
  synthetic calcitonin for, 275
  as transfusion reaction, 530
Hypercapnia
  see also Hypercarbia
  respiratory regulation affected by,
    26
Hypercarbia
  see also Hypercapnia
  hypothyroidism affecting ventilatory
    response to, 260
  neonatal response to, 482
  perinatal, 482
  perioperative management of, 51
Hyperchloremic acidosis
  as diabetic ketoacidosis complication,
    271
  metabolic, 216
Hypercholesterolemia, 105
Hypercoagulable state, pregnancy as,
    500
Hyperemic hypoxia, 62
Hyperglycemia, 269
  as fight-or flight response, 280
  hyperosmolar nonketonic coma,
    associated with, 271
  necrotizing enterocolitis and, 493
Hyperkalemia, 215
  pathophysiology, 215
  renal acid-base balance and, 213
  succinylcholine causing, 375–376
  as transfusion reaction, 530
Hypermagnesemia, 217
  calcitonin release triggered by, 275
Hypernatremia, 213
  diabetes insipidus associated with,
    255
  pathophysiology, 213
  polyuria and, 237
  therapy, 213
Hyperosmolality, 271
Hyperosmolar nonketonic coma
    (HNKC), 271–273
Hyperparathyroidism, 260–261
Hyperphosphatemia, 261
Hyperpigmentation, 389
Hyperplasia
  and hyperthyroidism, 257
  postnatal pulmonary, 480
Hyperpyrexia, 147
Hyperreflexia, autonomic, 298–299
Hypersensitivity pneumonitis, 50

Hypersplenism, 248
Hypertension, 105–106
  acute tubule necrosis and, 229
  American College of Obstetricians
    and Gynecologists' definition,
    504
  anesthetic management of patients
    with, 106
  antihypertensive drugs, 106, 507–508
  arterial, obesity and, 66
  chronic, 293, 504
  etiology, 105–106
  as fight-or flight response, 280
  as hypercalcemia sign, 260
  hypercarbia resulting in, 51
  intracranial, 183–185, 189
  and intracranial aneurysms, 181
  as ischemic heart disease risk factor,
    105
  ketamine affecting, 323
  malignant, pheochromocytoma with,
    266
  and mineralocorticoid excess, 263
  naloxone causing, 330
  obesity and, 65, 67, 144
  pheochromocytoma with, 266
  portal, 247
  in pregnancy, 56, 504–510
  pregnancy-induced, 504–510
  in primary aldosteronism, 263
  pulmonary, see Pulmonary
    hypertension
  refractory, of cyclosporin, 387
  renal blood flow and, 200
Hypertext markup language, 442
Hypertext transfer protocol, 442
Hyperthermia
  as hyperosmolar nonketonic coma
    sign, 272
  malignant, see Malignant
    hyperthermia
  in neuroleptic malignant syndrome,
    299
Hyperthyroidism, 257–258
  in pregnancy, 511–513
Hypertrophic adenoids, in infants, 483
Hypertrophic cardiomyopathy, 111–112
Hypertrophic obstructive
    cardiomyopathy, 110
Hypertrophic skin changes, 389
Hypertrophic tonsils, 483
Hyperuricemia, 270
Hyperventilation
  absence seizures precipitated by, 167
  and alveolar concentrations, 48
Hypnotics
  central nervous system affected by,
    163
  for chronic pain, 557
Hypoadrenalism, 265

Hypoalbuminemia, 247
Hypoaldosteronism, 204–205
Hypobaric exposure, see Altitude
Hypocalcemia, 215
  acute, 261, 262
  acute tubule necrosis and, 229
  chronic, 261
  effects, 215
  and hyperphosphatemia, 261
  hypomagnesemia associated with, 217
  hypoparathyroidism associated with,
    261
  pathophysiology, 215
  therapy, 261, 262
Hypocarbia, 51
Hypochloremia, 216
Hypogastric omphalocele, neonatal,
    494
Hypoglycemia, 269
  hypothyroidism and, 259, 260
  symptomatic, 269
Hypoglycemic agents
  enzyme induction caused by, 244
  oral, kidney failure affecting, 234
Hypokalemia, 214–215
  effects, 215
  glucocorticoid excess and, 262
  in heat stroke, 147
  hypomagnesemia associated with, 217
  and mineralocorticoid excess,
    263–264
  pathophysiology, 214–215
Hypomagnesemia, 216–217
  hypoparathyroidism and, 261
Hyponatremia, 213–214
  hypomagnesemia associated with, 217
  hypothyroidism and, 260
  mechanical ventilation caused by, 238
  pathophysiology, 213–214
  therapy, 214
Hypoparathyroidism, 261–262
Hypophosphatemia
  as diabetic ketoacidosis complication,
    271
  hyperparathyroidism and, 260
  hypomagnesemia associated with, 217
Hypophysectomy
  pituitary diabetes insipidus following,
    256
  supplement cortisol during, 262
Hypopituitarism, 254–255
Hypoproteinemia, 568
Hyporeflexia, 269
Hypotension
  amrinone causing, 92
  anaphylaxis causing, 391, 392
  arginine vasopressin and, 209
  autonomic hyperreflexia from, 298
  as cistracurium side effect, 360
  d-tubocurarine causing, 370

induced, *see* Induced hypotension
narcotics causing, 393
necrotizing enterocolitis and, 493
profound, local anesthetics causing, 351
protamine causing, 394
pulmonary vascular resistance and, 19
thiopentone causing, 318
vancomycin causing, 394
Hypothalamic-pituitary-adrenal suppression, 265
Hypothalamus
    arginine vasopressin and, 209
    temperature regulation by, 294
Hypothermia, 294–295
    categorization of, 295
    as cerebral protection, 178, 179, 181
    clinical effects, 295
    as hyperosmolar nonketonic coma sign, 272
    and hypothyroidism, 259, 260
    and intracranial aneurysms, 181
    intraoperative, aging and, 141
    as liver transplantation complication, 249
    mechanisms of loss, 294–295
    near-drowning with, 77
    in neonates, 486
    neuromuscular blockade affected by, 356
    as transfusion reaction, 530–531
Hypothyroidism, 259–260
    in pregnancy, 513
Hypoventilation
    alveolar, hypercarbia due to, 51
    obesity hypoventilation syndrome, 66, 67–68, 145
    in premature babies, 484
Hypovolemia
    arginine vasopressin and, 209
    as induced hypotension contraindication, 293
    and mineralocorticoid excess, 263
    polyuria and, 237
    and pulmonary atresia, 492
Hypovolemic shock
    in burn injuries, 568
    renal blood flow and, 200
Hypoxemia
    altitude and, 61
    asthma in pregnancy and, 55
    chronic, obesity and, 66
    in infants, 497–498
    with metabolic acidosis, 491
    and near-drowning, 77
    obesity and
        chronic hypoxemia, 66
        postoperative, 69–70, 147
        perioperative management of, 51–52

in sarcoidosis, 59
Hypoxia, 62–63
    altitude and, 17, 62–63
    alveolar, 17
    definitions, 62–63
    in diaphragmatic hernia, 490
    fetal breathing and, 481
    global, 17
    hypothyroidism affecting ventilatory response to, 259, 260
    in laryngotracheobronchitis, 496
    as liver transplantation complication, 249
    in near-drowning, 77
    in near-drowning and arrhythmias, 78
    neonatal bradycardia due to, 485
    neonates, 482, 484
    perinatal, 482
    pulse oximetry as monitor, 409–410
    renal blood flow and, 200
    respiratory regulation affected by, 27
Hypoxic drive, enflurane depressing, 311
Hypoxic pulmonary vasoconstriction, 17
Hypoxid hypoxia, 62
Hysteresis, 13

Iatrogenic injury, hypothyroidism as, 259
I-bands, 87
IBW, *see* Ideal body weight (IBW)
ICP, *see* Intracranial pressure
ICU admissions
    indications in near-drowning, 78–79
    of obese patients, 147
Ideal body weight (IBW), 143–144
IgE antibodies
    and latex/natural rubber reactions, 394
Ignition temperature, 429
Ileal carcinoid tumor, 268
Ileus, hypothyroidism causing, 259
Iliac arteries, 87
Imaging systems, 445–447
    see also specific imaging techniques
    resolution of, 445
IM drugs, in obese persons, 68, 146
Imidazole ring structure, 341
Imipramine, 31
Immunological disorders
    see also specific disorders
    acute kidney failure caused by, 228
    anesthetics causing, 541
Immunosuppression
    in kidney failure therapy, 236, 530
    as liver transplantation complication, 249
    in transfusions, 530
Immunosuppressive drugs, 386–389

Impedances, 432
    in ultrasound, 420–421
Imperforate anus, neonatal, 493
Implicit awareness, 159
Incompetent patients, 578–579
Increment, 463
Indefinite integral, 466
Independent contractor, 573
Independent events, 451
Induced hypotension, 292–294
    urologic effects, 237
    via isoproterenol, 91
Inductance, 432
Induction
    of coma, 164
    in congenital heart disease, 128
    enzyme, 244
    in hypothyroidism, 260
    in intracranial aneurysms, 180–181
Intravenous agents, *see* Intravenous induction agents
    of labor, 56
    during labor and delivery, 129
    in neonatal myelomeningocele, 495
    in obese patients, 69, 146
    in pheochromocytomas, 267
    in Pierre-Robin sequence, 495
    in pregnant patients, 128, 129
    rate of, 308
Indwelling bladder catheters, 293
Inert gas washout, 220
Infant respiratory distress syndrome, 53
Infants
    see also Neonates
    anesthetizing, Mapleson D, E and F for, 44
    d-tubocurarine in, 370
    pancuronium in, 367
    pipecuronium in, 368
    premature, *see* Premature infants
    vecuronium in, 372
Infection(s)
    see also specific types of infections
    chronic intracranial hypertension caused by, 183
    as diabetic ketoacidosis complication, 271
    Hemophilus influenza, 496
    hyperbaric oxygen therapy for, 74, 75
    hyperosmolar nonketotic coma, associated with, 271
    hyperosmolar nonketotic coma, concurrent with, 272
    of lungs, 28
    lungs as defensive mechanism against, 28
    from near-drowning, **79**
    nebulizers causing, 54
    necrotizing, 74, 75
    from neonatal myelomeningocele, 495

Infection(s), *continued*
    as subarachnoid bolt complication, 418
    transfusion-transmitted, 529–530
    in transplantation recipients, 386
    as ventriculostomy complication, 417
Infectious hepatitis, 245
Inference, 448
    on population means, 452–457, 457–459
Inferior mesenteric artery, 87
Inferior mesenteric ganglia, 280
Inferior vena cava interruption, 115
Infinite series, 469–470
Inflammation
    see also specific types of inflammation
    anti-inflammatory agents, *see* Anti-inflammatory agents
    small airway obstruction in infants caused by, 481
Informed consent, 573–574
    in controlled human clinical trials, 462
Infrared, 442
Infrarenal aortic cross-clamping, 238
Inhalation agents
    see also specific inhaled anesthetics
    central nervous system affected by, 164
    as cerebral protection, 178
    characteristics of, **309**
    effect on systems, **309**
    in elderly persons, 142
    hyperthyroidism and, 258
    intraoperative awareness and, 159
    urologic system, effects on, 228
Inhalation anesthetic agents
    in burn injuries, 569
    in infants, 484
    nondepolarizing muscle relaxants affected by, 356
    in pulmonary atresia, 492
Inhalation burns, 568
Injection port, 407
Innervation
    of epiglottis, 4
    of eye, 571
    of heart, 86, 282, 484–485
    of kidney, 195
    of larynx, 4–5
    of mouth, 3
    myocardial, 86
    of neonatal heart, 484–485
    of pharynx, 4
    of trachea, 5
Inotropic drugs, 90–92
    see also specific inotropes
    adrenergic receptor activities, 90–91
    as cardiac drug in pregnancy, 130

Inotropy, 88
Input impedance, 432
Insoluble anesthetics, 48
Insomnia, 63
Inspiration
    and airway resistance, 16
    chest x-ray of, 8
    conditioning of inspired air, 27
Inspiratory capacity (IC), 11
    in pregnancy, 500
Inspiratory flow rate, 53
Inspiratory pressure measurement, 412–413
Inspiratory reserve volume (IRV), 10
    in pregnancy, 500
Inspired and expired gas measurement, 406–408
Inspired concentrations, 46–47
Institutional review board (IRB), 424
Insulators, electric charge of, 431
Insulin, 276
    function of, 276
    as glomerular filtration rate marker, 220
    inhibition of secretion, 276
    lack of, diabetic ketoacidosis from, 269–271
    magnesium balance affected by, 216
    renal potassium balance and, 214
    stimulation of secretion, 276
Insulin dependent diabetes mellitus, 268
Insulin therapy
    in diabetic ketoacidosis, 271
    for hyperosmolar nonketotic coma, 273
    hypokalemia from, 271
Insurance and legal defense, 577
Integral calculus, 466
Integrated circuits, 433–434
Intensifying screen, in radiography, 446
Interfundibular atresia, 491
Intermediolateral cell column, 280
Intermittent hemodialysis, 236
Intermittent mandatory ventilation (IMV), 53
Internal carotid arteries
    aneurysm of, 255
    cerebral vasculature, 151
Internal intercostal muscles, 13
International Organization for Standardization, 428
Internet, 440–442
Internet Activities Board, 441
Internet registry, 441
Interspinous ligaments, 153
Interstitial nephritis
    acute kidney failure caused by, 232
    allergic, 223
Interstitium, 23

Intervertebral disks, 152
Intervertebral ligaments, 153
Intestinal tract, 281
Intoxication, in near-drowning, 78
Intra-abdominal pressure, obesity and, 67, 144
Intra-aortic balloon counterpulsation, 104
Intra-arterial injection
    of methohexitone, 319
    of promethazine, 344
    of thiopentone, 318
Intracardiac shunt, 47–48
Intracranial aneurysms, 179–182
    symptomatic, *see* SAH
Intracranial hypertension, 183–185
    in craniosynostosis, 189
Intracranial mass, 565
Intracranial pressure, 183
    as electroconvulsant therapy contraindication, 565
    enflurane affecting, 311
    flumazanil affecting, 163
    hypertension, *see* Intracranial hypertension
    measurement of, 417–419
    near-drowning affecting, 77–78
    normal, 417
    opioids affecting, 163
    safety standards for measurement devices, 428
    succinylcholine increasing, 376
    thiopentone decreasing, 317
Intradural tumor, 173
Intragastric pressure, 376
Intramuscular drugs, in obese patients, 68, 146
Intraocular pressure
    ketamine increasing, 323
    succinylcholine increasing, 376
Intraoperative blood salvage, 534
Intrapulmonary shunt, 47–48
Intrathoracic cancer, 115
Intrathoracic reflexes, 27
Intrauterine growth retardation, 55
Intravascular volume
    depletion, in hyperosmolar nonketotic coma, 271, 272
    hypothyroidism and, 260
    repletion, for diabetes insipidus management, 255
Intravenous anesthetics, 331–345
    see also specific anesthetics
Intravenous drugs, in elderly persons, 142
Intravenous hydration, 128
Intravenous induction agents, 317–330
    see also specific agents
    central nervous system affected by, 164

Intravenous pyelogram (IVP), 196
Intravenous SBE prophylaxis, 110
Intraventricular septum, 491–492
Intrinsic clearance, 244
Intrinsic cord syndrome, 172
Intrinsic sympathomimetic activity, 95
Intubation
    awake, *see* Awake intubation
    chest x-ray of tube position, 8
    endotracheal, *see* Endotracheal
        intubation
    fiberoptic, *see* Fiberoptic intubation
    nasal sinus drainage impeded by, 3
    neonatal bradycardia due to, 485
    oral, 50, 51
    for supraglottitis, 497
    traumatic, arytenoid cartilage
        dislocated during, 4
    vocal cords damaged by, 4
Invasive arterial blood pressure
        measuring technique, 415–416
Invasive monitors, in burn injuries,
        569
Investigational device exemption
        (IDE), 424
In vitro fertilization (IVF), 523
In vitro tests, 391–392
Iodine
    deficiency of, 259
    exogenous, 275
    and thyroid hormone synthetic
        pathways, 274
Iodotyrosine residues, 274
Iohexol, 220
Ion channel blockers, 178
Ion detector, 406
Ionization, 306
Ionization chamber, 406
Iothalamate, 221
Ipratropium bromide, 33
Iron
    deficiencies of, 537, 538
    stores of, 224
IR radiator detectors, 435
Irritant receptors (sensory nerves), 26
ISA, 95
Ischemia
    acute kidney failure caused by,
        229–230
    cerebral, 297
    and intracranial hypertension, 183
    myocardial, 293
    transient, 177
    ventricular function and, 89
Ischemic heart disease, 105
    death rate, 105
    ketamine and, 323
    risk factors, 105
Islet of Langerhans, 253–254
Isoetharine, 32–33

Isoflurane, 312–313
    central nervous system affected by, 164
    as nonflammable, 429
    urinary system, effects on, 228
Isolated patient connection, 427
Isolated power systems, 425–426
Isoproterenol, 287
    see also Isuprel
    as bronchodilator, 32
    as inotrope, 91
Isuprel
    see also Isoproterenol
    as vasodilator, 480

Jackson-Rees system, 45
Jaffe reaction, 221
Jaundice, 248
Jaw malformation, 51
Jejunum, 216
Jet nebulizers, 54
Joule, 432
J receptors, 26
Junctional arrhythmias, 375
Junctional premature beats, 123
Junctional rhythm, 123
    halothane affecting, 310
Juxtaglomerular apparatus (JGA)
        components, 195

Ketamine
    in burn injuries, 569
    central nervous system affected by,
        164, 323
    hypothyroidism and induction with,
        260
    as IV induction agent, 322–323
    muscle relaxants, interaction with,
        356
    urologic system, effects on, 228
Keterolac, 339
Ketoacidosis, diabetic, 269–271
Ketones
    in diabetic ketoacidosis, 270
    in urinalysis, 219
Kidney failure, 228–236
    anticholinesterase for, 380
    bleomycin dosage in, 389
    chronic, 232, 261
    complications of, 232–235
    hypoparathyroidism and, 261
    pancuronium in, 367
    pharmacologic effects of, 233–235
    protein binding and, 307
    therapy for, 235–236
Kidneys, 194
    aging and, 195
    anephric state, 237
    blood pressure control by, 89
    cortex, 194, 196
    dopamine affecting, 92

endocrine functions, 210–211
glomerular filtration barriers, *see*
        Glomerular filtration
infections of, 239
innervation, 195
location, 194
loop of Henle, 194
medulla, 194, 196
metabolic functions, 210–211
norepinephrine reducing blood flow
        to, 91
physiology, 196–218
preoperative evaluation, 239
proximal tubule, *see* Proximal tubule
renal artery supply to, 87
size, 194
sympathetic nervous system affecting,
        281
trauma to, 236, 239
tubules, *see* Tubules
vasculature, 87, 195
Kidney stones, 239
King-Denborough syndrome, 298
Kussmaul's respirations, 269
Kyphoscoliosis
    in Duchenne type muscular
        dystrophy, 60
    lung compliance reduced with, 13

Labetalol, 95, 286, 289
    in pregnancy, 131
    for pregnancy-induced hypertension,
        507–508
Labor and delivery
    see also Labor and delivery;
        Pregnancy
    anesthetic management during,
        56–57
    autonomic hyperreflexia from, 298
    Cesarean section, *see* Cesarean
        section
    induction during, 129
    induction of labor, 56
    mitral regurgitation and, 133
    mitral stenosis and, 132
    neonatal pulmonary blood flow at, 17
    oxytocics in, 501–502
    phases of labor, 503
    physiology of labor, 503
    preterm, tocolytics for, 502
    prolonged labor, by theophylline, 55
    pulmonary hypertension and, 138
    Tetralogy of Fallot and, 136
    vaginal delivery, *see* Vaginal delivery
Lack system, 44, **44**
Lactate, 270
Lactic acidosis, 271
Laminar flow, 15, 100
Laparoscopy, 525
Laryngeal edema, 391

Laryngoscopy
  in infants, 483
  neonatal bradycardia due to, 485
  obesity interfering in, 67
Laryngospasm
  and asphyxia in near-drowning, 76
  in infants, 483
Laryngotracheobronchitis, 496
Larynx, 4
  in infants, 483
  innervation, 4–5
  obesity affecting, 67, 145
Laser, 442
Laser surgery, 563
Latex sensitivity, 394
  and pediatric meningomyelocele, 187
Lecithin, 481
Lecithin-sphingomyelin ratio, 503
LeFort I fractures, 3
LeFort II fractures, 3
LeFort III fractures, 3
Left atrium, 83–84
Left bundle branch block, 121–122
Left coronary arteries, 86
Left lobar and segmental bronchi, 5
Left ventricle, 84
  diaphragmatic muscles and, 83
  drainage into coronary sinus, 86
  electrical assist system, 104
  in neonate, 484
  obesity and compliance, 144
  pulmonary circulation as reservoir,
    87
Left ventricular end diastolic pressure,
    obesity and, 67, 144
Legal defense, 577
Legal liability, 573
Let-go current, 426
Leukemia, 539–540
  acute lymphocytic, 388
Leukocytosis
  in diabetic ketoacidosis, 270
  in neuroleptic malignant syndrome,
    300
Leukotrienes, 30–31, 391
LeVeen shunt, 248
Levodopa
  abrupt withdrawal from, 299
  central nervous system affected by,
    166
  as neuroleptic malignant syndrome
    treatment, 300
Levorphanol, 336, 550
Liability insurance, 577
Lidocaine, 352
  as antidysrhythmic, 93
  cardiac effects of, 347, 351
  as cerebral protection, 178
  for chronic pain, 556
  as diprivan pretreatment, 321

  as etomidate pretreatment, 322
  in pediatric life support, **499**
Lifestyle, and ischemic heart disease,
    105
Ligaments, intervertebral, 153
Ligamentum flavum, 153
Light sources, for transducer, 435
Lignocaine, 31
Limited consent, 574
Linear integrated circuits, 434
Linear regression, 459–460
Lipid disorders, 321
Lipid enzymes, 254
Lipid metabolism, in hepatic system,
    242
Lipid solubility
  and blood-placental barrier, 501
  and local anesthetic potency, 349
Lipophilic drugs, obesity affecting, 67,
    145
Lipoproteinemia, obesity and, 67, 145
Liquid oxygen, 36
Lithium
  cistracurium interacting with, 361
  kidney failure affecting, 235
  muscle relaxants interacting with, 355
Lithium batteries, 444
Lithotripsy
  and incidence of air embolism, 174
  outside operating room, 563
Litigation involving consent, 574
Liver
  age, and function of, 141
  blood flow in, 87
    aging and, 141
    norepinephrine reducing, 91
    phamacokinetics affected by, 244
  enlargement as cirrhosis sign, 248
  excretory actions of, 243
  fetal, 479
  sympathetic nervous system affecting,
    281
Liver failure, 248
  acute, in heat stroke, 148
  drug metabolism and, 248
  pancuronium used in, 367
  protein binding and, 307
Liver function tests, 243–244
  in neuroleptic malignant syndrome,
    300
Liver transplantation, 249
  and incidence of air embolism, 174
Living will statutes, 579
Lobes of lung, 9, 10
Local anesthetics, 346–352
  cisatracurium interacting with, 361
  ester-allergic reactions, 393
  frequency-dependent blockade, 347
  muscle relaxants interacting with, 355
  nerve fiber classification, 347–348

  in ophthalmic surgery, 572
  pregnancy, sensitivity in, 501
  true allergic reactions, 393
Local area networks (LAN), 438–440
Local spinal anesthetic, 153
Local tissue acidosis, 349
Long incubation hepatitis, 245
Loop diuretics, 224–227
  see also specific diuretics
Loop of Henle, 194
Lorazepam, 342
Lorraine-Smith effect, 75
Lower extremities, aortic supply to, 87
Lower motor neuron lesions, 356
Lown-Ganong-Levine syndrome, 125
Low radio frequency (RF), 442
Lumbar puncture
  for coma, 169
  in intracranial aneurysms, 179
Lumbar vertebrae, 152
Lung(s), 4–7
  abscesses, computed tomography of,
    10
  as blood filter, 28
  as blood reservoir, 27
  compliance, left ventricular, 144
  elastic properties of, 13
  expansion and contraction, 12
  extracellular fluid volume, 27
  fluid exchange in, 27
  foreign substances handled by, 31
  gas transfer to, 47
  hormones and vasoactive compounds
    processed by, 29
  infected, oxygen consumption and, 28
  lobes of, 9, 10
  near-drowning affecting, 77
  oxidation metabolism and, 28–29
  particulate filtration, 28
  positron emission tomography of, 446
  protease released from, 29
  protease transport, involved in, 29
  seawater aspiration, 77
  vasculature, 7, 9, 87
Lung cancer
  metastatic, hypopituitarism caused
    by, 254
  vital capacity (VC) and, 12
Lung scan, 115
Lung volumes
  in infants, 483–484
  spirometry, 11
Lusitropy, 89
LVEDP, see Left ventricular end
    diastolic pressure
Lymphatics, 7
Lymph node enlargement, 58
Lymphocytic hypophysitis, 255
Lymphomas, 389
Lysosomal enzymes, 223

Macroshock, 426
Magill circuit, 44
Magnesium
  balance in urologic system, 216–217
  cistracurium, drug interactions with, 361
  parathyroid hormone and, 275
  for pregnancy-induced hypertension, 508
Magnesium sulfate, 502
Magnetic resonance imaging, 447
  for coma, 169
  full-body imager, 447
  in glucocorticoid excess, 262
  outside operating room, 563–564
  partial-body imager, 447
  permanent pacemaker as contraindication, 103
  renal blood flow measurement, 220
  time constants, 447
Mahaim pathway, 125
Mainframe gateways, 440
Major cardiovascular vessels, 83–87
Major causalgia, 559
Major depressive disorders, 565
Malabsorption, 261
Malignancies
  pheochromocytomas, 266
  transfusion-related immunosuppression, 530
Malignant hypertension, 266
Malignant hyperthermia, 296–298
  atracurium, use in, 359
  mivacurium use in, 365
  neuromuscular blockade affected by, 357
  pancuronium used in, 367
  rocuronium and, 369
  succinylcholine causing, 376, 377
Mandibular fractures, 3
Mandibular retrognathia, 495
Manic states, 565
Mannitol, 165
  central nervous system affected by, 165
  as osmotic diuretic, 227
Manometer, 101
Mantle fibers, 347
MAOIs, *see* Monoamine oxidase inhibitors (MAOIs)
Mapleson breathing system, 43–45
Mask ventilation, 490
Massive pulmonary embolus, 114
Mass lesions, 10
Mass spectrometry, 176
Mass spectroscopy, 406–407
Mast cells, 6
Master-servant relationship, 573
Maternal age, ART affected by, 523
Maxillares sinus, 3

Maximum inspiratory pressure (MIP; P_1max), 413
Mean arterial pressure, 293
Mean averages, 449
Mean blood pressure, 89
Mean deviation, 449
Mean pulmonary artery pressure (MPAP), 18
Mean right atrial pressure, neonatal, 485
Mean value for integral, 465
Mechanical circulatory assist devices, 104
Mechanical disorders, PVR and, 19
Mechanical ventilation, 238
Mechanomyography, 384
Mechanoreceptors, 27
Meconium aspiration
  neonatal resuscitation due to, 498
  postnatal, 480
Median averages, 449
Mediastinal structures
  chest x-ray of, 8, 9–10
  computed tomography of, 10
Medical device amendment, of Federal Food Drug and Cosmetic Act, 423–424
Medical experts, legal, 575
Medical malpractice, 575–576
Medical negligence, 574–575, 575–576
Medical records, 576
Medium radio frequency (RF), 442
Medulla oblongata, 25
Megaloblastic anemia, 538
Memory, in microprocessors, 437
Memory impairment, 259
Meninges, spinal, 153–154
Meningomyelocele, pediatric, 185–187
  Arnold-Chiari malformation and, 186, 494
Menorrhagia, 259
Mental retardation, 261
Meperidine
  central nervous system affected by, 163
  kidney failure affecting, 235
  as opiate agonist, 550
  as opioid agonist, 335–336
  seizures and, 168
Mepivicaine, 352
Meprobamate, 244
Mercuric oxide batteries, 444
Mesothelium, 7
Metabolic acidosis
  elevated anion gap, 269
  hyperchloremic, 216
  ketoacidosis, diabetic, 269–271
  in near-drowning, 78
  necrotizing enterocolitis and, 493
  phosphaturia accompanying, 270

Metabolic osmotics, 227
Metabolic requirements, cerebral, 177–178
Metabolic system
  craniosynostosis and, 189
  hyperthyroidism affecting, 258
  hypothermia affecting, 295
  kidney failure affecting, 233
  kidney function, 210–211
  and liver transplantation, 249
  obesity and, 66, 144
  respiratory exchange ratio (R) changes and, 24
Metabolism
  cerebral blood flow and, 156
  hepatic, *see* Hepatic metabolism
  in malignant hyperthermia, 296
  of narcotics, 548–549
  thyroid as mediator of, 252
Metals, electric charge of, 431
Metaproterenol, 32
Metaraminol
  as alpha$_1$ agonist, 285
  as vasoconstrictor, 98
Metastatic disease
  breast cancer, 254
  as liver transplantation contraindication, 249
  lung cancer, 254
  pheochromocytomas as, 266
Methacholine, 289
Methadone, 550
Methanol, 170
Methemoglobinemia, 351
Methohexital, seizures and, 168
Methohexitone, 318–319
Methoxamine, 285
Methylparaben, 351
Methylprednisolone, **277**
Methylxanthine agents, 34
Metoclopramide
  kidney failure affecting, 235
  for pulmonary aspiration, 527
Metoclopramide dopamine antagonist, 527
Metocurine, **363**–364
  histamine release from, 393
  as nicotinic antagonist, 291–292
Metolazone, 226–227
Metoprolol, 95, 289
Metubine, **363**–364
Mexiletine, 93
  for chronic pain, 556
Microcells, 443
Microcomputer, 436–437
Microprocessor, 436–437
Microscopic urinalysis, 219
Microshock, 426
Microsomal enzyme system, 141
Microvilli, 7

Microwave, 442
Midazolam, 341–342
  as IV induction agent, 324–325
Midbrain periaqueductal gray matter,
    159
Middle nasal concha, 3
Milrinone, 92
Mind-body dualism, 543
Mineralocorticoid excess, 263–264
Mineralocorticoids, 275–276
  aldosterone, see Aldosterone
  functions of, 275
Minor causalgia, 559
Miosis, 281
Mithramycin, 260
Mitochondria, 88
Mitral regurgitation, 109
  in pregnancy, 132–133
Mitral stenosis, 108
  in pregnancy, 131–132
Mitral valve, 84
Mitral valve prolapse, 109–110
  in pregnancy, 133
Mivacron, see also Mivacurium
  hepatic disease affecting, 356
Mivacurium, **364**–365
  see also Mivacron
  as nicotinic antagonist, 291–292
M-line, 87
M mode, in ultrasound, 421
Mobile phase, 407
Mobitz heart block, 121
Mode averages, 449
Modified Blalock-Taussig shunt,
    491–492
Modified Starling equation, 201
Modular components, 437
Modulation transfer function (MTF),
    445
Molecular forces, 14
Molecular size, blood-placental barrier
    and, 501
Molecular weight, 245
Monoamine oxidase inhibitors
    (MAOIs), 166
Morbidity rates, 448
Morbid obesity, 65, 143
  operative procedures for, 65
  psychopathology in, 67, 145
Morphine
  central nervous system affected by,
    163
  clearance, 333
  controlled-release preparation, 549
  as exogenous toxin, 170
  kidney failure affecting, 235
  as opiate agonist, 549
  as opioid agonist, 333
Morphology
  brain, 151

prenatal, 481
spinal cord, 153
synapses, 161
Mortality
  in acute tubule necrosis, 229
  in malignant hyperthermia, 296
  in neuroleptic malignant syndrome,
    300
  in pregnancy-induced hypertension,
    507
Mortality rates, 448
Motor end plate, 353
Motor evoked potentials (MEP), 156
Motor nerves, 282
Motor nerve terminal, 353
Motor pathways, 160
Mountain sickness, acute, 63
Mouth, 3–4
  innervation, 3
  obesity and decreased opening of, 67
Mucosa membranes, 394
Multiorgan failure, 300
Multiple correlation, 461
Multiple defendants, 577
Multiple myeloma, 540
Multiple regression, 460
Multiple sclerosis, 173
Multiplicative law, 450
Murmur, in air embolism, 176
Muscarinic antagonists, 33–34, 99, 291
  see also specific antagonists
Muscarinic receptors, 282, 283
  agonists, 289–291
  antagonists, see Muscarinic
    antagonists
Muscle contraction
  in malignant hyperthermia, 297
  pilomotor, 281
Muscle relaxants
  see also neuromuscular blockade
  allergic reactions to, 393
  anaphylactic reactions to, 393
  for burn injuries, 569
  central nervous system affected by, 164
  in elderly persons, 142, 357
  histamine release, 393
  ideal properties, 357
  in local anesthetics-induced seizure
    treatment, 350–351
  neuromuscular junction, 353–354
  nondepolarizing, central nervous
    system affected by, 164
  skeletal, for chronic pain, 557
  succinylcholine, see Succinyl choline
Muscles
  abdominal, 13, 146
  aging and, 140
  of chest, 12, 13
  creatinine production and muscle
    mass, 220–221

development of, vital capacity (VC)
    and, 12
  of eye, 485
  smooth muscle activity, 159
Muscle spasms, 59
Muscular diseases
  see also specific diseases
  affecting respiratory system, 59–61
  dystrophies, 60–61
Muscular dystrophy, 357
Muscular pain, 376
Muscular rigidity, 299
Musculoskeletal pain, 115
Musculoskeletal system
  hypothermia affecting, 295
  metabolism, increases in, 296
Myalgias, 269
Myasthenia gravis
  anticholinesterase for, 380
  atracurium, use in, 359
  neuromuscular blockade affected by,
    356
Myasthenic syndrome, 356
Mydriasis
  as fight-or flight response, 280
  sympathetic nervous system affecting,
    281
Myelinated fibers, 347, 348
Myelination, 347–348
Myelinolysis, 214
Myelodysplasia, neonatal, 494–495
Myelomeningocele, neonatal, 494–495
Myelopathy, 171
Myeloproliferative diseases, 539–540
Myocardial blood supply, 86, 89
Myocardial contractility
  enflurane decreasing, 311
  halothane decreasing, 310
  in neonates, 484
Myocardial contraction, 426
Myocardial depression, 394
Myocardial dysfunction, 293
Myocardial infarction
  acute, 272, 520
  as anesthetic emergency, 391
  as electroconvulsant therapy
    contraindication, 565
  obesity and, 65
  pulmonary embolus differentiated,
    115
Myocardial innervation, 86
Myocardial ischemia, 293
Myocardial necrosis, 32
Myocardial perfusion, 89
Myocardial perfusion scintigraphy,
    102–103
Myocardium, fetal, 484
Myoclonic movements
  diprivan causing, 321
  etomidate causing, 322

ketamine causing, 323
Myoclonic seizures, 167
Myoclonus, 319
Myocytes, cardiac, 87
  in neonates, 484
Myogenic theory, 89
Myoglobinuria, 300
Myometrium, 131
Myosin filaments, 87
Myotactic reflexes, 160, 259
Myotonic contractures, 60–61
Myotonic dystrophies, 60–61
  atracurium use in, 359
Myotonus, 319
Myxedema coma, 259

Nadolol, 94, 288
NaHCO$_3$
  in anaphylaxis treatment, 392
  in diabetic ketoacidosis, 271
Nalbuphine, 551
Nalorphine, 336
Naloxone
  as IV induction agent, 329–330
  as opioid antagonist, 329–330,
    336–337, 551
Naltrexone, 336, 337–338, 551
Narcotics
  see also Opioids
  for burn injuries, 569
  as chronic pain treatment, 545–552
  IV, urinary system affected by, 228
  kidney failure affecting, 235
  reactions to, 393
Nasal cavity, 3
Nasal fiberoptic intubation, 51
Nasal sinuses, 3
Nasogastric tube, in infants, 483
National Fire Protection Association,
  428
National Science Foundation, 441
Natural death acts, 579
Natural logarithmic function, 468
Natural rubber, allergic reactions to,
  394
Nausea
  in cirrhosis, 248
  as diabetic ketoacidosis sign, 269
  etomidate causing, 322
  from opioid drugs, 547
  as opioid side effect, 332
Near-drowning, 76–80
Nebulizers, 54
NEC, in premature infants, 490,
  493–494
Necrosis
  acute tubule, 229–230
  clostridial myonecrosis, see
    Clostridial myonecrosis
  cortical, 229

hyperbaric oxygen therapy for, 74, 75
  myocardial, 32
  necrotizing infections, 74, 75
  osteoradionecrosis, 74, 75
  radionecrosis, 74, 75
Necrotizing enterocolitis, in premature
  infants, 490, 493–494
Negligence, medical, 574–575
Neonates, 479
  see also Infants
  cardiac system, 484–485
  congenital heart disease, 126–128
  d-tubocurarine in, 370
  emergencies in, 490–495
  fluid balance in, 218
  heart of, 127, 484–485
  hemoglobin, 488–489
  hemolysis in, 515
  neuromuscular blockade in, 357
  physiology, 481–490
  respiratory system, 481–484
  resuscitation of, 497–**499**
  retinopathy, 485–486
  sodium balance in, 213
  thermal regulation in, 486–487
  transcutaneous Po$_2$ monitoring, 411
Neoplasms, see Tumor(s)
Neospinothalamic tract, 159
Neostigmine
  acid-base balance and, 356
  as anticholinesterase, 290
  neonatal bradycardia due to, 485
Neostigmine block, 379
Nephrectomy, 238
Nephritis, 239
Nephrogenic diabetes insipidus, 256
Nephrotoxicity
  of cyclosporin, 387
  fluoride-induced, 312
Nerve bundle, 347–348
Nerve fibers, 347–348
Nerve roots, 186
Nerve stimulators
  characteristics of, 382
  neuromuscular blockade monitoring,
    382–383
  pattern of stimulation, 382–383
  recording of response, 383–384
  train-of-four stimulation, 383
Nervous system
  see also specific systems
  pulmonary vascular resistance
    influenced by, 18
Network interface card, 439
Network operating systems (NOS), 440
Neural impulse conduction blockade,
  346–347
Neural membrane, 346
Neural tube defects, see Arnold-Chiari
  malformation

Neurogenic stimuli, 26
Neuroleptic malignant syndrome,
  299–300
Neurologic disorders
  see also specific neurologic disorders
  as hyperosmolar nonketotic coma
    sign, 272
  hyperthyroidism causing, 258
  hypothyroidism causing, 259
  as kidney failure complication, 232
  in premature infants, 490
  respiratory system affected by, 59–61
Neuromuscular blockade
  see also muscle relaxants
  applications, 381–382
  classification of, 354–357
  clinical monitoring, 381
  factors affecting, 355–357
  kidney failure affecting, 235
  monitoring, 381–387
  in obese patients, 147
  reversal of, 378–381
Neuromuscular junction
  components, **353**–354
  monitoring in obese patients, 69, 146
Neuromuscular system
  desflurane affecting, 314
  diseases of
    neuromuscular blockade affected
      by, 356
    pancuronium used in, 367
  enflurane affecting, 312
  halothane affecting, 310
  isoflurane affecting, 312–313
  malignant hyperthermia affecting,
    297–298
  sevoflurane affecting, 315
Neuromuscular transmission, 162–163
Neuronal polarization, 161–162
Neuronal transmission, 160–162
Neurons
  afferent, 279
  aging affecting, 141
  classification of, 161
  composition, 160–161
  lower motor neuron lesions, 356
  parasympathetic, 281
  polarization, 161–162
  structure, 160–161
  sympathetic, 280
  transmission by, 160–162
  upper motor neuron lesions, 356
Neuropathic pain, 558–559
Neurosurgery, 174
Neurotoxicity, 351
Neurotransmitters
  see also specific neurotransmitters
  of autonomic nervous system, 90, 282
  and blood flow control, 90
  classification, 161

Neutrophil chemotactic factor, 391
Newborn respiratory distress syndrome, 481
New York Heart Association functional classification, 115–116
Nickel cadmium batteries, 444
Nicotinamide, 268
Nicotinic receptors, 283
  agonists, 289
  antagonists, 291–292
Nifedipine, 96
Nimbex, *see* Cistracurium
Nitrates, 99
Nitric oxide (NO)
  for persistent pulmonary hypertension, 480
  as vasoactive compound, 29
Nitroglycerine, 97
  central nervous system affected by, 165
  urologic effects of, 238
Nitroprusside
  for acute autonomic hyperreflexia, 299
  kidney failure affecting, 235
  urologic effects of, 238
Nitrous oxide
  air embolism and, 176–177
  avoidance in congenital lobar emphysema, 493
  central nervous system affected by, 164
  concentration effect of, 49
  critical pressure, 43
  critical temperature of, 42–43
  fentanyl and, 328
  as fire hazard, 429
  liquefied, 42
  pressure gauge for, 42–43
  Rotameter measurement of, 398
  shunts affecting uptake of, 48
  vapor, 42
NO, 29, 480
N_2O, *see* Nitrous oxide
Nociceptive pain, 551–552
Nocturia, 239
Nodule, hyperfunctioning, 257
Non-A hepatitis, 245, 249
Non-B hepatitis, 245, 249
Noncompartmental approach, 304
Nonconvulsive status epilepticus, 168
Nondepolarizing muscle relaxants, 354, 357–373
  see also specific relaxants
  acid-base balance and, 356
  antibiotics increasing action of, 355
  burns affecting, 357
  central nervous system affected by, 164
  electrolytes affecting, 356
  hypothermia affecting, 356
  inhalational anesthetic agents affecting, 356

Nondiscriminatory medical care, 578
Nonhealing wounds, hyperbaric oxygen therapy for, 74, 75
Noninsulin dependent diabetes mellitus, 268
Nonlinear regression, 460
Nonnarcotic analgesics, 552–553
  see also specific nonnarcotic analgesics
Nonpharmacologic chronic pain treatment, 543–544
Nonselective beta agonists, 32
Nonselective beta antagonists, 94
Nonsignificant-risk-device study, 424
Nonsteroidal anti-inflammatory drugs, 338–339
  see also specific drugs
  acute kidney failure caused by, 232
  characteristics, 338
  for chronic pain, 552–553
  indications, 338
  pharmacokinetics, 338, 553
  platelet transfusions and, 532
  side effects, 338–339
Noradrenaline
  see also Norepinephrine
  as vasoactive compound, 30
Norcuron, *see* Vecuronium
Norepinephrine, 282
  see also Noradrenaline
  adrenal medulla releasing, 280
  as alpha agonist, 284–285
  as inotrope, 91
  neonatal thermoregulation and, 486
  as neurotransmitter, 280, 283
  as vasopressors, 165
Normal (Gaussian) distribution, 452
Normovolemic hemodilution techniques, 190
Nortriptyline, 31
Nose, 3
  breathing through, neonates, 482–483
  nasal cavity, 3
Nostrils, 498
NSFnet, 441
N trials, 451
Nuclear medicine scan
  of urologic system, 196
Nucleus ambiguus, 25
Nucleus pulposus, 152
Nucleus retroambiguus, 25
Numeric continuous data, 449
Numeric discrete data, 449
Nutrition
  in ascites therapy, 248
  hypothyroidism from inadequate, 259
  in kidney failure therapy, 235
  maternal, and pediatric meningomyelocele, 185
Nystagmus, 323

Obesity, 143
  airway affected by, 67, 145
  anesthesia risk and, 64
  as arteriosclerosis risk factor, 105
  and awake fiberoptic intubation, 51
  cardiovascular effects, 66–67, 144
  definition, 66, 143–144
  endocrine effects of, 66, 67, 144
  gastrointestinal effects of, 66, 67, 144
  general and regional anesthesia combined, 69, 147
  incidence, 64
  induction, 69, 146
  intraoperative management, 68–69
  morbid obesity, *see* Morbid obesity
  pathophysiologic changes, 66, 144–145
  pharmacokinetics/dynamics effect, 66, 67, 145
  premedication, 68, 146
  preoperative investigation, 68
  psychologic effects of, 66, 67, 145
  pulmonary effects of, 66, 144
  regional anesthesia, 69, 146–147
  respiratory system and, 64–70
  and supine position, *see* Supine position
  vital capacity (VC) and, 12
Obesity hypoventilation syndrome, 66, 67–68, 145
Oblique muscles, 13
Obstetrics, 56
  see also Labor and delivery; Pregnancy
  cardiovascular system in, 129–139, 500
  and incidence of air embolism, 174
  maternal-fetal physiology, 501–504
  mivacurium use in, 365
  pancuronium used in, 367
  and respiratory diseases, 56
  use of ephedrine in, 98
  vecuronium in, 372
Obstructive apnea, in infants, 489–490
Obstructive disorders
  acute kidney failure caused by, 228
  airway, *see* Airway obstruction
  apnea, in infants, 489–490
  of bladder neck, 344
  of cystic duct, 247
  hypertrophic obstructive cardiomyopathy, 110
  of pulmonary arteries, 13
  of pulmonary blood flow, 126
Obstructive lung disorders, 49–50
  asthma, *see* Asthma
  chronic bronchitis, *see* Chronic bronchitis
  chronic obstructive pulmonary disease, *see* Chronic obstructive pulmonary disease (COPD)

emphysema, *see* Emphysema
lung compliance reduced with, 13
near-drowning, mechanism of, 76–77
pulmonary vascular resistance and, 19
Occupational Safety and Health Administration (OSHA), 578
Occupational therapy, 544
Ocular disorders
  benzodiazepines causing, 340
  fentanyl causing, 327
  hyperthyroidism causing, 258
  sympathetic nervous system and, 281
Ocular oxygen toxicity, 76
Oculocardiac reflex, 572
Oculomotor (III) nerve, 571
OHS, 66, 67–68, 145
Oligemia, pulmonary, 480
Oliguria, 218, 237
  definition, 237
  in near-drowning, 78
  pathophysiology, 237
  perioperative fluid management, 237
  urine flow rate in, 218–219
Omphalocele, neonatal, 494
One-compartment model, 305
One lung ventilation, 51
Oocyte harvest, 524
Open breathing system, 43
Open heart surgery, 155
Open scavenging systems, 38, **39**
Open System Interconnection (OSI), 439
Operating room table, obese patients in, 68–69, 146
Operational amplifiers, 434, **436**
Ophthalmic nerve, 570
Ophthalmic surgery, 570–572
Opiate receptors, 545
Opiates, platelet transfusions and, 532
Opioid agonist-antagonist, 336, 551
Opioid agonists, 333–336, 549–551
  see also specific agonists
Opioid antagonists, 336–338
  see also specific antagonists
  pure antagonists, 336
  structure, 336
Opioid receptors, **331**–332
  agonist-antagonist, 336
  analgesic potency and, 331
  pure antagonist, 336
  sites of, 331
  spinal cord level, 331
  supraspinal, 331
Opioids, 331–332
  see also Narcotics
  Addison's disease, increased sensitivity to, 264
  central nervous system affected by, 163
  in elderly persons, 142

in pregnancy, 56
Opitropium bromide, 34
Optical fiber
  connecting local area network, 440
  for transducer, 435
Optical filters, for transducer, 435
Optical transducers, 101
Oral absorption, of opioids, 332
Oral administration, of narcotics, 548
Oral antiacid, in obese patients, 68
Oral intubation
  fiberoptic, 51
  perioperative management of, 50
Ordinary differential equations, 467
ORG 9487, **372**–373
Organ blood flow and autoregulation, 89
Organophosphates, 290–291
Orolaryngeal secretions, 323
Orthodromic conduction, 161–162
Oscillometry, 414
Oscillotonometry, 414
Osmolality
  specific gravity and, 222
  urinalysis, 219
  urine concentration, measure of, 222
Osmolar intake, 218–219
Osmolarity, 222
Osmolar load, 219
Osmotic diuretics, 227
Osmotic pressure, 222
Ostensible agency, 573
Osteomyelitis, 74
Osteopenia, 260
Osteoporosis, 565
Osteoradionecrosis, soft tissue, 74, 75
Ostwald solubility coefficient, 41
Otic ganglia, 282
Ovarian trauma, 523
Overpressure, 46–47
Ovulation enhancement, 523–524
Oxidative metabolism, 28–29
Oxidative phosphorylation, 28
Oxitropium bromide, 34
Oxycodone, 550
Oxygen
  angina and demand for, 99
  carriage of, 535
  critical temperature of, 43
  erythropoietin controlled by, 223–224
  hemoglobin, bound to, *see* Oxyhemoglobin
  need due to altitude, 62
  pregnancy increasing demand, 500
  transport of, *see* Oxygen transport
Oxygen, compressed
  for acute asthma in pregnancy, 56, 500
  in anaphylaxis treatment, 392
  as fire hazard, 429, 430

in heat stroke, 148
hyperbaric oxygen therapy, *see* Hyperbaric oxygen therapy
in operating room, 37
for persistent pulmonary hypertension, 480
in Pierre-Robin sequence, 495
postoperative, for obese patients, 147
for premature babies, 484
retinopathy of prematurity and, 485–486
Rotameter, measurement via, 398
supply of, 36–37
toxicity, 75–76
Oxygen, liquefied (O_2), 36–37
Oxygen-derived free radicals, 29
Oxygen-hemoglobin dissociation curve, 23
Oxygen in blood gas, 20
  methods of carrying O_2, 70
  transport of, 22–24
  uploading capacity of HbF and HbA, 488
Oxygen reserve, in infants, 484
Oxygen saturation
  fetal, 479
  neonatal, 489
Oxygen tension (P_{O_2}), 157
  bench top analyzer, 402–404
  continuous in vivo arterial blood gas monitor, 405
  fetal, 479
  hypoxia and, 62–63
  neonatal, 489
  point-of-care analyzers, 404
  renal, 223–224
  transcutaneous monitoring, 410–411
Oxygen transport, 22–24
  diffusion into interstitium and cells, 23–24
  neonatal, 22–24, 489
  uptake, 22
Oxyhemoglobin, 70, 489
  in neonate, 488
Oxymorphone, 550
Oxytocics, 274, 501–502

P_{50}, neonatal, 488, 489
Pacemaker, permanent, 103
$PaCO_2$, 481
Pagers, 443
PAH, 219, 220, 221
Pain
  abdominal, 248
  afferent pain pathways, 159, 279
  chest, 115
  electricity causing, 426
  flank, 239
  generalized pain disorders, 558–562
  muscular, 376

Pain, *continued*
  musculoskeletal, 115
  neuropathic, 558–559
  nociceptive, 551–552
  skeletal, 260
  sympathetic mediated, 559–561
Pain management
  chronic pain, 543–558
  postoperative, in obese patients, 146, 147
Pain on injection
  from diazepam, 324
  diprivan causing, 321
  etomidate causing, 322
Paleospinothalamic tract, 159
Palliation, 387
Palmar erythema, 248
Palpitations, 32
Pancreas, 253–254
  function of, 276
  glucagon secreted by, 276
  inhibition of secretion, 276
  insulin secreted by, 276
  stimulation of secretion, 276
  transplantation of, 273
Pancreatitis, acute, 261
Pancuronium, **366**–367
  hepatic disease affecting, 356
  as nicotinic antagonist, 291
PaO$_2$
  fetal, 479
  postnatal, 480
PAP, *see* Pulmonary artery pressure (PAP)
Paper drapes, as combustible, 429
Para-aminohippurate
  clearance, 219
  extraction, 220
  secretion of, 221
Paracentesis, 248
Paracervical block, 524
Parainfluenza 3, 496
Paralysis
  Guillain-Barré syndrome, 60
  of respiratory muscles, 12, 426
Paraplegia, 172
Paraquat toxicity, 31
Parasellar tumor, 254
Parasympathetic ganglia, 281–282
Parasympathetic nerves, 281
Parasympathetic nervous system, 281–282
  and blood flow control, 90
  energy-conserving/building responses, 281
  myocardial, 86
  in neonates, 485
  organs affected by, 282
Parasympathetic neurons, 281
Parasympathomimetics, 289–291

Parathyroid, 252
Parathyroidectomy, 260
Parathyroid hormone, 275
  effects of, 205
  hyperparathyroidism and, 260
  kinetics, 205
  renal effects, 205
    acid-base balance, 212
    calcium balance, 215
    magnesium excretion, 216
    phosphate balance, 216
    renal vascular resistance, 200
    tubular function, 205
Paravertebral ganglia, 280
Parenchyma, pulmonary
  aging and, 140
  lung compliance reduced with, 13
  rheumatoid nodules in, 58
Parenchymal liver disease, 247
Parenteral absorption, 332
Paroxysmal supraventricular tachycardia, 123
Partial convulsion, 166–168
Partial correlation, 461
Partial derivatives, 467
Partial differentiation, 464–465
Partial thrombin time (PTT), 242
Particular solution, in differential equation, 467
Particulate filtration, 28
Parties in lawsuit, 576
Partition coefficient, 41, **42**
  anesthetic gas transfer proportional to, 47
Partnerships, 577
Pascal's law, 35, 61
Passive diffusion, 306
Passive regurgitation, 526
Passover water humidifiers, 53–54
Pathologic reflexes, 160
Patient-applied risk current, 427
Patient care vicinity, 427
Patient connection, 427
Patient positioning
  and incidence of air embolism, 176
  in induced hypotension, 293
  in neonatal myelomeningocele, 495
  supine position, *see* Supine position
Patient safety, 423–430
  electrical safety, 425–428
  new medical devices, 423–424
Pavulon, *see* Pancuronium
Peak airway pressure, 391
Peak expiratory flow rate (PEFR), 15
  preoperative evaluation, 50
Peak inspiratory pressure (PIP), 412
Peak respiratory pressure, 53
Pediatrics, 479–499
  see also Neonates, Infants, Premature infants

  atracurium in, 359
  cerebral arteriovenous malformations, 182
  cistracurium use in, 361
  gamma knife used in, 567
  respiratory emergencies, 496–497
Pellagra, carcinoid-related, 268
Pelvic nerve, 279
Penalties, legal, 573
Peñaz, 414–415
Penicillins
  allergic reactions to, 394
  kidney failure affecting, 235
Pentamidine, 235
Pentazocine, 336, 551
Pentobarbital, 317
Percutaneous transhepatic cholangiography, 247
Perfusion pressure, 89
  cerebral, 318
Periaqueductal gray matter, 159
Peribulbar injection, 571–572
Pericardial effusion, 113
  hypothyroidism causing, 259
  lung compliance reduced with, 13
  tamponade from, 113–114
Pericarditis, 113
Pericardium, 113
  function, 113
  relation to heart, 83
Perinatal adaptation, 482
Periodic breathing, in infants, 484
Periorbital edema, 259
Peripartum cardiomyopathy, 137
Peripheral nervous system, in pregnancy, 501
Peripheral opiate receptors, 545
Peripheral temperature measurement, 295
Peripheral vascular resistance
  in neonates, 484
  in pregnancy, 500
Peristalsis, increased, 281
Peritoneal dialysis, 236
Persistent fetal circulation, 480, 482
Persistent fetal hypertension, 480
Persistent pulmonary hypertension, 490
Personal data assistant, 443
PET, 220, 446
PGD$_2$, 31
PGE$_1$, 31, 480
PGE$_2$, 31
PGF$_{2\alpha}$, 20, 31
PGG$_2$, 31
PGH$_2$, 31
pH
  assisted reproductive technologies affected by, 523
  bench top analyzers of, 403

continuous in vivo arterial blood gas monitor, 405
in diabetic ketoacidosis, 270
of fetal scalp, 503–504
point-of-care analyzers, 404
urinalysis, 219
Pharmacodynamics, 305
  changes in
    aging and, 142
    as cerebral protection, 178–179
    obesity and, 66, 67, 145
Pharmacokinetics, 304
  changes in
    aging and, 142
    as cerebral protection, 178–179
    obesity and, 66, 67, 145
Pharyngeal innervation, 4
Phased array transducers, 421
Phase II muscle relaxant, 354–355
Phenobarbital
  as exogenous toxin, 170
  as seizure treatment, 167
Phenothiazines
  kidney failure affecting, 235
  neuroleptic malignant syndrome from, 299
Phenoxybenzamine, 286
Phentolamine
  as alpha antagonist, 286
  as vasodilator, 97–98
Phenylbutazone, 244
Phenylephrine
  as alpha$_1$ agonist, 285
  as cardiac drug in pregnancy, 130
  as vasoconstrictor, 98, 349
  as vasopressor, central nervous system affected by, 165
Phenytoin
  as antidysrhythmic, 93
  kidney failure affecting, 235
  in pregnancy, 131
  as seizure treatment, 167
Pheochromocytoma, 266–267
  anesthetic management, 514
  in pregnancy, 514–515
Phlebitis, 115
Phosphate
  balance in urologic system, 216
  in diabetic ketoacidosis, 270, 271
  parathyroid hormone and, 275
Phosphatidylglycerol (PG), 481
Phosphaturia, 270
Phosphodiesterase inhibitor, 92
Phospholipid-azprotein complex, 481
Photomultiplier, 435
Photo resistor, 435
Phototube, 435
Physical dependence, on opioid drugs, 546–547

Physically demanding, obese persons as, 67, 145
Physical therapy, 544
Physostigmine, 290
Pia mater, spinal, 153
Pickwickian syndrome, 66, 67–68, 145
Pierre-Robin sequence, 495
Piezoelectric crystals, 420, 434
PIH, 504–510
Pilocarpine, 289
Piloerection, 280
Pilomotor muscle contraction, 281
Pindolol, 95, 288
Pin Index Safety System, 38, **39**
"Pink puffer", 49
Pipecuronium, **367**–368
Pitocin, 502
Pituitary, 252
  dysfunction of, 265
    see also specific disorders
    hypofunction, 259
    irradiation, 262
    microsurgery, 262
Pituitary apoplexy, 254
Pituitary diabetes insipidus, 256
Pituitary hormones, 274
Pituitary tumor
  acromegaly associated with, 256
  hypopituitarism caused by, 254
  hypothyroidism associated with, 259
Placebos, clinical trials using, 462
Placenta, retained, 521
Placenta accreta, 517
Placental abruptio, 520
Placental transfer, 501
Placenta percreta, 521
Placenta previa, 516–517
Planar process technology, 433
Plasma
  frozen, transfusion of, 532–533
  oxygen dissolved in, 70, 489
Plasma creatinine, 220
Plasma glucose, 221
Plasma histamine level, 392
Plasma norepinephrine levels, 140
Plasma proteins, 306
Plasma pseudocholinesterase concentration, 500
Plateau pressure (P$_p$), 412
Platelet activating factor, 391
Platelet count, 242
Platelet plug formation, 119
Platelets, 532
  disorders involving, 540
  sympathetic nervous system affecting, 281
  transfusion of, 532
Pleura, 7
  rheumatoid nodules on, 58

Pleural cavities
  chest x-ray of, 9, 10
  computed tomography of, 10
Pleural effusion
  in ascites, 248
  lung compliance reduced with, 13
  in rheumatoid disease, 58
Pleural fluid, 7
Pneumatic compression, intermittent, 115
Pneumonia
  lung compliance reduced with, 13
  as postoperative complication, 52
  pulmonary embolus differentiated, 115
  surfactant deficiencies associated with, 481
Pneumonitis
  acute lupus, 57
  hypersensitivity, 50
  as transesophageal fistula complication, 492
Pneumotachometer, 10, 400–401
Pneumotaxic center, 25
Pneumothorax
  chest x-ray of, 9
  computed tomography of, 10
  loculated, 10
  pulmonary embolus differentiated, 115
  subtle, 10
PO$_4$, see Phosphate
Point-of-care analyzers, 404
Poisson probability distribution, 451
Polarity, drug excretion affected by, 245
Poliomyelitis
  lung compliance reduced with, 13
  vital capacity (VC) and, 12
Polyarteritis, 19
Polycythemia
  in congenital heart disease, 127
  postnatal, 480
Polydipsia
  as diabetic ketoacidosis sign, 269
  as hypercalcemia sign, 260
  primary, polyuria differentiated, 256
Polyethylene gloves, 394
Polyglandular syndrome, 266
Polymeric devices, 429
Polyneuropathy, 259
Polynomial regression, 460
Polypeptide insulin, 276
Polyuria, 237
  diabetes insipidus associated with, 255, 256
  as diabetic ketoacidosis sign, 269
  differential diagnosis, 256
  effects, 237
  as hypercalcemia sign, 260
  pathophysiology, 237
  preoperative evaluation, 239

Polyvinyl gloves, 394
Pons, pneumotaxic center in, 25
Population distribution, 452
Population life table, 448
Population means, inference on, 452–457, 457–459
Porphyria
    acute intermittent, 318
    methohexitone causing, 319
    variegate, 318
Portal hypertension, 247
Portal vein, 241
Positive end expiratory pressure, 413
    and critical care ventilators, 53
Positron emission tomography, 446
    renal blood flow measurement, 220
Posteriorcord syndrome, 173
Posterior longitudinal ligament, 153
Posterior pituitary hormones, 274
Postganglionic parasympathetic nerves, 282
Postganglionic sympathetic nerves, 282, 283
Postirradiation complications, 254
Postnatal circulation, transition to, 480
Postoperative apnea, 490
Postoperative complications
    anesthesia-related, 52
    apnea, 490
    hypopituitarism caused by, 254
Postpartum bleeding, 521–523
Postpartum hemorrhage, treatment of, 56
Postsynaptic receptors
    alpha$_1$ adrenoreceptors, 90
    alpha$_2$ adrenoreceptors, 284
    beta$_1$ adrenoreceptors, 91
    beta$_2$ adrenoreceptors, 91
    depolarizing muscle relaxants binding to, 373
Posttetanic facilitation, 383
Posttetanic facilitation count, 383
Posttraumatic dystrophy, 559
Potassium
    in diabetic ketoacidosis, 270, 271
    excretion of
        calcitonin and, 275
        in primary aldosteronism, 263
    as hyperosmolar nonketonic coma therapy, 273
    hypokalemia, see Hypokalemia
    point-of-care analyzers, 404
    renal acid-base balance affected by, 212–213
    urologic system, balance in, 214–215
Potassium-sparing diuretics, 227–228
Potts shunt, 491
Power density, of batteries, 444–445
Power series, in infinite series, 469–470
Pralidoxime, 290

Prazosin, 286
Prednisolone, **277**
Prednisone, **277**
    as anaphylaxis prophylaxis, 392
    as immunosuppressive, 387
Preeclampsia
    acute kidney failure caused by, 230
    cardiovascular system in, 505
Preejection phase of cardiac cycle, 259
Preexcitation syndromes, 124–125
Preganglionic parasympathetic nerves, 282
Preganglionic sympathetic nerves, 282
Pregnancy
    see also Obstetrics
    asthma in, 54–57, 500
    bupivacaine in, 351
    cardiac disease in, 129–130, 134–137
    cardiac drugs in, 130–131
    cardiovascular changes, 129
    complications of, 504–523
    congenital heart disease in, 134–137
    diazepam in, 324
    as electroconvulsant therapy contraindication, 565
    labor and delivery, see Labor and delivery
    physiology of, 500–501, 510
    protein binding in, 307
    respiratory disease in, 54–57
    respiratory failure during, 57
    symptoms in, 129–130
    valvular heart diseases in, 131–134
Pregnancy-induced hypertension, 504–510
Preload increase, obesity and, 66, 144
Premarket approval, 423, 424
Premarket notification, regarding new devices, 423–424
Premature infants
    fatigue of respiratory muscles, 490
    hypoxia, response to, 482
    perinatal adaptations in, 482
    retinopathy of prematurity and, 486
    surfactant deficiencies associated with, 481
Premedication
    see also specific premedicants
    in hypothyroidism, 260
    in induced hypotension, 293
    of obese patients, 68, 146
Preoperative hemodilution, 534
Preponderance of evidence, 574
Pressure, 101, 412
    cardiac, 88
    equilibrium of gas and liquid pressures, **40**–41
    gastric, 526
    gauges, see Pressure gauges
    gauge vs absolute, 101

    hydrostatic, 17, 54
    intra-abdominal, obesity and, 67, 144
    intraocular, 323, 376
    measurement of, 37, 101
Pressure control ventilation, 53
Pressure/flow relationships, 15
Pressure gauges, 37–38, 101
    anaeroid gauge, 101
    on anesthesia machines, 37
    Bourdon tube type, **38**, 101
    color coded by gas, 38
    diaphragm gauge, 101
    manometer, 101
    for nitrous oxide, 42–43
    transducers, 101, 415, 428
Pressure support ventilation, 53
Pressurized, heated vaporizers, 35, 36
Prilocaine, 351
Primary adrenocortical insufficiency, 264
Primary aldosteronism, 263
Primary batteries, 444
Primary hyperparathyroidism, 260
Primary hypoparathyroidism, 261
Primidone, 167
Probability, 450–452
Probability distribution, 451
Procainamide
    as antidysrhythmic, 93
    cistracurium interacting with, 361
    kidney failure affecting, 235
Procoagulants, 540–541
Professional negligence, 575–576
Progesterone concentrations, 501
Prolonged nonventilation, 13
Promethazine, 343–344
Propafenone, 94
Propionic acid derivatives, 552
    see also specific derivatives
Propofol
    central nervous system affected by, 164
    as cerebral protection, 178
    in elderly persons, 142
    reactions to, 393
    seizures and, 168
Propoxyphene, 550
Propranolol, 94
    as beta antagonist, 288
    pulmonary circulation, taken up in, 31
Prostaglandin F$_2$
    as oxytocin, 502
Prostaglandins, 391
    and obstetric management, 56
    as oxytocin, 502
    as vasoactive compound, 30–31
Prostaglandins (E series)
    for congenital heart disease, 480
    as oxytocin, 502

for pulmonary atresia, 491
    renal vascular resistance and, 199
Prostatic hypertrophy, 344
Prostatic resection complications, 238
Prostatitis, 223
Protamine, 393–394
Protease transport, 29
Protein
    hepatic metabolism of, 242
    intake of, glomerular filtration rate
        and, 202
    urinalysis, 219
Protein binding
    aging and, 142, 307
    blood-placental barrier and, 501
    and kidney failure, 233, 307
    and liver failure, 307
    of local anesthetic, 349
    pharmacokinetics and, 244
    in pregnancy, 307
Proteinuria, 504
Proteolytic enzymes, 254
Prothrombin time (PT), 540
    tests of, 242, 244
Proventil, *see* Albuterenol
Proximal tubule, 194, 203
    acid-base balance and, 211–212
    brush border enzymes of, 223
    and carbonic anhydrase inhibitors,
        224
    injury to, 223
    phosphate absorption, 216
    potassium balance and, 214
    sodium balance and, 213
Pruritus
    diprivan for, 320
    fentanyl causing, 328
    as opioid side effect, 332, 547
Pseudocholinesterase, 374
    genetic variants of, **375**
    plasma concentration during
        pregnancy, 500
    succinylcholine and, 374
Pseudohypertrophic muscular
        dystrophy, 60, 298
Pseudohypoparathyroidism, 261
Pseudopseudohypoparathyroidism, 261
Psia, 37
Psig, 37
Psychiatric therapy, 564–566
Psychological dependence, 547
Psychologic disturbances
    in craniosynostosis, 189
    obesity and, 66, 67, 145
    recall of intraoperative events as, 159
Psychosis, 260
Psychosocial problems, 65
Psychosomatic disorders, 565
Psychotherapy, 543–544
PTH, *see* Parathyroid hormone

Public Health Service, 423
Pulmonary angiography, 115
Pulmonary arterial occlusion pressure
        (PAOP), 67
Pulmonary arteries, 7, 83
    anesthetic gas uptake in, 47
    atresia with intact intraventricular
        septum, 491–492
    baroreceptors, 27
    chest x-ray of, 8, 9
    left, 83
    obstruction, lung compliance reduced
        with, 13
Pulmonary artery catheter (PAC), **416**
Pulmonary artery flotation catheter, 69
Pulmonary artery pressure (PAP), 16
    for air embolism, 176
    neonatal, 485
    pulmonary vascular resistance
        influenced by, 18
Pulmonary aspiration
    obesity and, 67, 144
    in pregnancy, 525–528
    types of aspirates, 526
Pulmonary blood flow
    at birth, 17
    perinatal, 482
    post natal, 480
Pulmonary circulation, 16–18
    in congenital heart disease, 126
    drugs taken up in, 31
    hydrostatic pressure differences, 17
    inequality of distribution, 16–18
    multiple functions of, 87
Pulmonary edema, 54
    cardiac/hydrostatic, 54
    high-altitude, 63
    as kidney failure complication, 232
    naloxone causing, 330
    neurogenic, 54
    as supraglottitis complication, 497
    surfactant deficiencies associated
        with, 481
    transfusion-related deaths from, 249
    vital capacity (VC) and, 12
Pulmonary embolectomy, 115
Pulmonary embolism, 114–115
    as anesthetic emergency, 391
    in Guillain-Barré syndrome, 60
    hypercarbia due to, 51
    hyperosmolar nonketotic coma,
        concurrent with, 273
    pulmonary vascular resistance and,
        19
Pulmonary embolus syndrome, 114
Pulmonary fibrosis, 50
    lung compliance reduced with, 13
    pulmonary vascular resistance and, 19
Pulmonary function tests
    preoperative evaluation, 50

pulse oximetry, 409–410
    in rheumatoid disease, 58
    in sarcoidosis, 59
    in systemic lupus erythematosus, 58
Pulmonary hyperplasia, postnatal, 480
Pulmonary hypertension
    congenital heart disease and, 480
    in diaphragmatic hernia, 490
    idiopathic, postnatal, 480
    mitral stenosis in pregnancy and, 132
    neonatal, 485
    obesity and, 67, 144
    persistent, 480, 490
    in pregnancy, 132, 138–139
Pulmonary infarction, 114
Pulmonary infections, 60
Pulmonary oligemia, postnatal, 480
Pulmonary oxygen toxicity, 75
Pulmonary secretions, 281
Pulmonary shunts, 48
Pulmonary system
    cirrhosis affecting, 248
    disease as electroconvulsant therapy
        contraindication, 565
    sympathetic nervous system affecting,
        281
Pulmonary thromboembolism, 520
Pulmonary tissue pressures, 16
Pulmonary toxicity, 389
Pulmonary tree, 568
Pulmonary valve, 83
    hypoplastic, 491
Pulmonary valve cusps, 491
Pulmonary valvotomy, 491
Pulmonary vascular pressures, 16
Pulmonary vascular resistance (PVR),
        18–19
    influences on, 18
    neonatal, 484, 490
    perinatal, 482
    postnatal, 480
Pulmonary vasoconstriction
    catastrophic, 394
    hypoxic, 17
    postnatal, 480
Pulmonary veins, 7
    chest x-ray of, 9
    engorgement of, 13
Pulsed ultrasound, 421, 422
Pulsed-wave technology, 422
Pulse oximetry
    as hypoxia monitor, 409–410
    interference, 409–410
    limitations, 409
    in obese patients, 69, 146
    in ophthalmic surgery, 571
    principle, 409–410
Pulsus paradoxus, 113
Punitive damages, 575
Pupillary constriction, 281

Pupillary dilation
    as fight-or flight response, 280
    sympathetic nervous system affecting,
        281
Pure sensory neuropathies, 173
PVCs, obesity and, 67, 144
PVR, *see* Pulmonary vascular resistance
    (PVR)
Pyelonephritis, 232
Pyloric stenosis, neonatal, 493
Pyramidal tract, 160
Pyridostigmine, 290
Pyrrole derivatives, 552
    see also specific derivatives

QT syndrome, prolonged, 125
    hypoparathyroidism and, 261
Quadrate lobe, 241
Quadriplegia, 172
Quantal theory, 162
Quantum radiation detectors, 435
Quaternary anticholinergic, 34
Quinidine
    as antidysrhythmic, 92–93
    cistracurium interacting with, 361
    in pregnancy, 131

Racemic epinephrine, 496
Radial artery, 87
Radiation
    gamma knife using, 567
    neonatal heat exchange via, 487
Radiation detectors, 435
Radioactive microspheres, 220
Radioallergosorbent test, 392
Radiocontrast media
    acute kidney failure caused by,
        230–231
    allergic reactions to, 394
Radio frequency (RF), 442
Radiography, 445–446
    of systemic lupus erythematosus,
        57–58
Radionecrosis, soft tissue, 74, 75
Radionuclide cerebral blood flow study,
    185
Radionuclide flow scan, 220
Radionuclide scan
    cerebral, for coma, 169
    as thyroid function test, 252
Radionuclide scintigraphic imaging,
    102
Rales, 115
Random access memory, 437
Randomization, 461–462
Random variable, 451
Random variables and distributions,
    451–452
Ranitidine, 527–528
Ranks, in statistics, 449

Rapid computed tomography, 446
Rapid eye movement (REM)
    fetal breathing occurring during, 481
    neonatal apneic pauses during, 484
    periodic breathing in preterm babies
        during, 484
Rash, 360
RAST, *see* Radioallergosorbent test
Rastelli procedure, 492
RBF, *see* Renal blood flow
Reactive airway disease, *see* Asthma
Read-only memory, 437
Real-time scan, 422
Real-time scan, in ultrasound, 421
Rebleeding, 180
Rebreathing, 43
    and breathing systems, 44
Receptors
    acetylcholine, 162–163, 283
    adrenergic, *see* Adrenergic receptors
    alpha, *see* Alpha adrenoreceptors
    atrial natriuretic peptide, 206–207
    of autonomic nervous system, 283
    baroreceptors, *see* Baroreceptors
    beta, *see* Beta adrenoreceptors
    dopamine, 91–92, 283
    J receptors, 26
    mechanoreceptors, 27
    stretch, 90
    thyroid hormone, activity based on,
        274
Rechargeable alkaline-manganese
    dioxide batteries, 444
Recipient alloimmunization, 250
Rectal absorption, of opioids, 332
Rectal administration, of narcotics, 548
Rectus abdominous muscles, 13
Recurrent laryngeal nerve, 4
Red blood cells, 219
Red cell membrane, 538–539
Redirector software, 440
Red man's syndrome, 394
Reentry in rhythm disorders, 120
Reflection, in ultrasound, 420–421
Reflex(es)
    airway, 141–142
    Bainbridge, 27
    and blood pressure control, 89
    Hering-Breuer inflation, 25
    intrathoracic, 27
    myotactic, *see* Tendon reflexes
    oculocardiac, 572
    pathologic, 160
    spinal, 160
    tendon, 160, 259
Reflex sympathetic dystrophy, 160,
    559
Refractometer, 223
Refractory hypertension, 387
Refusal of treatment, 578

Regional anesthesia
    coagulation disorders and, 542
    in elderly persons, 143
    general anesthesia combined with, 69
    general anesthesia compared
        in elderly persons, 143
        in obese patients, 146
    in hypertensive patients, 106
    neonatal bradycardia risk reduced
        with, 490
    neonatal postoperative apnea risk
        reduced with, 490
    in obese patients, 69, 146–147
    in ophthalmic surgery, 570–572
    for pheochromocytoma in pregnancy,
        514–515
    in transvaginal aspiration, 524
    urologic effects of, 228
Reglan, 527
Regression
    and cytotoxins, 387
    in statistics, 459–461
Rejection reaction, controlling,
    386–389
Relative humidity, 42
Renal acid-base balance, 211–213
Renal artery, 87, 195
Renal blood flow, 196–201
    anesthesia effects, 201
    burn injuries affecting, 568
    in cardiopulmonary bypass, 239
    diprivan decreasing, 320
    diseases affecting, 200
    distribution, 196
    drug effects on, 200–201, 310
    halothane affecting, 310
    induced hypotension affecting, 238
    ketamine increasing, 323
    measurement of, 219–220
    mechanical ventilation affecting, 238
    methohexitone decreasing, 319
    regulation of, 196–197
    surgical effects, 201
    thiopentone affecting, 318
Renal drug elimination
    obesity affecting, 67, 145
    of opioids, 322
Renal excretion
    of aldosterone, 216
    calcitonin and, 275
    of magnesium, 216
    of naloxone, 329
Renal insufficiency
    in aging, 141
    in near-drowning, 78
    oliguria, *see* Oliguria
    perioperative fluid management, 237
Renal metabolism, of narcotics, **549**
Renal oxygen tension, 223–224
Renal pelvis, 195

Renal perfusion pressure, 196–197
Renal plasma flow, 196–201
  distribution, 196
  effective, (eRPF), 219–220
  in pregnancy, 501
Renal system
  desflurane affecting, 314
  disorders of
    see also specific disorders
    atracurium use in, 359
    mivacurium use in, 365
    neuromuscular blockade affected
      by, 356
  enflurane affecting, 312
  halothane affecting, 310
  hypothermia affecting, 295
  isoflurane affecting, 312–313
  malignant hyperthermia affecting,
    297
  methohexitone affecting, 319
  nonsteroidal anti-inflammatory drugs
    affecting, 338
  NSAIDs affecting, 552
  in pregnancy, 501
  pregnancy-induced hypertension
    affecting, 506
  sevoflurane affecting, 315
Renal vascular resistance, 197–200
Renal vasoconstriction, 568
Renarcotization, 330
Renin-angiotensin system, 90
  and renal vascular resistance,
    197–198
Renin secretion, 281
Resedation, 326
Residual sedation, 324
Residual volume (RV), 11, 12
Resistance, 431
  airway, 15–16
  in cardiovascular system, 100–101
  as circuit element, 432
  to flow through tube, 100
  vascular, see Vascular resistance
Resistive transducers, 101
Resistivity, 431
Resolution, 445
Respiration
  see also Breathing
  in infants, 484
  regulation of, 25–27
Respiration monitoring
  of anesthetic depth, 159
  in ophthalmic surgery, 571
Respiratory acidosis, 21
  in near-drowning, 78
  neuromuscular blockage and, 356
Respiratory bronchioles, 6
Respiratory center, 25–26
  apnea of prematurity and, 489
  arterial blood, 26

chemical control, 25, 26
damage of, 26
dorsal respiratory group, 25
Hering-Breuer inflation reflex, 25
location, 25–26
neonatal, 482
pneumotaxic center, 25
temperature and, 26
vasomotor center, 26
ventral respiratory group, 25
voluntary control, 26
Respiratory depression
  fentanyl causing, 328
  in infants, 497–498
  from opioid drugs, 146, 547
Respiratory distress
  near-drowning causing, 78
  in neonatal diaphragmatic hernia,
    490
  in tracheoesophageal fistula, 492
Respiratory distress syndrome
  adult, see Adult respiratory distress
    syndrome
  newborn, 481
Respiratory exchange ratio (R), 24
Respiratory failure, during pregnancy,
    57
Respiratory gas pressures, **65**
Respiratory paralysis
  electricity causing, 426
  vital capacity and, 12
Respiratory rate
  in infants, 484
  opioids affecting, 332
Respiratory system, 3–12
  see also specific structures
  acid base, 20–21, 356
  aging affecting, 140–141
  airway resistance, 15–16
  anaphylaxis affecting, 391
  benzodiazepines affecting, 340
  blood gas, 20
  compliance, see Compliance,
    respiratory
  desflurane affecting, 314
  diazepam affecting, 324
  diprivan affecting, 320
  disorders of, 49–80
    see also specific disorders
    pediatric emergencies, 496–497
  droperidol affecting, 344
  enflurane affecting, 311
  etomidate affecting, 322
  fentanyl affecting, 327
  gas transport, 21–24
  halothane affecting, 310
  hypothyroidism affecting, 259
  intrathoracic reflexes and, 27
  isoflurane affecting, 312–313
  ketamine affecting, 323

malignant hyperthermia affecting,
    297
  mechanics, 12–13
  methohexitone affecting, 319
  midazolam affecting, 325
  near drowning, 76–80
  neuromuscular blockade and, 356
  obesity and, 66, 144
  perinatal adaptation, 482
  physics of, 35–49
  physiology, 10–31
  in pregnancy, 500
  pregnancy-induced hypertension
    affecting, 505
  prenatal development, 481
  sevoflurane affecting, 315
  spirometry, 10–12, 401
  surface tension, 14
  ventilation-perfusion, 16–20
  work of breathing, 16
Restlessness
  local anesthetics causing, 350
Restrictive cardiomyopathy, 112–113
Restrictive lung disease
  hypersensitivity pneumonitis, 50
  pulmonary fibrosis, see Pulmonary
    fibrosis
  sarcoidosis, 50
  spirometry of, 12
  systemic sclerosis, 50
Resuscitation, of neonates, 497–**499**
Reticulocyte count, 224
Retinal detachment
  as electroconvulsant therapy
    contraindication, 565
  scleral buckling for, 486
Retinal hemorrhages, 63–64
Retinol binding protein, 223
Retinopathy of prematurity, 485–486
Retractions, 496
Retractor pressure, prolonged, 293
Retrobulbar hemorrhage, 572
Retrobulbar injection, 571
Retrognathia, 495
Retrolental fibroplasia, 55
Reversal of neuromuscular blockade,
    378–381
Rewarming, 296
Reynold's number, 100
Rh, ABO incompatibility, 515–516
Rhabdomyolysis, 296
Rheumatic heart disease, 129
Rheumatoid arthritis, 4
Rheumatoid diseases, 58
  arthritis, 4
Rheumatoid nodules, 58
Rh immune globulin, 515
Rhythm disorders, see Dysrhythmias
Rib elevation, 12
Rifampicin, 244

Right arterial catheter, positioning, 177
Right atrium, 83
  pathways and conduction through, 85
Right bundle branch block, 121
Right coronary arteries, 89
Right lobar and segmental bronchi, 5
Right to privacy, 573
Right ventricle, 83
  blood flow requirements, 89
  drainage into anterior cardiac veins, 86
  in neonate, 484
Ring, in local area networks, 438
Risk current, 427–428
Ritodrine, 288
  as tocolytic, 502
Rocuronium, **368**–369
  as nicotinic antagonist, 291–292
Rotameter, 100–101, 398
RPF, *see* Renal plasma flow
RPP, 196–197
Rubber, allergic reactions to, 394
Rule of correspondence, 463
Rule of "9's", 568

Sacral vertebrae, 152
SAH, 179–180
Salbutamol, 32
Salicylic acid derivatives, 552
  see also specific derivatives
Saline, normal, 270
Salivation, increased, 281
Salmeterol, 33
Saltatory conduction, 161–162
Sample inlet, in mass spectroscopy, 406
Sarcoid, hypopituitarism caused by, 254
Sarcoidosis, 50, 58–59
Sarcolemma, 87
Sarcomas, 388
Sarcomere, 87
Sarcoplasmic reticulum, 87
  in fetus, 484
Satellites, 442
Satellite telecommunications network, 444
Saturated vapor pressure, 40
Scalene muscles, 12
Scalp blood sampling, fetal, 503–504
Scalp electroencephalogram, 154
Scaphoid abdomen, 490
Scar tissue, 51
Scavenging systems, 38–**40**
Schizophrenia, 565
Scintigraphic imaging, 102–103, 103
Scleroderma, 19
Sclerosis
  pulmonary vascular resistance and, 19
  systemic, 50
Scopolamine, 291

Scuba diving
  air embolism caused by, 71–72
  decompression sickness, 71–73
Sealed lead batteries, 444
Seawater aspiration, 77
Secondary adrenocortical insufficiency, 265
Secondary aldosteronism, 263
Secondary batteries, 444
Secondary hyperparathyroidism, 261
Second-degree heart block, 121
Second gas effect, 48–49
Second heart sound, 115
Sedation
  in obese patients, 68, 146
  in ophthalmic surgery, 572
  in transvaginal aspiration, 524
Sedatives
  central nervous system affected by, 163
  for chronic pain, 557
Seizures, 167
  see also Convulsions
  analeptics causing, 166
  anesthetic considerations, 168
  eclampsia, 504
  electroconvulsant therapy producing, 564–566
  local anesthetics-induced, treatment of, 350–351
  in ophthalmic surgery, 572
  treatment, 167–168
Selective beta-adrenergic agonists, 32–33
  see also specific agonists
Self-determination, 578–579
Semiclosed breathing system, 43
Semiclosed scavenging systems, 38–39
Semiconductors, 432–433
Semiopen breathing system, 43
Separate counsel, 577
Sepsis
  acute kidney failure caused by, 230
  in burn injuries, 568
  imperforate anus as risk for, 493
  renal blood flow and, 200
Septic shock
  amniotic fluid embolism differentiated, 520
  renal blood flow and, 200
Septostomy, balloon atrial, 491
Sequence, in infinite series, 469
Serotonin, 267, 391
  see also 5-Hydroxytryptamine
  carcinoid syndrome from overproduction of, 267
  renal blood flow affected by, 200
Serotonin antagonists, 268
Serum creatinine, 221
Serum hepatitis, 245, 246

Serum lipids
  elevated, 105
  obesity and, 67, 144
Serum protein, in aging, 142
Server software, 440
Settlement offers, 576
Sevoflurane, 315–316
  central nervous system affected by, 164
  urinary system, effects on, 228
SG, 222–223
Shock
  as diabetic ketoacidosis complication, 271
  hypovolemic, 200, 568
  macroshock, 426
  microshock, 426
  septic, 200, 520
  spinal, 172
Short stature, 261
Shoulder-hand syndrome, 559
Shunt(s)
  anesthetic uptake affected by, 47–48
  Blalock-Taussig, 491
  intracardiac, 47–48
  intrapulmonary, 47–48
  LeVeen, 248
  modified Blalock-Taussig, 491–492
  obesity and, 144
  Potts, 491
  pulmonary, 48
  right-to-left, in neonatal diaphragmatic hernia, 490
  shunt equation, 19
  and ventilation/perfusion ratio, 19
  VP, in craniosynostosis, 189
  Waterson, 491
Shunt equation, 19
Si, 433
Sickle cell disease, 536
Sickle cell trait, 536
Sick sinus syndrome, 123
Sigmoid curve in pharmacodynamics, 305
Signal-to-noise ratio (S/N), 445
Significant risk device study, 424
Silver oxide batteries, 444
Single blind trials, 462
Single cuff system, 414
Single photon emission computed tomography (SPECT), 446
Sinoatrial (SA) node, 85
  conduction, halothane affecting, 310
Sinus bradycardia, 122–123
  succinylcholine causing, 375
Sinus tachycardia, 122
Site of surgery, 52
Skeletal abnormalities, 538
Skeletal muscle relaxants, 557
Skeletal nerves, 282

Skeletal pain, 260
Skin, 568
    anaphylaxis affecting, 391
    atracurium affecting, 359
    bleomycin affecting, 389
    electricity affecting, 426
    malignant hyperthermia affecting, 297
    noxious stimuli, autonomic
        hyperreflexia from, 298
    sympathetic nervous system affecting,
        281
Skin grafts/flaps, 74, 75
Skin tests, 391–392
Skull deformities, 189
Skull films, 169
Sleep disorders
    insomnia, 63
    somnolence, 260
Slurred speech, 350
Small bronchi, 6
    obstruction in infants, 481
Smoking
    as arteriosclerosis risk factor, 105
    cessation as preoperative
        preparation, 50
    cigarettes, 105
    fetal breathing affected by, 481
Soda lime
    as carbon dioxide absorbent, 46
    sevoflurane decomposing into,
        315–316
Sodium
    balance in urologic system, 213–214
    hypernatremia, see Hypernatremia
    hyponatremia, see Hyponatremia
    retention, 263
Sodium bicarbonate, **499**
Sodium channels, 347
Sodium excretion
    atrial natriuretic factor (ANF) and,
        90
    mechanical ventilation affecting, 238
Sodium ion
    in diabetic ketoacidosis, 270
    local anesthetics and permeability of,
        346
Sodium nitroprusside, 96–97
    central nervous system affected by,
        165
Soft palate, 4
    in neonate, 482
Soft tissue
    chest x-ray of, 8
    necrotizing infections, 74, 75
Software, 437
    for LAN protocol, 438
    for network operating systems, 440
    statistic analysis programs, 448
Solubility, 40–41
    of gases, 41

gas vs liquid, pressures of, **40**–41
    of solids, 41
Solubility coefficients, **40**–41
Soluble anesthetics, 48
Solute balance in lungs, 27
Solute diuresis, 256
Solution, in differential equation, 467
Somatomammotropic hormones, 274
Somatosensory evoked potentials
        (SSEP), 156
Somatostatin, 268
Somnolence, 260
Sonography, see Ultrasound imaging
Sotalol
    as antidysrhythmic, 95
    as nonselective beta antagonist, 94
Spasm(s)
    bronchospasm, see Bronchospasm
    laryngospasm, 76, 483
    methohexitone causing, 319
    of muscle, 59
    vasospasm, 180
Specific compliance, in newborns, 484
Specific gravity measurement, 222–223
Speed of onset, 348–349
Sphenoid sinus, 3
Sphenopalatine ganglia, 282
Sphygmomanometer, 413–414
    safety standards, 428
Spider angiomas, 248
Spina bifida, 394
Spinal anesthesia, 153
Spinal artery, anterior, 87, 154
Spinal artery, posterior, 87, 154
Spinal blockade, 299
Spinal cord, 153–154
    blood supply to, 87, 154
    complete transection of, 172–173
    hemisection of, 173
    lesions of, 171–173, 298–299
        vital capacity (VC) and, 12
    sympathetic nervous system neurons
        from, 280
Spinal cord level opioid receptors, 331
Spinal cord opiate receptors, 545
Spinal meninges, 153–154
Spinal nerves, 153
Spinal pathways, 159–160
Spinal reflexes, 160
Spinal shock, 172
Spine
    cervical, in obese persons, 67, 145
    curvatures of, 153
Spinothalamic tract, 159
Spinous processes, 152
Spirometry, 10–12, 401
    for gas volume measurement, 401
Spironolactone, 227
    in ascites therapy, 248
    kidney failure affecting, 234

Splanchnic nerve, 279
Spleen, 281
    enlarged, 248
Spontaneous abortion, 513
Spontaneous respiration, 53
Spontaneous ventilation, 51
Spread, in statistics, 449
Spread sheet programs, 448
Squamous cell carcinoma, 389
SSEPs, 293
Stagnant hypoxia, 62
Standard deviation, 449
Standard error of mean (SE), 449
Standards of care, 575
Star, in local area networks, 438
Starling equation, modified, 201
Static charge
    as Rotameter problem, 398
    spark from, 429
Static recoil, 14
Stationary phase, 407
Statistic analysis programs, 448
Statistics, 448–462
    summarization of data, 449
    variability of clinical measurement,
        450
Status epilepticus, 168
    phenytoin as treatment, 167
Statute of limitations, 576
Steam burns, 568
Stellate ganglia, 86, 280
Stellate ganglion block, 125
Stenosis
    aortic, see Aortic stenosis
    aqueduct, see Arnold-Chiari
        malformation
    mitral, see Mitral stenosis
    pulmonary artery, 491
    pyloric, in neonates, 493
Sternocostal surface, 83
Sternomastoid muscles, 12
Steroids
    see also specific steroids
    for acute asthma in pregnancy, 56
    as anaphylaxis treatment, 392
    as immunosupressive/antirejection
        drug, 387
    perioperative, hypothyroidism and,
        260
Stoichiometric concentrations, 429
Stomach, 281
Stomatitis, 389
Strabismus, 186
Stress
    arginine vasopressin and, 209
    assisted reproductive technologies
        affected by, 523
Stretch receptors, 90
Stridor, postoperative, 261
Strip craniectomy, 189

Stroke volume (SV)
  neonatal, 485
  obesity and, 66
Subarachnoid blocks
  in pregnancy
    gestational diabetes, 511
    pregnancy-induced hypertension, 509
    primary pulmonary hypertension and, 139
  in transvaginal aspiration, 524
Subarachnoid bolt, 418
Subclavian artery, 87
Subcritical hypoxia, 62
Subcutaneous injection, 318
  heparin, 70, 147
Subglottic space, 9
Submassive pulmonary embolus, 114
Succinylcholine
  antibiotics and, 355
  atracurium interacting with, 359
  burns affecting, 357
  central nervous system affected by, 164
  electrolytes affecting, 356
  hepatic disease affecting, 356
  histamine release from, 393
  malignant hyperthermia triggered by, 296
  at neuromuscular junction, 353–354
  as nicotinic antagonist, 291–292
  obesity and, 145
Suctioning, in neonatal resuscitation, 498
Sudden death
  in high-altitude pulmonary edema, 63
  obesity and, 65, 67, 144
Sudden infant death syndrome, 490
Sudeck's atrophy, 559
Sufentanil
  central nervous system affected by, 163
  as IV induction agent, 328–329
  as opiate agonist, 551
  as opioid agonist, 334
Sulfonamides, 231
Superficial coronary arteries, 89
Superficial femoral arteries, 87
Superhigh radio frequency (RF), 442, 443
Superior laryngeal nerve, 4–5
Superior lateral nasopharynx, 3
Superior mesenteric artery, 87
Superior mesenteric ganglia, 280
Superior nasal concha, 3
Superior vena cava
  chest x-ray of, 8
  right atrium and, 83
Supine position
  of obese patients, 66, 67

cardiovascular effects, 66, 144
  postoperative, 147
  pulmonary effects, 66, 144
  use of regional anesthesia, 69
  in pregnancy, 500
Supraglottitis, in children, 496–497
Suprarenal aortic cross-clamping, 238
Suprasellar tumor, 254
Supraspinal opiate receptors, 545
Supraspinal opioid receptors, 331
Supraspinous ligaments, 153
Surface tension, 14
  surfactant, 14
Surfactant, 481
  fetal development, formed late in, 14, 481
  surface tension and, 14
  synthesis of, 29
Suxamethonium, 485
Swallowing, 4
Sweating
  belladonna alkaloids inhibiting, 99
  hypercarbia resulting in, 51
  sympathetic nervous system increasing, 281
Sympathetic activation, 159
Sympathetic ganglia, 86, 280
Sympathetic mediated pain (SMP), 559–561
Sympathetic nervous system, 279–281
  anatomy of, 280
  and blood flow control, 90
  fight-or flight responses, 280
  myocardial, 86
  neonatal heart, innervation of, 484–485
  organs affected by, 280–281
Sympathetic stimulants, 258
Sympathetic tone, 259
Symptomatic intracranial aneurysms, 179–180
Synapses, 161
Synapsis, 280
Synaptic cleft, 353
Synchronous data link control, 440
Syncope, 125
Synthetic function, 242
Synthetic oxytocin, 502
Syringomyelia, 172
Systemic arterial supply, 7
Systemic circulation, 86–87
Systemic lupus erythematosus, 57–58
Systemic shunts, 48
Systemic toxicity, 350
Systemic vascular resistance
  enflurane decreasing, 311
  halothane and, 310
System memory, in microprocessors, **437**
Systole, 88

Systolic function, 89
Systolic pressure, 89
  neonatal, 485

Tabes dorsalis, 173
Tachycardia
  baroreceptor-mediated reflex, 310
  beta-adrenergic agonists, adverse effect of, 32
  d-tubocurarine causing, 370
  fetal, 503
  as fight-or flight response, 280
  hypercarbia resulting in, 51
  paroxysmal supraventricular, 123
  as pulmonary embolism sign, 115
  reflex, hydralazine causing, 98
  sinus, 122
  ventricular, 104, 124
Tachyphylaxis, 98
Tachypnea
  from cardiac/hydrostatic pulmonary edema, 54
  in pulmonary atresia, 491
  as pulmonary embolism sign, 114–115
Tagamet, 527–528
Tamponade, 113–114
Taylor's series, 470
TDMA, 443
Tec vaporizers, 35
TEE, 421
Television, blanking time of, 445
Temperature
  aging and regulation of, 141
  in burn injuries, 569
  and cerebral blood flow control, 157
  and combustion, 429
  critical, 42–43
  ignition, 429
  measurement of, 295, 434–435
  obese patients, intraoperative maintenance in, 69, 146
  respiratory control and, 26
Temperature-compensated, variable-bypass vaporizers, 35, 36
Temporal lobe epilepsy, 166
Tendon reflexes, 160
  relaxation of, and hypothyroidism, 259
Teratogens
  corticosteroids as, 55
  in craniosynostosis, 189
Terazosin, 286
Terbutaline, 32, 288
  as tocolytic, 502
Terminal bronchioles, 6
  prenatal branching of, 481
Termination of employment, 577
Testicular tumors, 389
Tetanus, 59–60
  as bacterial exogenous toxin, 171

in neuromuscular blockade
     monitoring, 383
Tetany, postoperative, 261
Tetracaine, 352
Tetracyclines, 235
Tetralogy of Fallot, in pregnancy,
     136–137
TGF, 199, 201
Thalassemias, 536–537
Thebesian veins, 86
Theophylline, 34
     for asthma in pregnancy, 55
     neonatal bradycardia and, 490
     neonatal postoperative apnea and,
        490
Thermal injury, 410
Thermistor, 434–435
Thermocouple, 434
Thermocouple temperature sensor,
     405
Thermoregulation
     in neonates, 486–487
     thyroid as mediator of, 252
Thermostasis, neonatal, 486
Thiazide diuretics, 227
     as acute hypocalcemia therapy, 262
Thick ascending limb, 194
     renal acid-base balance and, 212
     sodium balance and, 213
Thin ascending limb, 194
     renal acid-base balance and, 212
Thin descending limb, 194
     renal acid-base balance and, 212
Thiopental
     anaphylactoid reactions from, 393
     hyperthyroidism and, 258
     in local anesthetics-induced seizure
        treatment, 350–351
Thiopentone, 317–318
Thioxanthenes, 299
Third-degree heart block, 122
Thirst, in elderly persons, 218
Thoracic sarcoidosis, 58–59
Thoracic vertebrae, 152
Thorax, neonatal herniation into, 490
Three trials, 451
Threshold potential, 346–347
Thrombin time (TT), 541
Thrombocytopenia
     amrinone causing, 92
     autoimmune, 532
     cirrhosis, associated with, 248
     necrotizing enterocolitis and, 493
Thromboelastograph (TEG), 243
Thromboembolism, pulmonary, 520
Thrombolytic therapy, 115
Thrombophlebitis, 565
Thrombosis
     arterial, 271
     deep venous, 114

methohexitone causing, 319
Thromboxane
     renal blood flow affected by, 200
     TXA_2, 31
     as vasoactive compound, 30–31
Thyroglobulin, 274
Thyroid, 252
     calcitonin produced in, 275
     ectopic, 257
     electroconvulsant therapy and
        disease of, 565
     pregnancy affecting, 511–513
     thyroid hormone reserves in, 275
Thyroid cartilage, 4
Thyroid hormone
     activity based on receptors, 274
     blood flow and, 90
     fate of, 274
     feedback control, 274–275
     release of, 274
     reserves, 275
     synthetic pathways, 274
Thyroid storm, 258
     in pregnancy, 513
Tidal volume (Vt), 10
     enflurane decreasing, 311
     halothane decreasing, 310
     methohexitone decreasing, 319
     in newborns, 484
     in pregnancy, 500
     thiopentone decreasing, 318
Time division multiple access, 443
Time-position, in ultrasound, 421
Timolol, 288
Tinnitus, 350
Tissue uptake of anesthetic, 47
TLC, see Total lung capacity (TLC)
Tocainide, 93–94
     for chronic pain, 556
Tocolytics, 502
Tolazoline, 480
Tolerance, 546
Tongue, in neonate, 482
Tonic-clonic seizures, 167
     local anesthetics causing, 350
     phenytoin as treatment, 167
Tonic gamma efferent fibers, 160
Tonic seizures, 167
Tonsils, hypertrophic, 483
Tort law, 573
Total body water, 233
Total hip replacement, 174
Total lung capacity (TLC), 11
     aging and, 140
Total serum IgE, 392
Total solids meter, 223
Toxins
     dilated cardiomyopathy caused by,
        110–111
     exogenous, 170–171

Trachea, 5
     carina of, 5, 483
     chest x-ray of, 9
     in infants, 483
     inhalation burns injuring, 568
     innervation, 5
     shortened, 186
Tracheal constrictors, 31
Tracheoesophageal fistula, neonatal,
     492–493
Tracheostomy
     in burn injuries, 569
     pediatric, 495
     in Pierre-Robin sequence, 495
Tracrium, see Atracurium
Train-of-four stimulation (TOR), 383
Tranquilizers, 557
Transcendental functions, 468–469
Transcranial Doppler, 185
Transcutaneous CO_2 detection, 176
Transcutaneous nerve stimulator
     (TENS), 544
Transcutaneous PO_2 monitoring,
     410–411
Transdermal absorption, of opioids,
     332
Transdermal administration, of
     narcotics, 548
Transducers, 434–436
     extravascular, 415
     phased array, 421
     pressure measurement via, 415, 428,
        434
     in ultrasound, 420, 421
Transesophageal echocardiography,
     421
Transform analysis, 470–471
Transfusion reactions, 249–250, 530
Transfusion-related acute lung injury,
     530
Transfusion-transmitted diseases,
     249–250
     infections, 529–530
Transient apnea, 318
Transient ischemia, 177
Transitional flow, 14–15
Transit time blood flow rate
     measurement, 399–400
Transmembrane gradients of ions, 178
Transmembrane potential, 162
Transmucosal absorption, of opioids,
     332
Transmural pressure (TMP), 16
Transplacental absorption, of opioids,
     332
Transplantation
     and antirejection drugs, 386
     of kidney, 236
     of liver, 174
     of pancreas, 273

Transport
active, 306
among body compartments, 471–473
of carbon dioxide (CO_2), 24
drug, 87, 306
of elastase, 29
gas, 21–24
oxygen, 22–24, 489
protease, 29
tubular, 202–203
Transurethral surgery, 238
Transvaginal aspiration, ultrasound-
guided, 524–525
Transverse abdominous muscle, 13
Transverse processes, 152
Trapezoid approximation of definite
integral, 465
Trapped gas, 64
Trial, legal, 576–577
Tricuspid valve, 83
regurgitation, 491
Tricyclic antidepressants
central nervous system affected by,
166
kidney failure affecting, 235
Trifluoroacetic acid, 310–311
Trigeminal nerve, 297–298
Trigger point therapy, 544
Trigometric functions, 468–469
Trimethaphan, 97, 238
central nervous system affected by,
165
as nicotinic antagonist, 291
Trismus, 297–298
Trochlear (IV) nerve, 571
Tropomyosin, 87
Troponin complex, 87
True allergic reactions
to local anesthetics, 393
to protamine, 393–394
Trypsin, transport of, 29
Tuberculosis, 12
Tubular transport, 202–203
Tubules, 194
aging and, 195
connecting, 195, 203
distal, 194, 203
injury to
increased excretion as indication,
223
and measurement of RBF, 220
tests of, 223
lysosomal enzymes of, 223
measurement of function, 221–222
necrosis, acute kidney failure caused
by, 229–230
proximal, see Proximal tubule
regulation of function, 204–210
Tubuloglomerular feedback, 199
and glomerular filtration rate, 201

Tumor(s)
of adrenal gland, 262
of brain, 183
cancer, see Cancer
and cyclosporin, 387
dorsal extramedullary, 173
epidural, 173
gamma knife used on, 567
ileal carcinoid, 268
intracranial, 565
intradural, 173
parasellar, 254
pituitary, see Pituitary tumor
pseudohyperparathyroidism caused
by, 261
resection of, 268
suprasellar, 254
testicular, 389
Tungsten wire filament lamps, 435
Turbulent flow, 15, 100
Twisted pair cable, 440
Two-compartment model, 305
Two trials, 451
Tyrosine, 274

Ulnar artery, 87
Ultrahigh radio frequency (RF), 442
Ultrasonic flow rate measurement,
399–400
Ultrasonic nebulizers, 54
Ultrasound imaging, 420
cardiac function, monitoring of,
420–421
Doppler, See Doppler ultrasound
fetal ultrasound sonography, 186
transvaginal aspiration via, 524–525
of urologic system, 196
Underwriters Laboratories, Inc., 428
Unifascicular heart block, 121
Uniform probability distribution, 451
United States National Halothane
Study, 246
Univent, 51
Upper abdomen pneumonia, 52
Upper airway, 3–4
anomalies of, 51
obstructive apnea in infants,
489–490
suctioning, 498
supraglottitis as obstruction, 496
Upper motor neuron lesions, 356
Upper respiratory infection, 496
Uptake and distribution, 46–49
see also Distribution
in lungs, 47, 307, 308
rate of recovery, 308
Ureters, 195
Urethra, 195
transurethral surgery, 238
Urinalysis, 219

Urinary concentration, 218
of creatinine, 220
in elderly persons, 218
in neonates, 218
tests of, 222–223
Urinary retention, 332
Urinary tract infections, 239
Urine
dilute, 255
drug excretion in, 245
Urine flow rate (V), 218–219
mechanical ventilation affecting,
238
Urine glucose, 221
Urine output, 218
and hyperparathyroidism, 261
thiopentone affecting, 318
Urobilinogen, 243
Urologic system, 194–196
see also specific structures
acid-base balance, 211–213
calcium balance, 215
chloride balance, 216
drainage system, 195–196
general anesthetic effects, 228
hyperthyroidism affecting, 258
magnesium balance, 216–217
perioperative considerations,
237–239
pharmacology, 224–228
phosphate balance, 216
physiology, 196–218
potassium balance, 214–215
preoperative evaluation, 239
regional anesthetic effects, 228
sodium balance, 213–214
Urticaria, 391
U.S. Food and Drug Administration,
423–424
Uterine inversion, 521
Uteroplacental perfusion, 511
Uteroplacental unit, 506
Uterus
atony, 501–502
contractions of, 502, 523
enflurane affecting, 312
halothane affecting, 310
isoflurane affecting, 312–313
oxytocics, 274, 501–502
pregnancy-induced hypertension
affecting, 506
rupture of, 520–521
sympathetic nervous system relaxing,
281

Vacuum, 412
Vaginal delivery, 56–57
mitral regurgitation and, 133
mitral stenosis and, 132
Vagolytic effect, of glycopyrrolates, 99

Vagus (X) nerve
  afferent fibers in, 279
  heart, innervation of, 86, 282
  larynx, innervation of, 4–5
  as myocardial innervation, 86
Valproic acid
  adverse effect, 168
  as seizure treatment, 168
Valve replacement, 106
Valvotomy, pulmonary, 491
Valvular atresia, 491
Valvular heart disease
  see also specific diseases
  IV SBE prophylaxis, 110
  in pregnancy, 131–134
Vancomycin
  acute kidney failure caused by, 231
  allergic reactions to, 394
  kidney failure affecting, 235
Vaporizers, 35–36
V$_A$/Q, 19–20
Vascular occlusive disease, 293
Vascular pressure, 413–416
  pulmonary, 16
Vascular prostheses, 428
Vascular resistance
  peripheral, 484, 500
  pulmonary, see Pulmonary vascular
    resistance
  renal, 197–200
  systemic, 310, 311
Vascular system
  disorders of
    see also specific vascular disorders
    acute kidney failure caused by, 229
    as kidney failure complication, 232
    pulmonary vascular resistance and,
      19
  parasympathetic nervous system
    affecting, 282
  sympathetic nervous system affecting,
    280
Vasculature
  cardiovascular, aging and, 140
  cerebral, 151–152, 187
  of kidney, 87, 195
  of lung, 7, 9, 87
Vasoactive compounds
  endogenous, 29–31
  hormones, 29
  lungs processing, 29
Vasoconstriction
  arteriolar, 280
  hyperoxic, 71
  pulmonary, see Pulmonary
    vasoconstriction
Vasoconstrictors
  see also specific vasoconstrictors
  cardiovascular effects, 98
  local anesthetic as, 349–350

pulmonary vascular resistance
    influenced by, 18
Vasodilation, 282
Vasodilators
  see also specific vasodilators
  as angina therapy, 99
  cardiovascular effects, 96–98
  central nervous system affected by,
    165
  in pregnancy, 130
  pulmonary effects, 18, 29
Vasodilatory beta antagonists, 95
Vasomotor center, 26
Vasopressin
  arginine, see Arginine vasopressin
  polyuria and low level of, 237
  renal vascular resistance and, 200
Vasopressors, 165
Vasospasm, 180
VATER syndrome
  imperforate anus associated with, 493
  and tracheoesophageal fistula, 492
VC, 11, 12, 484
Vecuronium, **371**–372
  hepatic disease affecting, 356
  as nicotinic antagonist, 291–292
Venoconstriction, 281
Venodilation, 281
Venous access, in obese patients, 146
Venous air embolism, 174, 175
Venous blood
  lungs as filter, 28
  obese patients, access in, 69
Venous blood anesthetic, 47
Venous irritation, 319
Venous system
  myocardial, 86
  pulmonary circulation for filtration of
    venous drainage, 87
Ventilation
  in burn injuries, 569
  following craniosynostosis surgery,
    190
  mask, 490
  in neonatal resuscitation, 498
  patterns, 186
  volumes, aging and, 140
Ventilation-perfusion, 16–20
Ventilation-perfusion ratio (V$_A$/Q),
    19–20
Ventilators, anesthesia
  Bellows classification, 52
  classification, 52
  critical care, 53
  drive mechanism of, 52
  power source, 52
Ventolin, 32
Ventral respiratory group, 25
Ventricles
  cardiomyopathy and function of, 89

function of, 88–89
  left, see Left ventricle
  right, see Right ventricle
Ventricular fibrillation, 124
  anaphylaxis causing, 391
  due to near-drowning, 77
  electricity causing, 426
  epinephrine indicated by, 91
  in infants, 497–498
  succinylcholine causing, 375
Ventricular function, 88–89
Ventricular premature beats, 123–124
Ventricular septal defect, 134–135
Ventricular tachycardia, 124
  ablation for, 104
  drug therapy, 124
Ventriculitis, 417
Ventriculostomy, 417–418, 418
Venules, 7
Verapamil, 96
Vernitrol vaporizers, 35
Vertebrae, 152
Vertebral arch, 152
Vertebral arteries, 86
  cerebral vasculature, 151
Vertebral body, 152
Vertebral column, 152–153
Vertcbral processes, 152
Vertigo, 350
Very high radio frequency (RF), 442
Vessel rupture, 292–293
Vicarious liability, 573
Viral hepatitis, 245
Virtual telecommunications access
    method, 440
Viruses, transfusion-transmitted,
    529–530
Visceral smooth muscle, 332
Viscus, 298
Visual evoked potentials (VEP), 156
Vital capacity (VC), 11, 12
  in newborns, 484
Vital statistics, 448
Vitamin B$_{12}$ deficiency
  chronic anemia due to, 537
  posteriorcord syndrome caused by,
    173
Vitamin D, 210–211
  calcium balance affected by, 215
  parathyroid hormone increasing
    production, 275
Vitamin K absorption, 242
Vitrectomy, 486
Vocal cords, 4
  in infants, 483
  intubation, damaged by, 4
Volatile agent metabolism, in obese
    persons, 67, 145, 147
Volatile anesthetics
  blood system affected by, 541

Volatile anesthetics, *continued*
  central nervous system affected by,
    164
  triggering malignant hyperthermia, 296
Voltage, 431
  source of, 432
Volume assessment, 293
Volume expansion, 392
Volume of distribution, 305
  of narcotics, 548
Volume replacement
  in imperforate anus, 493
  in induced hypotension, 293
Vomiting
  in cirrhosis, 248
  as diabetic ketoacidosis sign, 269
  etomidate causing, 322
  from opioid drugs, 332, 547
  in pyloric stenosis, 493
Von Willebrand factor, 119
Von Willebrand's disease, 540
  platelet transfusions in, 532
VP shunts, 189
V/Q ratio, 20
  obesity and, 144

Warfarin, 115
Water and solute balance, 27–28
Water balance, 218
Water humidifiers, 53–54
Waterson shunt, 491
Watt, 432
Waveforms
  arterial, 415
  in electroencephalogram, 155
Weakness
  in cirrhosis, 248
  as diabetic ketoacidosis sign, 269
  as hypercalcemia sign, 260
Wegener's granulomatosis, 254
Wheatstone bridge circuits, **436**
White blood cells, urinalysis of, 219
White cell disorders, 539–540
White matter, 151
Wireless telecommunications, 442–444,
    443
Wire (noncellular) phones, 443
Withdrawal, from opioid drugs, **547**
Wolff-Parkinson-White syndrome,
    124–125
Work, 432

World Wide Web, 441–442
Wright Respirometer, 401
WWW consortium, 442

X-rays
  of cervical spine, 169
  of chest, *see* Chest x-rays
  of craniosynostosis, 189
  of skull, 169

Yellow ligament, *see* Ligamentum
    flavum
Yohimbine, 287

Zantac, 527–528
Zaroxolyn, *see* Metolazone
Z-bands, 87
Zemuron, *see* Rocuronium
Z-line, 87
Zona fasciculata, 253
Zona glomerulosa, 253
Zona reticularis, 253
Zygomatic arch fractures, 3
Zygote intrafallopian transfer (ZIFT),
    523

ISBN 0-07-033986-4

9 780070 339866